LONG-TERM MECHANICAL VENTILATION

LUNG BIOLOGY IN HEALTH AND DISEASE

Executive Editor

Claude Lenfant
Director, National Heart, Lung and Blood Institute
National Institutes of Health
Bethesda, Maryland

1. Immunologic and Infectious Reactions in the Lung, *edited by C. H. Kirkpatrick and H. Y. Reynolds*
2. The Biochemical Basis of Pulmonary Function, *edited by R. G. Crystal*
3. Bioengineering Aspects of the Lung, *edited by J. B. West*
4. Metabolic Functions of the Lung, *edited by Y. S. Bakhle and J. R. Vane*
5. Respiratory Defense Mechanisms (in two parts), *edited by J. D. Brain, D. F. Proctor, and L. M. Reid*
6. Development of the Lung, *edited by W. A. Hodson*
7. Lung Water and Solute Exchange, *edited by N. C. Staub*
8. Extrapulmonary Manifestations of Respiratory Disease, *edited by E. D. Robin*
9. Chronic Obstructive Pulmonary Disease, *edited by T. L. Petty*
10. Pathogenesis and Therapy of Lung Cancer, *edited by C. C. Harris*
11. Genetic Determinants of Pulmonary Disease, *edited by S. D. Litwin*
12. The Lung in the Transition Between Health and Disease, *edited by P. T. Macklem and S. Permutt*
13. Evolution of Respiratory Processes: A Comparative Approach, *edited by S. C. Wood and C. Lenfant*
14. Pulmonary Vascular Diseases, *edited by K. M. Moser*
15. Physiology and Pharmacology of the Airways, *edited by J. A. Nadel*
16. Diagnostic Techniques in Pulmonary Disease (in two parts), *edited by M. A. Sackner*
17. Regulation of Breathing (in two parts), *edited by T. F. Hornbein*
18. Occupational Lung Diseases: Research Approaches and Methods, *edited by H. Weill and M. Turner-Warwick*
19. Immunopharmacology of the Lung, *edited by H. H. Newball*
20. Sarcoidosis and Other Granulomatous Diseases of the Lung, *edited by B. L. Fanburg*
21. Sleep and Breathing, *edited by N. A. Saunders and C. E. Sullivan*
22. *Pneumocystis carinii* Pneumonia: Pathogenesis, Diagnosis, and Treatment, *edited by L. S. Young*
23. Pulmonary Nuclear Medicine: Techniques in Diagnosis of Lung Disease, *edited by H. L. Atkins*
24. Acute Respiratory Failure, *edited by W. M. Zapol and K. J. Falke*
25. Gas Mixing and Distribution in the Lung, *edited by L. A. Engel and M. Paiva*

26. High-Frequency Ventilation in Intensive Care and During Surgery, *edited by G. Carlon and W. S. Howland*
27. Pulmonary Development: Transition from Intrauterine to Extrauterine Life, *edited by G. H. Nelson*
28. Chronic Obstructive Pulmonary Disease: Second Edition, *edited by T. L. Petty*
29. The Thorax (in two parts), *edited by C. Roussos and P. T. Macklem*
30. The Pleura in Health and Disease, *edited by J. Chrétien, J. Bignon, and A. Hirsch*
31. Drug Therapy for Asthma: Research and Clinical Practice, *edited by J. W. Jenne and S. Murphy*
32. Pulmonary Endothelium in Health and Disease, *edited by U. S. Ryan*
33. The Airways: Neural Control in Health and Disease, *edited by M. A. Kaliner and P. J. Barnes*
34. Pathophysiology and Treatment of Inhalation Injuries, *edited by J. Loke*
35. Respiratory Function of the Upper Airway, *edited by O. P. Mathew and G. Sant'Ambrogio*
36. Chronic Obstructive Pulmonary Disease: A Behavioral Perspective, *edited by A. J. McSweeny and I. Grant*
37. Biology of Lung Cancer: Diagnosis and Treatment, *edited by S. T. Rosen, J. L. Mulshine, F. Cuttitta, and P. G. Abrams*
38. Pulmonary Vascular Physiology and Pathophysiology, *edited by E. K. Weir and J. T. Reeves*
39. Comparative Pulmonary Physiology: Current Concepts, *edited by S. C. Wood*
40. Respiratory Physiology: An Analytical Approach, *edited by H. K. Chang and M. Paiva*
41. Lung Cell Biology, *edited by D. Massaro*
42. Heart–Lung Interactions in Health and Disease, *edited by S. M. Scharf and S. S. Cassidy*
43. Clinical Epidemiology of Chronic Obstructive Pulmonary Disease, *edited by M. J. Hensley and N. A. Saunders*
44. Surgical Pathology of Lung Neoplasms, *edited by A. M. Marchevsky*
45. The Lung in Rheumatic Diseases, *edited by G. W. Cannon and G. A. Zimmerman*
46. Diagnostic Imaging of the Lung, *edited by C. E. Putman*
47. Models of Lung Disease: Microscopy and Structural Methods, *edited by J. Gil*
48. Electron Microscopy of the Lung, *edited by D. E. Schraufnagel*
49. Asthma: Its Pathology and Treatment, *edited by M. A. Kaliner, P. J. Barnes, and C. G. A. Persson*
50. Acute Respiratory Failure: Second Edition, *edited by W. M. Zapol and F. Lemaire*
51. Lung Disease in the Tropics, *edited by O. P. Sharma*
52. Exercise: Pulmonary Physiology and Pathophysiology, *edited by B. J. Whipp and K. Wasserman*
53. Developmental Neurobiology of Breathing, *edited by G. G. Haddad and J. P. Farber*
54. Mediators of Pulmonary Inflammation, *edited by M. A. Bray and W. H. Anderson*
55. The Airway Epithelium, *edited by S. G. Farmer and D. Hay*

56. Physiological Adaptations in Vertebrates: Respiration, Circulation, and Metabolism, *edited by S. C. Wood, R. E. Weber, A. R. Hargens, and R. W. Millard*
57. The Bronchial Circulation, *edited by J. Butler*
58. Lung Cancer Differentiation: Implications for Diagnosis and Treatment, *edited by S. D. Bernal and P. J. Hesketh*
59. Pulmonary Complications of Systemic Disease, *edited by J. F. Murray*
60. Lung Vascular Injury: Molecular and Cellular Response, *edited by A. Johnson and T. J. Ferro*
61. Cytokines of the Lung, *edited by J. Kelley*
62. The Mast Cell in Health and Disease, *edited by M. A. Kaliner and D. D. Metcalfe*
63. Pulmonary Disease in the Elderly Patient, *edited by D. A. Mahler*
64. Cystic Fibrosis, *edited by P. B. Davis*
65. Signal Transduction in Lung Cells, *edited by J. S. Brody, D. M. Center, and V. A. Tkachuk*
66. Tuberculosis: A Comprehensive International Approach, *edited by L. B. Reichman and E. S. Hershfield*
67. Pharmacology of the Respiratory Tract: Experimental and Clinical Research, *edited by K. F. Chung and P. J. Barnes*
68. Prevention of Respiratory Diseases, *edited by A. Hirsch, M. Goldberg, J.-P. Martin, and R. Masse*
69. *Pneumocystis carinii* Pneumonia: Second Edition, *edited by P. D. Walzer*
70. Fluid and Solute Transport in the Airspaces of the Lungs, *edited by R. M. Effros and H. K. Chang*
71. Sleep and Breathing: Second Edition, *edited by N. A. Saunders and C. E. Sullivan*
72. Airway Secretion: Physiological Bases for the Control of Mucous Hypersecretion, *edited by T. Takishima and S. Shimura*
73. Sarcoidosis and Other Granulomatous Disorders, *edited by D. G. James*
74. Epidemiology of Lung Cancer, *edited by J. M. Samet*
75. Pulmonary Embolism, *edited by M. Morpurgo*
76. Sports and Exercise Medicine, *edited by S. C. Wood and R. C. Roach*
77. Endotoxin and the Lungs, *edited by K. L. Brigham*
78. The Mesothelial Cell and Mesothelioma, *edited by M.-C. Jaurand and J. Bignon*
79. Regulation of Breathing: Second Edition, *edited by J. A. Dempsey and A. I. Pack*
80. Pulmonary Fibrosis, *edited by S. Hin. Phan and R. S. Thrall*
81. Long-Term Oxygen Therapy: Scientific Basis and Clinical Application, *edited by W. J. O'Donohue, Jr.*
82. Ventral Brainstem Mechanisms and Control of Respiration and Blood Pressure, *edited by C. O. Trouth, R. M. Millis, H. F. Kiwull-Schöne, and M. E. Schläfke*
83. A History of Breathing Physiology, *edited by D. F. Proctor*
84. Surfactant Therapy for Lung Disease, *edited by B. Robertson and H. W. Taeusch*
85. The Thorax: Second Edition, Revised and Expanded (in three parts), *edited by C. Roussos*

86. Severe Asthma: Pathogenesis and Clinical Management, *edited by S. J. Szefler and D. Y. M. Leung*
87. *Mycobacterium avium*–Complex Infection: Progress in Research and Treatment, *edited by J. A. Korvick and C. A. Benson*
88. Alpha 1–Antitrypsin Deficiency: Biology • Pathogenesis • Clinical Manifestations • Therapy, *edited by R. G. Crystal*
89. Adhesion Molecules and the Lung, *edited by P. A. Ward and J. C. Fantone*
90. Respiratory Sensation, *edited by L. Adams and A. Guz*
91. Pulmonary Rehabilitation, *edited by A. P. Fishman*
92. Acute Respiratory Failure in Chronic Obstructive Pulmonary Disease, *edited by J.-P. Derenne, W. A. Whitelaw, and T. Similowski*
93. Environmental Impact on the Airways: From Injury to Repair, *edited by J. Chrétien and D. Dusser*
94. Inhalation Aerosols: Physical and Biological Basis for Therapy, *edited by A. J. Hickey*
95. Tissue Oxygen Deprivation: From Molecular to Integrated Function, *edited by G. G. Haddad and G. Lister*
96. The Genetics of Asthma, *edited by S. B. Liggett and D. A. Meyers*
97. Inhaled Glucocorticoids in Asthma: Mechanisms and Clinical Actions, *edited by R. P. Schleimer, W. W. Busse, and P. M. O'Byrne*
98. Nitric Oxide and the Lung, *edited by W. M. Zapol and K. D. Bloch*
99. Primary Pulmonary Hypertension, *edited by L. J. Rubin and S. Rich*
100. Lung Growth and Development, *edited by J. A. McDonald*
101. Parasitic Lung Diseases, *edited by A. A. F. Mahmoud*
102. Lung Macrophages and Dendritic Cells in Health and Disease, *edited by M. F. Lipscomb and S. W. Russell*
103. Pulmonary and Cardiac Imaging, *edited by C. Chiles and C. E. Putman*
104. Gene Therapy for Diseases of the Lung, *edited by K. L. Brigham*
105. Oxygen, Gene Expression, and Cellular Function, *edited by L. Biadasz Clerch and D. J. Massaro*
106. Beta$_2$-Agonists in Asthma Treatment, *edited by R. Pauwels and P. M. O'Byrne*
107. Inhalation Delivery of Therapeutic Peptides and Proteins, *edited by A. L. Adjei and P. K. Gupta*
108. Asthma in the Elderly, *edited by R. A. Barbee and J. W. Bloom*
109. Treatment of the Hospitalized Cystic Fibrosis Patient, *edited by D. M. Orenstein and R. C. Stern*
110. Asthma and Immunological Diseases in Pregnancy and Early Infancy, *edited by M. Schatz, R. S. Zeiger, and H. N. Claman*
111. Dyspnea, *edited by D. A. Mahler*
112. Proinflammatory and Antiinflammatory Peptides, *edited by S. I. Said*
113. Self-Management of Asthma, *edited by H. Kotses and A. Harver*
114. Eicosanoids, Aspirin, and Asthma, *edited by A. Szczeklik, R. J. Gryglewski, and J. R. Vane*
115. Fatal Asthma, *edited by A. L. Sheffer*
116. Pulmonary Edema, *edited by M. A. Matthay and D. H. Ingbar*
117. Inflammatory Mechanisms in Asthma, *edited by S. T. Holgate and W. W. Busse*
118. Physiological Basis of Ventilatory Support, *edited by J. J. Marini and A. S. Slutsky*

119. Human Immunodeficiency Virus and the Lung, *edited by M. J. Rosen and J. M. Beck*
120. Five-Lipoxygenase Products in Asthma, *edited by J. M. Drazen, S.-E. Dahlén, and T. H. Lee*
121. Complexity in Structure and Function of the Lung, *edited by M. P. Hlastala and H. T. Robertson*
122. Biology of Lung Cancer, *edited by M. A. Kane and P. A. Bunn, Jr.*
123. Rhinitis: Mechanisms and Management, *edited by R. M. Naclerio, S. R. Durham, and N. Mygind*
124. Lung Tumors: Fundamental Biology and Clinical Management, *edited by C. Brambilla and E. Brambilla*
125. Interleukin-5: From Molecule to Drug Target for Asthma, *edited by C. J. Sanderson*
126. Pediatric Asthma, *edited by S. Murphy and H. W. Kelly*
127. Viral Infections of the Respiratory Tract, *edited by R. Dolin and P. F. Wright*
128. Air Pollutants and the Respiratory Tract, *edited by D. L. Swift and W. M. Foster*
129. Gastroesophageal Reflux Disease and Airway Disease, *edited by M. R. Stein*
130. Exercise-Induced Asthma, *edited by E. R. McFadden, Jr.*
131. LAM and Other Diseases Characterized by Smooth Muscle Proliferation, *edited by J. Moss*
132. The Lung at Depth, *edited by C. E. G. Lundgren and J. N. Miller*
133. Regulation of Sleep and Circadian Rhythms, *edited by F. W. Turek and P. C. Zee*
134. Anticholinergic Agents in the Upper and Lower Airways, *edited by S. L. Spector*
135. Control of Breathing in Health and Disease, *edited by M. D. Altose and Y. Kawakami*
136. Immunotherapy in Asthma, *edited by J. Bousquet and H. Yssel*
137. Chronic Lung Disease in Early Infancy, *edited by R. D. Bland and J. J. Coalson*
138. Asthma's Impact on Society: The Social and Economic Burden, *edited by K. B. Weiss, A. S. Buist, and S. D. Sullivan*
139. New and Exploratory Therapeutic Agents for Asthma, *edited by M. Yeadon and Z. Diamant*
140. Multimodality Treatment of Lung Cancer, *edited by A. T. Skarin*
141. Cytokines in Pulmonary Disease: Infection and Inflammation, *edited by S. Nelson and T. R. Martin*
142. Diagnostic Pulmonary Pathology, *edited by P. T. Cagle*
143. Particle–Lung Interactions, *edited by P. Gehr and J. Heyder*
144. Tuberculosis: A Comprehensive International Approach, Second Edition, Revised and Expanded, *edited by L. B. Reichman and E. S. Hershfield*
145. Combination Therapy for Asthma and Chronic Obstructive Pulmonary Disease, *edited by R. J. Martin and M. Kraft*
146. Sleep Apnea: Implications in Cardiovascular and Cerebrovascular Disease, *edited by T. D. Bradley and J. S. Floras*
147. Sleep and Breathing in Children: A Developmental Approach, *edited by G. M. Loughlin, J. L. Carroll, and C. L. Marcus*

148. Pulmonary and Peripheral Gas Exchange in Health and Disease, *edited by J. Roca, R. Rodriguez-Roisen, and P. D. Wagner*
149. Lung Surfactants: Basic Science and Clinical Applications, *R. H. Notter*
150. Nosocomial Pneumonia, *edited by W. R. Jarvis*
151. Fetal Origins of Cardiovascular and Lung Disease, *edited by David J. P. Barker*
152. Long-Term Mechanical Ventilation, *edited by N. S. Hill*

ADDITIONAL VOLUMES IN PREPARATION

Environmental Asthma, *edited by R. K. Bush*

Asthma and Respiratory Infections, *edited by D. P. Skoner*

Airway Remodeling, *edited by P. H. Howarth, J. W. Wilson, J. Bousquet, and R. Pauwels*

Respiratory-Circulatory Interactions in Health and Disease, *edited by S. M. Scharf, M. R. Pinsky, and S. Magder*

The Lung at High Altitudes, *edited by T. F. Hornbein and R. B. Schoene*

The opinions expressed in these volumes do not necessarily represent the views of the National Institutes of Health.

LONG-TERM MECHANICAL VENTILATION

Edited by

Nicholas S. Hill

Brown University School of Medicine
Rhode Island Hospital
Providence, Rhode Island

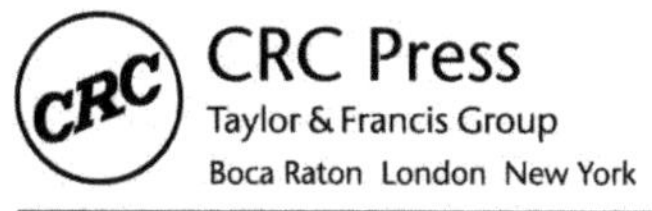

CRC Press is an imprint of the
Taylor & Francis Group, an **informa** business

CRC Press
Taylor & Francis Group
6000 Broken Sound Parkway NW, Suite 300
Boca Raton, FL 33487-2742

ISBN-13: 978-0-8247-0413-1 (hbk)
ISBN-13: 978-0-367-39816-3 (pbk)

Visit the Taylor & Francis Web site at
http://www.taylorandfrancis.com

and the CRC Press Web site at
http://www.crcpress.com

INTRODUCTION

In a volume titled *Advances in American Medicine* (1), Dr. Julius Comroe—certainly one of the most influential medical scientists of the last century—included the following among the many advances in pulmonary diseases and respiratory disorders:

1. Better understanding of the mechanical properties of the lungs and thorax.
2. Development and widespread use of quantitative measurement of O_2 and CO_2 tension, O_2 and CO_2 content, and pH of arterial blood.
3. Development of physiological tests as important aids to diagnosis and evaluation of therapy.

Although other advances are also listed, these three are particularly relevant to the subject of this volume.

At the end of the nineteenth century, the urge to perform intrathoracic surgery was clearly limited by the lack of respiratory support. This led to a number of approaches and devices that, from today's perspective, make us believe that those days truly belonged to another world! Just look! The first operation on human lungs was performed in a specially built negative pressure room that accommodated the patient, the surgeon, and his team. Years later, long-term respiratory support was made possible by the iron lung.

Today's world is, of course, quite different. The great advances listed by Dr. Comroe led to the development of a number of devices and to their application to the support and treatment of scores of patients. Long-term mechanical ventilation is clearly the result of years of basic physiological and clinical research. Among the success stories of the last century, this one ranks very high because of the many applications and benefits of the procedures.

However, long-term mechanical ventilation is not a therapy that can, or should, be used by everyone: a deep knowledge of its rationale and basis is required. That is what this volume will give to the reader and, more important, to the "user." But this book does much more: to borrow from the editor, it is "a stimulus for new ideas and future investigations." Dr. Nicholas S. Hill has brought together a cadre of contributors, from several countries, who are the leaders in the field of long-term mechanical ventilation. Together they represent the collective experience and knowledge of the field.

I am grateful to Dr. Hill and to his contributors for giving the Lung Biology in Health and Disease series of monographs the opportunity to present this volume.

Claude Lenfant, M.D.
Bethesda, Maryland

REFERENCE

1. Comroe JH. The heart and lungs. In: Bowers JA, Purcell EF, eds. Advances in American Medicine: Essays at the Bicentennial. New York: Josiah Macy Foundation, 1976: 484–535.

PREFACE

Long-term mechanical ventilation refers to ventilatory assistance for patients who require more than 6 hours of assisted ventilation daily for periods exceeding 21 days. Such patients include those unable to be liberated from mechanical ventilation after bouts of acute respiratory failure as well as those with severe ventilatory defects who undergo initiation of mechanical ventilation when they develop respiratory insufficiency prior to a respiratory crisis. These patients comprise a dynamic population; some succumb to their underlying illness or, occasionally, to complications of ventilation—and new patients enter the group on a daily basis. The number of such patients has been increasing steadily and their management has undergone a steady evolution in response to new knowledge and technology as well as changes in the insurance climate, which ultimately determines what resources are available to them. The purpose of this book is to provide a comprehensive and current reference for clinicians, reimbursement specialists, and others in the mechanical ventilation field on the state of knowledge regarding pathophysiology, clinical management, and reimbursement practices for long-term mechanical ventilation.

Chapter 1 provides an international perspective on the epidemiology of long-term mechanical ventilation, examining trends over recent years. Chapter 2 follows this evolutionary view, focusing on the development of sites of care for chronically ventilated patients within and outside of acute care hospitals. In particular, the development of the modern respiratory care unit is discussed as well as the continuing proliferation of long-term-care hospitals that specialize in the management of difficult-to-wean patients. Chapters 3 to 5 examine pathophysiological mechanisms contributing to the development of chronic respiratory failure. The critical role of the respiratory muscles and their interactions with the respiratory center that lead to alterations in the control of breathing are discussed in Chapter 3. Chapter 4 considers the impact of ventilatory dysfunction on sleep and vice versa, and the critical role of sleep-induced hypoventilation in the subsequent development of chronic respiratory failure. Chapter 5 then provides a perspective on important new insights into the role of the upper airway and glottis in determining the effectiveness of noninvasive ventilation.

Chapters 6 through 8 examine applications of long-term mechanical ventilation in patients with specific types of chronic respiratory failure. Chapter 6 covers the pathogenesis and management of chronic respiratory failure in patients with restrictive thoracic and central hypoventilatory disorders, emphasizing the role of noninvasive ventilation, which has had a revolutionary impact on the management of these patients. In Chapter 7, the ventilatory management of patients with chronic respiratory failure due to severe stable COPD—a topic that remains controversial because of the conflicting results of studies on the therapeutic value of noninvasive ventilation—is discussed. Because invasive ventilation still plays a role (albeit a diminishing one) in the management of patients with restrictive or obstructive pulmonary processes, it is included in the discussion. Long-term mechanical ventilation has also played an important role in the management of children with severe ventilatory defects, including those with congenital neuromuscular diseases, cystic fibrosis, and bronchopulmonary dysplasia. Chapter 8 considers applications of long-term mechanical ventilation in these patients, once again emphasizing the increasing role of noninvasive ventilation, but also considering the continuing need for invasive ventilation in some.

Despite the increasing use of noninvasive ventilation, invasive mechanical ventilation remains an option for patients who are poor candidates for noninvasive ventilation but desire chronic ventilatory assistance. Chapter 9 focuses on the knowledge and experience gained through management of such patients in the Chronic Ventilatory Demonstration Unit at Temple University. In particular, the need is emphasized for close attention to the function of the upper airway (including coughing and eating) for meticulous management to avoid the complications of chronic tracheostomy, and for considering psychosocial aspects of management that can be critical to the long-term success of invasive approaches. Paralleling the pragmatic approach taken in Chapter 9, Chapter 10 provides a practical perspective on the management of noninvasive ventilation for patients with chronic respiratory failure, an approach that has assumed increasing importance over the past decade in the management of patients receiving long-term mechanical ventilation.

An important development in the field of long-term mechanical ventilation has been the realization that patients with a high level of dependency on mechanical ventilatory assistance can still be managed noninvasively. Chapters 11 and 12 were written with this in mind. Chapter 11 describes an approach to the removal of tracheostomy tubes and conversion to noninvasive ventilation of patients previously considered dependent on invasive ventilation. Chapter 12 examines the critically important issue of secretion management in patients with severe cough impairment, a technique that renders noninvasive ventilation feasible in such patients.

Ideally, patients receiving long-term mechanical ventilation should be managed at home. Unfortunately, in most cases there are impediments to home management of long-term mechanical ventilator users, including limited caregiver availability and insufficient financial resources. Based on the experiences with management of children requiring long-term mechanical ventilation in Pennsylvania, Chapter 13 examines the reimbursement environment and some methods of dealing with the insufficiencies. Chapter 14 presents recent advances in ventilator technology for delivery of mechanical ventilation in the home that should enable better support of ventilator-dependent patients, particularly those with more sophisticated ventilator needs. These ventilators have the capability of providing breaths in many different modes and have sophisticated alarm and monitoring systems. In addition, some are very compact and permit improved mobility for ventilator users. In Chapter 15, a new approach to facilitating the management of patients outside the acute care hospital is discussed, as well as the formation of networks of ventilator users and providers for more efficient use of resources and empowerment relative to insurers.

For those long-term mechanical ventilator users who develop ventilator dependency following bouts of respiratory failure, trauma, or surgery, weaning remains a possibility, even if it proves lengthy and difficult. Specialized units have been developed to concentrate the effort of a skilled and experienced staff on the weaning of such patients. Chapter 16 describes the approach in one such unit at the Mayo Clinic in Rochester, Minnesota, that has reported very favorable success rates in the management of difficult-to-wean patients. Even if such patients are unable to wean entirely, rehabilitation can restore them to an optimal level of functioning. Chapter 17 presents the multidisciplinary approach that aims to maximize patient dependency by minimizing the amount of ventilatory assistance utilizing the least complicated and most economical means.

The field of outcomes research has evolved to provide tools for evaluating the results of medical interventions. Chapter 18 examines the outcomes of long-term mechanical ventilation applied invasively or noninvasively; this chapter is based largely on the results of the author's own work, as well as that of other large outcome studies mainly in Europe. Within the area of outcomes research, a new discipline has arisen to assess overall health status. The administration of questionnaires provides a tool for the determination of whether interventions enhance a patient's perception of life satisfaction and overall level of functioning. Chapter 19 discusses the use of recently developed questionnaires designed specifically to assess the impact of long-term mechanical ventilation.

The technological advances of the twentieth century have enabled medical practitioners in the developed world to support patients with chronic respiratory failure in ways never before feasible. More patients than ever before, with varying causes of their ventilatory impairment, can be sustained indefinitely using a variety of ventilatory techniques. Medical professionals caring for these patients aim to apply these techniques in the most effective and cost-conscious manner, based on recently acquired knowledge about the pathogenesis of chronic respiratory failure and steady advances in technology. These advances have been a blessing as well as a burden, as society has had to shoulder the large cost of supporting these often very needy ventilator-assisted individuals. This volume will serve as a comprehensive resource for practitioners devoted to the care of individuals receiving long-term mechanical ventilation as well as a stimulus for new ideas and future investigations. Only by continually expanding and refining our knowledge base and skills can we continue to improve the lives of the growing number of long-term ventilator users.

Nicholas S. Hill

CONTRIBUTORS

Monica Avendano, M.D. West Park Hospital and University of Toronto, Toronto, Ontario, Canada

John R. Bach, M.D., F.C.C.P., F.A.A.P.M.R. Professor, Department of Physical Medicine and Rehabilitation, University of Medicine and Dentistry–New Jersey Medical School, Newark, New Jersey

Giorgio Bertolotti IRCCS Istituto di Riabilitazione, Veruno, Italy

Mauro Carone IRCCS Istituto di Riabilitazione, Veruno, Italy

Bartolome R. Celli, M.D. Professor, Department of Pulmonary and Critical Care Medicine, St. Elizabeth's Medical Center, Boston, Massachusetts

Gerard J. Criner, M.D. Professor, Department of Pulmonary and Critical Care Medicine, Temple University School of Medicine, Philadelphia, Pennsylvania

Walter E. Donat, M.D. Department of Pulmonary Medicine, Rhode Island Hospital, Providence, Rhode Island

John J. Downes, M.D. Department of Anesthesia and Critical Care Medicine, The Children's Hospital of Pennsylvania, Philadelphia, Pennsylvania

Mark W. Elliott, M.D., F.R.C.P. (UK) Sleep and Noninvasive Ventilation Services, St. James's University Hospital, Leeds, England

Peter C. Gay, M.D. Associate Professor, Department of Pulmonary, Critical Care, and Sleep Medicine, Mayo Clinic and Mayo Foundation, Rochester, Minnesota

Allen I. Goldberg, M.D. Professor of Pediatrics, and Director, Loyola University Chicago, Pediatric Home Health, Loyola University Health Systems, Maywood, Illinois

Roger S. Goldstein, M.D. West Park Hospital and Professor of Medicine and Physical Therapy, Division of Respiratory Medicine, University of Toronto, Toronto, Ontario, Canada

Douglas R. Gracey, M.D. Chair, Division of Pulmonary and Critical Care Medicine, Mayo Clinic and Mayo Foundation, Rochester, Minnesota

Rosa Guell, M.D. Hospital Santa Creu I Sant Pau, Barcelona, Spain

Nicholas S. Hill, M.D. Professor of Medicine, Brown University School of Medicine, and Critical Care Services and Pulmonary Division, Rhode Island Hospital, Providence, Rhode Island

Rolf D. Hubmayr, M.D. Professor, Division of Pulmonary and Critical Care Medicine, Mayo Clinic and Mayo Foundation, Rochester, Minnesota

Paul W. Jones, B.Sc., M.B.B.S., Ph.D. Professor, Department of Physiological Medicine, St. George's Hospital Medical School, London, England

Robert M. Kacmarek, RRT, Ph.D. Harvard Medical School and Respiratory Care Services, Massachusetts General Hospital, Boston, Massachusetts

Patrick Leger, M.D. Croix Rousse Hospital, Lyon, France

Barry J. Make, M.D. Director, Emphysema Center and Pulmonary Rehabilitation, Division of Pulmonary Sciences and Critical Care Medicine, National Jewish Center for Immunology and Respiratory Medicine, Denver, Colorado

Martha M. Parra, M.S.N. The Children's Hospital of Pennsylvania, Philadelphia, Pennsylvania

Daniel O. Rodenstein, M.D., Ph.D. Head, Service de Pneumologie, Cliniques Universitaires Saint-Luc, Université Catholique de Louvain, Brussels, Belgium

Randall L. Rosenblatt St. Paul Medical Center and University of Texas Southwestern Medical School, Dallas, Texas

Anita K. Simonds, M.D. Sleep and Ventilation Unit, Royal Brompton and Harefield National Health Service Trust, London, England

W. Gerald Teague, M.D. Division of Pediatric Pulmonology, Department of Pediatrics, Emory University School of Medicine, Atlanta, Georgia

John M. Travaline, M.D. Associate Professor, Division of Pulmonary and Critical Care Medicine, Temple University School of Medicine, Philadelphia, Pennsylvania

Alice C. Tzeng, M.D. Research Fellow, Department of Physical Medicine and Rehabilitation, University of Medicine and Dentistry–New Jersey Medical School, Newark, New Jersey

Joseph Viroslav, M.D. St. Paul Medical Center and University of Texas Southwestern Medical School, Dallas, Texas

Martha S. Parra, M.S.N., The Children's Hospital of Pennsylvania, Philadelphia, Pennsylvania

Daniel O. Rodenstein, M.D., Ph.D., Head, Service de Pneumologie, Cliniques Universitaires Saint-Luc, Université Catholique de Louvain, Brussels, Belgium

Randall L. Rosenblatt, M.D., [illegible] University of Texas Southwestern Medical School, Dallas, Texas

Anita K. Simonds, M.D., Sleep and Ventilation Unit, Royal Brompton and Harefield National Health Service Trust, London, England

J. Gerald Teague, M.D., Division of Pediatric Pulmonology, Department of Pediatrics, Emory University School of Medicine, Atlanta, Georgia

[illegible] M. [illegible], M.D., Associate Professor, Department of Anesthesiology and Critical Care Medicine, Temple University School of Medicine, Philadelphia, Pennsylvania

[illegible] C. [illegible], M.D., [illegible], Department of Physical Medicine and Rehabilitation, University of Medicine and Dentistry of New Jersey–New Jersey Medical School, Newark, New Jersey

[illegible], M.D., St. Paul Medical Center and University of Texas Southwestern Medical School, Dallas, Texas

CONTENTS

LONG-TERM
MECHANICAL
VENTILATION

1

Epidemiology of Long-Term Ventilatory Assistance

BARRY J. MAKE

National Jewish Center for Immunology and Respiratory Medicine
Denver, Colorado

I. Introduction

The development of mechanical assistance to ventilation and its subsequent implementation as a routine part of medical practice represent the most important advance in respiratory care of the twentieth century. The application of such therapy has been life saving for acutely ill individuals with a wide variety of diverse conditions ranging from neurologic disorders such as polio to acute lung injury associated with severe medical illness. In addition, the use of endotracheal tubes has allowed control of the respiratory system during anesthesia and expanded the application of life-enhancing surgical procedures. Most often conceptualized as a short-term intervention, mechanical ventilation may nonetheless become a long-term treatment, particularly for individuals with underlying non-reversible medical conditions.

This chapter reviews the epidemiology of long-term mechanical assistance to ventilation. The first portion focuses on patients who are in acute care facilities and the second on patients who are in alternate settings (particularly the home) in different countries around the world.

II. Definition of Long-Term Ventilation

While it may be most satisfying to draw a clear distinction between the short-term and long-term use of mechanical assistance to ventilation, there is no universally accepted delineation of when the use of ventilation becomes long-term. Rather, multiple factors need to be considered before ventilation can be classified as chronic (Table 1) and the patient as unweanable from mechanical assistance to ventilation. Two scenarios illustrate the broad range of situations that must be included in any definition of long-term mechanical assistance to ventilation. In the first case, ventilatory assistance can clearly be considered long-term when instituted on a nonurgent basis for symptoms of daytime hypersomnolence and severe hypercapnia. Such a circumstance may occur in a patient with a chronic neurologic condition such as muscular dystrophy. The most appropriate method of initiating ventilatory assistance may be noninvasively using positive pressure ventilation via a nasal mask. On the other hand, the situation may be less clear in a patient with severe chronic obstructive pulmonary disease (COPD) intubated for an acute pneumonia. After three weeks of mechanical ventilation via an endotracheal tube and when the pneumonia has resolved, weaning may be progressing very slowly. Although the patient is off the ventilator for 8 hr each day, it may be unclear if the patient will wean completely or will require chronic ventilatory assistance.

A working definition of long-term ventilatory assistance is necessary in order to understand the patient population under discussion. Different definitions of chronic ventilatory dependency have been proposed (1–4). A 1991 survey by the American Association for Respiratory Care (AARC) suggested chronic ventilator dependency as "a patient who must receive mechanical ventilatory support for at least six hours of each 24 hour period and has been receiving mechanical ventilation for 30 days or more" (1). A Minnesota study used a similar definition (4). A statewide survey in Illinois defined long-term mechanically ventilated patients in the acute care hospital as individuals who had been

Table 1 Considerations in the Definition of Long-Term Mechanical Ventilatory Assistance

1. The reason ventilatory assistance was initiated
2. Underlying chronic medical conditions affecting the respiratory system including the bony thorax, peripheral and central nervous system, respiratory muscles, and lungs
3. The potential that ventilatory assistance can be discontinued
4. Duration of ventilatory assistance
5. Length of time each day ventilatory assistance is used

receiving ventilation for at least 3 wk and who appeared to be unweanable, and patients at alternate sites who were felt to require ventilation for the foreseeable future (3).

Any definition of long-term ventilatory assistance must take into account all the issues listed in Table 1. An acceptable working definition can be suggested:

> A long-term ventilator-assisted individual (VAI) is a person who requires mechanical ventilatory assistance for more than 6 hr a day for more than 3 wk after all acute illnesses have been maximally treated and in whom multiple weaning attempts by an experienced respiratory care team have been unsuccessful.

This definition does not denote the user of long-term use of mechanical ventilation as a "patient" but rather as an "individual" and the term "ventilator-assisted" replaces the more usual medical designation "ventilator-dependent." The subtle distinctions in terminology are designed to imply that the goal for patients who remain on mechanical ventilation following an acute illness often changes from a traditional acute medical model (reversing acute disease and weaning from the ventilator) to a long-term humanistic approach (improving quality of life and enhancing independence) (5,6). The length of time that the patient needs ventilatory support each day is set at 6 hr because many patients can be successfully treated with ventilatory assistance used only at night during sleep (a period of 6 to 8 hr). Since most patients can be removed from ventilatory support within 1 to 2 wk of the resolution of acute disorders, the use of mechanical ventilation for more than 3 wk may be considered long-term. However, long-term in this definition may not meet the needs of the increasingly competitive and financially restrictive medical environment in the United States. In addition, the time frame suggested in any definition may be misleading since the duration of mechanical ventilation alone may not be the most important factor in determining the site of continued care. Prior to the 3-wk time point, patients who have the potential to wean from ventilatory support are often transferred from the critical care unit to less intensive units in acute medical hospitals, to specialized weaning units, or even to other health care facilities. Mechanical ventilation should not be considered chronic unless all acute illnesses, particularly those related to the reason ventilation was initiated, have been maximally treated. Any proposed definition must be applicable not only to patients with an acute medical or surgical condition who fail to wean from mechanical ventilation but also to patients in whom ventilatory assistance is electively initiated for a chronic, underlying, respiratory system disorder. The use of continuous positive airway pressure (CPAP) for obstructive sleep apnea is not covered by the VAI definition given above and should be distinguished from the use of mechanical assistance for ventilation.

Individuals who are dependent on mechanical ventilation for prolonged periods of time present unique challenges to all sectors of the health care system. For physicians, management of the unusual medical needs of these individuals is often difficult and continued care in the home and alternate sites presents unfamiliar issues. Nursing staff need extensive evaluation skills to assess the respiratory, medical, and psychosocial needs of these patients. Discharge planners and case managers must determine the most appropriate site for long-term care based upon not only the medical and psychological needs of the patient but also issues of family support and the financial costs of care. Respiratory care professionals need to address the educational needs of patients and families to allow optimal long-term care. Medical insurers must develop funding mechanisms to assure cost-effective care.

III. Long-Term Ventilation in the Acute Care Hospital

The experience of critical care practitioners is that mechanical ventilation is not only one of the major reasons for patient treatment in intensive care units, but it is also one of the major reasons for prolonged stays in such units. Although the total number of patients who cannot be immediately weaned from mechanical ventilation may be relatively small, the total cost of caring for these patients is extraordinarily high.

One of the earliest studies of the prevalence of long-term ventilation in acute care hospitals was conducted in 1983 in Massachusetts (7). Extrapolation from the 147 patients in this statewide study who were ventilator dependent for longer than 3 wk suggested there were 6800 long-term ventilation patients in U.S. hospitals. The authors further estimated that these patients were accruing costs of $1.7 billion per year, or about 1.5% of total hospital costs in 1983.

The most complete and rigorous study of the prevalence of long-term VAIs in acute care hospitals was commissioned by the American Association for Respiratory Care (1). In December, 1990, telephone interviews were conducted with 300 respiratory care department managers and 100 pulmonary physicians. Long-term ventilator assistance was defined as patients requiring mechanical ventilation for ≥6 hr daily for ≤30 days. There was an average of 4.8 chronic ventilator patients in each facility, but the number of patients per hospital varied widely. Over half of the hospitals had no long-term ventilator patients, and 31% of hospitals (usually larger urban facilities) had 4 or more such patients. The number of patients per facility was related to hospital location and size; hospitals with over 400 beds had an average of 7.7 long-term ventilator patients, and large urban hospitals had an average of 6.6 long-term patients. Over half the patients were between the ages of 18 and 64, and 39% were age 65 or older. This 1990 survey found that 12% of patients remained hospitalized because of problems obtaining reimbursement for care at alternate sites and 17% were awaiting placement in other locations. The results of the AARC survey provided an estimate of approximately 11,419 chronic ventilator-dependent patients in U.S. hospitals and annual costs of $3.2 billion, figures twice that of the study 7 yr earlier (7).

There are few other studies to indicate if there have been any changes in the number or characteristics of VAIs in general acute care hospitals. The situation has become even more confusing in the United States due to the development of new terminology for the types of units in acute hospitals that manage ventilator-assisted individuals and an increasing number of alternate sites for care of these patients.

Studies from the late 1980s suggested that the costs for managing ventilator-dependent patients are not fully reimbursed by insurers in the United States (8–10). As a result of these findings, Medicare changed the payment categories for mechanically ventilated patients. Despite changes in reimbursement, respondents to the 1990 AARC report estimated that only 53% of charges were actually recovered by the hospitals from third party payers, although respiratory care department directors and physicians may not have had access to the most complete reimbursement information and cost data were not available.

With more widespread institution of managed care in the United States it is likely that reimbursement for the hospital care of patients requiring prolonged mechanical ventilation is even lower. It appears that the high costs for caring for ventilator-assisted individuals in acute care hospitals are not fully reimbursed; the costs must therefore be covered at least in part by the reimbursement for other lower-cost patients.

IV. Long-Term Ventilation Outside the Acute Care Hospital

A. Sites for Long-Term Care of Ventilator-Assisted Individuals

There has been a marked change in the facilities for medical care both within and outside the acute care hospital (for a more detailed discussion, see Chapter 2). Earlier discharge of patients from the acute care hospital has been fueled by the need to decrease health care costs. Alternate sites of care have been developed with the goal of not only weaning patients from mechanical ventilation but also of providing rehabilitation and reducing health care costs (6,11–16). Locations for ventilator-assisted individuals can be broadly divided into three categories—acute care, intermediate care, and long-term care (Table 2).

In recognition of the complexity and unique needs of ventilator-assisted patients, specialized respiratory care units in acute care hospitals have been developed to wean patients from mechanical ventilation (14,17–22). These units have been reported to have a lower nurse/patient ratio than critical care units and decrease costs by use of an experienced team to wean the patient. Medicare devel-

Table 2 Sites for Long-Term Care of Ventilator-Assisted Individuals

Acute Hospitals
Critical care units
Specialized respiratory care units
Long-term ventilator (weaning) units
Transitional care units
General medical/surgical units
Intermediate Care Facilities
Rehabilitation hospitals
Skilled nursing facilities
Transitional care units
Long-Term Care Environments
Home
Assisted living
Congregate living
Foster home care
Skilled nursing facilities

oped a 5-yr demonstration project to assess the efficacy of specialized respiratory weaning units (20–22). Unfortunately, this concept has received little subsequent attention due to the move to managed care and capitated hospital payments.

The goals of "intermediate" care facilities are to wean the patient from the ventilator and provide a transition to a more long-term site of care. These health care facilities provide a more limited range of services than acute care hospitals and thus have lower overhead and reduce health care costs. For-profit health care corporations in the United States (e.g., Vencor and Transitional Care) have expanded the number of long-term acute care hospitals, applied the concept to ventilator-assisted individuals and developed facilities in most major metropolitan areas. Rehabilitation hospitals provide similar services, and many specialize in a particular organ system, such as spinal cord injury or neurologic disorders. Skilled nursing facilities now admit patients following an acute hospitalization not with the goal of keeping the patient for the long term, but rather to transition patients from the hospital to the home. Many acute hospitals now have "transitional" care units and some are designated as skilled nursing facilities even though they share many resources with the acute care hospital.

The difficulty in discharging VAIs from acute care hospitals due to lack of resources in the community has been noted in earlier studies (5,23). The AARC reported an average of 5 wk to discharge a VAI from the hospital because of insufficient beds at alternate sites (1). Respiratory care department directors estimated that only 26% of VAIs were discharged home; 34% of hospital patients were discharged to a skilled nursing facility and 60% were sent to other long-term care medical environments (likely long-term care hospitals). Bone (23) reported that there was a long wait before patients were able to be discharged from acute care hospitals because of the limited number of nonacute health care facilities in the Chicago area. This study identified 50 to 80 patients awaiting transfer to the 33 long-term care beds that were available for VAIs in 1987. However, the reduced frequency of such reports in the more recent literature may reflect the increasing number of intermediate care sites, particularly long-term care hospitals, in the United States.

One of the largest experiences with mechanical ventilation in a long-term care facility in the United States has been reported from Barlow Hospital in Southern California (15). Of 1037 patients referred to this facility over 8 yr, 29% died, 56% were weaned from ventilation, and 15% were discharged on ventilators (27% of discharges were to home and the rest to extended care facilities). Earlier studies from another long-term respiratory unit reported that 24% of patients were discharged home and noted the cost effectiveness of this model of care (12,13). A report from one of the four participants in the Medicare ventilator-dependent demonstration program reported a very high survival rate of 95%, which may have been related to selective admission criteria (21,24).

B. Epidemiology of Long-Term Ventilation Outside the Acute Care Hospital

There are numerous factors that might be expected to influence the number of patients receiving long-term ventilation outside acute health care facilities (Table 3), and these factors are unique to each country (25). First and foremost, however, is the presence of a nationwide system to reliably and accurately collect such information. France has long had a national system to manage ventilator-assisted individuals using regional centers and prospectively collects and frequently reports national statistics on VAIs (26). More recently, the Scandinavian countries have developed registries to monitor the number of long-termVAIs (27–29). As noted by a recent Italian study, in which only 50% of centers responded to a questionnaire, surveys to assess prevalence of long-term ventilation often provide a less than optimal response (30).

Started in 1981 and expanding from the experience with polio survivors from the 1940s, the Association Nationale pour le Traitement A Domicile de l'Insuffisance Respiratoire Chronique (ANTADIR) has the largest reported experience with home ventilation and assists in the management of about 70% of home ventilator patients in France (26,31–35). France not only has the longest established system for home care but also the highest prevalence of home mechanical ventilation. Sweden and Switzerland have more recent registries and report a lower prevalence of home ventilation patients than France (28,36).

Table 3 Factors That May Affect The Prevalence of Long-Term Ventilator-Assisted Individuals Outside Acute Care Hospitals

Definition of long-term ventilator assistance
Prevalence of chronic disorders requiring long-term ventilation
Neuromuscular disorders
Tuberculosis sequelae
Physician issues
Knowledge and experience with long-term ventilation
Number and distribution of physicians experienced in home care of VAIs[a]
Patient selection criteria
Medical opinion regarding long-term ventilation
Initiation of mechanical ventilation
Continuation of long-term ventilation
Patient preferences
Initiation of mechanical ventilation
Continuation of long-term ventilation
Programs for ventilator-assisted individuals
Presence of regional referral/specialized care centers
Number and availability of health care professionals experienced in home care of VAIs
Population density
Home health care
Presence of organized home care system
Presence of home care resources
Availability and type of health care professionals
Availability of home caregivers
Distance of patient residence from medical center
Type of health care system
Nationalized health care
Health care financing
Presence of home care reimbursement for care of VAIs

[a]VAIs, ventilator-assisted individuals.

The organizational structure for care of VAIs in the home is an important factor influencing the ability to discharge patients and thus influences the prevalence of home care for these patients. Fully integrated regional systems may be expected to enhance the potential for home care for VAIs. The French experience is a case in point; France has the most comprehensive home care program for VAIs to go along with its highest reported prevalence of long-term ventilation in the home. A working group of the European Respiratory Society and International Union Against Tuberculosis and Lung Disease has outlined details of many national home care programs (36), and others have also reviewed the similarities and differences in respiratory home care in different countries (34,37,38). Rigaud-Bully has indicated that there are three different types of models of the organization and financing of home care for VAIs (25):

1. The discharging hospital furnishes home equipment and supplies (most Scandinavian countries, Great Britain [39,40] and Austria),
2. Private sector management of VAIs with the hospital only providing medical follow-up (Spain, Italy, Germany, Switzerland, and the United States), and
3. Specialized community-based organizations manage most aspects of home ventilation (France has a nonprofit organization while Canada utilizes private companies).

While there is a wide range in the prevalence of VAIs in the home (Table 4), surveys in different countries over the past two decades have revealed some universal features concerning home mechanical ventilation:

1. The use of noninvasive positive pressure ventilation (NPPV) has increased to the point where it is now much more common than invasive ventilation in the home, and patients with tracheostomies are less frequently encountered.
2. The number of patients receiving mechanical ventilation both in the home and at sites outside the acute care hospital is increasing.

Table 4 Worldwide Prevalence of Long-Term Ventilator Assistance Outside the Hospital

Country	Year	Prevalence (per 100,000 population)
France (25)	1995	16
Denmark (27,29)	1995	3.5
	1999	7.8
Sweden (27,29)	1995	5.5
	1999	8
Finland (27,28)	1995	2.4
	1999	4
Iceland (27,28)	1995	6.7
	1999	20
Norway (27,28)	1995	2.3
	1999	5.5
Italy (30)	1995	3.2
United States (4)	1992	4.9

3. Patients with neuromuscular and skeletal disorders represent the largest group at home, and COPD patients are encountered less frequently.
4. There are an increasing number of reports of children receiving ventilatory assistance in the home.

United States

In an attempt to gather nationwide information about VAIs, the National Center for Home Mechanical Ventilation enlisted the aid of home equipment companies over a 5-yr period from 1989 to 1994 (41). Reports were received on a total of 560 VAIs, 93% of whom resided in the home. The mean age was 43.0 ± 24.7 (standard deviation) at the time of enrollment and 25% were ≤21 yr old. Neuromuscular disorders were the most common reasons for needing ventilatory assistance in both adults (62%) and children (60%). Mechanical ventilation via tracheostomy was required in 86% of patients. The study supported the contention that home ventilation was successful despite a high degree of ventilatory support. Daily ventilator use was high; 45% used ventilation continuously. While 38% of VAIs did not require nursing assistance, 39% required some form of daily assistance from a paid health care provider. The use of paid health care workers may be related at least in part to the large number of patients requiring continuous ventilatory assistance. Despite the high ventilatory requirements, the duration of home ventilation was 5.0 ± 4.2 yr and 21% had been at home for >6 yr.

Surveys in two different states in the United States conducted during the 1980s and repeated in the 1990s (4,42,43) provide some information about the changing epidemiology of long-term ventilation. These studies surveyed VAIs outside the acute care hospital and provided estimates of the nationwide prevalence. A Massachusetts survey in 1983 identified 147 long-term VAIs (requiring mechanical ventilation for more than 3 wk); 62% were in acute care hospitals, 22% were in chronic hospitals, and 14% were at home (42). This study estimated a total long-term ventilator-assisted population in the United States of at least 6573. A subsequent survey in Massachusetts in 1995 of patients ventilated for over 20 days yielded similar results and did not show an increase in prevalence of long-term ventilation (43).

Cross-sectional surveys of VAIs in Minnesota in 1986, 1992, and 1997 defined long-term ventilation as ≥6 hr of ventilatory assistance per day for ≥30 days, and noted an increasing number of VAIs over these 11 yr (4,44). The investigators surveyed long-term care facilities and home durable medical equipment dealers. The difficulty in clearly identifying patients as requiring ventilatory assistance rather than therapy for sleep apnea led the investigators to exclude all patients on bilevel positive pressure ventilation in the earlier years, but in 1997, patients "receiving" bilevel positive pressure ventilation were included, as long as there was a backup rate. The most common diagnoses were neuromuscular disorders, and there were almost equal numbers of patients with polio, cervical trauma, amyotrophic lateral sclerosis, and muscular dystrophy.

Polio was the most prevalent diagnosis in the 1986 and 1992 surveys, but had declined in the 1997 survey and was no longer as prevalent as cervical trauma or muscular dystrophy, probably related to attrition as the polio population ages. The amyotrophic lateral sclerosis group had also declined in 1997, for unclear reasons. There was a 110% increase in the number of VAIs in Minnesota between 1986 and 1992, and a further 42% increase in 1997 (103, 216, and 306 VAIs identified in each of the 3 yr, respectively). During the period between 1986 and 1992, the number of VAIs in the home increased more rapidly than those in long-term care facilities; the number of long-term care facility patients increased from 20 to 75 (an increase of 275%), and the number of home care patients increased from 83 to 141 (70% increase). The proportion of patients at home and in long-term care facilities remained steady between 1992 and 1997. The increased prevalence of VAIs in these sites between 1986 and 1992 may have been related to the increase in available resources; the number of facilities caring for VAIs increased from one to four and the number of home medical equipment companies assisting in care of VAIs increased from 5 to 12. While the mean duration of mechanical ventilation was 3 yr, nine patients had received ventilatory support for over 20 yr. The duration of ventilation varied considerably in different diagnostic groups. Polio patients had the longest duration of mechanical ventilation, while patients with COPD had the shortest.

Perhaps the most remarkable finding of the Minnesota surveys was the increase in the proportion of VAIs using noninvasive ventilation in the 1997 survey. Noninvasive ventilation, mainly in the form of noninvasive positive pressure ventilation, accounted for 47% of the increase in VAIs between 1992 and 1997 and 16% of all ventilator users in the 1997 survey. The exclusion of patients using CPAP or bilevel positive pressure ventilation from the 1986 and 1992 surveys undoubtedly led to an underestimation of VAIs using noninvasive ventilation in the earlier surveys and magnified the increase. Nonetheless, this trend almost certainly reflects an increased use of NPPV by VAIs nationwide, as more practitioners recognize its advantages over invasive ventilation in properly selected patients (44).

An extensive study in Illinois in 1990 identified 453 VAIs (3). Long-term ventilation was defined as greater than 3 wk with the likelihood of continued prolonged ventilatory support. Of these patients, 45% were at home with an additional 32% in acute care hospitals. The major identified barriers to discharge were reimbursement issues, lack of information about discharge planning and long-term facilities, and the need for environmental modifications for children. These factors appear to support calls for a regional system of specialized centers with expertise and experience to manage long-term ventilator patients both in the hospital and at home (31,45).

The number of children at home appears to be increasing. In the Minnesota study, the number of patients ≤10 yr old increased from 15 in 1986 to 48 in 1992 (4). Twenty-two percent of all VAIs in 1992 were 10 yr old or less. There are also an increasing number of reports of the use of noninvasive ventilation in children (46,47).

Canada

A 1995 survey in Ontario, Canada, identified 114 long-term ventilation users (48).The most common diagnoses were kyphoscoliosis (41% of all patients) and myopathies (26%). Forty-seven percent of the subjects in this study received ventilatory support via a tracheostomy. Over a third of patients (36%) used ventilation only at night, 44% used ventilation nocturnally and occasionally during the day, and 18% required ventilation continuously (>22 hr per day). An interesting aspect of the results was the finding that 44% of the VAIs had never been married, 40% were married at the time of the survey, and an additional 16% were either separated, divorced, or widowed. Although only 28% were totally independent in their own care and an additional 33% could partially care for themselves, 89% resided in their own home. A significant number of VAIs (19%) in this study were employed at least part time; 12% were students, 10% were homemakers, and 19% had retired due to their disability.

Scandinavian Countries

Prevalence figures for VAIs in the home are available for 1995 and 1999 (see Table 4) and demonstrate a marked increase in the number of such patients. A 30% increase per year in the number of home ventilator patients has been noted in Denmark from 1990 to 1999 and a 15 to 20% increase per year in Sweden (28,29).

Denmark has developed a regional system of care for VAIs with one specialized center in the east and one in the western part of the country, and a centralized system is also in place in Iceland. Norregaard recently reported on 20 children in Denmark receiving home ventilation (47).

In Sweden, there are similar numbers of patients in three major diagnostic groups—postpolio, neuromuscular diseases, and thoracic deformities. Only 25% of patients have a tracheostomy, and two age peaks, 20 to 30 and 60 to 70, are noted among long-term ventilator patients in Sweden (28).

Italy

A 1-year survey from 1995 to 1996 in Italy identified a total of 1842 long-term VAIs (30). However, the resulting prevalence of 3.2 per 100,000 population should be considered only a rough estimate because 50% of 115 centers surveyed failed to respond. Moreover, 486 of the patients were reported to be using CPAP, and thus it is unclear if these patients were being treated only for sleep apnea rather than for ventilatory failure. Although most of the patients receiving home mechanical ventilation (31%) in Italy, had neuromuscular diseases, 27% of home patients had COPD. The most frequent neuromuscular disorders were muscular dystrophy (56% of all neuromuscular patients), spinal muscular atrophy (13%) and amyotrophic lateral sclerosis (11%). Noninvasive positive pressure ventilation was by far the most common method of ventilatory support in the home and was reported as the modality in 81% of patients; only 16% of patients had a tracheostomy. The survey identified a number of difficulties in arranging home ventilation in Italy, including obtaining appropriate supplies, wide geographic distribution of patients, collaboration with local physicians, patient adherence, understaffing, high costs, and follow-up medical care. Family and social problems prevented a substantial number of patients from receiving home ventilation. The majority of costs associated with home ventilation were reimbursed by the Italian National Health Service although less than optimal delivery and reimbursement policies presented barriers to obtaining drugs and supplies in the home.

France

At the end of 1990, there were a reported 17,862 patients treated at home for complex respiratory disorders; of the 4066 VAIs, 45% were using noninvasive support (26). The French experience has been described in numerous publications including one of the first studies of long-term survival of patients on home ventilation and has provided subsequent survival information (33,49). In 1998 there were approximately 12,550 patients receiving home ventilation (35). The majority of patients were treated with noninvasive methods of ventilation but about 3000 patients (23%) had tracheostomies.

C. Costs of Long-Term Ventilation Outside the Acute Care Hospital

A number of reports have indicated that the costs for long-term mechanical ventilation in acute care hospitals are high and can be reduced by discharging patients to facilities with less resources (4,50–53). Hospitalized long-term VAIs in the United States were estimated to cost $1.7 billion per year in 1983 dollars, and based upon the 1990 AARC study, the daily cost was estimated to be $3.2 billion (1,52). A 1983 Massachusetts study suggested that 40% of VAIs in acute care hospitals were potential candidates for transfer to lesser care sites (52). Reported costs of VAIs in intensive care units vary widely (3,51).

The costs for home care depend largely on the independence of the patient and the need for paid health care providers. The presence of a tracheostomy and the need for suctioning may also affect home care costs because of regulations in some states that prevent unlicensed attendants from performing endotracheal suctioning. From an analysis of eight selected cases, 1986 costs in Minnesota were found to be $19,351 per month in long-term care units and $6557 per mo at home compared with $64,513 in intensive care units (4). These results should be viewed with the recognition that only two of the eight patients had licensed nurses, three others had unlicensed personal care attendants, and three had only family caregivers. In a 1992 New York study, reimbursement in long-term care facilities was noted to be $718.80 per day and community care as $235.13 (52). All home care patients in the New York study were receiving noninvasive ventilation without a tracheostomy. The 30 VAIs studied required continuous ventilatory assistance and had been in the home for an average of 12.9 yr. The average cost for the personal care attendants employed by the patients and reimbursed by Medicaid was $191 per day.

The most extensive economic analysis of long-term VAIs in the home assessed both direct and indirect costs (54). This cross-sectional survey of 239 VAIs in 37 states noted an average monthly cost of $7642 per VAI. Caregiver burden was very high with an average of 12.0 ± 7.5 hr spent each day by caregivers and resulting decrease in caregiver leisure time. Utilization of home health care professionals was high (average of $5365 per mo), and only 13.8% of patients did not use home health services.

V. Conclusion

The epidemiology of long-term ventilation is changing as the prevalence of long-term mechanical ventilation rises throughout the developed world and noninvasive positive pressure support via nasal interfaces is applied more widely in non-emergency settings. Ventilator-assisted individuals may be managed in the home setting provided adequate resources for long-term care are in place. However, comprehensive outpatient programs are not available in all countries.

Despite the increasing use of noninvasive ventilation, there is still a substantial population of patients who are receiving long-term ventilation via tracheostomy following initial management in intensive care units of acute care hospitals. These high-cost and high-resource-utilizing patients present unique challenges to the health care system. A 1998 Consensus Conference Report from the American College of Chest Physicians concluded that additional data were required on the costs, survival, complications, physiologic features, quality of life and outcomes of VAIs in intermediate and long-care facilities (6). Without such information readily available to physicians, other health care professionals, and discharge planners, it is difficult to determine the optimal site of care for long-term ventilator-assisted individuals.

References

1. A Study of Chronic Ventilator Patients in the Hospital. Dallas: American Association of Respiratory Care, 1991.
2. Stoller JK. Establishing clinical unweanability. Resp Care 1991; 36:186–198.
3. Goldberg AI. The ventilator-assisted individuals study. Chest 1990; 98:428–433.
4. Adams AB, Whit J, Marcy T. Surveys of long-term ventilatory support in Minnesota: 1986 and 1992. Chest 1993; 103:1463–1469.
5. O'Donohue WJ Jr, Giovannoni RM, Goldberg AF, et al. Long-term mechanical ventilation: Guidelines for management in the home and alternate community sites. Chest 1986; 90:1S–37S.
6. Make BJ, Hill NS, Goldberg AI, et al. Mechanical ventilation beyond the intensive care unit: Report of a consensus conference of the American College of Chest Physicians. Chest 1998; 113:289S–344S.
7. Make B, Dayno S, Gertman P. Prevalence of chronic ventilator dependency. Am Rev Respir Dis 1986; 133:A167.
8. Douglas PS, Rosen RH, Butler PW, Bone RC. DRG payment for long-term ventilator patients: Implications and recommendations. Chest 1987; 91:413–417.
9. Douglas PS, Bone RC, Rosen RL. DRG payment for long-term ventilator patients—Revisited. Chest 1988; 93:629–31.
10. Gracey DR, Gillespie D, Nobrega F, Naessens JM, Krishan I. Financial implications of prolonged ventilator care of Medicare patients under the prospective payment system. Chest 1987; 91:424–27.
11. Nochomovitz ML, Montenegro HD, Parran S, Daly B. Placement alternatives for ventilator-dependent patients outside the intensive care unit. Resp Care 1991; 36: 199–204.
12. Indihar FJ, Forsberg DP. Experience with a prolonged respiratory care unit. Chest 1982; 81:189–192.
13. Indihar FJ, Walker NE. Experience with a prolonged respiratory care unit revisited. Chest 1984; 86:616–620.
14. Bone RC, Balk RA. The noninvasive respiratory care unit: A cost-effective solution for the future. Chest 1988; 93:390–394.
15. Scheinhorn DJ, Hassenpflug-Stern M, Heltsley DJ. Post-ICU mechanical ventilation treatment of 1,123 patients at a regional weaning center. Chest 1997; 111:1654–1659.
16. Make B, Gilmartin M, Brody JS, Snider GL. Rehabilitation of ventilator-dependent persons with lung disease: The concept and initial experience. Chest 1984; 86:358–365.
17. Elpern EH, Silver MR, Rosen RL, Bone RC. The noninvasive respiratory care unit: Patterns of use and financial implications. Chest 1991; 99:205–208.
18. Popovich J. Intermediate care units: Graded care options. Chest 1991; 99:4–5.
19. Krieger BP, Ershowsky P, Spivack D, Thorstenson J, Sackner MA. Initial experience with a noninvasive respiratory monitoring unit as a cost-saving alternative to the intensive care unit for Medicare patients who require long-term ventilator support. Chest 1988; 93:395–397.

20. O'Donohue WJ Jr, Branson RD, Hoppough JM, Make BJ. Criteria for establishing units for chronic ventilator-dependent patients in hospitals. Respir Care 1988; 33: 1044–1046.
21. Gracey DR, Viggiano RW, Naessens JM, Hubmayr RD, Silverstein MD, Koenig GE. Outcomes of patients admitted to a chronic ventilator-dependent unit in an acute-care hospital. Mayo Clin Proc 1992; 67:131–136.
22. Criner GJ, Kreimer DT, Pidlaoan L. Patient outcome following prolonged mechanical ventilation via tracheostomy. Am Rev Respir Dis 1993:A874.
23. Bone RC. Long-term ventilator care: A Chicago problem and a national problem. Chest 1987; 92:536–539.
24. O'Donohue WJ Jr. Chronic ventilator-dependent units in hospitals: Attacking the front end of long-term problem. Mayo Clin Proc 1992; 67:198–200.
25. Rigaud-Bully C. Comparison of the methods of organization of home mechanical ventilation in different countries. In: Robert D, Make BJ, Leger P, Goldberg AI, Paulus J, Willig T-N, eds. Home Mechanical Ventilation. Paris: Arnette Blackwell, 1995; 27–35.
26. Muir JF, Voisin C, Ludot A. Home mechanical ventilation (HMV)—national insurance system (France). Eur Respir Rev 1992; 2:418–421.
27. Midgren B. Home respiratory care in Scandinavia. Nord Med 1995; 110:142–144.
28. Midgren B. Presentation of a national register on home mechanical ventilation. Acta Anaesthesiol Scand 1999; 43:28.
29. Jacobsen E. Nordic incidences and prevalences of persons treated with home mechanical ventilation. Acta Anaesthesiol Scand 1999; 114:27.
30. Gasperini M, Clini E, Zaccaria S. Mechanical ventilation in chronic respiratory insufficiency: Report on an Italian nationwide survey. Monaldi Arch Chest Disor 1998; 53:394-399.
31. Goldberg AI. Home care for life-supported persons: Is a national approach the answer? Chest 1986; 90:744–748.
32. Robert D, Fournier G, Thomas L, Gérard M, Chemorin B, Bertoye A. Indications tea la ventilation chronique a domicile par tracheotomie del'insuffisance chronique non parapytique. Rev Fr Mal Respir 1979; 7:353–355.
33. Robert D, Gérard M, Leger P, et al. Domicilliary mechanical ventilation by tracheostomy for chronic respiratory failure. Rev Fr Mal Resp 1983; 11:923–936.
34. Leger P. Organization of home respiratory care in Europe. In: Simonds AK, ed. Non-invasive Respiratory Support. London: Chapman and Hall, 1996:150–157.
35. ANTADIR (Association Nationale pour le Traitement A Domicile de l'Insuffisance Respiratoire Chronique) 1998 Observatory; Annual Report. Vol 1. ANTADIR, 1999; 120.
36. Fauroux PH, Muir JF. Home treatment for chronic respiratory insufficiency: The situation in Europe in 1992. Eur Respir J 1994; 7:1721–1726.
37. Pierson DJ. Home respiratory care in different countries. Eur Respir J 1989; 2:630S–636S.
38. Goldberg AI. Mechanical ventilation and respiratory care in the home in the 1990's: Some personal observations. Respir Care 1990; 35:247–259.
39. Goldberg AI, Faure EAM. Home care for life supported persons in England: The responaut approach. Chest 1984; 86:910–914.

40. Simonds AK. The home ventilatory care network. In: Simonds AK, ed. Non-invasive Respiratory Support. London: Chapman and Hall, 1996; 143–149.
41. Glenn K, Make B. National center for home mechanical ventilation: Report to the board, 1994:1–34.
42. Make B, Dayno S, Gertman P. Prevalence of chronic ventilator-dependency. Am Rev Respir Dis 1986; 133:A167.
43. Harris J, Haughton J, Celli B. A survey of ventilator dependent patients in Massachusetts, 1995. Am J Respir Crit Care Med 1997; 155:A411.
44. Adams AB, Shapiro R, Marini JJ. Changing prevalence of chronic ventilator-assisted individuals in Minnesota: Increases, characteristics, and the use of noninvasive ventilation. Respir Care 1998; 43:643–649.
45. Goldberg AI. The regional approach to home care for life-supported persons. Chest 1984; 86:345–346.
46. Teague WG, Fortenberry JD. Noninvasive ventilatory support in pediatric respiratory failure. Resp Care 1995; 40:86–96.
47. Norregaard O. Acute and long term non-invasive ventilation in infants and children. Acta Anaesthesiol Scand 1999; 43:26.
48. Goldstein RS, Psek JA, Gort EH. Home mechanical ventilation: Demographics and user perspectives. Chest 1995; 108:1581–1586.
49. Muir J-F, Girault C, Cardinaud J-P, Polu J-M, Group tFCS. Survival and long-term follow-up of tracheostomized patients with COPD treated by home mechanical ventilation: A multicenter French study in 259 patients. Chest 1994; 106:201–209.
50. Sivak ED, Cordasco EM, Gipson WT. Pulmonary mechanical ventilation at home: A reasonable and less expensive alternative. Respir Care 1983; 28:42–49.
51. Wagner D. Economics of prolonged mechanical ventilation. Am Rev Respir Dis 1989; 140:S14–S18.
52. Make BJ, Gilmartin ME. Care of ventilator-assisted individuals in the home and alternative sites. In: Burton GG, Hodgkin JE, Ward JJ, eds. Respiratory Care: A Guide to Clinical Practice. Philadelphia: Lippincott, 1991; 669–690.
53. Bach JR, Intintola P, Alba AS, Holland IE. The ventilator-assisted individual: Cost analysis of institutionalization vs rehabilitation and in-home management. Chest 1992; 101:26–30.
54. Sevick MA, Kamlet MS, Hoffman LA, Rawson I. Economic cost of home-based care for ventilator-assisted individuals: A preliminary report. Chest 1996; 109:1597–1606.

2

Sites of Care for Long-Term Mechanical Ventilation

WALTER E. DONAT

Rhode Island Hospital
Providence, Rhode Island

NICHOLAS S. HILL

Brown University School of Medicine
Rhode Island Hospital
Providence, Rhode Island

I. Introduction

Patients who require long-term ventilatory assistance consume a disproportionate share of health care resources. In an effort to control health care costs, there is increasing economic pressure to manage such patients in settings other than acute medical or surgical intensive care units (ICUs). It is ironic that the impetus for development of the modern ICU was the development of technology that led not only to the survival of acutely ill patients in respiratory failure, but also to an increasing population of patients who were chronically dependent on the same technology. As the technology becomes ever more sophisticated, the ICU has evolved into a setting for the support of patients with multiorgan system failure, some of whom will never be liberated from the technology that enables them to survive.

Patients with multisystem organ failure who require complex ventilator strategies and invasive hemodynamic monitoring as well as vasoactive drug therapy demand a very high level of vigilance from nursing and medical staff. On the other hand, those with respiratory failure but stability of other organ systems may require less intensive monitoring and can often be managed in a less costly environment. Such patients might require a brief period of observation and management in a medical ICU, but then can be safely and effectively followed in a less sophisticated environment where the major focus is on respiratory care. Nevertheless, the optimal location for such ventilator-assisted individuals (VAIs) remains unclear, and sufficient data to guide placement decisions are not yet available in most circumstances. This chapter explores different loci available for the placement of the VAI beyond the intensive care unit setting, considering patient admission guidelines, relative costs, and resources available in the various settings.

II. Sites of Care for Ventilator-Assisted Individuals

Many sites are potentially available for the placement of VAIs. In the absence of sufficient information on outcomes, however, no standard recommendations

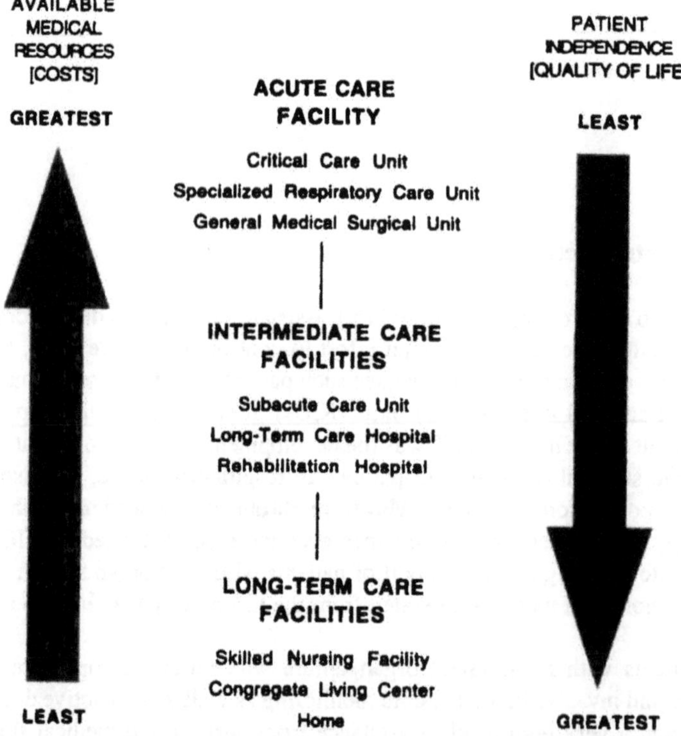

Figure 1 Potential sites of care for ventilator-assisted individuals shown as a continuum from the acute to the long-term settings. Centers at the top require the greatest resources, but off the least independence, whereas those at the bottom have the least resources, but offer the greatest independence. From Ref. 1, with permission.

can be made as to the optimal location for such patients. What is clear is that economic pressures and shortages of acute ICU beds have made it necessary to discharge such patients from the ICU setting. This has led to the creation of a variety of settings appropriate for VAIs, such as intermediate care facilities, dedicated respiratory care units, skilled nursing facilities, and free-standing long-term care hospitals. The choice of any particular unit is often an arbitrary determination dictated by the patient's needs and local or regional resource availability, patterns of referral, and reimbursement issues. No matter what type of unit is chosen or specific care recommended, the main goals of management for VAIs are universal and include the following: 1) to provide a safe environment that optimizes the individual's potential for weaning and/or rehabilitation, 2) to improve the patient's physical and physiologic function by a multidisciplinary approach, 3) to extend life, and 4) to provide cost-effective care (1).

As yet there has been no standardized classification of sites available for long-term ventilatory care. For the purposes of this chapter, sites are grouped into 3 main categories; acute care facilities, intermediate care facilities, and long-term care facilities (Figure 1) (1,2). Obviously, the more acutely ill patient will be managed in the acute care setting whereas the most long-term ventilatory-dependent patient without comorbid disease will tend to be managed in a chronic care setting or home. Due to inadequate reimbursement, problems are encountered in many regions in placing VAIs who have no prospect for weaning or returning home. Also, there is much overlap between different sites of care and considerable regional variation in resource availability and management practices. It is fair to say that the development of such a hierarchy of respiratory care facilities is still in evolution.

III. Acute Care Settings

Acute care hospitals are designed to care for patients with acute medical illnesses. These hospitals have evolved at least three designated locations where ventilator-dependent patients may receive care. The first setting, developed some 30 years ago, is the medical intensive care unit. Economic costs and pressures for ICU beds led subsequently to the creation of specialized respiratory care units or non-invasive respiratory care units (3,4). In addition, as the demands for these specialized beds has increased, many of the more stable, chronic ventilator-dependent patients who are unable to be placed elsewhere are, of necessity, assigned to a general medical/surgical unit.

A. Critical Care Units

The critical care unit has the greatest capability for invasive and noninvasive monitoring and the highest nurse/patient ratio in the hospital, averaging 1:1 to 2:1. These units are most beneficial to patients in the first several days to several weeks of respiratory failure when they might require technologically advanced forms of mechanical ventilation or might exhibit hemodynamic instability and require invasive monitoring. For many patients, indeed probably the majority of patients with uncomplicated respiratory failure secondary to chronic obstructive pulmonary disease (COPD) or neuromuscular diseases, the ventilator management is usually far less sophisticated. Such patients rarely need 1:1 nursing. On the other hand, in a critical care setting, a disproportionate amount of physician and nursing effort is given to patients with multiorgan system failure, adult respiratory distress syndrome (ARDS), or sepsis syndrome. For the patient with chronic respiratory illness due to COPD or neuromuscular disease, a multimodal approach involving respiratory therapy, physical and occupational therapy, nutrition support services, and psychiatric services is more appropriate for weaning followed by eventual rehabilitation and discharge. This approach is also suited to patients who have suffered prolonged mechanical ventilation due to catastrophic medical or surgical illnesses, such as those recovering from prolonged bouts of respiratory failure due to ARDS or pneumonia with sepsis.

The resources of the critical care unit are best devoted to the hyperacute and acute phases of the patient's hospitalization. The focus of the critical care team is not on patients who have suffered prolonged respiratory failure and need a slow and concentrated effort in order to effect successful weaning. The needs of these patients may, in fact, be last on the priority list in a busy critical care unit. Thus, the critical care unit delivers high-cost care that may not be appropriate for the needs of long-term VAIs.

B. Specialized Respiratory Care Units

The need for cost containment and the recognition that patients with prolonged respiratory failure have unique care demands have led to the creation of specialized respiratory care units (3). These units exist as part of an acute care hospital. They lack the invasive monitoring capabilities of the critical care unit, but they generally offer bedside and telemetry noninvasive monitoring of heart and respiratory rate, pulse oximetry, noninvasive blood pressure, and occasionally, end-tidal carbon dioxide (CO_2) (4). In some units, arterial lines are permitted as well as CVP monitoring, but pulmonary artery catheters are usually not an option. Still other units specify minimal requirements for monitoring, lacking even telemetry capability (5). The focus of these units is to provide a safe environment for ongoing ventilator care as well as for intensive multidisciplinary efforts to wean and liberate the patient from mechanical ventilation.

Information has become available about specialized respiratory care units for VAIs. Indihar and Walker (6) reported their experience with a prolonged respiratory care unit (PRCU) in St. Paul, MN. This unit opened on a trial basis in 1979 and the first 3.75 yr of experience were reported in 1984. As summarized in Tables 1 and 2, the unit has 29 beds with an overall occupancy rate of 93%. Of 178 cases admitted over 45 mo, the average length of stay was 146 days (range 2 to 831 days). The allocation of nursing and respiratory therapy staff was stratified depending on the care needs of the patients. Level I allocated one registered nurse (RN), one licensed practical nurse (LPN), and one nursing assistant to six patients and one respiratory therapist to 10 patients. Level IV allocated one RN, one LPN, and one nursing assistant to three patients and one respiratory therapist to four patients. All patients required physical therapy.

The majority of patients carried the diagnosis of chronic obstructive pulmonary disease (67%). A variety of other illnesses accounted for the remainder, although 99% of patients had more than one diagnosis. Of 182 discharges from the prolonged respiratory care unit, 39% of the patients died, and another 24% were discharged home. However, 26% of patients had to be transferred either back to the intensive care unit (24%) or to other specialty care units due to an exacerbation of their underlying disease process. Only 4% of patients were sent to nursing homes and only 2% were eligible for rehabilitation services elsewhere.

The authors felt that the majority of these respiratory patients were too complicated and their care too costly for routine nursing home placement. However, a substantial cost saving was demonstrated when compared with the intensive care setting. Substantial savings were due to bulk purchasing of supplies and medications, unit-based ventilator and respiratory equipment, a permanently assigned respiratory therapist, and less utilization of laboratory and x-ray services.

Table 1 PRCU: 3.75 Years in Overview

Beds	29
Occupancy rate	93%
Average length of stay	146 days
Range length of stay	2–831 days
Total cases	178 cases
Average daily census	
1980	16.7
1981	23.8
1982	27.0
1983	27.0
Admissions (by physician type)	
Internists	69%
Family practitioners	20%
Pulmonary specialists	11%

Source: Ref. 6.

Table 2 Primary Diagnoses of PRCU Patients (1982 Discharge Data)

Diagnosis	Patient distribution (%)
Chronic airway obstruction	57
Emphysema	10
Asphyxia	6
Malignant neoplasm	6
Quadriplegia	6
Cerebrovascular disease	3
Muscular dystrophy	3
Anoxic brain damage	3
Pneumonia, pulmonary fibrosis, dyspnea, convulsions	1% each
99% of the patients had more than one diagnosis	
82% had more than two diagnoses	
51% had more than three diagnoses	

Source: Ref. 6.

Cordasco et al. (7) reported on 99 long-term ventilatory-dependent patients cared for in a specialized respiratory care unit within a tertiary care hospital. They divided these patients into rehabilitative (50 patients) or custodial (49 patients) groups. Twenty-five patients were eventually weaned from mechanical ventilation: 24 of these were in the rehabilitative group and only 1 from the custodial patient group. There were 74 survivors and 25 deaths. All but one of the deaths occurred in the custodial patient group. Thirty patients required ongoing mechanical ventilation: 20 in the rehabilitative group requiring only part-time mechanical ventilation and 10 in the custodial group requiring full-time mechanical ventilation.

Gracey reported his initial experience with a chronic ventilator-dependent unit in an acute care hospital in 1992 (5) and this was updated in 1995 (8). The initial series reported on the outcomes of 61 patients admitted to the chronic ventilator-dependent unit, most of whom had been ventilator-dependent for at least 21 days. Some were admitted sooner if it appeared that prolonged weaning would be inevitable. The unit applied a multidisciplinary approach to the management of patients with respiratory failure, with all patients undergoing an evaluation by the rehabilitation and nutritional services. Psychosocial support was provided when necessary. The nurse/patient ratio in the unit averaged 1:2.5

compared with 1:1 or 1:2 in the intensive care unit. Before admission to the unit, all patients were required to undergo tracheostomy, have rehabilitation potential, and be medically stable enough so that electrocardiographic monitoring was not required.

Conditions associated with prolonged respiratory failure among patients admitted to the unit are given in Table 3. Chronic obstructive pulmonary disease was the most frequent underlying diagnosis, occurring in 28 patients. Neuromuscular disorders and restrictive lung disease accounted for prolonged respiratory failure in 18 patients. Of the 61 patients admitted, 3 died before discharge. Of the survivors, 50 were weaned entirely from the ventilator and another 5 remained on nocturnal ventilation. Forty-six (75%) patients were eventually discharged home, 35 of whom were discharged directly and 11 others who were transferred to a rehabilitation center, another hospital, or chronic care facility prior to discharge home (Table 4). Only 12 patients (20%) remained institutionalized. A substantial savings was realized when the authors compared the cost and reimbursement in the chronic ventilator-dependent unit with that in the intensive care units.

In 1995 Gracey reported on outcomes of a larger series of 129 patients from the same ventilator-dependent unit (VDU) (8). This, again, was a highly selected population of patients who had chronic ventilatory failure but, nevertheless, had significant rehabilitation potential. With the exception of two patients, all the patients were originally cared for in other medical or surgical units in an acute care hospital. In this series of patients, 83 of 132 admissions (63%) suffered

Table 3 Major Underlying Diagnoses Contributing to Ventilator Dependence in 61 Mayo Patients in the Chronic Ventilator-Dependent Unit (Jan 2, 1990, through June 30, 1991)

	No. of patients		
Major diagnosis	Surgical (N = 40)	Medical (N = 21)	Total (N = 61)
COPD[a]	23	5	28
Neuromuscular disorder	3	7	10
Restrictive lung disease	3	5	8
Postoperative respiratory failure	7	0	7
Acute lung injury	4	1	5
Heart disease	0	2	2
Other	0	1	1

[a] COPD, chronic obstructive pulmonary disease.
Source: Ref. 5.

Table 4 Dismissal Location of 61 Mayo Patients in the Chronic Ventilator-Dependent Unit (Jan. 2, 1990 through June 30, 1991)

	Patients	
Dismissal location	No.	%
Home		
Dismissed directly	35	57
Rehabilitation then home	8	13
Another hospital or rehabilitation unit then home	3	5
Chronic-care facility		
Dismissed directly	9	15
A medical floor of our hospital then chronic-care facility	2	3
Remains in unit	1	2
Died in hospital	3	5
Total	61	100

Source: Ref. 5.

from respiratory failure secondary to a complication of a surgical condition. The average duration of ventilator dependence before admission to the ventilator-dependent unit was 37 ± 22 days. Patients averaged 67 ± 36 days in the hospital with 31 ± 20 days in the ventilator-dependent unit. Thirteen of 132 patients (9.8%) died within the hospital. Of the 119 patients discharged from the unit, 68 patients (57%) were discharged directly home while 23 patients (19%) were transferred to a rehabilitation hospital or another hospital unit prior to discharge home. Eventually, 91 out of the 119 discharged patients (77%) were able to return home (Table 5). Sixteen patients (13%) required nocturnal ventilation. Of 22 patients discharged to a nursing home, all had been weaned from the ventilator. The short- and long-term survival rates were quite good and the 24-mo survival rate was 72%. When compared with historical controls (pre-VDU patients), there was a significant reduction in mortality but much of this reduction was attributable to selection bias.

Elpern et al. (4) described their experience with a noninvasive respiratory care unit in an acute care hospital. This was an 11-bed unit with the capacity to care for eight patients receiving continuous ventilation. Criteria for admission were that patients require specialized respiratory monitoring and support and be hemodynamically stable. The nurse to patient ratio was 1 RN to 3 patients during the day shift and 1 RN to 5 patients on the evening and night shifts. Extensive

Table 5 Ventilator-Dependent Unit Patient Outcomes, 119 Discharges

Discharge destination	Patients No.	%
Home	91	77
Directly home	68	57
Physical medicine and rehabilitation → home	18	15
Other hospital unit → home	5	5
Nursing home	22	18
Home hospital → home	4	3
Home hospital → nursing home	2	2
Total	119	100

Source: Ref. 8.

noninvasive monitoring was available including oximetry and end-tidal CO_2 monitors. However, arterial or pulmonary artery catheters were not permitted. Patients could be ventilated through translaryngeal endotracheal tubes or tracheostomy.

Of 136 patients cared for in the noninvasive respiratory care unit, 107 (78%) of the patients received mechanical ventilation for an average of 16.2 days. The average length of hospitalization was 26.6 days. Approximately 25% of the patients were not considered weanable and were admitted to the unit for custodial or terminal care. Forty-five patients (33%) were discharged home, four of whom required mechanical ventilation. Seventy-two patients (53%) died during their hospitalization. The high percentage of deaths reflected the unselected patient population. When compared with the medical intensive care unit, the average cost per ventilator day in the noninvasive respiratory care unit averaged almost one-third less (Table 6). The authors concluded that the noninvasive respiratory

Table 6 Comparison of Costs: NRCU vs MICU[a]

	No. ventilator days	Total costs	Average cost per ventilator day
NRCU	554	$657,976	$1,188
MICU	411	$1,300,424	$3,164

[a] NRCU, noninvasive respiratory care unit; MICU, medical intensive care unit.
Source: Ref. 3.

care unit was an important step in providing quality care at substantial cost savings.

In summary, specialized respiratory survival units can provide excellent outcomes with regard to the percentage of patients weaned and the rate of discharge home. These outcomes can be achieved at substantial cost savings in comparison with ICUs. However, the lack of controlled trials or specific patient selection criteria weaken the strength of evidence from the available published reports. Although the favorable impact on patient outcomes reported for these units cannot be considered proven, it appears very likely that they improve efficiency of resource utilization in comparison with ICUs. Their development in acute care hospitals large enough to provide a steady flow of patients is encouraged.

C. General Medical or Surgical Units

The third placement option for patients with prolonged ventilator dependence within acute care hospitals is assignment to a general medical or surgical unit as an alternative to ICU care. However, the needs of a ventilator patient may be substantial, and this may have an adverse impact on the routine functioning of a busy medical or surgical unit. Proper training and in-servicing must be available to nursing and ancillary staff for the care of such patients. Unfortunately, the placement of ventilator patients on general medical or surgical wards may be haphazard and dictated by pressure for beds in intensive care units or by the lack of alternative sites in the community. It is probably best to reserve this option for only the most stable patients, or the terminally ill who are not to be resuscitated (1).

IV. Intermediate Care Facilities

A. Subacute Care Units

Subacute care units (sometimes referred to as ''post–acute care units'') provide for patients whose needs for medical care and monitoring are less than those offered by an ICU, but are too complex for a skilled nursing facility. These units may exist as part of an acute care hospital, or may be part of a rehabilitation hospital or other intermediate care facility. They provide a higher level of monitoring, intravenous (IV) therapy, skilled nursing care, and rehabilitation care than long-term care facilities. The focus of subacute care units may or may not be on chronic ventilator-dependent patients, with some units excluding those with no potential to wean from mechanical ventilation. Daily nursing care in these units generally includes 3 to 8 hr by an RN with an additional 2 hr of nursing assistant care (1,9).

Over the past 15 yr, specialized care centers have emerged to provide long-term and intermediate care for the VAIs. Some are for-profit centers, such as those managed by Vencor, Inc. (Nashville, TN), a national corporation that owns free-standing hospitals devoted to the care of patients with chronic and subacute respiratory failure, as well as those with other rehabilitation needs. Other large for-profit corporations have rehabilitation as their focus, such as Mediplex Rehab (Sun Health, Inc.), which provides for general rehabilitation needs but also accepts chronic ventilator-dependent patients. The impetus for the growth of these centers had been the diagnosis-related group (DRG) exempt status for rehabilitation hospitals that provide for patients whose average length of stay exceeds 25 days. In theory, providing care for such patients in these centers is less costly than in an acute care hospital, but confirmatory financial data are unavailable (1).

The structure of for-profit subacute weaning centers is extremely sensitive to changes in the reimbursement system. The Budget Balancing Act of 1997 made sweeping changes in reimbursements for these centers. The DRG-exempt system was replaced with a capped payment system referred to as Resource Utilization Groups (RUGs) that is based on needs assessments for nursing care, occupational therapy, physical therapy, nutritional support, and so on. Reimbursement for respiratory therapy time was bundled into coverage for nursing time. As a consequence, caring for ventilator-dependent patients, even those with a prospect for weaning, has become less profitable. These centers have either closed ventilator beds, accepted fewer ventilator-dependent patients, or expanded their rehabilitation services to make up for reduced revenues accruing from care of VAIs.

B. Long-Term Ventilator Hospitals or Units

These facilities provide for long-term ventilator-dependent patients. Their role overlaps with the subacute care unit in that patients may be medically complex. They differ in that they are more often not-for-profit or government-supported and are more likely to accept VAIs with little or no prospect for weaning. Generally, these types of units accept patients who have been ventilator-dependent for at least 3 to 6 wk. Typically, patients will have had a tracheostomy as well as a feeding gastrostomy tube placed prior to entry. The focus of these units is to optimize the functional status of each patient by a multimodal treatment plan that includes rehabilitation services, nutritional services, and respiratory care. Many patients originally felt to be unweanable have been successfully weaned in these centers.

Scheinhorn et al. (10) reported on 421 patients admitted to a 49-bed, DRG-exempt, not-for-profit, regional weaning center over a 36-month period. The major focus of the hospital was to accept ventilator-dependent patients and provide two different levels of care. A general care unit provided a nurse/patient ratio of 1:4 to 1:5 with a respiratory therapist/patient ratio of 1:7, and a 6-bed ICU was available where the nurse/patient ratio was 1:1 to 1:2 and the respiratory therapist/patient ratio was 1:3 to 1:4. Critical paths specifically designed for this patient population were used.

The etiology of ventilator dependency for patients in Scheinhorn et al.'s report is given in Table 7. Of the 421 patients, 116 (28%) died, and of the survivors, 212 (70%) were eventually liberated from the ventilator. Approximately half of the patients who were weaned from the ventilator were discharged home. The 1-yr survival was 28%. The authors determined that the care in the regional weaning center was $1500 per day less costly than ICU care and $208 per day less costly than care in a noninvasive respiratory care unit attached to an acute care hospital.

Bagley and Cooney (11) reported on 278 patients admitted to a regional weaning unit opened in 1988 to care for long-term ventilator-dependent patients. The care provided was primarily custodial, but it was subsequently found that many patients admitted with chronic respiratory failure had a potential to wean. A formal weaning program was established in 1991. The authors emphasize that regardless of an individual patient's potential for weaning, the goal of therapy was always to provide the highest level of functional capability. All patients admitted were required to have a tracheostomy and, whenever possible, a feeding gastrostomy or jejunostomy. Patients had to be hemodynamically stable and could not be receiving concurrent dialysis. No admission decisions were based on prognosis, weaning potential, or rehabilitation potential. Weaning trials did not begin until strength and nutritional status improved, at the discretion of the pulmonologist. Of the 278 patients admitted, 38% were liberated from the ventilator, 47% died and 20% were eventually discharged home. The authors report that for the fiscal year 1995, the average cost per day was approximately $630.

C. Rehabilitation Hospitals

All ventilator-dependent patients should receive some form of physical therapy and occupational therapy. Such therapy can be provided in long-term care hospi-

Table 7 Etiology of Ventilator Dependency in a Regional Weaning Center

	Patients	
Category	No.	%
Chronic lung disease	103	24.5
Acute lung disease	134	31.8
Postoperative	99	23.5
Cardiac disease	21	5.0
Neurologic disease	33	7.8
Other	21	5.0
Unable to determine	10	2.4

Source: Ref. 10.

tals as well as in subacute care units or noninvasive respiratory care units. However, an outgrowth of the mission of rehabilitation hospitals has been the extension of services to ventilator-dependent patients. All patients must be able to meet the requirement of participating in rehabilitation for at least 3 hr per day. This will not be possible for many patients with prolonged ventilator dependency. Many of the for-profit hospitals are based on a rehabilitation model, seeking to wean or rehabilitate and then to discharge the patient to home or another chronic care facility. Unfortunately, financial and outcome data on long-term ventilated patients treated at rehabilitation hospitals are not available at this time.

V. Long-Term Care Facilities

These facilities include skilled nursing facilities, congregate living centers and, ideally, home. The more stable patients who are chronically dependent on ventilatory assistance will eventually gravitate to these options. Many of these patients will have exhausted their insurance-covered length of stay at acute care hospitals or rehabilitation hospitals and have already failed multiple attempts at weaning. Therefore, these facilities serve to provide custodial care in a safe and secure environment. Resources generally are not available for providing complex medical care or weaning trials.

A. Skilled Nursing Facilities

At this time, most skilled nursing facilities do not readily accept ventilator-dependent patients. However, occasional nursing homes and convalescent centers have accepted such patients. The problem is that reimbursement for care remains low and there has been no incentive for skilled nursing facilities to take on additional liability and strain already limited resources. From a patient perspective, however, the skilled nursing facility may provide a safe, caring environment at a lower cost than similar care in the home setting. Resources such as registered nurses, nursing assistants, and respiratory therapists are shared among many patients. Patients who are so limited in their ventilator dependence that they are unable to participate in basic activities of daily living may do better in a skilled nursing facility than at home. Moreover, skilled nursing facilities can assume the burden of care which would otherwise fall on the patient's family or primary caregiver.

B. Congregate Living Centers

These facilities function much like group homes for patients with psychiatric needs. They are located in private residences or apartments. Responsibility is shared among the residents who contract separately for nursing care, respiratory therapy, and physical therapy. These facilities are more common in Europe than in the United States (2).

C. Home Care

Discharge home is a desirable option for patients with chronic respiratory failure and is discussed in more detail in Chapter 14. The most important factor in the successful home discharge is the presence of a family willing to learn and assume a large portion of the patient's care. Prior to discharge home, a great deal of planning and coordination is required in order to facilitate transfer to the home setting. A home respiratory care company needs to be contacted early in the discharge planning phase. Most of the basic instruction is provided in the acute care setting or specialized care unit. The patient and family must acquire a working knowledge of ventilators, oxygen equipment, and humidifiers. Routine tracheostomy care and proper suctioning techniques must also be taught. Provision for enteral nutrition, gastrostomy, or jejunostomy care must also be established. Financial resources are, unfortunately, usually limited and the division of labor must therefore be apportioned among patient self-care, family caregiver(s), skilled nurses, and home health aide(s) (5). Every patient will have unique requirements so that care plans must be individualized.

The cost estimates for home care vary greatly depending on the types of services provided (12). In a 1991 report by Indihar, the cost estimate was $8265 per year. If the family was the principal provider of care with the help of licensed practical nurses 8 hours per day, the cost rose to $25,870 per year. If the services of a registered nurse were required 8 hours per day, the cost rose to $34,655 per year. If supervisory care was required for 24 hours per day, then the home cost estimates exceeded $100,000 per year, more expensive than costs in some long-term care facilities. Home care for VAIs may be extremely stressful for families and the lack of third party reimbursement may pose a prohibitive financial burden. Unfortunately, these concerns prevent many VAIs from returning home. Therefore, patients who are suitable for home care will likely be those who are most independent and require the least amount of ancillary services. Patients requiring only nocturnal ventilation, particularly those receiving noninvasive ventilation, are more likely to have successful home placement.

VI. Perspectives on Placing VAIs in Care Facilities

Characteristics of the sites of care discussed above are summarized in Table 8. Although three main categories—acute, intermediate, and long-term care facilities—have evolved, it should be apparent that there is considerable overlap among the different sites. For example, a patient who has stabilized after a bout of respiratory failure and is undergoing weaning trials would be a candidate for

Table 8 Characteristics of Sites of Care for Ventilator-Assisted Individuals

Sites	Nurse:patient ratio	Monitoring capabilities	Charges/day	Other considerations
Acute care				
Intensive care unit	1:1–1:2	Invasive	$3,000–5,000	Only acute care
Respiratory care unit	1:2.5–1:5	Noninvasive, some arterial lines	$1,200–2,000	For weaning, stabilization, and further placement
General med/surg ward	1:5–1:8	Noninvasive	$500–1,000	For stable, unweanable patients without placement options, or terminal care
Intermediate care				
Subacute (or "postacute") care unit				
For profit	1:3–1:8	Noninvasive	$300–500	For weaning patients, not-for-profit may accept some with little or no weaning potential
Not for profit	1:3–1:8	Noninvasive	$300–500	
Long-term ventilator hospitals	1:4–1:7	Noninvasive	$500–750	
Rehabilitation hospitals	1:4–1:7	Noninvasive	$500–1,000	For patients with rehabilitation potential, able to participate >3 hr/day
Long-term care				
Skilled nursing facilities	Variable	Minimal	$160–450	Few beds available, may be appropriate for stable chronic ventilator-dependent patients
Congregate living centers	Variable	Minimal	ND[a]	
Home care	Variable	Minimal	up to $500[b]	The most desirable site for most, but depends on patient needs, caregiver availability, and financial resources

[a] ND, no data.
[b] Cost varies widely depending on need for skilled nursing (cost approximately $20/hr).

Table 9 Criteria for Transferring Patients from ICU to a Subacute or Intermediate Site, or from Intermediate Care to a Skilled Nursing Facility (SNF) or Home

	ICU to intermediate care	Intermediate care to SNF or home
Medical stability	Nonrespiratory organ dysfunction stabilized (i.e., no uncontrolled cardiac arrhythmias, hemorrhage, sepsis, etc.)	Nonrespiratory organ dysfunction stable for 1 to 2 wk.
Respiratory stability[a]	Safe and secure airway, oxygenation adequate on $F_{IO_2} \le 0.6$, PEEP $\le$ 10 cm H_2O No need for sophisticated ventilator modes (i.e., inverse ratio, high frequency, etc.) Frequency of suctioning/treatments depends on capabilities of unit	Stable settings on mechanical ventilator with tracheostomy or noninvasive ventilation; no need for frequent suctioning/treatments. Oxygenation adequate on $F_{IO_2} \le 0.4$, PEEP $\le$ 5 cm H_2O.
Neuropsychiatric stability	Noncomatose, or if comatose, prognosis for recovery	Willing and able to participate in care or has capable caregivers. No major affective disorders that preclude participation in care.
Monitoring needs	Noninvasive monitors, i.e., oximetry, EKG No need for central hemodynamic monitoring or frequent (i.e., <1–2 hr) vital sign checks	Intermittent noninvasive monitoring; EKG telemetry unnecessary.

[a] F_{IO_2}, fraction of inspired oxygen; PEEP, positive end-expiratory pressure.

transfer to a respiratory care unit within the acute care facility, a free-standing for-profit or not-for-profit subacute facility, a long-term ventilator hospital, or a rehabilitation facility. The choice among them will be made based on multiple considerations, including the regional availability of different sites, bed availability within the sites, the prospects for rapid versus slower weaning, rehabilitation needs of the patient and the capability to participate in rehabilitation, insurance resources, patient and family desires, and caregiver preferences.

Although numerous factors should be considered in placing patients, certain guiding principles should also be observed. Most importantly, patients' needs for medical and nursing care, monitoring, and rehabilitation should be met as much as possible. Second, assuming patients' needs are met satisfactorily, care should be delivered in a cost-efficient manner. For example, as soon as a patient has stabilized sufficiently to be managed outside of the expensive ICU environment (Table 9), transfer should be arranged. Third, the site of care should be the one that optimizes the patient's rehabilitation, not necessarily weaning potential. On the other hand, there are numerous examples of patients who have weaned successfully after several months at a chronic ventilator hospital (11). Therefore, the ability to wean should be reassessed periodically. Finally, returning patients to their homes is usually the most desirable option. It is important for caregivers to be realistic, however, and not force home placement on patients or caregivers who are reluctant, unprepared, or incapable of administering proficient home care.

Observation of these principles should assist in making appropriate placement decisions. It is acknowledged, however, that limitations on resource availability often force caregivers to compromise these principles, and the best possible option may be less than ideal.

VII. Summary and Conclusions

The increasing number of VAIs is a phenomenon of modern technology. Increasing knowledge regarding respiratory failure and advances in ventilator technology mean that more patients can be sustained with ventilator support than ever before. Unfortunately, as is the case with many technologically driven phenomena, the advances in technology create unanticipated problems and outstrip the services available to deal with them. This has certainly been the case with regard to ventilator technology.

Over the past two decades, the effort to deal most efficiently and effectively with VAIs has spawned a wide range of locations for care. These are aimed at moving patients out of ICUs when their acute medical problems have been stabilized (noninvasive respiratory units within acute care hospitals, or free-standing intermediate care facilities). Alternatively, if prolonged medical attention is required because of failure to wean despite a potential for rehabilitation, some locations aim to provide effective rehabilitation services (long-term or rehabilitation hospitals). In addition, some long-term facilities have space allocated for VAIs who have no potential to wean or return home. Unfortunately, these patients usually quickly deplete their financial and insurance resources and may be very difficult to place because of the limited reimbursements available through Medicaid.

The large regional differences in the availability of the different types of facilities and the large differences among individual patients make it difficult to provide firm, specific recommendations on optimal placement. Also, because of the constantly evolving nature of sites available, partly in response to changes in reimbursement practices, it is difficult to acquire outcome or cost data on many of the options currently available. The greatest amount of published information pertains to noninvasive specialized respiratory units within acute care hospitals. Although uncontrolled, highly selected, and largely out of date, these data support the development of such units to provide favorable outcomes at a lower cost than in an ICU.

The need for facilities to care for VAIs is likely to increase in the future. For many, if not most, discharge home will not be a realistic possibility. Reimbursement policies will continue to be a major determinant of the nature of facilities available. From the clinician's perspective, it is hoped that noninvasive respiratory units in acute facilities will be reimbursed adequately, the growth of long-term hospitals with rehabilitation potential will be encouraged, and facilities to care for VAIs with no potential of returning home will be expanded, so that such patients spend less time occupying more expensive and less appropriate beds in acute care facilities. Ideally, cost should not be the sole factor in determining the site of chronic ventilator care. Resources should be matched to patient needs on an individual basis.

References

1. Make BJ, Hill NS, Goldberg AI, Bach JR, Dunne PE, Heffner JE, Keens TA, O'Donahue WJ, Oppenheimer EA, Robert D. Mechanical ventilation beyond the intensive care unit: Report of a consensus conference of the American College of Chest Physicians. Chest 1998; 113(suppl):289S–344S.
2. Make BJ, Gilmartin M. Care of the ventilator-assisted individual in the home and alternative community sites. In: Hodgkin JE, Connors GL, Bell CW, eds. Pulmonary rehabilitation: Guidelines to success. 2nd ed. Philadelphia: Lippincott, 1993; 359–391.
3. Bone RC, Balk RA. Noninvasive respiratory care unit: A cost effective solution for the future. Chest 1988; 93:390–394.
4. Elpern EH, Silver MR, Rosen RL, Bone, RC. The noninvasive respiratory care unit. Patterns of use and financial implications. Chest 1991; 99:205–208.

5. Gracey DR, Viggiano RW, Naessens JM, Hubmayr RD, Silverstein MD, Koenig GE. Outcomes of patients admitted to a chronic ventilator-dependent unit in an acute-care hospital. Mayo Clin Proc 1992; 67:131–136.
6. Indihar FJ, Walker NE. Experience with a prolonged respiratory care unit—Revisited. Chest 1984; 86:616–620.
7. Cordasco EM Jr, Sivak ED, Perez-Trepichio A. Demographics of long-term ventilator-dependent patients outside the intensive care unit. Cleve Clin J Med 1991; 58: 505–509.
8. Gracey DR, Naessens JM, Viggiano RW, Koenig GE, Silverstein MD, Hubmayr RD. Outcome of patients cared for in a ventilator-dependent unit in a general hospital. Chest 1995; 107:494–499.
9. Joint Commission for Accreditation of Healthcare Organization (JCAHO). Accreditation Manual for Home Care. Vol 1. Oakbrook Terrace, IL: JCAHO, 1993.
10. Scheinhorn DJ, Artinian BM, Catlin JL. Weaning from prolonged mechanical ventilation. The experience at a regional weaning center. Chest 1994; 105:534–539.
11. Bagley PH, Cooney E. A community-based regional ventilator weaning unit. Development and outcomes. Chest 1997; 111:1024–1029.
12. Indihar FJ. Cost comparison of care for chronic ventilator patients. Chest 1991; 99: 260–263.

3

Pathogenesis of Chronic Respiratory Failure and Effects of Long-Term Mechanical Ventilation on Respiratory Muscle Function

BARTOLOME R. CELLI

St. Elizabeth's Medical Center
Boston, Massachusetts

I. Introduction

The worldwide poliomyelitis epidemic in the middle of the twentieth century resulted in many cases of ventilatory failure. An ingenious, albeit palliative, answer to this type of ventilatory failure was the development of the iron lung, an external negative pressure ventilator that saved the lives of countless patients who developed respiratory failure during the epidemic. Assisted ventilation was instituted not to restore the function of the motor neurons, but to take over the work of the failing muscles. Even though poliomyelitis is now very infrequent in the developed parts of the world, the use of ventilators has increased and the machines have evolved in sophistication and capability. Close to half of all patients admitted to intensive care units require mechanically assisted ventilatory support. Almost all the ventilatory support currently uses positive rather than negative pressure, but the overall aims and principles remain the same: to be as unobtrusive and effective as possible. In addition, the incorporation of microprocessor technology to mechanical ventilation has resulted in a giant leap forward in the way machines can operate under difficult and frequently changing physiologic conditions. Respiratory patterns can be altered to satisfy an individual patient's needs and to fulfill specific therapeutic goals.

Fundamentally, ventilation depends upon the ability of the respiratory pump to move air in and out of the gas exchange portion of the lung. The respiratory muscles serve as the vital link between the different components of the pump: the respiratory centers, the conducting nerves, and, ultimately, the lung itself (1–5). The respiratory muscles contract during the breathing cycle, thereby changing the anatomical configurations of the chest wall by displacing its components, so that air can move in and out of the lungs. This chapter systematically analyzes the overall anatomic and physiologic arrangements of the respiratory muscles. It points out how, under a variety of clinical conditions, the ventilatory control lapses, and muscles fail to ventilate the lungs, the final result of which is ventilatory failure with hypoxia and, frequently, hypercapnia. It specifically addresses the clinical application of these concepts in relation to mechanical ventilation and its use in chronic ventilatory failure.

II. Anatomic Considerations

There are many muscles that participate in ventilation, and they can be divided into those that are inspiratory in action and those that, by their anatomic arrangement, are predominantly expiratory in function (4,5). In turn, the inspiratory muscles are divided into ones that actively contribute to inspiratory pressure generation during regular tidal breathing (the so-called primary muscles of respiration) and the accessory muscles, which are activated to participate in ventilation under conditions of increased ventilatory demand.

There are also muscles that participate in breathing but whose function is not primarily to displace the rib cage or abdomen. These muscles, located in the upper airways, act to prevent the collapse of the conduits and, in this way, facilitate airflow (1–3). The pharyngeal constrictor muscles, genioglossus, and neck strap muscles all increase patency of the pharynx, while the laryngeal abductor muscles open the vocal cords. The activation of these muscles must be synchronized, and actually precedes the contraction of the inspiratory muscles.

The diaphragm is the most important muscle of inspiration. It has a central noncontractile tendon from which muscle fibers radiate down and outward to attach to the lower rib cage and the first three lumbar vertebrae. During contraction, the diaphragm assists lung inflation through three mechanisms. First, it uses the abdomen as a fulcrum, thereby expanding the rib cage. Second, the diaphragm helps inflation because of the cephalocaudal orientation of its fibers and the curvature of its shape (2). This anatomic arrangement expands the rib cage as the fibers shorten. The curvature of the diaphragm approximates the shape of a hemisphere with a radius, r. Laplace's law for a sphere states that $P = 2T/r$, where P is the pressure inside the sphere and T is the tension in the wall. If T is maintained constant and the diaphragm flattens, its curvature will decrease, r will increase and, by definition, P must decrease. Third, the diaphragm transmits the increase in abdominal pressure during contraction to the rib cage, through its zone of apposition (6). This action also has an expansive action on the rib cage.

Patients with chronic obstructive pulmonary disease (COPD) characteristically develop lung hyperinflation, causing an increase in the resting volume of the ribcage (4,5,7). It is believed that hyperinflation reduces diaphragmatic strength by shortening of the diaphragmatic fibers, which places the muscle at a suboptimal point on its length-tension curve. However, studies have demonstrated that when diaphragmatic fibers are experimentally shortened, the muscles adapt by dropping sarcomeres and achieving a new optimal length, so that each bundle is capable of generating its maximal tension for that new length (8,9). It can therefore be implied that the decreased diaphragmatic pressure-generating capacity in COPD patients is either due to anatomic and mechanical derangement or to contractile dysfunction, and not to simple length-tension changes. Patients with neuromuscular diseases also often have dysfunctional respiratory muscles. Regardless of the nature of the disease, the end result is the presence of decreased respiratory muscle strength with conditions of increased respiratory loads.

The other primary inspiratory muscles are the external intercostals, the parasternal part of the internal intercostals, the triangularis sterni, and the scalene. They are activated during tidal breathing in normal individuals, but significantly increase their participation in ventilation during increases in ventilatory demand (10,11). They play a particularly important role in diseases characterized by hyperinflation such as COPD because they undergo less anatomic shortening, and therefore operate at a lesser mechanical disadvantage than the diaphragm. On the other hand, the true "accessory muscles," i.e., the sternomastoid, subclavian, pectoralis minor and major, serratus anterior, upper and lower trapezius, and latissimus dorsi, are usually inactive during normal breathing but may become increasingly important under special circumstances. These include strenuous exercise and severe increases in ventilatory load, as may be seen in kyphoscoliosis, thoracoplasty, and diaphragmatic paralysis.

There are other muscles that are not thought to be respiratory in nature, such as the muscles of the shoulder girdle (12). These muscles have dual actions that include fixing the upper rib cage, partaking in upper torso positioning, and elevating the upper extremity. They may also exert a pulling action on the rib cage, when they contract and are fixed at their extrathoracic anchoring point. Because of this, patients with severe COPD will often find relief to their dyspnea when they lean on a surface and fix their shoulder girdle.

The respiratory muscles have functions other than breathing. They also participate in very complex functions, such as speaking and singing (1,13). This requires the simultaneous activation of the inspiratory and expiratory muscles. In other instances, synchronous expulsive maneuvers will be needed to achieve other functions, such as sneezing, vomiting, and defecating. The expiratory muscles may also need to act in concert to facilitate parturition and micturition. Unique aspects of the respiratory system are the sneezing and coughing reflexes. These maneuvers require an initial deep inspiratory effort, followed by closure of the glottis and a forceful contraction of the diaphragm and the abdominal muscles. When the upper airways suddenly open, the increased intra-abdominal pressure results in an explosive expiratory effort. This sudden increase in peak flow helps clear the upper airways and is very important for the management of secretions. Conditions that result in impaired coughing (i.e., neuromuscular diseases) frequently lead to the accumulation of secretions in the lungs, leading to development of atelectasis. The retained secretions may become infected and this, in turn, worsens respiratory function and increases ventilatory demand.

A. Physiologic Principles

Two basic principles control the behavior of muscles when subjected to physiologic stimuli. These are applicable to muscles in general, including the respiratory muscles. The first principle is that the muscle generates more force as it lengthens until it reaches an optimal length (Fig. 1). Stretching the muscle beyond this length decreases strength, until the muscle fiber breaks. More importantly, as the resting length of a muscle shortens (which occurs in diseases that cause lung hyperinflation), the force-generating capacity for a given electrical stimulus decreases. In the case of the respiratory muscles, if a similar pressure is required to maintain ventilation, then the only possible compensatory mechanism is the

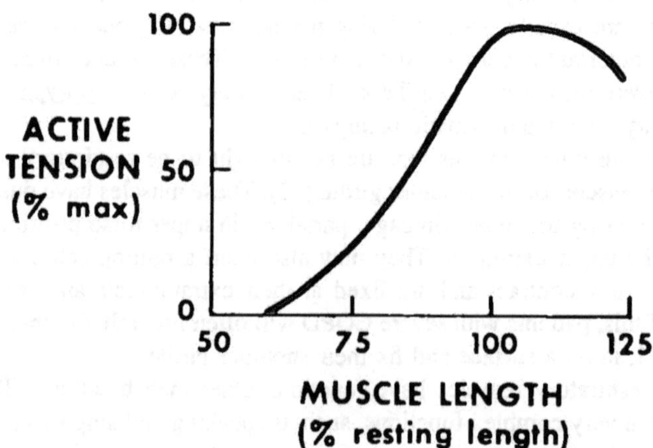

Figure 1 The force that a muscle is able to generate decreases with muscle shortening. Conversely, muscle force increases as the muscle lengthens.

recruitment of more muscle fibers, i.e., increasing the motor output of the central nervous system, and then increasing the firing rate to the muscle.

The second principle, represented in Figure 2, is that the capacity of the muscle to generate force decreases as the velocity of contraction increases (i.e., increased respiratory rate) (14). Although of limited clinical importance normally because of the relatively low speed of contraction of the respiratory muscles, this property it may become important at very fast breathing rates, or in patients whose respiratory ailment is associated with very short inspiratory times. Under resting breathing conditions, the velocity of contraction and the inspiratory muscle force generated amount to about 5% of their maximal capacity. Up to 50% of maximal force or velocity can be sustained for prolonged periods of time (hours) (15).

B. Skeletal Muscle Cell Types

Skeletal muscles are composed of different types of muscle fibers. Based upon histochemical staining they have been divided into types I, IIa, and IIb. Type I fibers have a high oxidative capacity and a low concentration of glycolytic enzymes. They are referred to as "slow twitch" fibers because when activated, they develop a slow rise in force. Physiologically, they are the first to be recruited during muscle activation, because they generate low levels of force and are fatigue resistant. Type IIb fibers, referred to as "fast twitch" fibers, have a low oxidative capacity and a high concentration of glycolytic enzymes. They are the

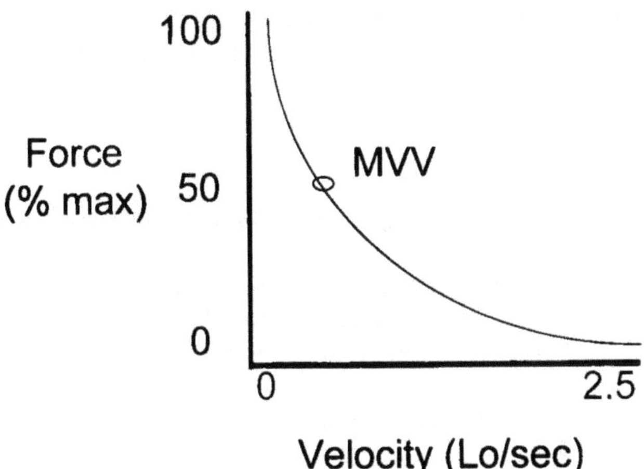

Figure 2 The force that a muscle generates decreases with more rapid velocity of contraction. This relationship is curvilinear as shown and has increasing importance in the most extreme conditions.

last to be recruited, generate the optimal level of force quickly, and may also fatigue rapidly. Type IIa fibers have moderate enzyme concentrations and are intermediate with respect to fatigability. The diaphragm is composed of approximately 50% Type I and 50% type II fibers, enabling it to withstand the enduring work it has to perform over an individual's lifetime (2,3). The fiber composition of the skeletal muscles bears an important relation to their response to training. In the case of the respiratory muscles, an increasing number of motor units are recruited with increasing ventilatory loads, with the type I, IIa, and IIb fibers being recruited in a sequential fashion.

The effects of training on fiber composition vary, depending on the method of training utilized. Endurance training increases the myoglobin content, the capillary density, the mitochondrial density, and the oxidative enzyme capacity of type I fibers. In contrast, strength training increases fiber size (i.e., muscle hypertrophy) with little or no effect on enzyme concentration. Animal studies using biopsy specimens of the ventilatory muscles before and after different forms of training have shown the aforementioned training effects on the diaphragm and other inspiratory muscles. It is now becoming evident that there is a continuum of the fiber composition of type II muscle cells, rather than two distinct groups.

The actual mix of fibers in the respiratory muscles of patients with clinical disease is less well characterized. The best information has come from biopsies of the diaphragms of patients with severe COPD undergoing lung volume reduction surgery (16). Histochemistry and molecular biology techniques were used to evaluate the differences in content of heavy chain myosin between patients and normals. Diaphragms from COPD patients had more heavy chain myosin than controls. This was interpreted as the consequence of a continuous mechanical load on the diaphragm, leading to a shift toward more fatigue-resistant (type I) muscle fibers. There is very little information in other stable nonmyopathic clinical conditions.

III. Metabolic and Energy Demands of Respiratory Muscles

The respiratory muscles behave like mechanical devices, consuming energy and producing work, both of which are measurable. Skeletal muscle efficiency is estimated to be about 25%, whereas respiratory muscle efficiency varies from 2 to 24%. It is well accepted that a lack of energy supply, in the form of insufficient oxygen and substrate, results in muscle failure. To provide nutrition to a working diaphragm, blood flow to the diaphragm increases as the diaphragm vasculature dilates (17–19). It follows that under conditions of decreased blood supply, when the energy demand outstrips the supply, the respiratory muscles will fail.

Blood flow to the diaphragm has been studied during phrenic nerve stimulation. As opposed to limb muscles, where the duty cycle (duration of contraction) is relatively constant, the duty cycle of the respiratory muscles can vary. The duty cycle is considered to be important because, during contraction, the blood flow is either partially or completely interrupted, with flow restitution occurring during the relaxation phase. The first comprehensive studies quantifying the relationship between diaphragmatic blood flow (Qdi) and the duty cycle were published by Bellemare et al. (17,20,21). In those studies, diaphragmatic blood perfusion was related to the product of the pressure generated by the diaphragm (Pdi), and the duty cycle (duration of the inspiration as a fraction of the duration of the respiratory cycle [Ti/Ttot]). This mathematical product, the tension (or pressure) time index (TTdi for the diaphragm), has been very useful to define the physiological behavior of the loaded diaphragm.

Bellemare et al. described a parabolic relation between TTdi and Qdi. Diaphragmatic perfusion rises up to a TTdi value of 0.20, then declines. Earlier studies had shown that the endurance time of the diaphragm when breathing against resistance was also related to the product of force developed and the duty cycle, and that time to task failure was predictable (19). If the breathing load is maintained at a TTdi of approximately 0.20, the time to fatigue is about 1 hr. On the other hand, at TTdi of 0.30, the time to task failure is about 15 minutes. Interestingly, a much higher Pdi (70% of Pdi max) can also be sustained for 1 hr, provided that the duty cycle is decreased to 0.30, which gives more perfusion time (TTdi remains at 0.21). The effect of high tension is offset by the shorter duty cycle. The concept of a "pressure threshold" is, in reality, valid only if Ti/Ttot is 0.40 to 0.45. The concept of a "threshold" TTdi, below which task failure does not develop, and above which it will eventually occur, was developed by Bellemare and Grassino and is graphically displayed in Figure 3 (21). It should be noted that these results apply to the prevailing experimental conditions from which the data were obtained (i.e., constant perfusion pressure and square pressure wave). Regardless of the conditions, the results emphasize the relevance of blood perfusion to the maintenance of diaphragm contractility (17,22).

For a given TTdi, endurance can be shorter or longer, depending on perfusion pressure. If perfusion pressure is increased, endurance is prolonged. In shock, TTdi task failure develops at a TTdi lower than 0.15 to 0.20. In addition, respiratory rate can also affect respiratory muscle perfusion. Faster frequencies increase Qdi for a given TTdi, since in normal humans Qdi is linearly related to the respiratory muscles' oxygen consumption. Other conditions may also influence diaphragmatic perfusion. For example, hypoxemia increases blood supply to the diaphragm. The aforementioned mechanisms seem to be adaptive in COPD, where both a fast respiratory rate and a lower tidal volume (faster, shallow breathing) may help to preserve muscle performance.

The cellular mechanisms by which blood flow regulates muscle contractility are not only related to the delivery of oxygen (O_2) and other substrates, but also to the washout of different catabolites. An example is the accumulation of

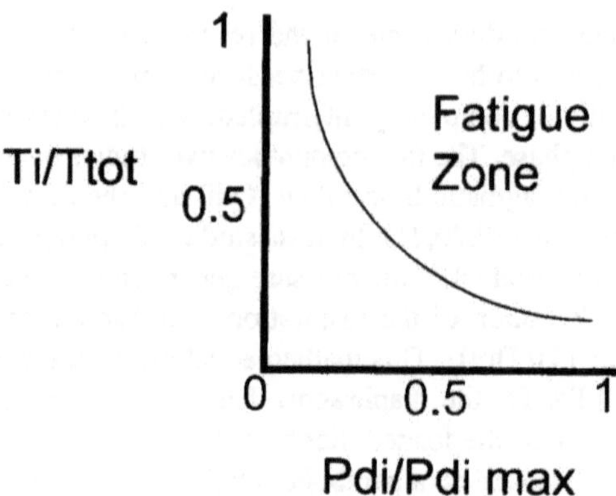

Figure 3 The graphical expression of the tension time index (TTdi) of patients with COPD. The force that the diaphragm generates with each breath (Pdi) as a function of the maximal pressure the diaphragm can generate (Pdi max) and the ratio of the duration of inspiration (Ti) as a function of the total duration of a respiratory cycle (Ttot) are the most important variables that contribute to the genesis of fatigue. Patients with COPD are breathing close to the fatigue threshold. With exercise, they may move toward the fatigue zone, where the load can only be held for a limited period of time.

inhibitors of muscle contractility such as phosphorus and hydrogen ions that occurs during anaerobic metabolism. These arise from the reliance on creatine kinase and myokinase for adenosine triphosphate (ATP) synthesis from adenosine diphosphate (ADP).

IV. Neural Control and Coordination

The diaphragm and the other respiratory muscles are controlled by central motor neurons that normally maintain rhythmic breathing (1–3). The muscles of the upper airways are innervated by lower cranial nerves (ninth, tenth, eleventh, and twelfth). The innervation of the other muscles depends on their anatomic location and, in descending order, includes the sternocleidomastoid, supplied by the spinal accessory nerve (eleventh cranial nerve) with roots from cervical 1 and 2 (C1 and C2) levels; the diaphragm, supplied by the phrenic nerves with roots from C3 to C5; and the parasternal intercostal, supplied by the intercostal nerves. The abdominal muscles, which are mainly expiratory in action, are supplied by motor neurons arising from thoracic 8 (T8) to lumbar 2 (L2) levels.

Given the wide array of neurons that may participate in ventilation, a great degree of coordination is needed to maintain efficient and appropriate ventilation. Unique to the respiratory system is the fact that the cortex can voluntarily override natural rhythmic automatic breathing. The system usually functions smoothly, because during quiet breathing we use primarily the diaphragm, the scalene, and some intercostals (1,12). With increased ventilatory loads, "accessory muscles" increase their participation in ventilation, and actually become important muscles of respiration. Apart from their potential role in respiration, some of the "accessory" muscles participate in other functions (12). For example, the upper torso and shoulder girdle muscles assist in positioning the upper extremities, abdominal muscles help with speech, defecation, and parturition. Therefore, in situations in which these muscles are being used for nonventilatory work, it is important that they maintain a high degree of coordination. When incoordination occurs, either because of an increased load or because of competing control integration, the resulting dysfunction can compromise the patient with underlying lung disease. Patients with severe COPD performing unsupported arm exercise develop early thoracoabdominal dyscoordination and fatigue (12). This type of exercise causes dyssynchrony between the rib cage and the diaphragm-abdomen, because of the competing output from the centers controlling respiratory and tonic activities of the accessory ventilatory muscles.

V. Respiratory Muscle Fatigue

During sustained exertion, the maximal force or velocity of shortening of a muscle eventually decreases (22–24). This exertional loss of the capacity to generate maximal force, recoverable during rest, is defined as *muscle fatigue* (24). The theoretical mechanisms causing fatigue are many. These include adaptation of the motor cortex, which may decrease its output in an attempt to preserve motor function (central fatigue), and inability of the sarcomere microfibers to translate the central output into a functional effective contraction (peripheral fatigue) (22,24). Since the concept of fatigue is a temporary loss of force, maximal force must be measured two or more times during the trial period. Task failure is defined as the inability of the muscle to continue to perform at a given prefixed target level (work, force, tidal volume, or increased ventilation) (23). Although fatigue precedes task failure, task failure does not necessarily follow fatigue. Task failure of the respiratory muscles occurs when they lose the capacity to generate the force required to sustain normal alveolar ventilation. Muscle injury is defined as a structural change in the sarcolemma or sarcoplasm, and is usually induced by fatiguing contractions, sustained for long periods of time (several hours), as may happen to the respiratory muscles during airway obstruction (25–27). Recovery from injury takes several days, giving place to muscular remodeling in which, in addition to muscle repair, there are changes in the quality of the muscle's structural or contractile proteins. Finally, muscle weakness is a permanent loss of force, regardless of its origin.

A. Mechanisms of Respiratory Muscle Fatigue

Breathing tasks that are "sustainable" rely on the recruitment of fatigue-resistant fibers (type I) using oxygen to generate ATP. By themselves, type I fibers will generate no more than 30% of the maximal force, but are able to sustain force for prolonged periods of time. Greater force (about 40 to 50% of max) limits muscle perfusion and may deprive all muscle cell types of adequate O_2 delivery and catabolite removal. Less force allows adequate perfusion of "fatigue-resistant" type I fibers, so that breathing is sustained for life. Excessive loads alter the chemical composition of the muscular interstitial space (e.g., potassium [K^+] and hydrogen ions [H^+] accumulate) and these provide neural feedback to the respiratory center. This may be perceived as the unpleasant sensation of unsustainable effort or dyspnea. In some circumstances, the central controller output may decrease in an effort to minimize respiratory muscle dysfunction (central fatigue). This mechanism is supported by the observation that the force of the diaphragm increases when an involuntary maximal electrical stimulus is applied to the phrenic nerves of subjects after fatiguing breathing loads (3,20).

Several techniques are available to monitor the mechanisms of muscle fiber function relevant to fatigue. Electromyography (EMG) is used to measure membrane excitability related to changes in the sarcolemma polarity induced by nerve stimulation (28–31). Membrane excitation is relevant to fatigue because it is a key mechanism to liberate calcium ions (Ca^{2+}) from the sarcoplasmic reticulum, which is necessary for contraction of the sarcomere. An EMG signal showing a decrease in the ratio of the force generated during sustained muscle contractions at constant length indicates fatigue because it reflects failure of the muscle contraction mechanism relative to the neural output. The frequency domain analysis of the EMG provides information about the velocity of propagation of potentials along the fibers, through calculation of the frequency power spectrum. The EMG signal contains a spectrum ranging from low (20 to 100 Hz) to high (100 to 1000 Hz) frequencies. Fatiguing muscle fibers, while exerting high force, show a shift toward the low frequency component of the total spectrum. A shift in the frequency power spectrum occurs early in a fatiguing contraction (within a minute of loading), and may serve as a predictor of task failure.

Muscle biopsies and nuclear magnetic resonance (NMR) spectroscopy have also been used to monitor metabolic changes in contracting muscle. While these techniques have been of great value to study limb muscles, their use in respiratory muscles is much more limited. Biopsies of the diaphragm are impractical because of its relatively inaccessible anatomic location, whereas NMR spectroscopy is difficult because of the constant movement that characterizes respiratory muscle function. Phosphorus was the earliest and has been the most frequently used atom to measure high-energy phosphates (ATP, ADP, P2r or pH). The carbon atom (magnetic resonance spectroscopy) has also been used to label substrates such as glucose, acetate, and pyruvate.

Magnetic resonance spectroscopy of sodium and potassium atoms permits the monitoring of intracellular ionic compositions, both of which have great significance in the propagation of membrane potential and intracellular and extracellular water movement in muscle tissue. Cine magnetic resonance imaging (MRI) is a recent technological development that has been applied to visualize dynamic internal events, such as the beating of the heart or displacement of the diaphragm. Intense muscular exercise results in an accumulation of Pi and an increase in H^+, both affecting pHi and the cells' capacity to generate ATP (14,18). Metabolic changes leading to muscle fatigue may soon be amenable to in vivo measurements.

B. Respiratory Muscle Fatigue in Human Subjects

Some of the studies on respiratory muscle fatigue measured the total duration during which a given force could be sustained and were actually measures of the time to task failure, or endurance (15,19). Once task failure occurs, we can assume that it was preceded by a fatiguing contraction pattern. The evolution of maximal force as a function of time has been well documented in studies of fatiguing contractions. Two major types of tasks have been used to elicit fatigue of the respiratory muscles: 1) breathing against high inspiratory (or expiratory) resistance and 2) sustaining maximal voluntary ventilation under isocapnic conditions. The resistive breathing protocol consists of setting a target Pdi or mouth pressure, duty cycle, and breathing frequency. The target is held until task failure occurs while $Paco_2$ is maintained at a normal level. Fewer studies have also used breathing resistance without specifying a breathing pattern (i.e., the subjects choose their own pattern of breathing). Under these conditions, $Paco_2$ is allowed to fluctuate; in general, it increases considerably when resistance is high and decreases when resistance is low. Overall, the results of resistive breathing experiments have shown that a pressure swing of about 50% of maximum force sustained at a duty cycle of 0.4 could be endured for 1 hr or longer.

A few studies have evaluated fatigue in accessory respiratory muscles or abdominal muscles. Task failure was well documented in these studies, and we can infer that fatigue must also have occurred. In resistive breathing, the pattern of contraction consists of slow velocity, high force, small shortening, and high intramuscular pressure. The development of muscle fatigue has been documented by measuring the force frequency curves of the diaphragm before and after task failure (22). All studies have shown decreases in maximal inspiratory pressure following resistive breathing that ended in task failure. Thus, we can conclude that fatigue of the respiratory muscles in human subjects occurs during experimental loaded breathing (32).

The model of fatigue caused by inspiratory resistance breathing may also apply to some clinical conditions such as heavy snoring or sleep apnea, in which peak pleural pressures of 40 to 60 cm H_2O have been reported (33). Such conditions are, however, prevalent for short periods (minutes), followed by unloading (airway opening), and are unlikely to cause clinically relevant fatigue.

Expiratory resistive breathing causes fatigue of abdominal muscles, and this happens in severe expiratory airway obstruction. Patients with COPD develop Pdi swings of 10 to 15 cm H_2O at rest, and these increase to 20 cm during exercise; pressures that are close to 50% of their maximum Pdi (34). High intramuscular tension limits muscle blood perfusion and leads to failure (1–3). In COPD, the measured Pdi may underestimate the intramuscular tension, because the flat diaphragm is far less effective in developing intrathoracic pressure due to a defective coupling with the rib cage. Further, the greater radius of curvature caused by the flattening increases diaphragm tension by Laplace's law (2,3). However, it is not certain that diaphragm perfusion is impaired in COPD. The degree of activation of the diaphragm in patients with COPD during resting breathing is about three times higher than in normal subjects. Further, recent studies show that activation of the diaphragm in COPD can rise to 85% of maximal during moderate exercise. These observations support the idea that diaphragmatic intramuscular tension is high in COPD patients, which may not be evident from Pdi measurements (32).

Besides resistive breathing, a second method used to induce respiratory muscle fatigue is to ask normal subjects to sustain the maximal voluntary ventilation (MVV) as long as they can, which is usually a very short period of time (about 30 sec). Normal subjects can sustain a V_E of about 55 to 60% of their MVV for periods of 20 min or longer. Such levels of ventilation are seen in aerobic sports such as marathon running, skiing, and biking (23). During MVV, the muscles contract at high speed with relatively low force and undergo large changes in length with every breath.

In order to assess fatigue of the diaphragm at high levels of minute ventilation, the Pdi has been measured by applying single electrical pulses of 10 and 20 Hz ("twitch" Pdi) to the phrenic nerves of normal subjects before and after exercise at 85 or 95% of their $V_{O_2}max$ (ventilation in the range of 80 to 120 l/min, respectively) (32). Decreases in the twitch Pdi, volitional Pdi max, and a reduction in the relaxation rate were observed after exercising at 95% of $V_{O_2}max$, but no difference was found after exercising at 85% $V_{O_2}max$. Studies of Pdi max following a marathon run also resulted in decreases in volitional Pdi max (32). It is therefore reasonable to assume that fatigue of the diaphragm develops when V_E is held at high percentages of the MVV. How these observations relate to patients with neuromuscular disease or COPD is unclear.

In summary, the loss of force of the respiratory muscles leading to fatigue occurs in human subjects. This becomes evident when subjects are sustaining either 50% of their maximal force or 50% of their maximal voluntary ventilation.

Fatigue occurring at lower ventilatory rates has not been well documented. The development of monitoring parameters to show evidence of more subtle degrees of muscle dysfunction in both normal and diseased subjects remains an exciting challenge.

VI. Respiratory Muscle Rest

Based on the evidence accumulated, we can conclude that when the respiratory muscles have to work against a large enough load, they fatigue. As we have seen, this has been shown to occur both in normal volunteers and in patients with acute respiratory failure but remains unproven in patients with chronic stable respiratory diseases. In those patients in whom respiratory muscle fatigue has developed, continuation of the load will result in ventilatory failure and, if left unabated, in death. The typical situation is that of patients on mechanical ventilation who fail to wean. In these cases, reinstitution of mechanical ventilation reverses the symptoms and improves the breathing pattern and arterial blood gases (35).

We know from clinical experience that the majority of the patients who survive respiratory failure will be weaned from mechanical ventilation as the underlying lung pathologic process reverses (36). Part of the reversal is thought to be due to resting of respiratory muscles, provided by ventilatory assistance. Perhaps even more compelling than the findings obtained from patients with acute respiratory failure is the vast experience gathered from multiple trials of mechanical ventilation in patients with primary neuromuscular conditions (37–42). In some of these trials, intermittent mechanical ventilation aiming to improve symptoms and arterial blood gases has also resulted in improvement in respiratory muscle force. As established by an expert NIH panel, improvement in respiratory muscle strength after rest represents the best evidence of respiratory muscle fatigue (24). However, it is possible that more than one mechanism is responsible for the beneficial changes observed after mechanical ventilation. These include improvement in blood gases with an increase in oxygen supply and improved removal of detrimental metabolites including carbon dioxide (CO_2), reversal of the "central" component of fatigue, or improvement in "peripheral" muscle fatigue.

VII. Mechanical Ventilation and Restrictive Diseases

The institution of mechanical ventilation in animals and normal human volunteers decreases respiratory rate, pressure time index of the respiratory muscles (a surrogate of metabolic work), and the neuromuscular output to the diaphragm (42–44). This leads to reversal of the power spectral analysis EMG changes that are characteristic of muscle fatigue, with a shift from lower to faster frequency components. These observations support the application of chronic intermittent mechanical ventilation to patients with ventilatory failure thought to be due to progressive respiratory muscle fatigue, even though mechanical ventilation is instituted primarily to treat the nighttime hypoxemia and hypercapnia of chronic respiratory failure (45,46). When these patients improve, it is hard to tease out the effects of chronic intermittent mechanical ventilation on respiratory muscle function from those resulting from correction of the blood gas abnormalities.

There is ample evidence that chronic mechanical ventilation applied to patients with chronic restrictive pulmonary diseases either via tracheostomy or using noninvasive methods, improves symptoms, arterial blood gases, and functional capacity (37–42,45,46). We studied maximal respiratory muscle strength (P_I max and P_E max) as well as transdiaphragmatic pressure using the double balloon technique in three patients with bilateral diaphragmatic paralysis before and 1 to 4 mo after intermittent mechanical ventilation (47). Mechanical ventilation not only improved symptoms, but it also increased indexes of respiratory muscle strength (Fig. 4), supporting the concept of reversal of respiratory muscle fatigue. The increase in respiratory muscle strength was associated with an improvement in functional status, indicating that the improvement was not confined to physiologic measurements but extended to clinically significant outcomes as well. Although these results are supportive, they do not conclusively prove the presence of respiratory muscle fatigue as the only, or even the predominant, factor

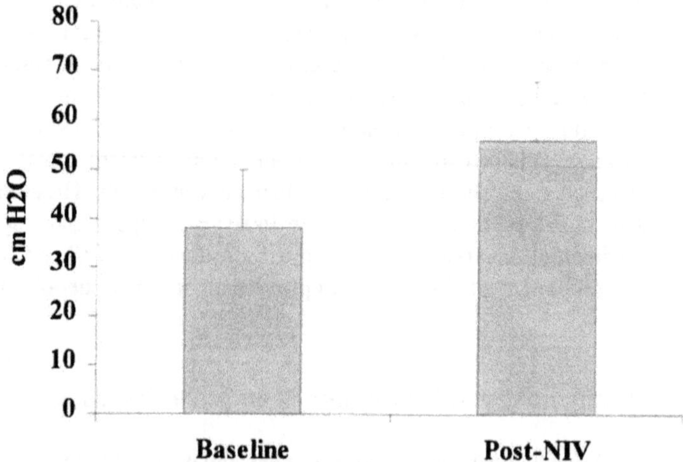

Figure 4 Maximal inspiratory pressure before (baseline) and after noninvasive mechanical ventilation (post-NIV) in three patients with bilateral diaphragmatic paralysis. The significant improvement suggests reversal of muscle fatigue. (Adapted from Ref. 47.)

in the genesis of these patients' respiratory failure. The improved respiratory muscle strength could also have been due to better effort related to improved sleep or to overall improvement in blood gases.

VIII. Acute on Chronic Respiratory Failure

Several uncontrolled trials of noninvasive ventilation (NIV) in acute on chronic respiratory failure suggested a role for respiratory muscle unloading and resting (41). This has been confirmed in several randomized trials using noninvasive mechanical ventilation (48–51). These trials evaluated different outcomes, including rate of intubation, length of ICU and hospital stay, dyspnea, and mortality. Although not all showed the same results in the most important outcomes, such as mortality, there was uniform agreement that respiratory muscle resting using noninvasive positive pressure ventilation was effective in reversing acute respiratory failure. The patients most likely to benefit from NIV were those with elevated $Paco_2$, who were able to cooperate with the caregivers and with no other important co-morbid problems (sepsis, severe pneumonia, cardiovascular collapse, arrhythmias). Interestingly, none of these trials evaluated respiratory muscle function per se, so it is impossible to determine if the effect is due to resting of the muscles or to the support provided to the whole system as the basic pathologic process is being treated.

IX. Mechanical Ventilation in Chronic Stable COPD

The possibility that the respiratory muscles of patients with severe COPD breathe with a pattern close to the fatigue threshold has led numerous investigators to explore the therapeutic role of resting the muscles with noninvasive negative and positive pressure ventilators (24). Short-term studies have shown that the diaphragmatic EMG in patients with COPD can be suppressed with mechanical ventilation. Several subsequent studies reported improvement in symptoms, but most of these initial studies were uncontrolled in design (52). On the other hand, the longer-term controlled trials using either form of ventilation showed no benefit in most of the outcomes studied (53–56). One recent trial showed a benefit of nasal positive pressure mechanical ventilation on quality of life and arterial blood gases in patients with stable COPD, but there was no change in pulmonary function (57). Unfortunately, no respiratory muscle function was evaluated. In the largest study to date, exercise tolerance, arterial blood gases, frequency of decompensation, and pulmonary functions were similar in treated and untreated patients (54). A recent study, which has only been reported as an abstract, found no difference in 1-yr mortality, rate of exacerbation, and hospitalization between patients with chronic stable COPD randomized to noninvasive nasal ventilation or usual care (58). In addition, none of the studies found evidence of improvement in respiratory muscle strength or endurance. To date, there is no evidence that intermittent respiratory muscle resting for stable patients with COPD improves respiratory muscle function. In contrast, when such a patient develops an acute decompensation, especially with elevated $Paco_2$, a trial of noninvasive positive pressure ventilation may rest fatigued respiratory muscles and help prevent intubation with its consequences. More studies will define the population that may best benefit from these techniques.

X. Conclusion

If the respiratory pump is faced with a large enough load, it will fail. Fatigue of the respiratory muscles, with or without a central component, has been shown to occur during experimental conditions, and is thought to be a very important contributor to ventilatory failure. In patients with acute respiratory compromise, the institution of mechanical ventilation results in restoration of more normal function, likely because of the reparative effects of resting. In contrast, evidence that fatigue plays a role in the stable patient with chronic respiratory conditions is much weaker and remains an area of needed research. From the results of several studies that have evaluated mechanical ventilation in patients with neuromuscular diseases, some contribution of respiratory muscle fatigue to the overall clinical picture is likely. In patients with chronic stable COPD, the evidence for presence of fatigue is limited at best. The advent of less-invasive tools, such as MRI, may allow a proper characterization of the role that fatigue plays in the development of ventilatory failure in patients with chronic respiratory diseases.

References

1. Epstein S. An overview of respiratory muscle function. Chest Clin North Am 1994; 15:619–639.
2. Rochester DF. The diaphragm: Contractile properties and fatigue. J Clin Invest 1985; 75:1397–1402.
3. Roussos CH, Macklem PT. The respiratory muscles. N Engl J Med, 1982; 307:786–797.
4. Tobin M. The respiratory muscles in disease. Clin Chest Med 1988; 9:263–286.
5. Celli BR. Respiratory muscle function. Clin Chest Med 1986; 7:567–580.
6. Mead J. Functional significance of the area of apposition of diaphragm to ribcage. Am Rev Respir Dis 1979; 119:31–32.
7. Martinez F, Couser J, Celli B. Factors influencing ventilatory muscle recruitment in patients with chronic airflow obstruction. Am Rev Respir Dis 1990; 142:276–282.
8. Supinsky GS, Kelsen SG. Effects of elastase-induced emphysema on the force-generating ability of the diaphragm. J Clin Invest 1982; 70:978–988.

9. Farkas G, Roussos C. The diaphragm in emphysematous hamsters: Sarcomere adaptability. J Appl Physiol 1983; 54:1634–1640.
10. DeTroyer A, Estenne M. Coordination between ribcage muscles and diaphragm during quiet breathing in humans. J Appl Physiol 1984; 57(3): 899–906.
11. Moxham J, Wiles C, Newman D, Edwards RHT. Sternomastoid function and fatigue in man. Clin Sci 1980; 5:433–468.
12. Celli BR, Rassulo J, Make B. Dyssynchronous breathing during arm but not leg exercise in patients with chronic airflow obstruction. N Engl J Med 1986; 314:1485–1490.
13. DeTroyer A, Sampson M, Sigrist S, et al. How the abdominal muscles act on the ribcage. J Appl Physiol 1983; 54(2):465–469.
14. Vollestad N. Changes in activation, contractile speed, and electrolyte balances during fatigue. In: Roussos C, ed. The Thorax. New York: Dekker, 1996; 235–253.
15. Tenney S, Reese RE. The ability to sustain great breathing efforts. Resp Physiol 1968; 5:187–201.
16. Levine S, Kaiser L, Leferovich L, et al. Cellular adaptation in the diaphragm in chronic obstructive pulmonary disease. N Engl J Med 1997; 337:1799–1804.
17. Bellemare F, Wright D, Lavigne C, Grassino A. Effect of tension and timing of contraction on the blood flow of the diaphragm. J Appl Physiol 1983; 54:1597–1606.
18. Hussain S. Regulation of ventilatory muscle blood flow. J Appl Physiol 1996; 81(4): 1455–1468.
19. Roussos C, Macklem P. Diaphragmatic fatigue in man. J Appl Physiol 1977; 43: 189–197.
20. Bellemare F, Bigland Ritchie B. Central components of diaphragm fatigue assessed by phrenic nerve stimulation. J Appl Physiol 1987; 62:263–277.
21. Bellemare F, Grassino A. Effect of pressure and timing of contraction on human diaphragmatic fatigue. J Appl Physiol 1982; 53(5):1190–1195.
22. Aubier M, Farkas G, DeTroyer A, Roussos C. Detection of diaphragmatic fatigue in man by phrenic stimulation. J Appl Physiol 1981; 50:538–544.
23. Clanton TL. Respiratory muscle endurance in humans. In: Roussos C, ed. The Thorax. New York: Dekker, 1996; 1199–1230.
24. National Heart, Lung, and Blood Institute (NHLBI) workshop on respiratory muscle fatigue: Report of the respiratory muscle fatigue workshop group. Am Rev Resp Dis 1990; 142:474–480.
25. Bertocci LA. Emerging opportunities with nuclear magnetic resonance: Fatigue. Gandevia S et al., eds. New York: Plenum Press, 1995; 211–240.
26. Zhu E, Petrof B, Gea J, Comptois N, Grassino A. Diaphragm muscle fiber injury after inspiratory resistive breathing. Am J Respir Crit Care Med 1997; 155:1110–1116.
27. Esau S, Bellemare F, Grassino A, Permutt S, Roussos C. Changes in relaxation rate with diaphragmatic fatigue in humans. J Appl Physiol 1983; 54:1353–1360.
28. Eastwood PR, Hillman D, Finucaine K. Ventilatory responses to inspiratory threshold loading and rate of muscle fatigue in task failure. J Appl Physiol 1994; 76(1): 185–195.
29. Gross D, Grassino A, Ross W, Macklem P. EMG pattern of diaphragmatic fatigue. J Appl Physiol 1979; 46:1–7.

30. Sinderby C, Lindstrom L, Grassino A. Automatic assessment of electromyogram quality. J Appl Physiol 1995; 79:1803–1815.
31. Beck J, Sinderby C, Weinberg J, Grassino A. Effects of muscle to electrode distance on the human diaphragm EMG. J Appl Physiol 1995; 79:975–985.
32. Johnson B, Babcock M, Suman E, Dempsey J. Exercise induced diaphragmatic fatigue in healthy humans. J Physiol (Lond) 1993; 460:385–405.
33. Vinken W, Guilleminault C, Cosio M, Grassino A. Onset of diaphragmatic fatigue. Am Rev Resp Dis 1985; 135:372–377.
34. Ninane V, Rypens F, Yernault JC, DeTroyer A. Abdominal muscle use during breathing in patients with chronic airflow obstruction. Am Rev Respir Dis 1992; 146:16–21.
35. Cohen C, Zaigelbaum G., Grotz D, Roussos Ch. Clinical manifestations of respiratory muscle fatigue. Am J Med 1982; 73:308–316.
36. Yang KL, Tobin M. A prospective study of indexes predicting the outcome of trials of weaning from mechanical ventilation. N Engl J Med 1991; 324:1445–1450.
37. Splaingard ML, Frates RC, Jefferson LS, Rosen CL, Harrison GM. Home negative pressure ventilation: Report of 20 years of experience in patients with neuromuscular disease. Arch Phys Med Rehabil 1985; 66:239–242.
38. Bach JR, Alba A, Shin D. Noninvasive airway pressure assisted ventilation in the management of respiratory insufficiency due to poliomyelitis. Am J Phys Med Rehabil 1989; 68:264–271.
39. Mohr CH, Hill NS. Long term follow up of nocturnal ventilatory assistance in patients with respiratory failure due to Duchenne-type muscular dystrophy. Chest 1990; 97:91–96.
40. Claman DM, Piper A, Sanders MH, Stiller RA, Votteri RA. Nocturnal noninvasive positive pressure ventilatory assistance. Chest 1996; 110:1581–1588.
41. Bach JR, Alba A, Saporito LR. Intermittent positive pressure ventilation via the mouth as an alternative to tracheostomy for 257 ventilator users. Chest 1993; 103: 174–182.
42. Masa JF, Celli BR, Riesco J, Sanchez de Cos J, Disdier C, Sojo A. Noninvasive positive pressure ventilation and not oxygen may prevent overt ventilatory failure in patients with chest wall diseases. Chest 1997; 112:207–213.
43. Ambrosino N, Nava S, Bertone P, Fracchia C, Rampulla C. Physiologic evaluation of pressure support ventilation by nasal mask in patients with stable COPD. Chest 1992; 101:385–391.
44. Brochard L, Harf A, Lorino H, Lemaire F. Inspiratory pressure support prevents diaphragmatic fatigue during weaning from mechanical ventilation. Am Rev Respir Dis 1989; 139:513–521.
45. Garay SM, Turino GM, Goldring RM. Sustained reversal of chronic hypercapnia in patients with alveolar hypoventilation syndromes: long-term maintenance with noninvasive nocturnal mechanical ventilation. Am J Med 1981; 70:269–274.
46. Curran FJ. Night ventilation by body respirators for patients in chronic respiratory failure due to late stage Duchenne muscular dystrophy. Arch Phys Med Rehabil 1981; 62:270–274.
47. Celli BR, Rassulo J, and Corral R: Ventilatory muscle dysfunction in patients with bilateral idiopathic diaphragmatic paralysis: Reversal by intermittent external negative pressure ventilation. Am Rev Respir Dis 1987; 136:1276–1278.

48. Brochard L, Isabey D, Piquet J, et al. Reversal of acute exacerbations of chronic obstructive lung disease by inspiratory assistance with a face mask. N Engl J Med 1990; 323:1523–1530.
49. Kramer N, Meyer T, Meharg J, Cece R, Hill NS. Randomized prospective trial of noninvasive positive pressure ventilation in acute respiratory failure. Am J Respir Crit Care Med 1995; 151:1799–1806.
50. Bott J, Caroll P, Conway J, et al. Randomized controlled trial of nasal ventilation in acute ventilatory failure due to obstructive lung disease. Lancet 1993; 341:1555–1557.
51. Brochard L, Mancebo J, Wysocki M, et al. Noninvasive ventilation for acute exacerbation of chronic obstructive pulmonary disease. N Engl J Med 1995; 333:817–822.
52. Braun N, Marino W. Effect of daily intermittent rest of respiratory muscles in patients with severe chronic airflow limitation. Chest 1984; 85:59.
53. Zibrak J, Hill NS, Federman E, et al. Evaluation of intermittent long-term negative pressure ventilation in patients with severe chronic obstructive pulmonary disease. Am Rev Respir Dis 1988; 138:1515–1520.
54. Celli, B, Lee H, Criner G, et al. Controlled trial of external negative pressure ventilation in patients with severe chronic airflow limitation. Am Rev Respir Dis 1989; 140:1251–1257.
55. Shapiro S, Ernst P, Gray-Donald K, et al. Effect of negative pressure ventilation in severe pulmonary disease. Lancet 1992; 340:1425–1428.
56. Strumpf D, Millman RP, Carlisle C, et al. Nocturnal positive-pressure ventilation via nasal mask in patients with severe chronic obstructive pulmonary disease. Am Rev Respir Dis 1991; 144:415–420.
57. Meecham-Jones J, Paul E., Jones P, Wedzicha J. Nasal pressure support ventilation plus oxygen compared with oxygen therapy alone in hypercapnic COPD. Am J Respir Crit Care Med 1995; 152:538–544.
58. Casanova C, Abreu I, Tos L, Soriano E, Fernandez M, Garcia I, Hernandez C, Acosta O. Nocturnal nasal ventilation with BIPAP in stable severe COPD. Am J Respir Crit Care Med 1996; 153:A605.

48. Brochard L, Isabey D, Piquet J, et al. Reversal of acute exacerbations of chronic obstructive lung disease by inspiratory assistance with a face mask. N Engl J Med 1990; 323:1523–1530.
49. Kramer N, Meyer T, Meharg J, Cece R, Hill NS. Randomized, prospective trial of noninvasive positive pressure ventilation in acute respiratory failure. Am J Respir Crit Care Med 1995; 151:1799–1806.
50. Bott J, Carroll MP, Conway JH, et al. Randomised controlled trial of nasal ventilation in acute ventilatory failure due to chronic obstructive airways disease. Lancet 1993; 341:1555–1557.
51. Brochard L, Mancebo J, Wysocki M, et al. Noninvasive ventilation for acute exacerbations of chronic obstructive pulmonary disease. N Engl J Med 1995; 333:817–822.
52. Braun N, Marino W. Effect of daily intermittent rest of respiratory muscles in patients with severe chronic airflow limitation. Chest 1984; 85:59S.
53. Zibrak JD, Hill NS, Federman EC, et al. Evaluation of intermittent long-term negative pressure ventilation in patients with severe chronic obstructive pulmonary disease. Am Rev Respir Dis 1988; 138:1515–1518.
54. Celli B, Lee H, Criner G, et al. Controlled trial of external negative pressure ventilation in patients with severe chronic airflow obstruction. Am Rev Respir Dis 1989; 140:1251–1256.
55. Shapiro SH, Ernst P, Gray-Donald K, et al. Effect of negative pressure ventilation in severe chronic obstructive pulmonary disease. Lancet 1992; 340:1425–1429.
56. Strumpf DA, Millman RP, Carlisle CC, et al. Nocturnal positive-pressure ventilation via nasal mask in patients with severe chronic obstructive pulmonary disease. Am Rev Respir Dis 1991; 144:1234–1239.
57. Meecham Jones DJ, Paul EA, Jones PW, Wedzicha JA. Nasal pressure support ventilation plus oxygen compared with oxygen therapy alone in hypercapnic COPD. Am J Respir Crit Care Med 1995; 152:538–544.
58. Lin CC. Comparison between nocturnal nasal positive pressure ventilation combined with oxygen therapy and oxygen monotherapy in patients with severe COPD. Am J Respir Crit Care Med 1996; 154:353–358.

4

Nocturnal Mechanical Ventilation

Effects on Sleep Quality and Control of Breathing

PETER C. GAY

Mayo Clinic and Mayo Foundation
Rochester, Minnesota

I. Introduction

Patients with severe chronic obstructive pulmonary disease (COPD) and restrictive lung diseases have an altered control of breathing that leads to disturbances of gas exchange and sleep quality. It is very difficult to precisely evaluate the neural control of breathing in humans, awake or during sleep. Therefore, studies try to approach this indirectly with assessments of gas exchange, pulmonary mechanics, and respiratory muscle responses. Most investigations have examined normal awake subjects, and small numbers of patients usually limit what has been shown for those with disease while asleep. In addition, conclusions about sleep and breathing with or without nocturnal mechanical ventilation must be made cautiously, especially when comparing different respiratory diseases.

Interpretations about the effect of nocturnal mechanical ventilation on sleep quality and control of breathing are often based on "before and after" findings. This indirect methodology leaves many unanswered questions about the true cause and effect or exact mechanisms proposed to explain the observations. With these caveats, our discussion is organized to include a general and brief discussion of the respiratory changes noted during sleep in normal adult subjects. We then review the appearance and significance of gas exchange abnormalities and the associated sleep quality in various respiratory disorders. Finally, we comment on the effect of nocturnal mechanical ventilation on sleep quality and gas exchange. This chapter concentrates primarily on nocturnal mechanical ventilation delivered *noninvasively* at the nose and/or mouth.

II. Control of Breathing in Normal Adults

Respiration during sleep can be described in terms of gas exchange and ventilatory effort by monitoring simple pulse oximetry and measures of airflow or respiratory muscle effort (e.g., spirometry, electromyography, or maximal respiratory pressures). Sleep is also characterized electroencephalographically to distinguish sleep stages (I to IV and rapid eye movement [REM]). The efficiency (total sleep time/total time in bed) and sleep fragmentation or arousals (change from a deeper to lighter stage of sleep or wakefulness) can also be noted (1,2).

The effect of sleep on breathing in normal adults has been studied with all of the above descriptors (3). A detailed description of normal sleep physiology was the subject of a previous volume in this series (4), but a brief overview is necessary here. In the adult, sleep typically proceeds in a cyclic fashion through various stages of non-REM with periods of REM sleep occurring every 90 to 120 min. There are distinctive behavioral and physiologic differences between REM and non-REM sleep that directly affect breathing control and sleep quality. Within REM sleep there are also distinctive forms called *tonic* and *phasic*. The tonic form is characterized by suppression of skeletal muscle tone, whereas the phasic form is distinguished by bursts of rapid eye movements with respiratory and other autonomic irregularities. Elaborate animal studies have investigated the complex neural integration that leads to the appearance of these sleep stages and associated breathing responses. What is known about human sleep has been acquired largely through indirect and inferential means (5,6).

A fundamental assumption for both normals and those with disease is that the same basic mechanisms that control breathing during wakefulness exist during sleep. What is thought to differ between wakefulness and sleep is the gain or magnitude of responses. The decreased consciousness during sleep has a blunting effect on most integrated feedback processes. Minute ventilation falls progressively to a minimum during REM sleep. This is explained by a reduction in tidal volume, while respiratory rate increases slightly (7). This leads to a small but significant reduction in Pa_{O_2} and a rise in Pa_{CO_2} during REM sleep, particularly phasic REM. The breathing pattern both in terms of frequency and tidal volume also becomes much more irregular.

Studies on the control of breathing during sleep in normals have shown wide variation in the arousal threshold to hypoxia (8). Half of the subjects studied in one report did not arouse at the preassigned safety limit of 70% oxygen saturation by pulse oximetry (Spo_2) regardless of sleep state. The ventilatory response to hypoxia was also reduced in all sleep states compared with wakefulness with the slope falling by 50% in REM. There are gender differences as well: women preserve the hypoxic ventilatory response in non-REM sleep significantly better than men do (9). Based on these findings, hypoxia appears to be a poor stimulus to arousal in normal individuals.

A similar blunting of the ventilatory response to hypercapnia occurs in sleeping subjects, although the gender differences seem to disappear (10). The changes in slope and intercept for minute ventilation vs. $Paco_2$ during different sleep stages are shown in Figure 1. The comparison of male and female responses for both hypoxic and hypercapnic responses is shown in Figure 2. At least for the hypercapnic response, the reduced slope during sleep may relate to peripheral as well as central adaptations. Others have shown that the contractility of the diaphragm for a given electrical stimulus is reduced in the presence of hypercapnia and that this promotes the rapid development of muscle fatigue and reduced ventilatory responsiveness (11).

Local lung receptor control mechanisms also modulate breathing in humans. These mechanisms have been extensively studied in animals, usually anes-

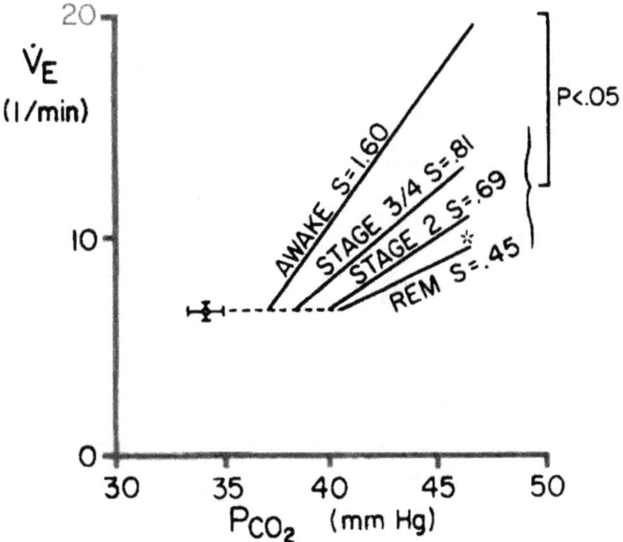

Figure 1 Mean minute ventilation/P_{ETCO_2} relationships for all 12 subjects, indicating the mean ± SEM resting minute ventilation/CO_2 point in the awake state. The hypercapnic ventilatory response is reduced in Stages 2 and 3/4 compared with that in wakefulness and is further decreased in REM sleep. $\dot{V}_E$, expired ventilation; *, $p < 0.05$ REM different from stage 2 and 3/4 sleep. (From Ref. 10.)

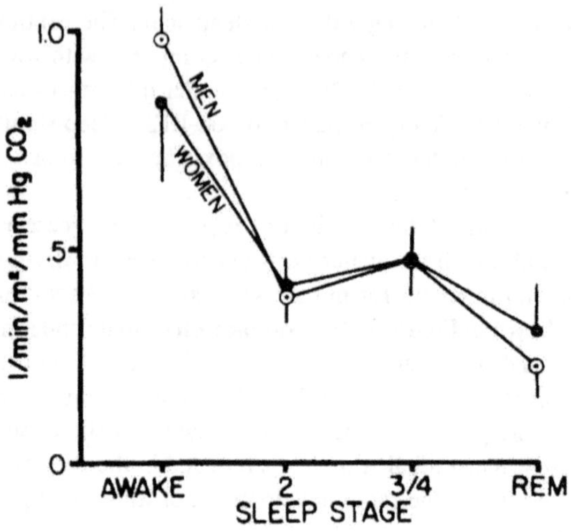

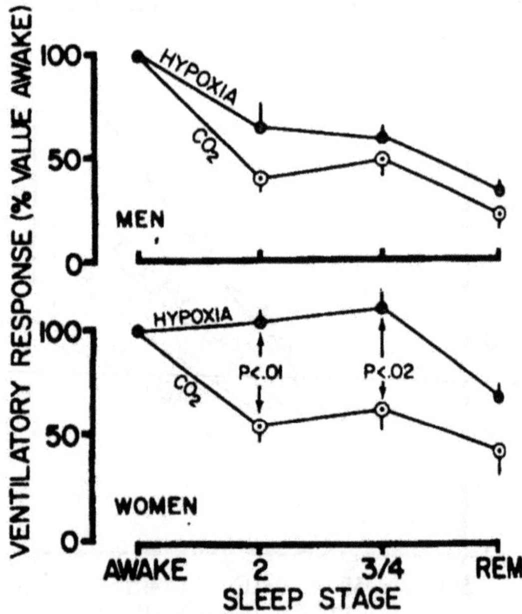

Figure 2 (Top) Hypercapnic ventilation responses are similar for men and women in all sleep stages. Mean ± SEM for six men and six women. (Bottom) Decreases in hypoxic and hypercapnic responses from the level in wakefulness in men and women. Mean ± SEM for six men and six women. Women preserve their hypoxic response in non-REM sleep significantly better than their hypercapnic response. In men, the decrements are similar. (From Ref. 10.)

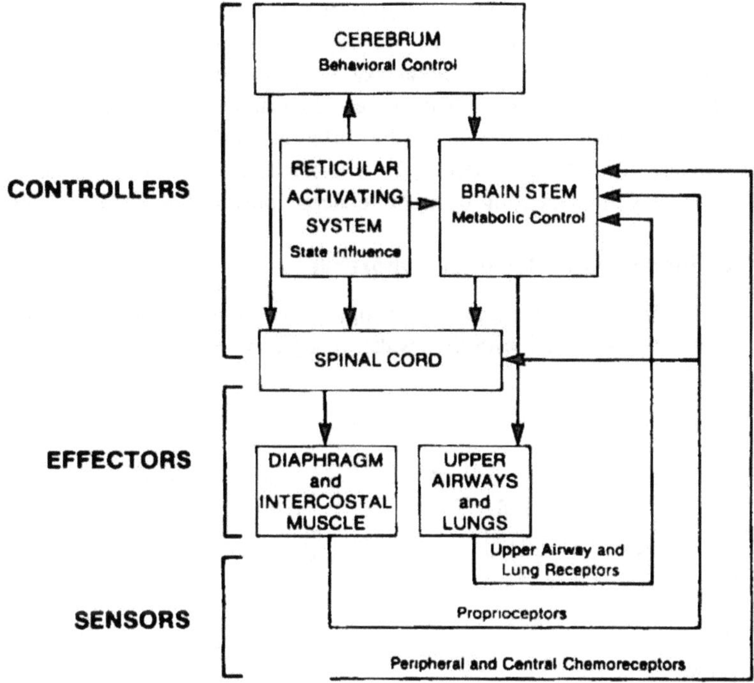

Figure 3 Schematic representation of the respiratory control system. (Modified from Ref. 3.)

thetized, where the influences appear to be both sleep-stage- and vagal-tone-dependent (12,13). The profound influence that upper airway changes have during sleep on the control of breathing is extensively discussed in Chapter 5. A general schematic of the mechanisms that control breathing during sleep is shown in Figure 3. All of the above studies support the finding that breathing responses to metabolic and chemical stimuli are generally depressed during sleep, and this is most apparent during REM sleep. Lung stretch responses are further discussed below in section V.

III. Nocturnal Gas Exchange in Patients with Respiratory Diseases

Nocturnal oxygen saturation monitoring provides the most easily obtained evidence of disturbed breathing during sleep in patients with respiratory disease. The most widely studied group of patients has been those with COPD who have long been known to have nocturnal hypoxemia during sleep (14–16). Studies show that patients with severe COPD may spend more than 20% of sleep time with oxygen saturation >5% below awake Sp_{O_2}. This occurs most profoundly during REM sleep (Fig. 4) (17). The degree of desaturation reported for COPD patients varies widely and is affected by different patient characteristics (e.g., "pink puffers" vs. "blue bloaters") in addition to how stringently the study excluded those with coexisting obstructive sleep apnea (OSA) (18).

A. Predictors of Nocturnal Hypoxemia

For patients with COPD, the maximal change in nocturnal oxygen saturation has been negatively correlated with the awake ventilatory response to hypercapnia;

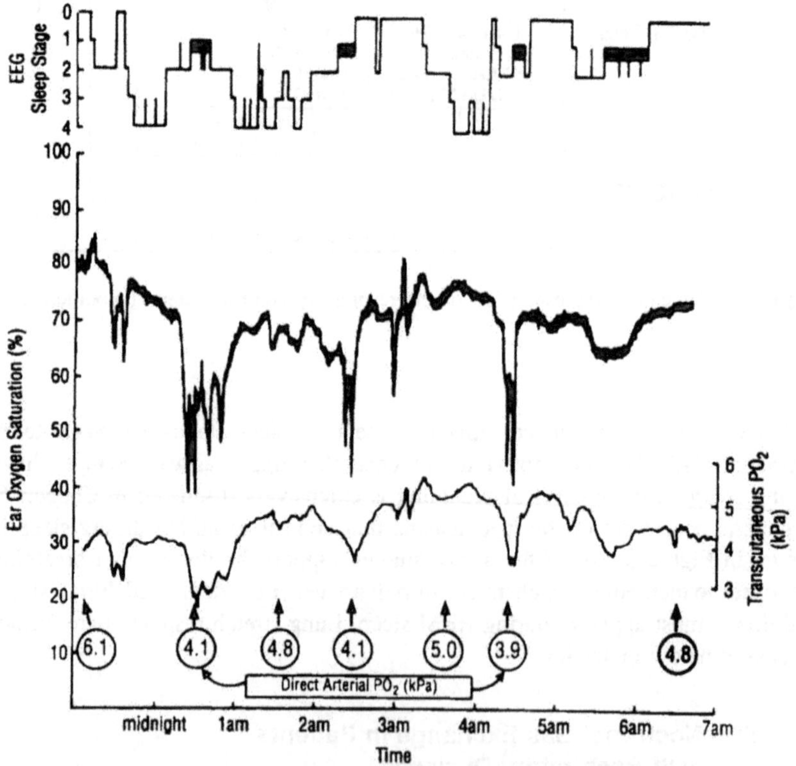

Figure 4 Overnight recordings of EEG sleep stage, in which thick black bands represent REM sleep; oxygen saturation; transcutaneous oxygen tension; and intermittently measured arterial oxygen tension in a 55-year-old male patient with chronic obstructive pulmonary disease. (From Ref. 17.)

this correlation is independent of sleep stage. Mean and maximal reductions in nocturnal oxygen saturation are also negatively correlated with awake oxygen saturation (14–16). Contrariwise, the hypoxic ventilatory response during wakefulness is not useful in predicting nocturnal oxygen saturation.

Pulmonary function testing has a low predictive value and correlates poorly with nocturnal hypoxemia, but moderate desaturation during exercise predicts a reduced nocturnal mean and nadir saturation (19). Awake oxygen saturation and the lowest saturation recorded during sleep usually correlate well, especially in patients with chronic bronchitis (''blue bloaters'') who are also prone to associated heart rhythm disturbances (20–22). The significance of nocturnal gas exchange problems for COPD patients is discussed below.

In patients with restrictive disease, the predictors and significance of hypercapnia and/or nocturnal hypoxemia vary, in part because many studies lump several disease categories together. For example, one would predict that the severity of inspiratory muscle weakness as determined by maximal inspiratory pressures (PiMax) would strongly correlate with nocturnal oxygen desaturation, but most studies find that this is untrue for neuromuscular disease (NMD) and kyphoscoliosis (KS) (23–26). Given further thought, however, this should not be surprising because gas exchange abnormality tends to be a late manifestation of NMD and usually does not emerge until the forced vital capacity (FVC) is severely reduced (27,28). On the other hand, the PiMax predicts survival in patients with specific diseases, such as amyotrophic lateral sclerosis (ALS) (29). In one study of patients with ALS, a PiMax with a magnitude threshold of <60 cm H_2O, was highly *sensitive* in the prediction of both nocturnal oxygen desaturation and survival (Fig. 5) (30).

Several authors have shown that awake and nocturnal oxygen desaturations worsen in patients with NMD as spirometrically determined lung volumes fall (23–30). The FVC may be the most specific spirometric predictor for nocturnal desaturation and survival in patients with restrictive thoracic diseases, particularly if the trend rather than the absolute value is examined (27,30). Maximal voluntary ventilation measurements may have similar utility (27,30).

B. Significance of Nocturnal Oxygen Desaturation and Worsening Hypercapnia in COPD

The significance of decreases in oxygen saturation and worsening hypercapnia during sleep in COPD patients remains controversial. The Nocturnal Oxygen Therapy Trial (NOTT) demonstrated improved survival with the continuous use of supplemental oxygen in a large population of COPD patients, which paralleled a reduced rate of progression for pulmonary hypertension (31,32). Fletcher et al. (33) investigated the effect of nocturnal desaturation (REM-related Spo_2 <85% for >5 min) on diurnal pulmonary hemodynamics in a smaller series of COPD

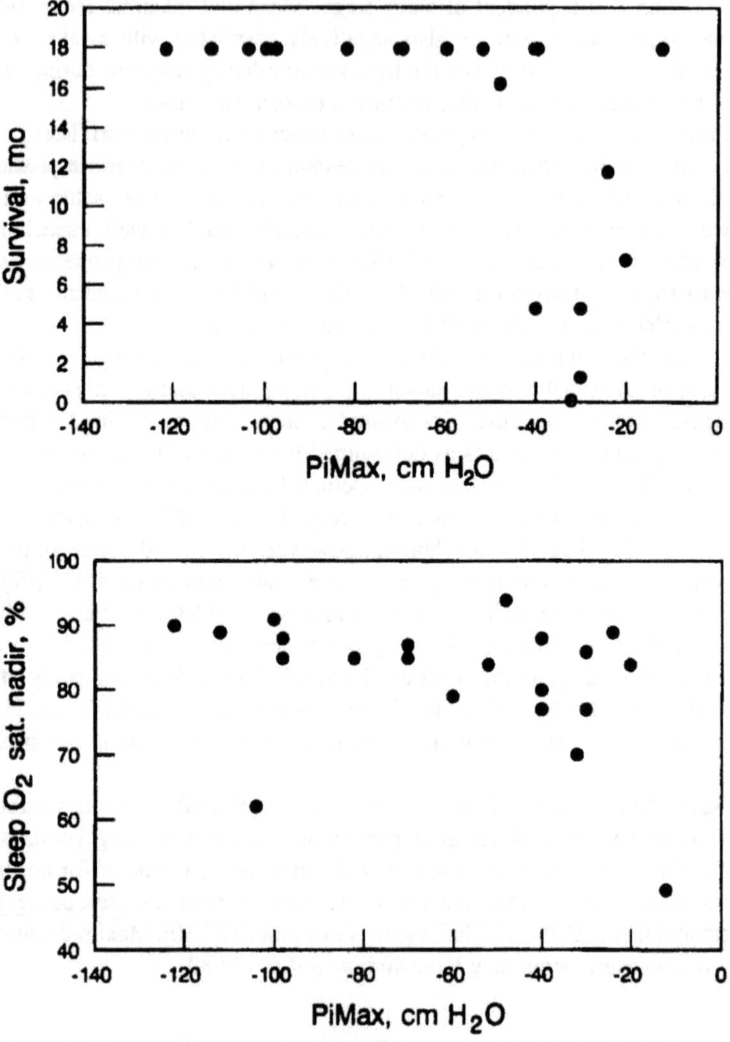

Figure 5 (Top) Survival time in months plotted against maximal inspiratory pressure (PiMax) for 21 patients with amyotrophic lateral sclerosis. All patients with a PiMax of more than −60 cm H_2O completed the 18-month study. (Bottom) PiMax plotted against nocturnal oxygen saturation (O_2 sat) nadir in 21 patients with amyotrophic lateral sclerosis. Note that all but one of the seven patients with a nocturnal oxygen saturation nadir of 80% or less had a PiMax of −60 cm H_2O or less, a sensitivity of 86%. (From Ref. 30.)

patients with daytime Pao_2 >60 mm Hg. They found a significant correlation between marked drops in oxygen saturation (especially during REM sleep) and the development of increased pulmonary vascular resistance and poorer survival (33). When oxygen was provided to these patients during sleep for 36 months, there was a fall in pulmonary artery pressure not seen in patients given sham treatment (34,35). In another large registry of patients with severe COPD given long-term oxygen therapy who later died, a full 20% expired during their sleep and 26% of those deaths were unexpected (36). A recently completed randomized, multicenter trial from Europe in 135 consecutive stable COPD patients with borderline awake hypoxemia failed to show any advantage in survival for the oxygen group after an average of 40 mo of oxygen use for 12 to 14 hr/day. One-third of all patients died in the first 3 yr and 6 patients in the oxygen group died suddenly at home (37).

The question of whether sleep-related desaturation (defined by >30% of the night at Spo_2 <90%) in COPD patients is associated with increased pulmonary artery pressures was recently reexamined (38). The $Paco_2$ combined with forced expiratory volume in 1 sec (FEV_1) correctly predicted the presence of nocturnal desaturation, which occurred in 82% of the total number of patients. Mean nocturnal oxygen saturation correlated with body mass index and $Paco_2$ but not with Pao_2. No single or combined variables predicted the presence of pulmonary hypertension. Although the need to treat awake Pao_2 <55 mm Hg is well accepted, the justification for oxygen treatment of patients with milder nocturnal oxygen desaturation, as defined by the studies above, is not clearly substantiated. The cost effectiveness of treatment in this group is therefore being called into question.

The presence of daytime hypercapnia in COPD patients (which, if present, assuredly worsens during sleep) is generally regarded as an indicator of a poorer prognosis. Patients with chronic bronchitis (who are more likely to have hypercapnia) have a higher mortality and are also more likely to die in the early morning than a control population (39). The prognostic significance of hypercapnia was called into question by an older longitudinal study of COPD patients. Survival was poorer with a lower nocturnal mean or nadir and awake Spo_2. Although a higher daytime $Paco_2$ value predicted more nocturnal hypoxia than expected from awake oxygen saturation values alone, increased $Paco_2$ levels did not affect the prediction of survival (40). The prognostic value of hypercapnia was also recently challenged by the observations from another large registry of patients with severe COPD or sequelae of tuberculosis given long-term oxygen over 8 yr. Patients with a $Paco_2$ level >45 torr had either the same (COPD patients) or better (TB patients) survival than those with a $Paco_2$ level <45 torr (41). The survival benefit was most apparent in former TB patients with restriction in the absence of severe airway obstruction, suggesting that hypercapnia may be protective in some patient subgroups (Fig. 6). However, a rise in $Paco_2$ in COPD pa-

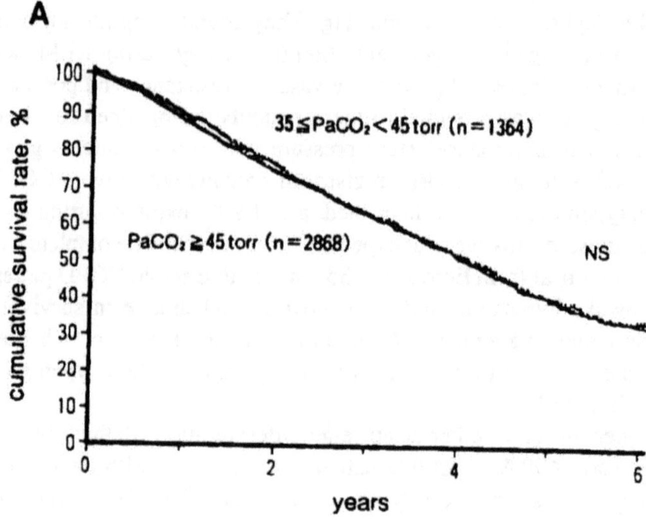

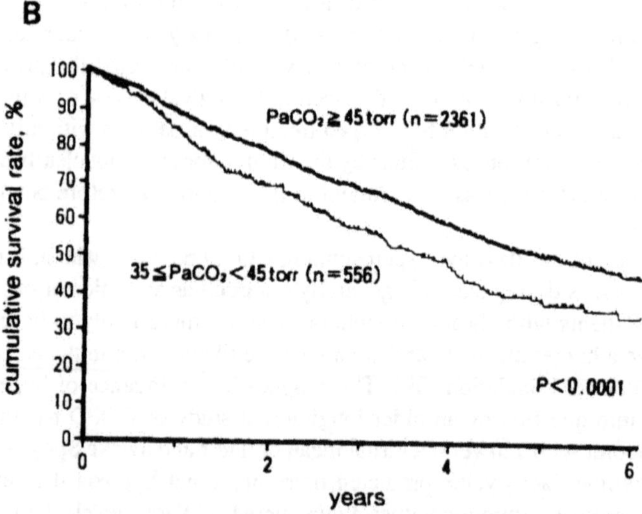

Figure 6 Cumulative survival curves by the level of $Paco_2$. (A) COPD. (B) Sequelae of pulmonary tuberculosis. NS, not significant. (From Ref. 41.)

tients in the first 6 to 18 mo of oxygen therapy was associated with a poorer prognosis and may identify those susceptible to daytime hypoventilation with supplemental oxygen that may be further exaggerated at night. This susceptibility to hypoventilation with oxygen supplementation may be particularly pronounced in NMD patients with diaphragm dysfunction (42).

C. Mechanisms for Nocturnal Oxygen Desaturation/Hypoventilation

The mechanisms for nocturnal oxygen desaturation in COPD and NMD patients are schematized in Figure 7. The major culprit that explains nocturnal desaturation is hypoventilation, which occurs primarily during REM sleep for all disease categories. For COPD patients, this is seen as hypopneas—few patients actually develop apnea (15,17). However, it should not be overlooked that patients with primary (such as COPD patients) or secondary (those with old polio and kyphoscoliosis) respiratory disease commonly harbor obstructive sleep apnea, particularly if they are obese (up to 15% of COPD patients) (21,44,45).

With either COPD or NMD patients, central drive during sleep is markedly depressed beyond that expected from the sleep state alone. As noted above, the evidence for decreased ventilatory responsiveness to hypoxia and hypercapnia supports this notion. Studies have been designed that specifically look at dia-

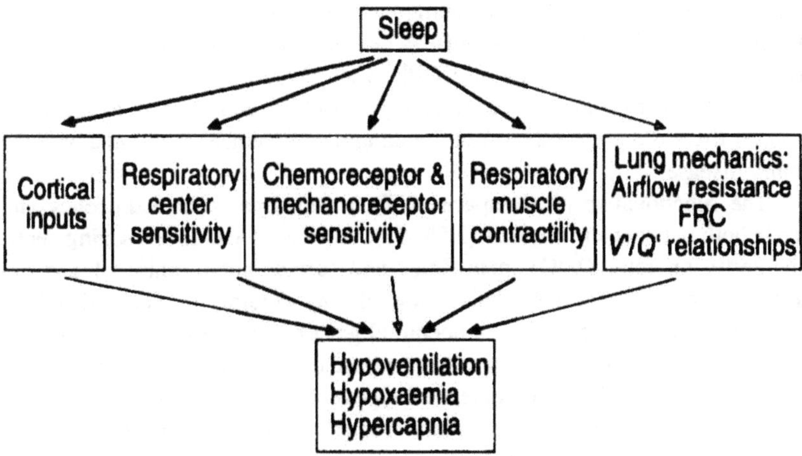

Figure 7 Schematic diagram of the effects of sleep on respiration. In each case, sleep has a negative influence, which has the overall impact of producing hypoventilation and/or hypoxemia and hypercapnia. FRC, functional residual capacity; $\dot{V}/\dot{Q}$, ventilation-perfusion ratio. (From Ref. 43.)

phragmatic output as a reflection of central drive using the measurement of P0.1, which is the pressure generated during the first 100 msec of an inspiratory effort (46). For many years, studies have confirmed that COPD patients, even those with acute respiratory failure, when compared with normal, have increased P0.1 values (associated with increased central drive). Respiratory insufficiency in COPD patients is thus caused not by a problem with respiratory drive but rather by the coupling distortion imposed by the increased load on the respiratory system (47,48). This finding of normal or increased central drive based on P0.1 has also been demonstrated for patients with ALS and other neuromuscular diseases, and the respiratory failure is explained by neuromechanical coupling dysfunction (29,49).

The increased load in COPD patients relates to the unfavorable configuration of the diaphragm associated with severe hyperinflation, as well as increased upper and lower airway resistance. In addition, the contributions of the intercostal and accessory muscles to ventilation are reduced in COPD and NMD patients, especially during REM sleep (50,51). Patients with COPD may actually exhibit abdominal paradox during sleep similar to neuromuscular patients with diaphragm muscle failure, emphasizing the relative weakness of the diaphragm in these patients (see Chapter 6) (52,53). If COPD patients are dependent on accessory muscle use, then the onset of REM with accompanying skeletal muscle hypotonia (as would occur in intercostal muscles) exacerbates hypoventilation (43).

Patients with chest wall deformities and neuromuscular diseases also have an increased load and work of breathing caused by reduction in chest wall and lung compliance (49,54). They would also be expected to have the same difficulty during REM sleep as patients with COPD when chest wall and other accessory muscles develop hypotonia. The accessory muscle dependence is exaggerated whenever there is a greater degree of diaphragm involvement associated with the primary disease.

The functional residual capacity (FRC) decreases with recumbency and sleep in both patients and normals (3,55–57). This could lead to worsening ventilation-perfusion ratio ($\dot{V}/\dot{Q}$) inequalities and further compromise of gas exchange, especially if the FRC falls below closing volume. Evidence that $\dot{V}/\dot{Q}$ mismatching plays a major role in nocturnal gas exchange abnormalities comes from a study in which COPD patients, who were categorized as major and minor sleep desaturators, had similar degrees of hypoventilation based on end-tidal CO_2 measurement (19). The authors therefore proposed that another mechanism must be considered, such as $\dot{V}/\dot{Q}$ mismatch. However, there is concern that end-tidal CO_2 in these patients does not accurately reflect arterial $Paco_2$ and the degree of hypoventilation (16).

Evidence against a major role for $\dot{V}/\dot{Q}$ mismatching in causing nocturnal hypoventilation in COPD patients comes from a study that used a body plethysmograph to provide more accurate measurements of lung volumes (58). Absolute lung volume did not change in this small group of patients constrained to sleep on their backs in an iron lung apparatus. Hypoventilation that was observed along with decreased inspiratory flow and tidal volume was explained by increased upper airway resistance and decreased central neuromuscular output (measured by P0.1). Hypoventilation is presumed to be the predominate mechanism in patients with either NMD or COPD. Ventilation-perfusion ratio mismatching likely remains less important unless significant basilar atelectasis is present, as is more commonly present in NMD or obesity hypoventilation syndrome patients.

The effect of sleep on upper airway resistance is discussed in detail in Chapter 5. This topic deserves some mention in this chapter, however, and is discussed below in section V.

IV. Sleep Quality in Patients with Primary and Secondary Respiratory Diseases

A. Chronic Obstructive Pulmonary Disease

A number of studies have summarized the general characteristics of sleep quality in COPD patients (16,20,21,59–61). When compared with normals, COPD patients report more difficulty falling and staying asleep and are more likely to regularly use hypnotics. These patients also have more daytime sleepiness and sleep fragmentation; the increased number of arousals correlates strongly with the level of nocturnal desaturation, especially during REM sleep (61). Patients with moderate COPD and milder awake hypoxemia do not seem to have either objective or subjective evidence of daytime sleepiness despite shorter total sleep time and numerous arousals. More severely obstructed and hypoxemic COPD patients have much less total sleep time, three times more frequent sleep stage changes, and less REM sleep (16). Although many of the arousals appear to be related to oxygen desaturation, this same study confirmed that supplemental oxygen had no effect on the reduced sleep time and increased sleep stage changes, despite an effective improvement in nocturnal oxygen saturation. Interestingly, most COPD patients have reported subjective improvement in sleep quality with oxygen. In a small study of exclusively hypercapnic and hypoxemic COPD patients ("blue bloaters"), oxygen at night significantly increased sleep time as well as the number and duration of REM periods (20). Other factors besides breathing may also disturb sleep in COPD and should not be forgotten. Gastroesophageal reflux that commonly exists as a co-morbid condition has also been shown to independently lead to increased arousals (60).

B. Neuromuscular Disease

Sleep quality in patients with neuromuscular disease has not been as systematically documented as that in COPD patients. Studies done in patients with kyphoscoliosis and/or postpolio syndrome show disturbed sleep with frequent desaturations (62). Those who also have either hypercapnia or coexisting OSA reveal reduced total sleep time and reduced REM time with severe hypoxemia (26,44,63).

In a study of patients with ALS, the need to look at many different factors that contribute to sleep disturbance was emphasized, including muscle cramps and pain from reduced mobility, swallowing problems, increased myoclonic activity, and anxiety or depression (64). Symptoms that best correlate with sleep-related breathing disturbance in these patients include orthopnea, "daytime sleepiness" (but not "morning headaches"), or "difficulty sleeping" (30,65,66). In general, sleep disturbance and nocturnal oxygen desaturation tend to follow the course of the disease with relatively good preservation of sleep quality until more severe breathing abnormality develops (30,65–67). Sleep-disordered breathing was reportedly most prominent in those patients with more severe bulbar involve-

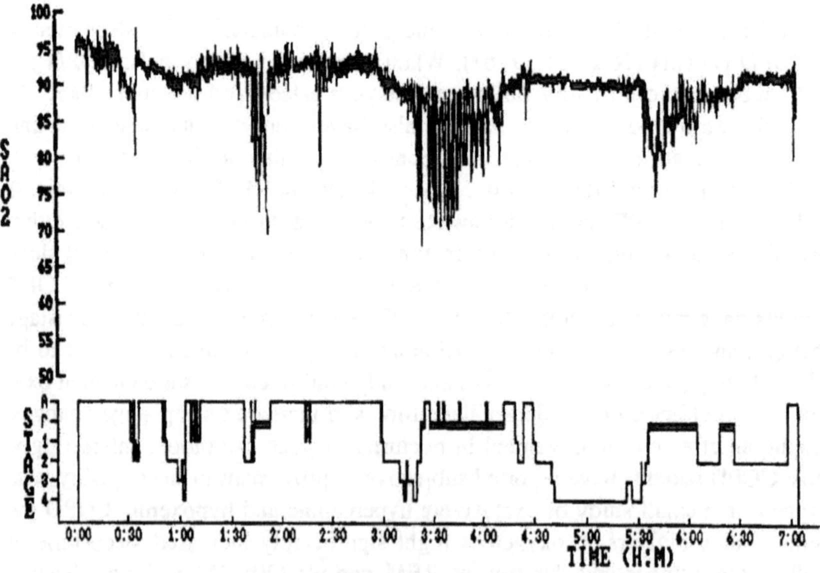

Figure 8 Overnight oxygen saturation profile in a patient with bulbar ALS with respiratory muscle weakness. Baseline saturation is normal. Significant, episodic nonapneic desaturation is apparent during REM sleep (A, awake; r, REM). (From Ref. 66.)

ment, in whom reduced sleep time, increased stage I time, more frequent arousals, and more nocturnal desaturations were noted compared with normal sleep (30,66). In these studies, obstructive events were occasionally noted, but clinically significant OSA was not seen even in the presence of notable bulbar dysfunction. Commonly, patients will report that they no longer snore, especially if there is significant weight loss and swallowing dysfunction. A classic example of an abnormal overnight tracing with marked REM desaturations (patient had normal awake saturation) is shown in Figure 8.

Patients with muscular dystrophy reportedly die more frequently at night and many may display significant sleep-related breathing disturbances despite little or no symptomology or abnormality in awake gas exchange (24,68,69). Conversely, patients with apparently milder disease may have markedly disturbed sleep, desaturation, and daytime hypersomnolence. This seems most likely to occur when early diaphragmatic involvement or coexisting OSA in obese patients is overlooked (70,71). The patients who display abdominal wall paradoxical breathing show greater desaturation in both REM and non-REM sleep and often have disturbed sleep-related symptoms (24,72). Sleep architecture is well preserved until the disease and breathing abnormality are more advanced (68). More severely affected patients with or without coexisting cardiomyopathy are also much more likely to have cardiac arrhythmias associated with nocturnal desaturations regardless of sleep stage (73).

V. Effect of Nocturnal Mechanical Ventilation on Sleep and Gas Exchange

The earliest work that stimulated interest in nocturnal mechanical ventilation (NMV) to treat patients with respiratory failure is best credited to Rochester and Braun (74). Interestingly, these authors' earliest studies were done to evaluate the control of breathing and response of the respiratory system to assisted breathing rather than to test NMV as a therapeutic alternative (74). For the purpose of this discussion, some general comments should be made about the responses of the respiratory system to the use of NMV in normal subjects and those with disease. This has also been discussed in a previous volume of this series (75).

The response of the respiratory system and hence, sleep quality and gas exchange depend to a large extent on the ventilator settings. As a simple example, an adequate inspiratory driving pressure may completely reverse the presence of diaphragmatic paradox associated with inspiratory muscle weakness in some patients (Fig. 9). Increases in inspiratory pressure or tidal volume settings also decrease respiratory rate, whereas increases in inspiratory flow rate at a given

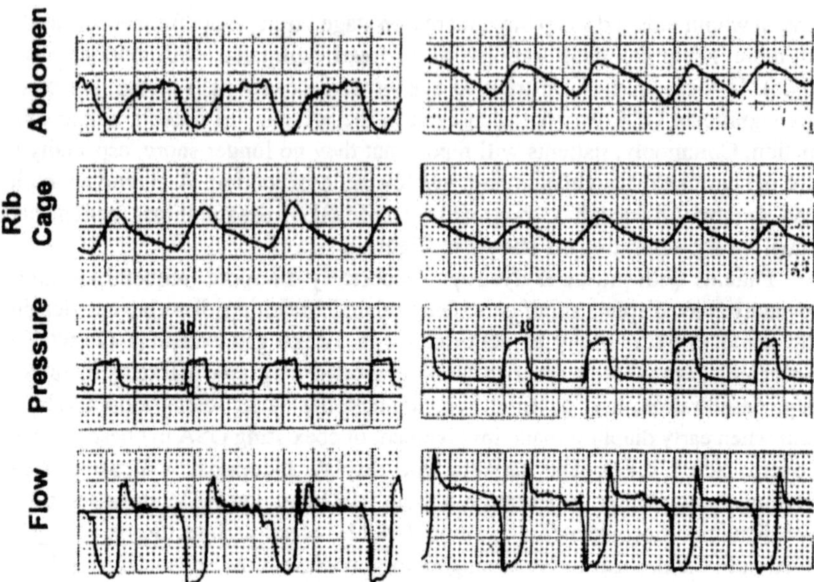

Figure 9 Abdominal and rib cage displacement, mask pressure, and flow are plotted against time at two different pressure settings (5 cm H_2O in left panels and 10 cm H_2O in right panels) in an awake patient with COPD. Note that the inverted abdominal signal consistent with abdominal paradox (left panel) reverses at the higher delivered pressure (right panel).

tidal volume in awake or sleeping normals receiving assisted ventilation through a mask raise breathing rates. These responses occur even in subjects denervated by way of trauma or lung transplantation (76–78). The rise in breathing frequency seen when the inspiratory flow rate is increased is associated with shortening of the inspiratory neural activation time of the respiratory muscles (79). In some subjects, however, the delivered pressure or rate may be excessive, and this leads to irregular or periodic breathing patterns with apnea and a worsening of arousals (80,81).

Evidence indicates that patients with restrictive lung disease perceive an improvement in sleep quality in association with more effective nocturnal ventilation. This observation comes from studies in which patients who were accustomed to NMV were temporarily withdrawn from treatment (82,83). One study was done in six patients with restrictive lung disease and daytime hypercapnia who were accustomed to NMV after they were withdrawn from nocturnal ventilatory support for a period of 1 wk (82). Despite no change in awake vital signs or arterial blood gases, daytime symptoms of sleep-disordered breathing returned, including daytime hypersomnolence, morning headache, decreased restfulness, fatigue, and energy loss. The nocturnal studies done following withdrawal of NMV revealed increased tachycardia, tachypnea, and oxygen desaturation. Reversal of daytime symptomology related to nocturnal hypoventilation has similarly been reported before and after treatment with both negative pressure ventilators and positive pressure ventilation delivered through a tracheostomy (84,85). Other than studies of symptom improvement, there are no formal polysomnographic data detailing sleep architecture and quality of sleep with chronic tracheostomy and NMV use.

The mechanisms for improved sleep and breathing with NMV could also be mediated by improved ventilation while awake. This is best shown in a study of sleep and ventilatory responsiveness to oxygen and carbon dioxide in a young patient with primary hypoventilation before and after treatment with NMV (86). Over a 3-mo period, there was a progressive improvement in awake gas exchange, ventilatory responsiveness, and $Paco_2$ in conjunction with less REM desaturation and sleep disruption. In patients with severe kyphoscoliosis, treatment with nasal NMV showed improvement in daytime symptoms and gas exchange despite continued significant sleep disruption associated with residual nocturnal desaturation (87). Although it is generally accepted that treatment must be given nocturnally to treat the period when breathing is expected to be most compromised, some evidence shows benefit with daytime mechanical ventilation therapy alone (88).

A significant concern related to the efficacy of NMV in sleeping patients is patient ventilator synchrony. Presumably, subjects that synchronize best with the ventilator secure optimal ventilatory assistance by coordinating both machine output and patient effort. One might also expect improvements in sleep quality when the ventilator is set to avoid machine overventilation during sleep, which causes abrupt changes in arterial CO_2 levels and ventilatory instability, contributing to arousals (89,90).

The above raises the question of what constitutes ideal ventilator settings. If effective minute ventilation alone is targeted, then some studies suggest that controlled ventilation with a higher frequency and lower tidal volume is preferred (81,91). The timing of the delivered breath appears to be crucial, however, as the preparedness of the upper airway is also a major determinant of optimal ventilation and sleep quality (92,93). A study was done to assess vocal cord function/interaction in a ventilator-dependent quadriplegic patient, and compared with two normal subjects during controlled ventilation using an iron lung respirator. The vocal cords closed during inspiration and created a large pressure gradient (12 to 19 cm H_2O) across the cords when the patient and the normal subjects relaxed and did not make an effort to coordinate with the respirator. Contrariwise, the cords opened widely during coordinated inspiration with large increases in flow and tidal volume when the subjects assisted with only a slight effort that was too small to increase transdiaphragmatic and esophageal pressure. This confirmed that the improved ventilation with the slight assistance was related to decreased inspiratory obstruction of the upper airway. Any chosen ventilator settings must therefore also take into account the effects on upper airway function as well.

Synchrony with the ventilator assistance may also be compromised by failure of the ventilator to sense and assist. This may lead to wasted or unassisted efforts with diminished ventilation. Occasionally, the ventilator may autocycle, delivering rapid repeated breaths that result in further mistimed or ineffective assistance. Graphic examples of all these events are shown in Figure 10.

Given the above problem in setting the ventilator, analyzing studies on the effects of NMV on sleep is difficult because few studies demonstrate that the methodology has incorporated the above considerations or that settings have been optimized. This is illustrated by the discrepant findings in severely hypercapnic COPD patients given NMV (94–98). Even in these carefully designed short- and long-term randomized clinical trials in which settings were usually pushed to "tolerance," mean inspiratory assist pressure levels ranged widely from 10 to 22 cm H_2O. Only at the highest mean pressure levels ($\geq$18 cm H_2O) was a mild but significant increase in sleep efficiency and total sleep time noted 95,98). As reported from several studies, sleep architecture and the number of arousals is usually unchanged before and after NMV but REM sleep percentage remains reduced when compared with data from normal older adults (96–99). Given that sleep stage changes occur more frequently with NMV treatment, it is not surprising that overall architecture and arousals may not improve despite increased total sleep time after NMV.

There are no randomized clinical trials that look at sleep in patients with NMD before and after NMV. These types of studies are unlikely to be forthcoming given the widely accepted efficacy of NMV in patients with restrictive disorders and general difficulty getting symptomatic NMD patients to participate in studies with sham arms. Several small studies however have reported that sleep quality improved in terms of architecture and efficiency with NMV when symptomatic patients with NMD and kyphoscoliosis were treated (83,100,101). One of these studies looked at the effects of 15-day nasal NMV treatment withdrawal on actual sleep quality in five patients with restrictive lung disease. Although patients had no change in sleep efficiency or percentage of REM sleep, the number of arousals and desaturations during REM sleep were much higher without NMV and daytime symptoms of dyspnea and morning headaches returned in most patients (83). With improved nocturnal gas exchange, the improvement in sleep efficiency and decreased time spent in lighter stages I and II sleep is much more dramatic than that seen for COPD patients. Although some patients can be

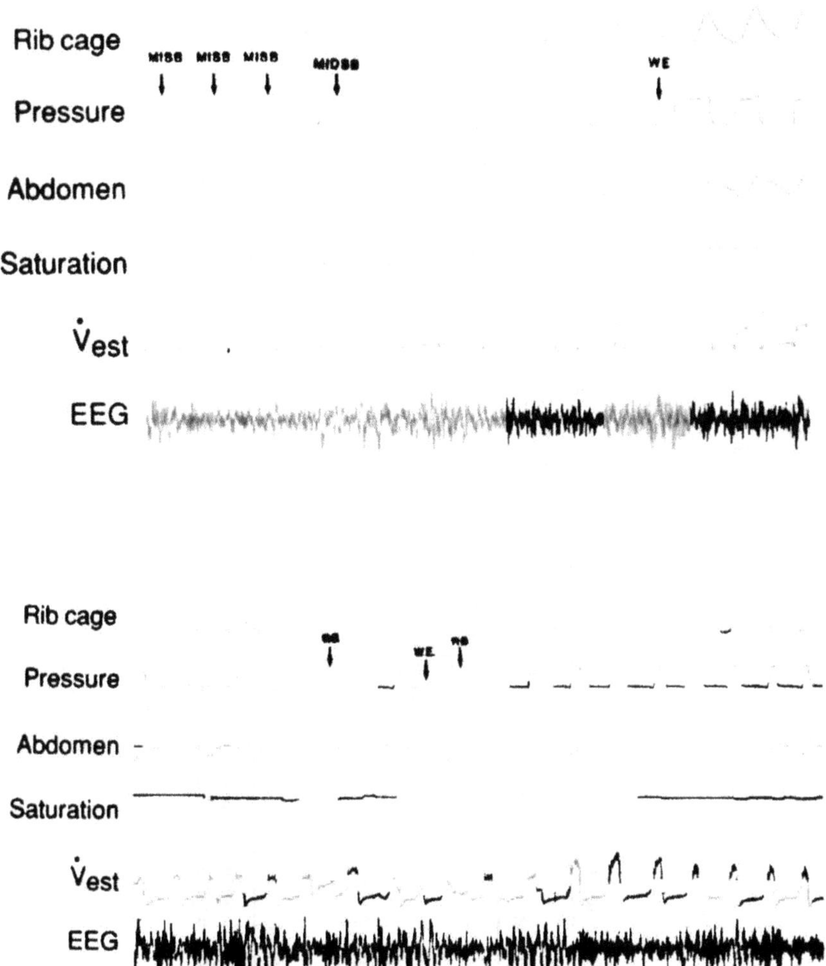

Figure 10 Rib cage and abdominal displacement, mask pressure, oxygen saturation, estimated machine flow (V̇est), and EEG are shown plotted against time in a sleeping subject. Appropriately timed breaths delivered either by the timed mode (MISB, machine initiated synchronous breath) or spontaneously triggered mode (all unlabeled breaths) are shown (top). Also note the failed triggering (WE, wasted efforts), auto-cycled or runaway breaths (RB) (bottom), and ill-timed breaths (MIDSB, machine initiated dyssynchronous breath) that result in reduced assistance of rib cage and abdominal displacement.

Table 1 Sleep Responses to NMV[a]

Reference	Author	N	Disease	Total sleep time	Efficiency	% REM	No. of Arousals
83	Masa Jimenez	5	Mixed restrictive	U	+	NC	+
100	Barbe	8	NMD	+	++	+	++
101	Ellis	7	Kypho	U	U	++	++
94	Strumpf	7	COPD	NC	NC	NC	U
95	Meecham-Jones	18	COPD	++	++	NC	U
96	Gay	10	COPD	NC	NC	−−	U
97	Lin	12	COPD	U	−	NC	U
98	Krachman	6	COPD	++	++	NC	NC

[a]Abbreviations: COPD, chronic obstructive pulmonary disease; Kypho, kyphoscoliosis; NMD, neuromuscular disease; NMV, nocturnal mechanical ventilation; ++, significantly improved; +, improved; NC, no change; − worse; −−, significantly worse; and U, unavailable.

initially supported with triggered pressure support modes, the best results are noted with full or partial timed breath settings (100,102).

Patients using nasal NMV may experience sleep disruption and desaturation associated with air leak through the mouth. Although there is no special reason to think this problem is unique to a specific subgroup of patients, two studies done in patients with kyphoscoliosis showed marked oral air leak associated with desaturation and sleep disruption especially during REM sleep. Increased arousals and desaturations occurred in all sleep stages despite maintenance of good overall mean oxygen saturation using either pressure or volume-targeted devices. Nevertheless, patients experienced a significant improvement of overall nocturnal ventilation and related daytime symptoms and some patients in the latter study that used the pressure-targeted devices appear to accommodate the leaks and have fewer arousals (87,103). The difficulty with air leak at the mouth may also explain why NMD patients without coexisting OSA do not tolerate higher expiratory pressures. This leads to reduced total sleep time and more arousals (104). Table 1 summarizes the changes in sleep after NMV treatment noted in several different studies for both NMD and COPD patients.

VI. Summary

Studies clearly need to be continued to further explain the true effect of NMV on sleep quality and control of breathing, both on an immediate and sustained basis. Until the mechanisms to explain the benefit of NMV for obstructive, restrictive, and mixed respiratory disease disorders are better known, the indications, idealized ventilator settings, and expected response will remain unclear. Despite the lack of hard evidence from randomized trials, NMD patients with sleep-related breathing abnormalities clearly have improved nocturnal and awake gas exchange. The amelioration of nocturnal oxygen desaturations, especially during REM sleep, probably contributes to the improvement in sleep quality observed in these patients during NMV treatment.

A select subgroup of COPD patients also appears to have improved sleep after treatment with NMV but specific characteristics that describe this subgroup well remain to be elucidated. The COPD patients with clear evidence of hypoventilation while awake as evidenced by daytime hypercapnia are a reasonable starting target group. Those COPD patients who also show continued sleep disruption or worsening hypercapnia and nocturnal hypoventilation despite oxygen therapy should be further investigated. Ultimately, we need to define optimal equipment design and settings in hopes of improving acceptance and willingness to continue long-term therapy for all types of appropriate patients likely to benefit from NMV.

References

1. Rechtschaffen A, Kales A. A Manual of Standardized Terminology, Techniques and Scoring System for Sleep States of Human Subjects. National Institutes of Health (NIH) Publication #204. Washington, DC: NIH, 1968.
2. American Thoracic Society (ATS) Consensus Conference: Indications and standards for cardiopulmonary sleep studies. Am Rev Respir Dis 1989; 139:559–568.
3. Phillipson EA. Control of breathing during sleep. Am Rev Respir Dis 1978; 118: 909–939.
4. Saunders NA, Sullivan CE, eds. Sleep and Breathing. 2nd ed. New York: Dekker, 1994.
5. Lydic RL, Baghdoyan HA. The neurobiology of rapid-eye movement sleep. In: Saunders NA, Sullivan CE, eds. Sleep and Breathing. 2nd ed. New York: Dekker, 1994.
6. Jones BE. Basic mechanisms of sleep-wake states. In: Kryger MH, Roth T, Dement WC, eds. Principles and Practice of Sleep Medicine. 2nd ed. Philadelphia: Saunders, 1994; 125–144.
7. Douglas NJ, White DP, Pickett CK, Weil JV, Zwillich CW. Respiration during sleep in normal man. Thorax 1982; 37:840–844.
8. Berthon-Jones M, Sullivan CE. Ventilatory and arousal responses to hypoxia in sleeping humans. Am Rev Respir Dis 1982; 125:632–639.
9. Berthon-Jones M, Sullivan CE. Ventilation and arousal responses to hypercapnia in normal sleeping humans. J Appl Physiol 1984; 57:59–67.
10. Douglas NJ, White DP, Pickett CK, Weil JV, Zwillich CW. Hypercapnic ventilatory response in sleeping adults. Am Rev Respir Dis 1982; 126:758–762.
11. Juan G, Calverley P, Talamo C, Schnader J, Roussos C. Effect of carbon dioxide on diaphragmatic function in human beings. N Engl J Med 1984; 310: 874–879.
12. Sullivan CE, Kozar LF, Murphy E, Phillipson EA. Primary role of respiratory afferents in sustaining breathing rhythm. J Appl Physiol 1978; 45:11–15.
13. Phillipson EA, Murphy E, Kozar LF. Regulation of respiration in sleeping dogs. J Appl Physiol 1976; 89:688–699.
14. Fleetham JA, Mezon B, West P, Bradley CA, Anthonisen NR, Kryger MH. Chemical control of ventilation and sleep arterial oxygen desaturation in patients with COPD. Am J Respir J 1980; 122:583–589.
15. Douglas NJ. Sleep in patients with COPD. Clin Chest Med 1998; 19:115–125.
16. Fleetham JA, West P, Mezon B, Conway W, Roth T, Kryger M. Sleep, arousals, and oxygen desaturation in chronic obstructive pulmonary disease. Am Rev Respir Dis 1982; 126:429–433.
17. Douglas NJ. Nocturnal hypoxemia in patients with chronic obstructive pulmonary disease. Clin Chest Med 1992; 13:524–532.
18. Fletcher EC, Miller J, Divine GW, Fletcher JG, Miller T. Nocturnal oxyhemoglobin desaturation in COPD patients with arterial oxygen saturation tensions above 60 mmHg. Chest 1987; 92:604–608.

19. Mulloy E, McNicholas WT. Ventilation and gas exchange during sleep and exercise in severe COPD. Chest 1996; 109:387–394.
20. Calverley PM, Brezinova V, Douglas NJ, Catterall JR, Flenley DC. The effect of oxygenation on sleep quality in chronic bronchitis and emphysema. Am Rev Respir Dis 1982 126:206–210.
21. Catterall JR, Douglas NJ, Calverley PMA, Shapiro CM, Brezinova V, Brash HM, Flenley DC. Transient hypoxemia during sleep in chronic obstructive pulmonary disease is not a sleep apnea syndrome. Am Rev Respir Dis 1983; 128:24–29.
22. Tirlapur VG, Mir MA. Nocturnal hypoxemia and associated electrocardiographic changes in patients with chronic obstructive airways disease. N Engl J Med 1982; 306:125–130.
23. Kramer NR, Hill NS, Millman RP. Assessment and treatment of sleep-disordered breathing in neuromuscular and chest wall disease. Clin Pulm Med 1996; 3:336–342.
24. Smith PEM, Calverley PMA, Edwards RHT. Hypoxemia during sleep in Duchenne muscular dystrophy. Am Rev Respir Dis 1988; 137:884–888.
25. Piper AJ, Sullivan CE. Effects of long-term nocturnal nasal ventilation on spontaneous breathing during sleep in neuromuscular and chest wall disorders. Eur Respir J 1996; 9:1515–1522.
26. Mezon BL, West P, Israels J, Kryger M. Sleep and breathing abnormalities in kyphoscoliosis. Am Rev Respir Dis 1980; 122:617–621.
27. Fallat RJ, Jewitt B, Bass M, Kamm B, Norris FH. Spirometry in amyotrophic lateral sclerosis. Arch Neurol 1979; 36:74–80.
28. Kaplan LM, Hollander D. Respiratory dysfunction in amyotrophic lateral sclerosis. Clin Chest Med 1994; 15:675–681.
29. Vitacca M, Clini E, Facchetti D, Pagani M, Poloni M, Porta R, Ambrosino N. Breathing pattern and respiratory mechanics in patients with amyotrophic lateral sclerosis. Eur Respir J 1997; 10:1614–1621.
30. Gay PC, Westbrook PR, Daube JR, Litchy WJ, Windebank AJ, Iverson R. Effects of alterations in pulmonary function and sleep variables in survival in patients with amyotrophic lateral sclerosis. Mayo Clin Proc 1991; 66:686–694.
31. Nocturnal Oxygen Therapy Trial. Ann Int Med 1980; 93:391–398.
32. Timms RM, Khaja FU, Williams, and the NOTT Group. Hemodynamic response to oxygen therapy in COPD. Ann Int Med 1985; 102:29–36.
33. Fletcher EC, Luckett RA, Miller T, Costarangos C, Kutka N, Fletcher JG. Pulmonary vascular hemodynamics in chronic lung disease patients with and without oxyhemoglobin desaturation during sleep. Chest 1989; 95:157–166.
34. Fletcher EC, Levin DC. Cardiopulmonary hemodynamics during sleep in subjects with COPD: The effect of short- and long-term oxygen. Chest 1984; 85:6–14.
35. Fletcher EC, Luckett R, Goodnight-White S, Miller CC, Qian W, Costarangos-Galarza C. A double-blind trial of nocturnal supplemental oxygen for sleep desaturation in patients with chronic obstructive pulmonary disease and a daytime Pao_2 above 60 mmHg. Am Rev Respir Dis 1992; 145(5):1070–1076.
36. Zielinski J, MacNee W, Wedzicha J, Ambrosino N, Braghiroli A, Dolensky J, How-

ard P, Gorzelak K, Lahdensuo A, Strom K, Tobiasz M, Weitzenblum E. Causes of death in patients with COPD and chronic respiratory failure. Monaldi Arch Chest Dis 1997; 52:43–47.

37. Gorecka D, Gorzelak K, Sliwinski P, Tobiasz M, Zielinski J. Effects of long-term oxygen therapy on survival in patients with chronic obstructive pulmonary disease with moderate hypoxemia. Thorax 1997; 52:674–679.
38. Chaouat A, Weitzenblum E, Kessler R, Charpentier C, Ehrhart M, Levi-Valensi P, Zielinski J, Delaunois L, Cornudella R, Moutinho dos Santos J. Sleep-related O_2 desaturation and daytime pulmonary haemodynamics in COPD patients with mild hypoxaemia. Eur Respir J 1997; 10:1730–1735.
39. McNicholas WT, Fitzgerald MX. Nocturnal deaths in patients with chronic bronchitis and emphysema. Brit Med J 1984; 289:878–892.
40. Connaughton JJ, Catterall JR, Elton RA, Stradling JR, Douglas NJ. Do sleep studies contribute to the management of patients with severe chronic obstructive pulmonary disease? Am Rev Respir Dis 1988; 138:341–344.
41. Aida A, Miyamoto K, Nishimura M, Aiba M, Kira S, Kawakami Y. Prognostic value of hypercapnia in patients with chronic respiratory failure during long-term oxygen therapy. Am Rev Respir Crit Care Med 1998; 158:188–193.
42. Gay PC, Edmonds LC. Severe hypercapnia after low-flow oxygen therapy in patients with neuromuscular disease and diaphragmatic dysfunction. Mayo Clin Proc 1995; 70:327–330.
43. McNicholas WT. Impact of sleep in respiratory failure. Eur Respir J 1997; 10:920–933.
44. Hsu AA, Staats BA. Postpolio sequelae and sleep-related disordered breathing. Mayo Clin Proc 1998; 73:216–224.
45. Lopata M, Onal E. Mass loading, sleep apnea, and the pathogenesis of obesity hypoventilation. Am Rev Respir Dis 1982; 126:640–644.
46. White DP. Occlusion pressure and ventilation during sleep in normal humans. J Appl Physiol 1986; 61:1279–1287.
47. Montes de Oca M, Celli BR. Mouth occlusion pressure, CO_2 response, and hypercapnia in severe chronic obstructive pulmonary disease. Eur Respir J 1998; 12: 666–672.
48. Aubier M, Murciano D, Fournier M, Milic-Emili J, Pariente R, Derenne JP. Central respiratory drive in acute respiratory failure of patients with chronic obstructive pulmonary disease. Am Rev Respir Dis 1980; 122:191–199.
49. Baydur A. Respiratory muscle strength and control of ventilation in patients with neuromuscular disease. Chest 1991; 99:330–338.
50. Johnson MW, Remmers JE. Accessory muscle activity during sleep in COPD. J Appl Physiol 1984; 57:1011–1017.
51. Newsom-Davis J, Loh L. Alveolar hypoventilation and respiratory muscle weakness. Bull Eur Physiopathol Respir 1979; 15:45–51.
52. Hudgel DW, Martin RJ, Capehart M, Johnson B, Hill P. Contribution of hypoventilation to sleep oxygen desaturation in chronic obstructive pulmonary disease. J Appl Physiol 1983; 55:669–677.
53. Meurice JC, Marc I, Series F. Influence of sleep on ventilatory and upper airway

response to CO_2 in normal subjects and patients with COPD. Am Rev Respir Crit Care Med 1995; 152:1620–1626.

54. De Troyer A, Borenstein S, Cordier R. Analysis of lung volume restriction in patients with respiratory muscle weakness. Thorax 1980; 35:603–610.
55. Hudgel DW, Devadetta P. Decrease in functional residual capacity during sleep in normal humans. J Appl Physiol 1984; 57:1319–1322.
56. Phillipson EA, Goldstein RS. Breathing during sleep in COPD. Chest 1984; 85S: 24S–30S.
57. Muller NL, Francis PW, Gurwitz D, Levison H, Bryan AC. Mechanism of hemoglobin desaturation during rapid eye movement sleep in normal subjects and in patients with cystic fibrosis. Am Rev Respir Dis 1980; 121:463–469.
58. Ballard RD, Clover CW, Suh BY. Influence of sleep on respiratory function in emphysema. Am Rev Respir Crit Care Med 1995; 151:945–951.
59. Orr WC, Shamma-Othman Z, Levin D, Othman J, Rundell OH. Persistent hypoxemia and excessive daytime sleepiness in chronic obstructive pulmonary disease (COPD). Chest 1990; 97:583–585.
60. Orr WC, Shamma-Othman Z, Allen M, Robinson MG. Esophageal function and gastroesophageal reflux during sleep and waking in patients with chronic obstructive pulmonary disease. Chest 1992; 10:1521–1525.
61. Cormick W, Olson LG, Hensley MJ, Saunders NA. Nocturnal hypoxaemia and quality of sleep in patients with chronic obstructive lung disease. Thorax 1986; 41: 846–854.
62. Sawicka EH, Branthwaite MA. Respiration during sleep in kyphoscoliosis. Thorax 1987; 42:801–808.
63. Guilleminault C, Kurland G, Winkle R, Miles LE. Severe kyphoscoliosis, breathing, and sleep: the "Quasimodo" syndrome during sleep. Chest 1981; 79:626–630.
64. Hetta J, Jansson I. Sleep in patients with amyotrophic lateral sclerosis. J Neurol 1997; 244:S7–S9.
65. David WS, Bundlie SR, Mahdavi Z. Polysomnographic studies in amyotrophic lateral sclerosis. J Neurol Sci 1997; 152S:S29–S35.
66. Ferguson KA, Strong MJ, Ahmad D, George CF. Sleep-disordered breathing in amyotrophic lateral sclerosis. Chest 1996; 110:664–669.
67. Minz M, Autret A, Laffont F, Beillevaire T, Cathala HP, Castaigne P. A study on sleep in amyotrophic lateral sclerosis. Biomedicine 1979; 30:40–46.
68. Barbe F, Quera-Salva MA, McCann C, Gajdos P, Raphael JC, de Lattre J, Agusti AG. Sleep-related respiratory disturbances in patients with Duchenne muscular dystrophy. Eur Resp J 1994; 7:1403–1408.
69. Cirignotta F, Mondini S, Zucconi M, Barrot-Cortes E, Sturani C, Schiavina M, Coccagna G, Lugaresi E. Sleep-related breathing impairment in myotonic dystrophy. J Neurol 1987; 235:80–85.
70. Culebras A. Sleep and neuromuscular disorders. Neurol Clinics 1996; 14:791–805.
71. Khan Y, Heckmatt JZ. Obstructive apneas in Duchenne muscular dystrophy. Thorax 1994; 49:157–161.

72. Smith PE, Edwards RH, Calverley PM. Ventilation and breathing pattern during sleep in Duchenne muscular dystrophy. Chest 1989; 96:1346–1351.
73. Carroll N, Bain RJ, Smith PE, Saltissi S, Edwards RH, Calverley PM. Domiciliary investigation of sleep-related hypoxemia in Duchenne muscular dystrophy. Euro Respir J 1991; 4:434–440.
74. Rochester DF, Braun NM, Laine S. Diaphragmatic energy expenditure in chronic respiratory failure: The effect of assisted ventilation with body respirators. Am J Med 1977; 63:223–232.
75. Hubmayr RD, Simon PM. Assessment of drive/muscle function. In: Marini JJ, Slutsky AS, eds. Physiological Basis of Ventilatory Support. New York: Dekker, 1998; 153–175.
76. Puddy A, Patrick W, Webster K, Younes M. Respiratory control during volume-cycled ventilation in normal humans. J Appl Physiol 1996; 80:1749–1758.
77. Mitrouska I, Bshouty Z, Younes M, Georgopoulos D. Effects of pulmonary and intercostal denervation on the response of breathing frequency to varying inspiratory flow. Eur Resp J 1998; 11:895–900.
78. Georgopoulos D, Mitrouska I, Bshouty Z, Anthonisen NR, Younes M. Effects of non-REM sleep on the response of respiratory output to varying inspiratory flow. Am J Respir Crit Care Med 1996; 153:1624–1630.
79. Fernandez R, Younes M. Effect of ventilator flow rate on respiratory timing in normal humans. Am J Respir Crit Care Med 1999; 159:710–719.
80. Morrell MJ, Shea SA, Adams L, Guz A. Effects of inspiratory support upon breathing in humans during wakefulness and sleep. Respir Physiol 1993; 93:57–70.
81. Parreira VF, Delguste P, Jounieaux V, Aubert G, Dury M. Rodenstein DO. Effectiveness of controlled and spontaneous modes in nasal two-level positive pressure ventilation in awake and asleep normal subjects. Chest 1997; 112:1267–1277.
82. Hill NS, Eveloff SE, Carlisle CC, Goff SG. Efficacy of nocturnal nasal ventilation in patients with restrictive thoracic disease. Am Rev Respir Dis 1992; 145:365–371.
83. Masa Jimenez JF, Sanchez de Cos Escuin J, Disdier Vicente C, Hernandez Valle M, Fuentes Otero F. Nasal intermittent positive pressure ventilation. Analysis of its withdrawal. Chest 1995; 107:382–388.
84. Goldstein RS, Molotiu N, Skrastins R, et al. Reversal of sleep-induced hypoventilation and chronic respiratory failure by nocturnal negative pressure ventilation in patients with restrictive ventilatory impairment. Am Rev Respir Dis 1987; 135: 1049–1055.
85. Hoeppner VH, Cockcroft DW, Dosman JA, Cotton DJ. Nighttime ventilation improves respiratory failure in secondary kyphoscoliosis. Am Rev Respir Dis 1984; 129:240–243.
86. Ellis ER, McCauley VB, Mellis C, Sullivan CE. Treatment of alveolar hypoventilation in a six-year-old girl with intermittent positive pressure ventilation through a nose mask. Am Rev Respir Dis 1987; 136:188–191.
87. Bach JR, Robert D, Leger P, Langevin B. Sleep fragmentation in kyphoscoliotic individuals with alveolar hypoventilation treated by NIPPV. Chest 1995;107:1552–1558.

88. Schonhofer B, Geibel M, Sonneborn M, Haidl P, Kohler D. Daytime mechanical ventilation in chronic respiratory insufficiency. Eur Resp J 1997; 10:2840–2846.
89. Olson EJ, Simon PM. Sleep-wake cycles and the management of respiratory failure. Curr Opin Pulm Med 1996; 2:500–506.
90. Hubmayr RD. The importance of patient/ventilator synchrony interactions during noninvasive mechanical ventilation. Acta Anaesthesiol Scand 1996; 109S:46–47.
91. Parreira VF, Jounieaux V, Delguste PE, Aubert G, Dury M, Rodenstein DO. Determinants of effective ventilation during nasal intermittent positive pressure ventilation. Eur Resp J 1997; 10:1975–1982.
92. Parreira VF, Jounieaux V, Aubert G, Dury M, Delguste PE, Rodenstein DO. Nasal two-level positive-pressure ventilation in normal subjects: Effects of the glottis and ventilation. Am J Respir Crit Care Med 1996; 153:1616–1623.
93. Parreira VF, Delguste P, Jounieaux V, Aubert G, Dury M, Rodenstein DO. Glottic aperture and effective minute ventilation during nasal two-level positive pressure ventilation in spontaneous mode. Am J Respir Crit Care Med 1996; 154:1857–1863.
94. Strumpf DA, Millman RP, Carlisle CC, Grattan LM, Ryan SM, Erickson AD, Hill NS. Nocturnal positive-pressure ventilation via nasal mask in patients with severe chronic obstructive pulmonary disease. Am J Respir Crit Care Med 1991; 144: 1234–1239.
95. Meecham-Jones DJ, Paul EA, Jones PW, Wedzicha JA. Nasal pressure support ventilation plus oxygen compared with oxygen therapy alone in hypercapnic COPD. Am J Respir Crit Care Med 1995; 152:538–544.
96. Gay PC, Hubmayr RD, Stroetz RW. Efficacy of nocturnal nasal ventilation in stable, severe chronic obstructive pulmonary disease during a 3-month controlled trial. Mayo Clin Proc 1996; 71:533–542.
97. Lin CC. Comparison between nocturnal nasal positive pressure ventilation combined with oxygen therapy and oxygen monotherapy in patients with severe COPD. Am J Respir Crit Care Med 1996; 154:353–358.
98. Krachman SL, Quaranta AJ, Berger TJ, Criner GJ. Effects of noninvasive positive pressure ventilation on gas exchange and sleep in COPD patients. Chest 1997; 112: 623–628.
99. Shore ET, Millman RP, Silage DA, Chung DC, Pack AI. Ventilatory and arousal patterns during sleep in normal young and elderly subjects. J Appl Physiol 1985; 59:1607–1615.
100. Barbe F, Quera-Salva MA, de Lattre J, Gajdos P, Agusti AG. Long-term effects of nasal intermittent positive-pressure ventilation on pulmonary function and sleep architecture in patients with neuromuscular diseases. Chest 1996; 110:1179–1183.
101. Ellis ER, Grunstein RR, Chan S, Bye PT, Sullivan CE. Noninvasive ventilatory support during sleep improves respiratory failure in kyphoscoliosis. Chest 1988; 94:811–815.
102. Guilleminault C, Philip P, Robinson A. Sleep and neuromuscular disease: Bilevel positive airway pressure by nasal mask as a treatment for sleep disordered breathing in patients with neuromuscular disease. J Neur Neurosurg Psych 1998; 65:225–232.

103. Meyer TJ, Pressman MR, Benditt J, McCool FD, Millman RP, Natarajan R, Hill NS. Air leaking through the mouth during nocturnal nasal ventilation: Effect on sleep quality. Sleep 1997; 20:561–569.
104. Elliott MW, Simonds AK. Nocturnal assisted ventilation using bilevel positive airway pressure: The effect of expiratory positive airway pressure. Eur Respir J 1995; 8:436–440.

5

The Upper Airway in Noninvasive Ventilation

DANIEL O. RODENSTEIN

Cliniques Universitaires Saint-Luc
Université Catholique de Louvain
Brussels, Belgium

I. Introduction

The notion of ventilation as the result of the action of a muscular negative pressure pump led to attempts to devise negative pressure breathing apparatuses during the first half of the nineteenth century (1). But more than 50 years earlier, positive pressure had been proposed as the means to force air into the lungs during resuscitation maneuvres (2). Animal experiments led to a still common complication of positive pressure ventilation: a fatal pneumothorax, which prompted the Académie Française and the Royal Humane Society to condemn this technique. Positive pressure ventilation resurfaced in 1952, when Lassen demonstrated that positive pressure manual (i.e., bag) ventilation through a tracheostomy tube was by far superior to negative pressure mechanical ventilation, the standard form of assisted ventilation at that time (3). The results were so extraordinary that negative pressure ventilation was almost completely abandoned worldwide, and the new concept of specialized units for the care of patients with transient life-threatening organ failure came to life (4). Manual bag ventilation was rapidly replaced by mechanical pumps, and the modern mechanical ventilator emerged (4).

A new application of positive pressure was introduced during the early 1980s, this time noninvasively, to treat obstructive apneas during sleep. The success of this technique was as extraordinary and rapid as the one that followed the Lassen experience. Sullivan et al. (5) used a continuous level of positive pressure from a blower connected to the spontaneously breathing patient through a nasal mask. After several years of increasing massive use with good acceptance and few serious complications, the same approach began to be widely used to provide mechanical intermittent positive pressure ventilation with volumetric portable ventilators to patients with neuromuscular diseases previously ventilated with negative pressure devices (6).

In the late 1980s, Sanders and Kern (7) introduced the next improvement in noninvasive positive pressure ventilation: the use of two different levels of fixed pressure, a higher one during inspiration and a lower one during expiration. Although devised for patients with obstructive sleep apnea, the development of two-level positive airway pressure ventilation (in essence a form of pressure support ventilation), provided a particularly comfortable form of ventilatory assistance when used in the spontaneous mode. This develpment contributed to the widespread use of noninvasive positive pressure ventilation that we know today (8–22).

All the respirators currently available for mechanical ventilation can be used either invasively through an endotracheal tube or a tracheostomy, or noninvasively through nasal or face masks or an oral connection. Similarly, most of the ventilatory modes available can be used with either an invasive or a noninvasive approach. In essence, what differentiates the invasive from the noninvasive approach is that the former bypasses the natural upper airway whereas the latter does not. This seemingly trivial difference has been shown to have unexpected consequences that must be understood and taken into account in order to make the best use of this extraordinarily useful form of assisted ventilation.

II. Apneas During Noninvasive Ventilation

The first main consequence of using a noninvasive approach is of course the occurrence of air leaks, which are avoided during invasive ventilation by the use of balloon-cuffed endotracheal or tracheostomy tubes. The most obvious leaks occur between the nasal or face mask and the skin. The other major source of leaks is the mouth when a nasal mask is used. The almost unavoidable existence of leaks makes it necessary to use volumes generally in excess of what is common in nonleaky invasive ventilation.

Several years ago we instituted noninvasive assisted ventilation in a young lady with acute on chronic respiratory failure. She had a congenital myopathy, compromising mouth occlusion because of masseter muscles weakness, and we expected large oral leaks. We therefore planned to use high delivered tidal volumes. During the polysomnographic control of the efficacy of noninvasive nocturnal assisted ventilation, we found episodes of deep falls in oxygen saturation (Sa_{O_2}), down to 60%, corresponding to complete abolition of respiratory movements of the chest wall. However, direct observation showed that, contrary to our expectations, this did not correspond to massive oral leaks (23). Such episodes of cessation of breathing movements were repetitive, occurred during sleep, in the absence of spontaneous respiratory efforts as shown by abolition of respiratory muscle electromyographic signal, lasted from 10 to 70 sec and ended with an arousal reaction that nearly coincided with the resumption of respiratory movements in synchrony with the respirator (Fig. 1). Most of these features reminded us of what can be seen in patients with obstructive sleep apnea (though in such patients spontaneous respiratory efforts usually persist). This similarity led us to

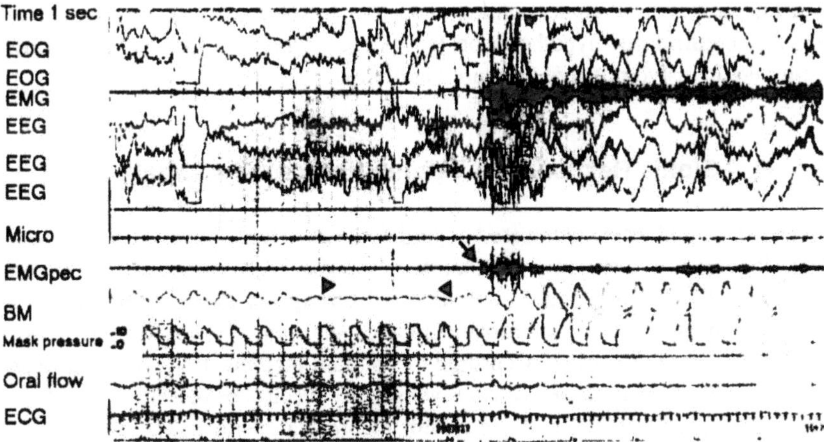

Figure 1 One-minute tracing of polysomnography in a patient with myopathy during noninvasive assisted ventilation. From top to bottom: Time in sec, electrooculogram (EOG), chin electromyogram (EMG), electroencephalogram (EEG), sound (Micro), pectoral muscle electromyogram (EMGpec), breathing movements of the thorax (BM), pressure in the nasal mask (Mask pressure), oral flow from a thermocouple (Oral flow), and electrocardiogram (ECG). At the start of the record, the patient is in stage 2 non-REM sleep. Note that after six breaths, breathing movements abruptly cease (left arrowhead on the BM tracing), whereas the ventilator continues to deliver its strokes (see Mask pressure tracing) and oral leaks increase slightly (see Oral flow tracing). After five strokes, breathing movements reappear (right arrowhead on the BM tracing). After 2 sec, an arousal reaction intervenes (arrow on the EMGpec tracing) and oral leaks cease. Note also that throughout the whole record, breathing movements are synchronous with the ventilator strokes.

postulate that during noninvasive positive pressure mechanical ventilation there was a closure site in the upper airway that intermittently abolished any entry of air into the lungs during the inspiratory strokes of volumetric ventilators (23). We excluded the pharynx as a candidate site because positive pressure ventilators can deliver high inspiratory pressures that would force the pharynx to open. The remaining candidate was the glottis. The glottis can actively open and close, it can resist very high pressure levels, and it had already been shown to be a possible obstacle to assisted ventilation during negative pressure assisted ventilation (24). We also postulated that the glottis could narrow or close in response to the absolute (or relative) hypocapnia induced by noninvasive ventilatory assistance. It had indeed been shown in animals that hypocapnia can result in activation of vocal cord adductors (25,26).

After verifying that the phenomenon of intermittent upper airway closure was not a particular feature of a particular patient [we were able to reproduce it in two of three patients on long-term home mechanical ventilation tested for it by trying to increase minute ventilation during sleep (23)], we decided to experimentally confirm our hypothesis on the glottic origin of upper airway closure during noninvasive positive pressure ventilation.

III. Glottic Response to Volumetric Controlled Ventilation

Seven healthy subjects volunteered to participate in a study on the effects of nasal intermittent positive pressure ventilation on the glottis, during both wakefulness and sleep (27–28). Sleep state was assessed through continuous recordings of electroencephalographic, electrooculographic, and chin electromyographic signals from surface electrodes according to standard methods (29). An electrocardiographic signal was recorded from two surface electrodes placed on the chest. One thermocouple in front of the mouth recorded oral flow. The electromyographic activity of the diaphragm was assessed from surface electrodes. An inductance plethysmograph calibrated with the isovolume technique allowed for the measurement of effective tidal volume (i.e., the tidal volume actually reaching the lungs, as opposed to the tidal volume actually delivered by the ventilator) and respiratory frequency, and thus of effective minute ventilation (as opposed to the minute ventilation actually delivered by the ventilator). Mask pressure was measured from a port in the nasal mask. Transcutaneous oxygen (O_2) saturation and pulse rate were obtained from the finger probe of a pulse oximeter. End-tidal carbon dioxide (CO_2) was sampled using a thin catheter passing through a small hole drilled in the nasal mask, and placed in the right nostril.

A thin (3.5-mm external diameter) fiberoptic bronchoscope was passed through a second orifice drilled in the nasal mask and, through the left nostril, into the pharynx. The tip of the bronchoscope was placed 2 to 3 cm above the vocal cords. The fiberoptic bronchoscope was connected to a color videocamera and to a videocassette recorder, and images were recorded throughout the experiment. The aperture of the glottis was assessed by measuring breath by breath the widest inspiratory angle formed by the vocal cords at the anterior commissure, a dimension closely related to glottic surface but much less affected by geometric and variable distance problems (30).

Subjects were connected through the nasal mask to a volumetric intermittent positive pressure ventilator, at a starting delivered ventilation close to 9 l/min. After recordings were obtained, delivered ventilation was increased by steps, first by increasing delivered tidal volume and then by increasing ventilator frequency, up to a maximum of 30 L/min. We tried to obtain stable recordings of all signals during each step, but this was not always possible because of the invasive nature of the study, with frequent swallowing and low-quality video images.

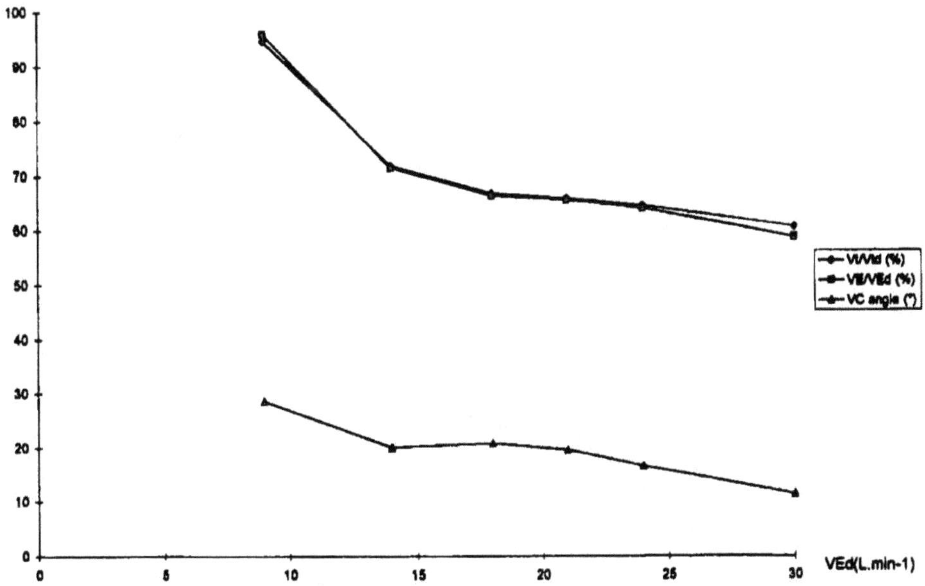

Figure 2 Evolution of glottic aperture (expressed as the value of the angle formed by the vocal cords at the anterior commissure), and of effective tidal volume, Vt (or minute ventilation, VE) expressed as a percentage of the delivered tidal volume, Vtd (or of the delivered minute ventilation, VEd) at increasing levels of delivered minute ventilation in an awake normal subject. Note that as the delivered minute ventilation increases, the glottis narrows, and the proportion of the delivered tidal volume (or of the delivered minute ventilation) effectively reaching the lungs decreases.

The main observations of the study were as follows: As the delivered ventilation was increased, the vocal cords narrowed progressively (and could completely close, resulting in a glottic apnea). This caused the proportion of the delivered tidal volume and delivered minute ventilation that effectively reached the lungs to progressively decrease (Fig. 2). The narrowing of the glottis resulted in a stepwise increase in airway resistance and in nasal mask pressure (Fig. 3). Sleep resulted in an enhancement in glottic narrowing for a given setting of the ventilator. For a given delivered tidal volume and ventilator frequency (and hence delivered minute ventilation), the glottis was almost always narrower during sleep than during wakefulness. This resulted in a lower tidal volume and minute ventilation, with a higher P_{ETCO_2}, during sleep than during wakefulness. In other words, the proportion of the delivered tidal volume and ventilation effectively reaching the lungs is decreased during sleep with respect to wakefulness. During most of the time, controlled mechanical ventilation resulted in reductions or complete abolition of the diaphragmatic electromyographic signal. When the dia-

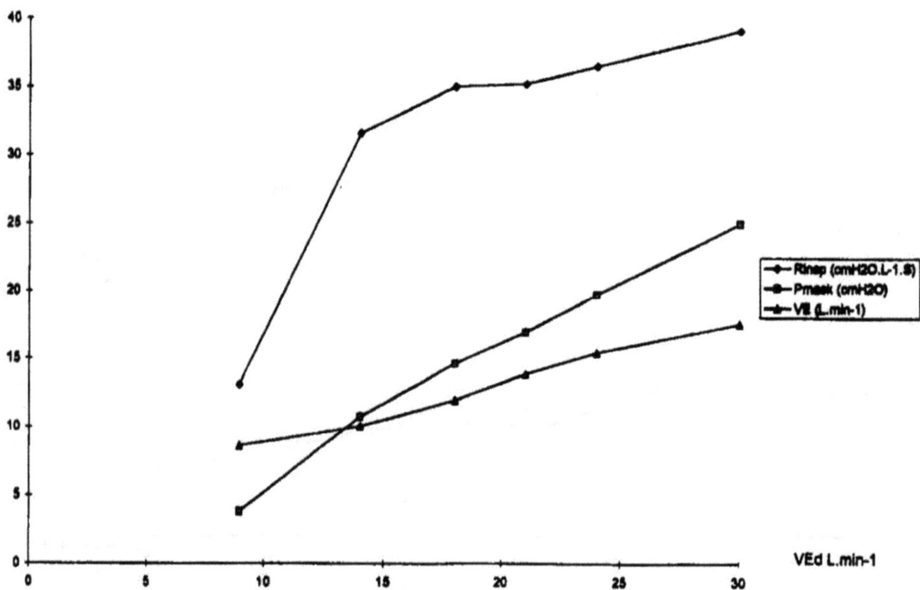

Figure 3 Evolution of the effective minute ventilation (VE), of pressure in the nasal mask (Pmask) and of the inspiratory airflow resistance (Rinsp) at increasing levels of delivered minute ventilation (VEd) in an awake normal subject. Note that as the delivered ventilation increases, airflow resistance increases, as does the positive pressure in the nasal mask. The increase in effective minute ventilation is always lower than each stepwise increase in delivered minute ventilation.

phragmatic electromyographic signal became present, for whatever reason (awakening from sleep for instance), the vocal cord angle increased (i.e., the glottis widened) to normal spontaneous breathing values (27).

These results were obtained using volumetric ventilators in the controlled mode so that the delivered tidal volume was imposed by the ventilator and was constant. The situation could be theoretically very different using positive pressure ventilators with two levels of positive pressure, the so-called "bilevel" ventilators (or pressure support ventilators). Indeed, with this type of machine, effective tidal volume is not imposed but depends on a complex interaction between the imposed inspiratory pressure, the inspiratory time (also imposed if the ventilator is used in the controlled mode), and the impedance of the respiratory system. The latter might be highly influenced by the airflow resistance of the upper airway, including the glottis (31).

IV. Glottic Response to Two-Level Positive Pressure Ventilation in the Controlled Mode

To sort out the effects of assisted mechanical ventilation on the glottis using two-level positive pressure ventilation in the controlled mode, we studied a group of six normal subjects during wakefulness and sleep. Inspiratory pressure was set at 10, then 15, and finally 20 cm H_2O, whereas expiratory pressure was maintained constant at 4 cm H_2O. The imposed respirator frequency was 17 breaths per minute, with an inspiratory/expiratory time ratio of 0.8. The experimental setting was essentially the same as in the previous study.

The main results showed that there was no consistent response of the glottis to two-level positive pressure ventilation in the controlled mode. Increases in inspiratory pressure could lead to narrowing or widening of the glottis, or there could be no change in glottic width with increasing levels of inspiratory positive airway pressure. The combination of an increase in the inspiratory pressure and a variable response of the glottis led to variable changes in the effective tidal volume and effective ventilation. These could increase, remain stable, or paradoxically decrease when inspiratory positive pressure was increased. Thus, an increase in applied pressure did not necessarily lead to an increase in effective ventilation. Sleep induced a further decrease in glottic width with respect to wakefulness for a given applied inspiratory pressure. As a consequence, effective ventilation was almost always lower during sleep than during wakefulness. The vocal cords could also show, during both wakefulness and sleep, an oscillatory pattern of widening and narrowing, culminating or not in total closure, leading to a cyclic variable amplitude of effective tidal volume that increased and decreased in a manner analogous to periodic breathing as can be observed with Cheyne-Stokes breathing. In contrast to Cheyne-Stokes breathing, however, it was not waxing and waning of respiratory drive that explained this periodic breathing pattern, but rather a progressive narrowing then widening of the vocal cords. In Cheyne-Stokes breathing, the central command to all respiratory muscles progressively decreases until there is total abolition of respiration for several seconds. The resumption of the central activity (resulting in mechanical activation of all respiratory muscles) is gradual, with a progressive increase until a maximal level is reached, leading again to a progressive decrease. Under our experimental conditions, vocal cord activity is also probably centrally determined. What differentiates periodic breathing secondary to vocal cord widening and narrowing from true Cheyne-Stokes respiration is that the former occurs in a setting of complete abolition of central command to the respiratory muscles, as assessed through diaphragmatic electromyography. Thus, there is a dissociation between the abolition of the central command to "respiratory pump" muscles and the activation of central command to vocal cord muscles, whereas in true Cheyne-Stokes respiration it is most likely that the waxing and waning of the central command applies to the whole of the respiratory musculature. When a cycle culminated in total closure of the vocal cords (this was exclusively the case during sleep), glottic obstructive apneas occurred that lasted 20 seconds on average. As in the previous experiment with controlled volumetric ventilation, the reappearance of the diaphragmatic electromyographic signal was always accompanied by widening of the glottis (31).

Thus, the use of two-level ventilators in the controlled mode led to unpredictable consequences on effective ventilation. Indeed, with increasing inspiratory pressure levels, the resulting increase in airflow resistance secondary to glottic narrowing could lead to a decrease in effective ventilation, or could be partially or totally offset by the higher inspiratory pressure, so that effective ventilation could remain unchanged or increase. The observation that reappearance of diaphragmatic activation led to a normal inspiratory glottic widening prompted the hypothesis that ventilators used in the spontaneous (or so-called "assist") mode could avoid glottic narrowing. In the spontaneous mode, it is the ventilated subject who initiates each breath by activation of his own respiratory muscles (and presumably of his own glottic abductors), thus maintaining a normal inspiratory abduction of the vocal cords.

V. Glottic Response to Two-Level Positive Pressure Ventilation in the Spontaneous Mode

To test this hypothesis, 10 normal subjects were studied during wakefulness and sleep using the same experimental setting as that previously used for the bilevel positive pressure ventilator in the controlled mode. The inspiratory pressure was set at 10, 15, and then 20 cm H_2O, whereas the expiratory pressure was kept at

Table 1 Data of Effective Minute Ventilation and Tidal Volume, Respiratory Frequency, and Vocal Cord Angle for the Group of Awake Subjects Studied on Noninvasive Ventilation with Two-Level Positive Pressure Ventilation in the Spontaneous Mode

	SP[a]	IPAP-10	IPAP-15	IPAP-20
VI, L/min	6.0 (1.6)	6.6 (2.0)	7.9 (3.0)	9.4 (3.7)
Vt, mL	484 (155)	456 (150)	659 (260)	914 (302)
f/min	13 (3)	15 (2)	12 (3)	10 (3)
VC angle, °	42 (5)	38 (9)	39 (11)	41 (10)

[a] SP, spontaneous unassisted breathing; IPAP, inspiratory positive airway pressure set at 10, 15, or 20 cm H_2O; VI, effective minute ventilation; Vt, effective tidal volume; f, respiratory frequency; VC angle, glottic aperture assessed through the measurement of the angle formed by the vocal cords at the anterior commissure. Figures are mean values, with standard deviations in parentheses.

4 cm H_2O. The switch from expiration to inspiration was flow-triggered, and was set at the most sensitive position (20 to 50 mL/sec).

As expected, the glottic width did not change with any level of positive inspiratory pressure with respect to the one observed during unassisted spontaneous breathing. However, minute ventilation only increased significantly (with respect to spontaneous breathing levels) at a positive inspiratory pressure of 20 cm H_2O. This was due to a decrease in respiratory frequency partially offsetting the increase in effective tidal volume at each increase in inspiratory pressure (Table 1). Apneas of the central type and independent of the glottic behavior (i.e., the glottis could close or remain open during these central apneas) were observed during both wakefulness and the rare moments of sleep available in this study. Similarly, periodic breathing of the central type was sometimes observed in wakefulness and sleep in three subjects (32). One may wonder whether this type of event (i.e., periodic breathing of the central type) would occur in patients with respiratory disease, to the extent that it may be much more difficult to induce overventilation in patients with mechanical impairments and high minute ventilation requirements than it is in the normal subjects we studied. However, if overventilation is induced in patients, this type of event will probably also occur.

VI. Controlled Versus Spontaneous Modes in Two-Level Positive Pressure Ventilation

It was thus confirmed that glottic narrowing in response to assisted ventilation could indeed be avoided using the spontaneous mode of assisted ventilation. However, the decrease in respiratory frequency in response to increased levels of inspiratory pressure (and effective tidal volume) did not grant higher levels of effective minute ventilation for the same inspiratory positive pressure in the spontaneous versus the controlled mode. To further understand the mechanisms for this, a group of eight normal awake and asleep subjects was studied under assisted ventilation with a two-level barometric positive pressure ventilator used both in the spontaneous and controlled modes. To facilitate the study, we decided not to use direct glottic observation. The fiberoptic bronchoscope was thus not used, but the rest of the experimental setup was similar to the previous ones. In the controlled mode, the ventilator was used with a frequency of 17 and then 25 breaths per minute, an inspiratory positive pressure of 15 cm H_2O and an expiratory positive pressure of 4 cm H_2O. The inspiratory/expiratory time ratio was fixed at 1. In the spontaneous mode, the inspiratory positive pressure was set at 10, 15, and then 20 cm H_2O, whereas the expiratory positive pressure was kept at 4 cm H_2O.

In the controlled mode during wakefulness, at a pressure of 15 cm H_2O, effective minute ventilation was 10.8 L/min at a respirator frequency of 17/min, and it was 11.8 L/min at a frequency of 25/min. In the spontaneous mode, effective minute ventilation was 9.8 L/min at 15, and 11.7 L/min at 20 cm H_2O of inspiratory pressure, respectively. During stage 2 non-REM sleep, effective minute ventilation was 8.4 L/min at an inspiratory pressure of 15 cm H_2O and frequency of 17/min (controlled mode), whereas it was only 7.0 L/min at the same inspiratory pressure level in the spontaneous mode. Moreover, periodic breathing and especially apneas were much more common in the spontaneous than in the controlled mode during sleep (33).

It thus appears that for a given inspiratory pressure, effective minute ventilation is higher when the ventilator is used in the controlled mode, at least if the frequency is fixed at 17/min or higher. The data confirmed that for a given setting of the ventilator, effective minute ventilation is generally lower during sleep in both the spontaneous vs. controlled modes. Finally, the use of the controlled mode during sleep avoids the occurrence of apneas, which are very common in the spontaneous mode, and are probably of the central type, independent of the glottis.

VII. How to Increase Effective Ventilation with Volumetric Ventilators in the Controlled Mode

Since the use of volumetric controlled ventilation leads to glottic narrowing that reduces effective ventilation to the lungs, we wanted to determine the best combination of ventilator settings that would optimize effective minute ventilation despite glottic narrowing. We studied a group of 10 normal subjects awake and asleep under controlled volumetric noninvasive positive pressure ventilation. As in the previous study, a fiberoptic bronchoscope was not used. Eight different combinations of tidal volume, ventilator frequency, and inspiratory/expiratory time ratios were successively applied, with a range of delivered tidal volumes of 850 to 1160 mL, of ventilator frequencies of 15 to 27/min, of delivered minute ventilation of 12.7 to 22.9 L/min, and of delivered inspiratory flows of 0.42 to 1.21 L/sec.

For a given delivered tidal volume and minute ventilation, increases in delivered inspiratory flows (i.e., reductions in inspiratory time) resulted in a higher effective tidal volume and minute ventilation up to a flow of about 0.85 L/sec. Further increases in the delivered inspiratory flow did not result in further increases in effective ventilation. For a given delivered minute ventilation, effective ventilation was higher if the delivered tidal volume was lower and the ventilator frequency higher, than if the delivered tidal volume was higher and the ventilator frequency lower. These observations applied to both wakefulness and sleep, and effective ventilation was almost always lower during sleep than during wakefulness for a given ventilator setting.

For a given delivered tidal volume, increases in ventilator frequency and delivered minute ventilation resulted in increases in effective ventilation up to a certain value. Beyond this level, further increases in frequency and delivered minute ventilation did not raise effective ventilation. In this study, periodic breathing was not very frequent, and apneas were never observed (34).

According to these results obtained in normal volunteer subjects, the settings allowing for the higher effective ventilation using a volumetric ventilator in the controlled mode are a delivered tidal volume of about 13 mL/kg body weight, a delivered inspiratory flow not exceeding 0.9 L/sec, and a ventilator frequency around 20 breaths/min. These results are close to the ones we observed in a group of 33 patients with various neuromusculoskeletal diseases and restrictive ventilatory defects treated with home noninvasive positive pressure volumetric ventilators. It should be noted that the settings of the ventilators had been determined in these patients by a trial-and-error process, in which ventilator frequency, delivered tidal volume, and inspiratory/expiratory time ratios had been progressively increased and decreased in order to obtain the best possible sleep quality and oxygen saturation without supplemental oxygen. These patients had been put on home noninvasive assisted ventilation before the results of the experimental study in the healthy subjects were available to us (34). It should also be noted that none of these patients had chronic airflow obstruction, and therefore none of them had an intrinsic end-expiratory pressure. In the presence of airflow obstruction, our recommendations must be taken very cautiously, since we use rather high respiratory frequencies, which could be detrimental in the presence of significant levels of intrinsic end-expiratory pressure.

VIII. Mechanism of the Glottic Response to Noninvasive Assisted Ventilation Applied Through the Nose

From a theoretical point of view, glottic narrowing could be a passive process (inhibition of glottic abductors), an active process (through activation of glottic adductors), or a combined process, in which abductors are partially or completely inhibited while adductors are activated. Disappearance of diaphragmatic inspiratory phasic activation (related to ventilatory hypocapnic inhibition) implies the disappearance of the inspiratory posterior cricoarytenoid phasic abduction (30), resulting in passive glottic narrowing (or absence of active glottic widening). It is known that passively induced hypocapnia results in activation of glottic adductors in both animals and humans (25,26,30). We have frequently observed episodes of "periodic breathing" with alternating progressive increases and decreases in effective tidal volume due to progressive widening, then narrowing, of the glottis. We have also observed periods of complete glottic closure, in which the glottis resisted positive pressures of 10 to more than 20 cm H_2O. We can therefore postulate that during noninvasive mechanical ventilation, glottic aperture depends most probably on a combined dynamic balance between inhibition of vocal cord abductors and activation of vocal cord adductors, which can vary from one ventilatory cycle to the next and can be influenced by different factors.

IX. Factors Influencing the Glottic Response to Noninvasive Ventilation

Throughout the above reported studies, a number of factors that may influence the response of the glottis to noninvasive assisted ventilation have been explored. These are briefly reviewed here.

A. Hypocapnia

Glottic narrowing could depend partly on hypocapnia. Indeed, noninvasive ventilation in our patients and normal volunteers aimed to increase effective minute ventilation and thus to decrease $Paco_2$ (irrespective of whether the starting level of $Paco_2$ was normal, as in the healthy volunteers, or increased, as in the patients in respiratory failure). To test the relationship between glottic aperture and $Paco_2$, we added CO_2 to the intake valve of the volumetric ventilator used in one of the studies in order to increase $Paco_2$ without changing the delivered volume or flow. In two of three awake subjects, the glottis partially widened, but without reaching the normal width. It did not widen at all in the third subject despite an end-tidal CO_2 of 45 mm Hg. During sleep, partial widening of the vocal cords was observed during CO_2 addition in 5 of 9 trials in three subjects (28). Glottic narrowing appears thus to depend, at least partly, on hypocapnia.

B. Vigilance State

Vigilance state has a noticeable effect on the response of the glottis to noninvasive assisted ventilation. For a given level of delivered minute ventilation (or tidal volume), the degree of glottic narrowing depends on the vigilance state. The glottis narrows more during sleep than during wakefulness in most of the comparisons that could be performed. The sleep-related enhanced glottic narrowing results in lower effective tidal volumes and effective minute ventilation levels during sleep than during wakefulness. This effect of sleep on the glottis is seen with both volumetric and barometric ventilators (28,31). Moreover, different sleep stages have different effects on the glottic response to assisted ventilation. For instance, using volumetric ventilators, at low levels of delivered ventilation the glottis narrows more in stage 2 non-REM sleep than in stages 3 and 4 non-REM sleep, whereas at higher levels of delivered ventilation the narrowing of the glottis is similar in stage 2 and in stages 3 and 4 non-REM sleep (28). Rapid eye movement sleep appears to inhibit glottic closure, but not enough data were available to confirm (or refute) this impression (34).

C. Neuromuscular Inhibition

Vocal cord abduction is part of the normal integrated neuromuscular mechanism of inspiration (35). Inspiratory muscles are activated in an orderly fashion, from the dilator alae nasi to the diaphragm (35). Inhibition of inspiratory activation will therefore, by necessity, abolish the glottic widening associated with inspiration. In turn, this ventilatory inhibition is partly dependent on hypocapnia, but may also depend on neuromechanical factors (see below) and on behavior-dependent cortical influences independent of ventilatory regulatory factors. For instance, during stable ventilation in awake subjects with narrowed glottides, reappearance of diaphragmatic activity in response to a noise was always accompanied by normal glottic widening (27).

D. Mechanical Factors

Our studies have shown that glottic aperture (and the resulting effective ventilation) is at least partly partly influenced by mechanical factors such as delivered flow and volume (27,34). Similar effects have already been observed in studies on the nonchemical influences on the respiratory muscles (36). This may be part of a general response of all inspiratory muscles to flow, temperature, or volume afferents arising from upper airway or intrathoracic receptors (37–44).

X. The Glottis, Noninvasive Ventilation, and Leaks

During noninvasive mechanical ventilation, glottic narrowing will increase airflow resistance, and this will lead to a lower effective tidal volume reaching the lungs. As a consequence, air flowing from the ventilator will leak outside the larynx. Leaks are known to be one of the most troublesome problems of noninvasive ventilation. Leaks can be classified as "external" (i.e., air leaking between the mask and the skin, or air entering through the nares and flowing out of the mouth) and "internal" (i.e., air flowing into the esophagus and the stomach, or air being accommodated in the compliant pharyngeal airway). The partitioning of the flow and volume of gas delivered by the ventilator on each mechanical inspiration between "useful" flow or volume effectively reaching the lungs and "useless" leaking flow and volume may depend to a large extent on glottic aperture, and is probably one of the major consequences of the glottic response to noninvasive ventilation that must be carefully considered when instituting mechanical ventilation in an individual patient. Although experimental data are lacking, clinical symptoms of gastric distension (such as epigastric pain, alleviated by eructation) are not infrequent in patients on long-term nocturnal noninvasive ventilation. Similarly, mouth and pharyngeal distension can be easily observed as a bulging out of soft tissues of the base of the mouth and the neck with each inspiratory positive pressure strike. Mouth and mask leaks have never been quantified, but we have already observed an increase in the deflections on the mouth thermocouple signal during glottic narrowing and closure (see Fig. 1). As far as the pharynx is concerned, we have calculated from data available in the literature that for pressures of 20 cm H_2O, the pharynx can accommodate from 20 to 130 mL of air (32).

XI. Conclusions

Noninvasive intermittent positive pressure mechanical ventilation poses the particular problem of adaptation of the upper airway structures to a totally unnatural ventilatory mechanism: positive pressure inspiration. The response of the glottis seems to depend on an array of behavioral, neuromuscular, chemical, and mechanical factors that must be understood and taken into account in order to avoid possible drawbacks and to obtain the best results of this revolutionary and life-saving form of ventilatory support. The notion that the glottis can effectively block the access of air into the lungs during noninvasive assisted ventilation has practical implications that should not be overlooked. Every practitioner concerned with noninvasive ventilation should remember that increasing the ventilator output (be it volume or pressure) does not necessarily lead to an increase in the amount of ventilation reaching the lungs of the patient, but that it can rather increase the amount of air leaking out of the lungs. It is surprising to realize that a patient's ventilation can be improved by decreasing the delivered tidal volume only after several attempts to improve it by increasing delivered tidal volume have proved vain. New ventilators are provided with screens that display huge amounts of information. One should remember that this information concerns the ventilator, not the patient. Good functioning of the ventilator does not guarantee, in the noninvasive realm, adequate ventilation of the patient. The glottis is at the center of this concept.

References

1. Woollman CHM. The development of apparatus for intermittent negative pressure respiration 1832–1918. Anaesthesia 1976; 31:537–547.
2. Colice GL. Historical perspective on the development of mechanical ventilation. In: Principles and practice of mechanical ventilation. Tobin MJ, ed. New York: McGraw Hill, 1994; 1–35.
3. Lassen HCA. A preliminary report on the 1952 epidemic of poliomyelitis in Copenhagen. Lancet 1953; Jan:37–41.
4. Severinghaus JW, Astrup P, Murray JF. Blood gas analysis and critical care medicine. Am J Respir Crit Care Med 1998; 157:S114–S122.
5. Sullivan CEF, Issa FG, Berthon Jones M, Eves L. Reversal of obstructive sleep apnoea by continuous positive airway pressure applied through the nares. Lancet 1981; Apr:862–865.
6. Ellis ER, Bye PTP, Bruderer JW, Sullivan CE. Treatment of respiratory failure during sleep in patients with neuromuscular disease. Positive-pressure ventilation through a nose mask. Am Rev Respir Dis 1987; 135:148–152.
7. Sanders MH, Kern N. Obstructive sleep apnea treated by independently adjusted inspiratory and expiratory positive airway pressures via nasal mask: Physiologic and clinical implications. Chest 1990; 98:317–324.
8. Pennock BE, Kaplan PD, Carlin BW, Sabangan JS, Magovern JA. Pressure support ventilation with a simplified ventilatory support system administered with a nasal mask in patients with respiratory failure. Chest 1991; 100:1371–1376.
9. Ambrosino N, Nava S, Bertone P, Fracchia C, Rampulla C. Physiologic evaluation of pressure support ventilation by nasal mask in patients with stable COPD. Chest 1992; 101:385–391.
10. Waldhorn RE. Nocturnal nasal intermittent positive pressure ventilation with bilevel positive airway pressure (BiPAP) in respiratory failure. Chest 1992; 101:516–521.
11. Appendini L, Patessio A, Zanaboni S, Carone M, Gukov B, Donner CF, Rossi A. Physiologic effects of positive end-expiratory pressure and mask pressure support during exacerbations of chronic obstructive pulmonary disease. Am J Respir Crit Care Med 1994; 149:1069–1076.
12. Meduri GU, Conoscenti PP, Menashe P, Nair S. Noninvasive face mask ventilation in patients with acute respiratory failure. Chest 1989; 95:865–870.
13. Meduri GU, Abou Shala N, Fox RC, Jones CB, Leeper KV, Wunderink RG. Noninvasive face mask mechanical ventilation in patients with acute hypercapnic respiratory failure. Chest 1991; 100:445–454.
14. Heckmatt JZ, Loh L, Dubowitz V. Night-time nasal ventilation in neuromuscular disease. Lancet 1990; 335:579–582.

15. Goldstein RS, De Rosie JA, Avedano MA, Dolmage TE. Influence of noninvasive positive pressure ventilation on inspiratory muscles. Chest 1991; 99:408–415.
16. Leger P, Bedicam JM, Cornette A, Reybet Degat O, Langevin B, Polu JM, Jeannin L, Robert D. Nasal intermittent positive pressure ventilation: Long-term follow-up in patients with severe chronic respiratory insufficiency. Chest 1994; 105:100–105.
17. Renston JP, DiMarco AF, Supinski GS. Respiratory muscle rest using nasal BiPAP ventilation in patients with stable severe COPD. Chest 1994; 105:1053–1060.
18. Simonds AK, Elliott MW. Outcome of domiciliary nasal intermittent positive pressure ventilation in restrictive and obstructive disorders. Thorax 1995; 50:604–609.
19. Bott J, Carroll MP, Conway JH, Keilty SE, Ward EM, Brown AM, Paul EA, Elliott MW, Godfrey RC, Wedzicha JA, et al. Randomised controlled trial of nasal ventilation in acute ventilatory failure due to chronic obstructive airways disease. Lancet 1993; 341:1555–1557.
20. Brochard L, Isabey D, Piquet J, Amaro P, Mancebo J, Messadi AA, Brun Buisson C, Rauss A, Lemaire F, Harf A. Reversal of acute exacerbations of chronic obstructive lung disease by inspiratory assistance with a face mask. N Engl J Med 1990; 323:1523–1530.
21. Ambrosino N, Foglio K, Rubini F, Clini E, Nava S, Vitacca M. Noninvasive mechanical ventilation in acute respiratory failure due to chronic obstructive pulmonary disease: Correlates for success. Thorax 1995; 50:755–757.
22. Kramer N, Meyer TJ, Meharg J, Cece RD, Hill NS. Randomised prospective trial of noninvasive positive pressure ventilation in acute respiratory failure. Am J Respir Crit Care Med 1995; 151:1799–1806.
23. Delguste P, Aubert-Tulkens G, Rodenstein DO. Upper airway obstruction during nasal intermittent positive-pressure hperventilation in sleep. Lancet 1991; 338:1295–1297.
24. Scharf SM, Feldman NT, Goldman MD, Haot HZ, Bruce F, Ingram RH. Vocal cord closure: A cause of upper airway obstruction during controlled ventilation. Am Rev Respir Dis, 1978; 177:391–397.
25. Bartlett D, Remmers JE, Gautier H. Laryngeal regulation of respiratory airflow. Respir Physiol 1973; 18:194–204.
26. Murakami Y, Kirchner A. Respiratory movements of the vocal cords. Laryngoscope 1972; 82:454–467.
27. Jounieaux V, Aubert G, Dury M, Delguste P, Rodenstein DO. Effects of nasal positive-pressure hyperventilation on the glottis in normal awake subjects. J Appl Physiol 1995; 79:176–185.
28. Jounieaux V, Aubert G, Dury M, Delguste P, Rodenstein DO. Effects of nasal positive-pressure hyperventilation on the glottis in normal sleeping subjects. J Appl Physiol 1995; 79:186–193.
29. Rechtschaffen A, Kales A. A Manual of Standardized Terminology, Techniques, and Scoring System for Sleep Stages of Human Subjects. Los Angeles: University of California at Los Angeles, 1968.
30. Kuna ST, McCarthy MP, Smickley JS. Laryngeal response to passively induced hypocapnia during NREM sleep in normal adult humans. J Appl Physiol 1993; 75: 1088–1096.
31. Parreira VF, Jounieaux V, Aubert G, Dury M, Delguste P, Rodenstein DO. Nasal

two-level positive-pressure ventilation in normal subjects: Effects on the glottis and ventilation. Am J Respir Crit Care Med 1996; 153:1616–1623.

32. Parreira VF, Delguste P, Jounieaux V, Aubert G, Dury M, Rodenstein DO. Glottic aperture and effective minute ventilation during nasal two-level positive pressure ventilation in spontaneous mode. Am J Respir Crit Care Med 1996; 154:1857–1863.
33. Parreira VF, Delguste P, Jounieaux V, Aubert G, Dury M, Rodenstein DO. Effectiveness of controlled and spontaneous modes in nasal two-level positive pressure ventilation in awake and asleep normal subjects. Chest 1997; 112:1267–1277.
34. Parreira VF, Jounieaux V, Delguste P, Aubert G, Dury M, Rodenstein DO. Determinants of effective ventilation during nasal intermittent positive pressure ventilation. Eur Respir J 1997; 10:1975–1982.
35. Strohl KP, Hensley MJ, Hallett M, Saunders NA, Ingram RH. Activation of upper airway muscles before onset of inspiration in normal humans. J Appl Physiol 1980; 49:638–642.
36. Henke KG, Arias A, Skatrud JB, Dempsey JA. Inhibition of inspiratory muscle activity during sleep: Chemical and non-chemical influences. Am Rev Respir Dis 1988; 138:8–15.
37. McBride B, Whitelaw WA. A physiological stimulus to upper airway recepetors in humans. J Appl Physiol 1981; 51:1189–1197.
38. Jammes Y, Barthelemy P, Delpierre S. Respiratory effects of cold air breathing in anesthetized cats. Respir Physiol 1983; 54:41–54.
39. Ukabam CU, Knuth SL, Bartlett D. Phrenic and hypoglossal neural responses to cold airflow in the upper airway. Respir Physiol 1992; 87:157–164.
40. Issa FG, Edwards P, Szeto E, Lauff D, Sullivan C. Genioglossus and breathing responses to airway occlusion: Effect of sleep and route of occlusion. J Appl Physiol 1988; 64:543–549.
41. Hwang JC, John WMSt, Bartlett D. Receptors responding to changes in upper airway pressure. Respir Physiol 1984; 55:355–366.
42. Van Lunteren E, Strohl KP, Parker DM, Bruce EN, Van de Graaff WB, Cherniak NS. Phasic volume-related feedback on upper airway muscle activity. J Appl Physiol 1984; 56:730–736.
43. Bolser DC, Lindsey BG, Shannon R. Respiratory pattern changes produced by intercostal muscle/rib vibration. J Appl Physiol 1988; 64:2458–2462.
44. Shannon R, Bolser DC, Lindsey BG. Medullary neurons mediating the inhibition of inspiration by intercostal muscle tendon organs? J Appl Physiol 1988; 65:2498–2505.

two-level positive-pressure ventilation in normal subjects. Effects of [illegible] ventilation. Am J Respir Crit Care Med 1996; 153:1615–1623.
52. Parreira VF, Delguste P, Jounieaux V, Aubert G, Dury M, Rodenstein DO. Glottic aperture and effective minute ventilation during nasal two-level positive pressure ventilation in spontaneous mode. Am J Respir Crit Care Med 1996; 154:1857–1863.
53. Parreira VF, Delguste P, Jounieaux V, Aubert G, Dury M, Rodenstein DO. Effectiveness of controlled and spontaneous modes in nasal two-level positive pressure ventilation in awake and asleep normal subjects. Chest 1997; 112:1267–1277.
54. Parreira VF, Jounieaux V, Delguste P, Aubert G, Dury M, Rodenstein DO. Determinants of effective ventilation during nasal intermittent positive pressure ventilation. Eur Respir J 1997; 10:1975–1982.
55. [illegible]
56. [illegible]
57. [illegible] J Appl Physiol 1991; 71: [illegible]
58. Jammes Y, [illegible] Respiratory effects of [illegible] ventilation in [illegible] Respir Physiol [illegible]
59. Bartlett D, Knuth SL, [illegible] Respir Physiol [illegible]
60. [illegible] J Appl Physiol 1988; [illegible]
61. [illegible] Respiration-dependent [illegible] upper airway pressure. Respir Physiol 1986; [illegible]
62. Van Lunteren E, Strohl KP, Parker DM, Bruce EN, Van de Graaff WB, Cherniack NS. Phasic volume-related feedback on upper airway muscle activity. J Appl Physiol 1984; 56:730–736.
63. [illegible] Respiratory pattern changes produced by intercostal muscle/rib vibration. J Appl Physiol 1988; 65:2459–2467.
64. Shannon R, Baker DC, Lindsey BG. Medullary neurons mediating the inhibition of inspiration by intercostal muscle tendon organs? J Appl Physiol 1988; 65:2498–2505.

6

Long-Term Mechanical Ventilation for Restrictive Thoracic Disorders

PATRICK LEGER

Croix Rousse Hospital
Lyon, France

NICHOLAS S. HILL

Brown University School of Medicine
Rhode Island Hospital
Providence, Rhode Island

I. Introduction

The first patients to receive home mechanical ventilation were those who suffered from restrictive thoracic disorders. The large number of ventilator-dependent polio survivors during the 1950s stimulated the organization of home care groups in Europe, particularly France, and in the United States. As will be demonstrated in this chapter, these patients and those with other types of restrictive thoracic disorders have improved survivals and a good quality of life when treated with long-term mechanical ventilation.

Long-term mechanical ventilation (LTMV) includes both noninvasive and invasive techniques. Although negative pressure ventilation had been the preferred form of noninvasive ventilation for most of the past century, since the late 1980s, noninvasive positive pressure ventilation (NPPV) has been the ventilatory method of first choice for LTMV, even preferred over tracheostomy ventilation. Although the use of invasive ventilation in the home has decreased as a consequence of the increasing use of NPPV, there remain some indications for invasive techniques as will be discussed later.

After briefly outlining the various restrictive thoracic disorders, the chapter reviews pathophysiologic characteristics that contribute to hypoventilation. Next, the general approach to patients is considered, followed by a discussion of indications for therapy, selection of patients, and main therapeutic options. Outcomes of therapy are discussed in general, and then the natural history and response to therapy of the major restrictive thoracic disorders that are treated with LTMV are considered specifically. The presentation is limited to adult patients, as Chapter 8 includes a detailed discussion of LTMV in children.

II. Disease Entities Classified as Restrictive Thoracic Disorders

The term restrictive thoracic disorders refers to a group of illnesses characterized by reduced lung volumes attributable to difficulties in expanding the chest wall. These fall into two main categories: those caused by increased chest wall stiffness (or elasticity), and those caused by respiratory muscle weakness (and too little force to adequately expand the chest wall) (Table 1). Often, these two basic pathophysiologic defects are combined, particularly in congenital neuromuscular syndromes that affect spinal muscles, leading to progressive scoliosis.

A third pathophysiologic category that causes chronic hypoventilation and

Table 1 Main Restrictive Diseases

Chest wall deformities
Idiopathic kyphoscoliosis >100°
Mutilating sequelae of tuberculosis: thoracoplasty, fibrothorax
Thoracic kyphosis
Pectus excavatum
Ankylosing spondylitis
Neuromuscular disorders
Cervical spinal cord injury (≥C4)
Anterior horn lesions
Sequelae of polio
Amyotrophic lateral sclerosis
Spinal muscular atrophy
Myopathies
Duchenne muscular dystrophy
Myotonic dystrophy
Metabolic myopathies: acid maltase deficiency
Neuropathies
Multiple sclerosis
Bilateral diaphragm paralysis
Impaired ventilatory control
Central alveolar hypoventilation
Obesity hypoventilation syndrome

is not strictly a restrictive thoracic disorder is central hypoventilation. This is included because there is overlap; a central component is often present when patients with restrictive thoracic disorders hypoventilate, and patients with obesity hypoventilation syndrome have a component of thoracic restriction. Also, all three categories are characterized by a lack of parenchymal lung involvement (with the exception of patients with sequelae of tuberculosis), which means that the therapeutic approach focuses on assisting the bellows rather than correcting oxygenation defects or overcoming defects in lung mechanics per se. Specifically excluded is a discussion of LTMV in restrictive lung diseases such as interstitial fibrosis for which there is essentially no literature, and application of which is thought to be an exercise in futility.

III. Pathophysiologic Factors Contributing to Respiratory Failure in Restrictive Thoracic Disorders

A. Reduction of Lung Volumes

Patients with restrictive respiratory disorders (Table 2) have significantly reduced lung volumes due to respiratory muscle weakness or paralysis and/or increased chest wall elastance caused by thoracic deformity. In thoracovertebral deformities, the asymmetric deformity of the thoracic cage is responsible for the restrictive ventilatory defect. This reduction affects total lung capacity (TLC) and functional residual capacity (FRC) proportionately more then residual volume (RV). In addition, if the restriction is present during early childhood, lung growth can be affected, with less alveolarization and, consequently, reduced lung sizes (1).

These abnormalities in static properties of the respiratory system compromise respiratory muscle function, as well. Because the lung volumes are low, the respiratory muscles occupy a relatively disadvantageous position on the length-tension curve. In neuromuscular disorders, the respiratory muscles are weak to begin with, but this is often complicated by the development of thoracic scoliosis that further reduces respiratory muscle efficiency and increases work of breathing. Measurements of inspiratory capacity (IC) and expiratory reserve volume (ERV) help to differentiate the effects on inspiratory versus expiratory muscle, as some myopathies have much greater effects on one versus the other. In general, when hypoventilation occurs, vital capacity (VC) has fallen below 1.2 liters. If hypercarbia is present in patients with VCs greater than this, other contributing factors should be sought (2).

B. Alterations in Respiratory Mechanics/Increased Work of Breathing

In patients with chest wall deformities, dynamic lung compliance averages about one-half of normal, whereas thoracic cage compliance is less than one-quarter

Table 2 Characteristics of the Main Restrictive Diseases

	Incidence*	Age of CRI	Characteristics of CRI	Cardiac involvement	Progressiveness
CHEST WALL DEFORMITIES					
Idiopathic scoliosis > 120°	↓↓	Usually > 50	Restrictive	Pulmonary hypertension	Very slow
Mutilating sequels of tuberculosis	↓↓	60–70 40, 50 years after TB	Restrictive and obstructive ± bronchiectasis	Pulmonary hypertension	Slow
NEUROMUSCULAR DISEASES					
Sequels of poliomyelitis	↓↓	50–60	Restrictive, variable motor handicap		Very slow
Spinal cord injury C1-C4	↑↑	Young adult	Restrictive		Very slow
Duchenne muscular dystrophy	↑↑	Male teenager	Restrictive ± swallowing disorders	Myocardiopathy	Progressive 5–10 years
Becker		Male young adult	Restrictive		Slow
Myotonic dystrophy		Adult	Restrictive + frequent sleep apnea	Cardiac rhythm disturbances	Slow
Metabolic myopathy		Adult	Restrictive, variable motor handicap		Slow
Limb girdle myopathy		Adult	± diaphragm involvement		Slow
Spinal muscular atrophy		Infant	Severe scoliosis		Variable
Amyotrophic lateral sclerosis	↑↑	50–60	Restrictive + swallowing disorders		Fast 1–5 years
IMPAIRED VENTILATORY CONTROL					
Central alveolar hypoventilation	Rare	Young male adult	Ventilatory control impairment	Pulmonary hypertension	Slow
Obesity hypoventilation syndrome	↑↑		Ventilatory control impairment ± restrictive ± OSAS	Pulmonary hypertension	Slow

*Incidence in Clinical Practice: Frequency of CRI and referral for evaluation or discussion of ventilatory support.

of normal (3). These abnormalities substantially increase the work of breathing. If these patients are to maintain normal tidal volume at a normal frequency, the work of breathing is at least five times greater than normal (4). To maintain minute ventilation and decrease the work of breathing, patients adopt a rapid shallow breathing pattern, reducing tidal volume to the same degree as they increase respiratory rate. However, the net effect of this is to increase the ratio of anatomic dead space to tidal volume, further increasing the minute volume necessary to maintain carbon dioxide (CO_2) homeostasis (5).

C. Muscle Force

Routine measurements of maximal inspiratory and expiratory force (PImax and PEmax) help to determine the relative degree of inspiratory and expiratory muscle involvement in the restrictive disorders. The PImax in normal healthy males is in excess of 120 cm H_2O and that for females approximately 90 cm H_2O (6). Values reduced to 25 cm H_2O or less indicate severe inspiratory muscle involvement, although the measurement is effort dependent and should be interpreted with caution. If accompanied by a VC <1.2 liters, the result signals the need for further clinical evaluation.

Expiratory muscle strength/function is assessed using the PEmax, which in normal healthy adults exceeds 150 cm H_2O, or peak cough flow, which exceeds 3 L/sec in patients with cough adequacy (7). The cough impairment caused by expiratory muscle weakness is compounded by inspiratory muscle weakness, because the low inspiratory capacity that results further diminishes expiratory airflow. The resulting tendency to secretion retention and atelectasis predisposes to frequent respiratory tract infections. Retained secretions also add to airway resistance and gas exchange abnormalities and may predispose to a hypercapnic decompensation. Although the measurement of PEmax, like that for PImax, is effort dependent, a PEmax <60 cm H_2O indicates severe expiratory muscle impairment. Especially in a patient who has limited inspiratory reserve, it indicates a high risk of respiratory failure in the face of respiratory infections.

D. Work of Breathing

The work of breathing in patients with restrictive thoracic disorders is drastically increased (8). The patient adopts a ventilatory pattern consisting of low tidal volumes and a proportionally increased respiratory frequency. This pattern allows the patient to maintain minute ventilation at a lower work of breathing, but increases the fraction of dead space ventilation and can induce alveolar hypoventilation. Before developing chronic hypoventilation, the patient will experience episodic hypoventilation during effort or during sleep, especially during rapid eye movement (REM) sleep.

E. Sleep-Disordered Breathing

Over the last decade, it has become evident that ventilatory failure in patients with restrictive thoracic disorders is preceded by sleep-related abnormalities in arterial blood gas tensions, in the form of oxygen desaturation associated with nocturnal hypoventilation (9) (Table 3). Sleep-disordered breathing appears early during the evolution of respiratory impairment and may have very important consequences. The symptoms of nocturnal hypoventilation—morning headache, fatigue, and hypersomnolence—often lead the patient to seek medical attention.

During REM sleep, the suppression of accessory muscle activity in addition to the mechanical disadvantage of the diaphragm results in alveolar hypoventilation (9). This is the predominant mechanism of hypoventilation in these patients, although central apnea or obstructive apneas and hypopneas have also been reported (10). The earliest and most severe oxygen desaturations occur during REM sleep because of the reduction in intercostal and accessory muscle tone and suppression of central drive that occur during this stage. Later, the hypoventilation and desaturations extend into non-REM sleep and ultimately diurnal respiratory failure results. Moreover, the hypoventilation and desaturations associated with sleep-disordered breathing contribute to arousals, inducing sleep fragmentation and decreasing the amount of time spent in REM or slow wave sleep (11,12).

This progressive deterioration of sleep quality occurs as the underlying restrictive process progresses, and underscores the need to closely monitor patients at risk of decompensation during sleep. Having low VCs (below 50% of predicted and symptoms suggesting hypoventilation identifies these patients (see below). If no daytime CO_2 retention is detected on blood gas analysis, these patients should undergo polysomnography to determine the severity of nocturnal gas exchange defects and exclude the presence of obstructive sleep apnea. If sustained desaturations are found, nocturnal noninvasive ventilation (not supplemental oxygen) should be administered (see below).

Table 3 Features of Sleep-Disordered Breathing in Patients with Restrictive Thoracic Disorders

Obstructive apneas and hypopneas
Frequent oxygen desaturations
Hypoventilation
Arousals and sleep fragmentation
Most prominent during REM sleep when upper airway and chest wall muscles become hypotonic
Diminished REM, slow wave sleep
Reduced sleep efficiency, quality

F. Central Ventilatory Drive

Chronic nocturnal hypoventilation induces a decrease in the sensitivity of the respiratory drive (13,14). It is hypothesized that the respiratory center sensitivity to CO_2 (or "CO_2stat") is reset by nocturnal hypoventilation in a progressive fashion. As nocturnal hypoventilation worsens, the CO_2stat becomes more tolerant of CO_2 retention, and daytime hypercarbia eventually develops. Retention of bicarbonate contributes to this process as metabolic compensation for the respiratory acidosis occurs. This abnormality of ventilatory control is sometimes referred to as "central fatigue" to distinguish it from peripheral muscle fatigue. It is thought that rather than maintain normocapnia at the cost of respiratory muscle exhaustion, the respiratory center permits hypercarbia that requires less work from the breathing muscles (15). Hence, although the ultimate cause of hypercarbia in these patients is the poor respiratory mechanics and increased work of breathing, this blunting of respiratory drive may be seen as a central compensation to preserve what muscle function remains.

G. Pulmonary Hypertension and Cor Pulmonale

Pulmonary hypertension and cor pulmonale occur frequently in hypoventilating, hypoxic patients with restrictive thoracic disorders (16). Pulmonary hypertension occurs in response to alveolar hypoxia, as the vascular bed constricts and structurally remodels in response to the hypoxic stimulus. The net effect of these changes is to decrease the effective radius of the pulmonary vascular bed, increase pulmonary vascular resistance, and promote the development of pulmonary hypertension. The development of cor pulmonale contributes to exercise limitation and detracts from the prognosis of restrictive thoracic disease if not aggressively treated. In hypoventilating patients, the therapy of choice is not oxygen supplementation, but rather ventilatory assistance in the form of noninvasive ventilation. Amelioration of the hypoventilation usually leads to prompt resolution of cor pulmonale and an improvement in prognosis (17).

H. Bulbar Function

In some forms of neuromuscular disease, such as the motor neuron diseases, bulbar dysfunction often precedes involvement of other respiratory muscles. Patients with bulbar dysfunction develop severe swallowing disorders and have problems with frequent aspiration. This predisposes to respiratory infection and detracts from the prognosis. As long as cough function is intact, some aspiration is tolerated, but the combination of swallowing dysfunction and severe expiratory muscle weakness spells disaster. In these patients, cough assistive techniques may be helpful but ultimately, tracheostomy will be necessary in patients who wish to maximize their chances for survival.

I. Co-Morbidity

Patients with old tuberculosis (TB) often have bronchiectasis and substantial airway obstruction. Chronic tobacco abuse and repetitive respiratory infections also contribute to airway hypersecretion and obstruction. In addition, some forms of neuromuscular disease, such as Duchenne muscular dystrophy (DMD), are associated with cardiomyopathy (18). Pulmonary function tests and echocardiograms should be obtained in such patients. Therapy directed at optimizing airway or cardiac function may be useful in ameliorating respiratory dysfunction.

IV. Evaluation of Patients with Restrictive Thoracic Disorders

As described above, the natural evolution of the restrictive thoracic disorders varies considerably among specific disorders, but with many, there is a progressive worsening of respiratory status with eventual respiratory failure. These are usually gradual processes and if not treated optimally, patients will suffer from a decrease in quality of life, sometimes for years before succumbing to the consequences of untreated respiratory failure. Because of the slow progression, the majority of these patients adapt their lifestyle to their pulmonary limitations, tolerating their respiratory insufficiency without major complaints for a long period of time.

Eventually, though, the limited respiratory reserve renders the patient susceptible to even minor respiratory insults. At that point, patients may present after developing an upper respiratory illness or with progression of their chronic hypoventilation, either of which may lead to a sudden decompensation and the need for hospitalization. Ideally, this scenario is averted if clinicians following these patients are sensitive to the signs and symptoms that signal impending decompensation. Also, patients need to be informed well in advance of that stage of their illness about the potential for respiratory problems and alerted to the signs and symptoms of respiratory decompensation. In addition, they should be informed about high-risk situations, such as respiratory infections or general anesthesia, and provided with a logical plan to cope with these situations.

A. Symptoms and Signs of Chronic Respiratory Failure

As listed in Table 4, perhaps the most common complaint for ambulatory patients with chest wall deformities is dyspnea on exertion. When restriction is advanced, these patients present with severe exercise limitation, even with the most minor of daily activities such as dressing or bathing. On the other hand, clinicians should not be reassured by the absence of dyspnea in nonambulatory neuromuscular patients. These patients are remarkable in that they may develop severe hypercar-

Table 4 Clinical Features of Hypoventilation

Shortness of breath during activities of daily living (nonparalyzed patient)
Nocturnal or early morning headaches
Poor sleep quality: insomnia, nightmares, frequent arousals, enuresis
Daytime fatigue and sleepiness, loss of energy
Decrease in intellectual performance
Loss of appetite
Orthopnea in disorders of diaphragmatic dysfunction
Loss of weight
Appearance of recurrent complications: respiratory infections
Cor pulmonale

bia in the complete absence of respiratory distress. Presumably, the inability to exert resulting from paralysis and the very slow onset of hypoventilation combine to mask the symptom of dyspnea. Rather, these patients develop morning headaches thought to be caused by increased intracerebral pressure resulting from CO_2-induced cerebral vasodilation. These headaches usually disappear after the patient awakens, when ventilation improves and CO_2 drops. Unfortunately, this symptom does not occur consistently with severe hypercapnia, and its absence does not exclude severe hypoventilation.

Other symptoms, related to the sleep disturbances described earlier, are helpful in signaling the development of hypoventilation. These include daytime hypersomnolence, fatigue, restless sleep, daytime irritability, personality changes, diminished intellectual performance and, occasionally, nocturnal enuresis. With advanced hypoventilation, these symptoms severely impair daytime function. Clinicians should be sensitized to these symptoms and avoid the impulse to administer hypnotics to these patients whose chief complaint may be "difficulty sleeping."

Other sleep-related symptoms that may occur in these patients include orthopnea and sudden awakening with dyspnea and/or choking. These suggest diaphragmatic involvement in patients with amyotrophic lateral sclerosis (ALS) or possible cardiac decompensation in patients with Duchenne muscular dystrophy. Another cause of nocturnal dyspnea and choking in ALS patients is inspiratory stridor related to vocal cord weakness (19).

Weight loss may also occur as a consequence of hypoventilation. The increased energy requirements of eating and digestion in combination with abdominal bloating may cause patients to experience dyspnea during or after meals, decreasing food intake as a result. In addition, the increased work of breathing seen in many of these patients may raise caloric needs. The combination of decreased caloric intake and increased caloric requirements may contribute to a wasting syndrome. Perhaps partly as a consequence of weight loss–related immune compromise and the progressive weakness of expiratory muscles, the occurrence of repeated respiratory infections should also alert clinicians to the possibility of decreased pulmonary reserve.

The most common signs of chronic respiratory failure are related to the cardiovascular consequences of sustained hypoventilation and alveolar hypoxia: pulmonary hypertension and cor pulmonale (16). Auscultation over the pulmonic area may reveal an increased intensity of the pulmonic component of the second heart sound (P_2). As cor pulmonale advances, a murmur of tricuspid regurgitation may be audible, and a right ventricular impulse or (with marked right ventricular dilatation) heave may be palpable. Jugular venous distension and lower extremity edema or even ascites may develop in advanced cases. Other signs of chronic hypoventilation less often seen include papilledema, thought to be related to elevated intracranial pressure. Pulmonary hypertension and cor pulmonale are seen commonly on presentation in patients with chest wall disorders, but are not as frequently encountered in patients with neuromuscular disease unless they present with severe hypoventilation.

Other possible signs include abdominal paradox in patients with diaphragmatic weakness. The assessment of thoracoabdominal coordination in the supine position should be a routine part of the physical examination in patients with restrictive thoracic disorders. Auscultation over the larynx with deep breathing is also useful to elicit evidence for vocal cord weakness, particularly in ALS patients. Evidence of cardiomyopathy should also be sought in neuromuscular disorders that affect the cardiac muscles, such as Duchenne muscular dystrophy, but signs may be absent until the process is advanced.

It is also well to keep in mind that symptoms are only apparent in retrospect, after patients have had a favorable response to ventilatory assistance. This may be related to denial or the fact that the onset of respiratory impairment is insidious, giving patients time to adapt to each decrement in function. For this reason, the patient's spouse or family should be queried about specific signs and symptoms, such as changes in activity level or dyspnea, or in breathing during sleep. Also, the astute clinician should have a low threshold for performing tests, particularly arterial blood gases, to evaluate the possibility of incipient hypoventilation.

B. Pulmonary Function Testing

Pulmonary function testing (PFT) is an essential component of the evaluation and follow-up of patients with restrictive thoracic disorders. Testing can be done in a fully equipped pulmonary function laboratory or a screening can be done in a clinic using a hand-held spirometer. Full PFT including lung volumes should be done at least initially to confirm the presence of restriction, and forced vital capacity (FVC), peak expiratory flow, forced expiratory volume in 1 sec (FEV_1), and maximal inspiratory and expiratory pressures should be obtained during follow-up visits. In patients suspected of diaphragm weakness or paralysis, FVC should be performed in the sitting and supine positions. A drop in FVC of greater than 25% supine compared with upright indicates significant diaphragm weakness and a nocturnal evaluation is recommended (20).

Measured values are compared with normal predicted values based on age, height, sex, and ethnic group. However, selecting the appropriate predicted values for patients with severe scoliosis can pose challenges because of the difficulty in estimating height in paralyzed patients with numerous contractures. This can result in a gross under- or overestimations of the respiratory handicap. Maximal inspiratory and expiratory pressures may also be misleading and must be interpreted with caution because of the effort dependence of the test. Nonetheless, these can be useful in following the progression of neuromuscular syndromes, and peak expiratory flow and pressures may be helpful in assessing the integrity of the cough mechanism. Overall, the FVC is usually the most useful and reliable test.

In patients with neuromuscular disease, PFT should be done at least annually or more frequently depending on the severity of impairment and the expected natural history of the disease. In ALS patients, for example, the rate of progression may necessitate PFT three or four times yearly. For chest wall deformities, baseline PFT should be obtained at the time the patient comes to medical attention. Subsequent yearly tests are used to establish the rate of progression. Some of these patients need closer follow-up with the possibility of fusion surgery in mind. Close supervision is recommended if the angle of curvature is >100°, when patients usually experience dyspnea on exertion. An angle exceeding 120° will usually cause hypoventilation (8,17). However, some patients have very stable disease and are not apt to develop problems until late in adulthood, so less frequent follow-up is acceptable. In general, restrictive patients should be followed closely and screened for evidence of hypoventilation when their FVC falls below 1.5 liters or 50% of predicted or their PImax falls below 30 to 60 cm H_20 or 30 to 50% of predicted (21).

Occasionally, special studies are helpful in assessing respiratory muscle function in patients with restrictive thoracic disorders. When bilateral diaphragm paralysis is suspected, measurement of transdiaphragmatic pressure is the most accurate way of assessing diaphragmatic function. However, this is an invasive test necessitating the placement of esophageal and gastric balloons in patients who may have severely weakened cough muscles. Most often, the bedside examination and upright and supine FVCs suffice to make the diagnosis. These may be difficult to interpret in obese patients, in whom balloon studies may be helpful. Fluoroscopy of the diaphragms and diaphragmatic electromyograms should not be relied upon to make the diagnosis of bilateral diaphragm paralysis.

C. Cough

Because expiratory muscle strength is preserved and airway resistance is normal, cough function is usually intact in patients with chest wall deformities unless inspiratory capacity is very severely reduced. By contrast, cough is often ineffective in neuromuscular disorders because of inspiratory, pharyngeal and expiratory muscle weakness (7). Poor cough effectiveness predisposes to secretion infection and difficulty during respiratory infections.

Cough effectiveness can be evaluated using pulmonary function testing. Maximal expiratory pressure can be measured using the same manometer that is used for inspiratory pressure. When PEmax falls below 60 cm H_2O, cough effectiveness is generally very reduced. In addition, peak expiratory flow can be measured as an index of cough effectiveness, with a value exceeding 160 L/min thought to be favorable (22). Even if this value is obtained only after assisted cough maneuvers, it still suggests that secretion removal will be effective (22). Identifying poor cough effectiveness allows the respiratory clinician to identify patients who could benefit from assisted coughing, allowing an early teaching program to be implemented.

D. Gas Exchange

Arterial blood gases (ABGs) are indicated when FVC falls to <1.2 L or the patient develops symptoms of hypoventilation. The threshold for obtaining arterial blood gases should be low because symptoms may be very subtle and some patients hypoventilate well before the FVC drops severely. This occurs because of sleep-related breathing abnormalities or a component of central hypoventilation. An elevation in serum bicarbonate should also lead to blood gas analysis. Alternatives to ABGs include blood gases on earlobe capillary blood samples that correlate well with ABG results (23). Pulse oximetry is insensitive to mild to moderate increases in $Paco_2$ in patients with normal lungs, and end-tidal and transcutaneous Pco_2 measurements lack sufficient accuracy to replace blood gases (24).

E. Nocturnal SpO_2/Polysomnography

Nocturnal recordings are indicated in all patients who have symptoms of nocturnal hypoventilation but do not have daytime hypoventilation. In addition, they are recommended in asymptomatic patients with FVC <1 to 1.5 L and/or maximal inspiratory pressure <30 to 60 cm H_2O. Substantial sleep-disordered breathing can occur well before the clinical indicators of hypoventilation. On the other hand, symptomatic patients with daytime hypoventilation do not have to wait for a sleep study before initiating therapy because the results are unlikely to alter the therapy, and a delay could be deleterious. Sleep-related hypoventilation is invariably present in patients with daytime hypoventilation and there is no need to prove it with polysomnography unless obstructive sleep apnea is suspected.

Ideally, evaluation of nocturnal hypoventilation should include measurements of Spo_2 and transcutaneous or end-tidal Pco_2 as part of a full polysomnogram. This allows a detailed assessment of the breathing patterns contributing to hypoventilation, nonobstructive hypoventilation, or central or obstructive apneas and/or hypopneas, as well as an analysis of sleep quality (e.g., the presence of arousals leading to sleep fragmentation). The results may also help to guide the selection of initial pressures, especially if obstructive apneas require a certain minimal expiratory pressure for elimination. Due to the complexity, cost, and variable availability of full polysomnography, however, more limited studies may be necessary to screen patients. Nocturnal polysomnography may be more important after initiation when problems with adaptation are encountered.

F. Other Assessments

Other kinds of assessment may be useful in the initial evaluation of patients with restrictive thoracic disorders. Evaluation of the musculoskeletal system by physical and occupational therapists may enhance overall patient functioning. Specific limitations may be identified, with prescriptions of exercises given to maintain strength and flexibility. The occupational therapist may devise ways for the patient to put the mask on and remove it or attach the ventilator to a wheelchair. Evaluation by a speech therapist of swallowing function may be useful when deciding on noninvasive versus invasive ventilation or whether or not to have a gastric tube placed. A nutritional evaluation is indicated in patients with histories of weight loss or gain.

V. Indications and Contraindications for Long-Term Mechanical Ventilation in Patients with Restrictive Thoracic Disorders

A. Indications for Long-Term Mechanical Ventilation

The main indication for beginning LTMV in restrictive patients is the presence of symptoms of chronic hypoventilation in conjunction with a gas exchange disturbance (Table 5). If the patient has significant daytime hypoventilation ($Paco_2$ >45 mm Hg) or evidence of sustained nocturnal hypoventilation (Spo_2 <88% for more than 5 consecutive min) even in the absence of daytime hypoventilation, LTMV is indicated. In addition, an FVC below 50% of predicted in a symptomatic patient serves as an indication. The latter indication is of most importance in patients with rapidly progressive neuromuscular syndromes such as ALS, in which earlier initiation allows more time for adaptation. However, there is little evidence to support this criterion in slowly progressive restrictive processes, and it should be considered a "soft" or "possible" indication in the absence of any

Table 5 Indications for Noninvasive Ventilation*

1. Symptoms consistent with sleep disruption or hypoventilation
2. Gas exchange disturbance
   a. Daytime hypoventilation ($PaCO_2 > 45$ mm Hg) or
   b. Nocturnal hypoventilation (O_2sat < 88% for > 5 consecutive minutes)
3. Severe pulmonary dysfunction (FVC < 50% predicted) (mainly for rapidly progressive neuromuscular diseases)
4. Repeated hospitalizations for respiratory exacerbations
5. No contraindications to noninvasive ventilation (see Table 7)

*Criteria 1–3 are recognized as criteria for reimbursement by Medicare in the United States.

gas exchange disturbance. The guidelines listed in Table 5 parallel those proposed by a recent consensus conference on the use of noninvasive ventilation (25) and have been adopted by the Health Care Financing Agency that sets reimbursement guidelines for Medicare in the United States. Some authors have recommended using PImax <60 cm H_2O as an additional guideline for initiating LTMV in symptomatic patients, but reliance on this measure is discouraged because of its dependence on patient effort.

Another possible indication for LTMV is an acute bout of respiratory failure. Such a bout in restrictive patients is indicative of poor reserve and there is a high risk of recurrence. Unless there is rapid and complete reversal and the patient is left with at least some reserve, LTMV should be considered. If a patient has not been started after an initial bout, LTMV should be initiated after recurrent bouts. Also, patients who are unable to wean entirely after a bout of acute respiratory failure after should be started on LTMV.

B. Contraindications to Long-Term Mechanical Ventilation

Although LTMV can be initiated in many patients with respiratory failure, ideally, it should be reserved for patients who have some potential for rehabilitation. Thus, patients with vegetative states or terminal diseases with little or no prospect for recovery are not good candidates for LTMV. Patients who are medically unstable, agitated and uncooperative, or severely depressed are poor candidates and have difficulty leaving the acute care environment unless these conditions improve. However, deciding on whether or not such patients should be placed on LTMV often raises difficult ethical issues, which are discussed in more detail later in the chapter.

The relative contraindications for LTMV listed in Table 6 interfere with the potential for rehabilitation and returning home. Patients who lack motivation for recovery and have no interest in managing their own affairs are much less

Table 6 Relative Contraindications to Long-Term Mechanical Ventilation

Terminally ill patient or vegetative state
Absence of patient motivation
Absence of financial resources
Absence of family and social support
Medically unstable
Agitated or uncooperative
Depression

likely to respond to rehabilitation or succeed in the home environment. A lack of financial resources or family/caregiver support may also preclude discharge home, although such patients can be supported in chronic care facilities for long periods of time. Preferably, though, LTMV patients are sent home whenever possible. Discharge home is desirable because of fewer and less serious infectious complications than in hospitalized patients, lower costs unless around-the-clock skilled nursing is required (24), and the preference of most patients for living at home. Unfortunately, laws precluding the use of nonprofessional but trained personnel from performing suctioning at home (raising costs) and the reluctance of many insurers to cover more than 12 hr of nursing coverage per day renders discharge home impossible for many adult LTMV patients.

C. Timing of the Initiation of Long-Term Mechanical Ventilation

Some investigators have proposed that by providing intermittent rest, early initiation of LTMV before the onset of symptoms or gas exchange abnormalities would retard the deterioration of respiratory muscle function (25). However, in a controlled study by Raphael et al. testing this hypothesis (26), patients with Duchenne muscular dystrophy begun early on nasal ventilation had a higher mortality than those given standard therapy without ventilatory assistance. Although this study has been criticized for not monitoring patient compliance and including more patients with cardiomyopathies in the treatment than in the control group, the results have dimmed the enthusiasm for early initiation.

On the other hand, the evidence is strong to support the initiation of NPPV in symptomatic patients with nocturnal hypoventilation, even before the onset of daytime hypoventilation. Masa et al. (27) found that nocturnal gas exchange and symptoms were substantially improved when restrictive patients with nocturnal but no daytime hypoventilation were begun on noninvasive ventilation. Thus, the current consensus view is that patients should not be started on LTMV unless they have symptoms attributable to hypoventilation, partly because compliance with the therapy is likely to be poor unless patients are motivated by the desire for symptom relief. On the other hand, there is no need to await the onset of daytime hypoventilation if nocturnal hypoventilation (as evidenced by sustained oxygen desaturations) is demonstrable. One additional caveat is that patients who have severe daytime hypoventilation ($Paco_2$ >50 to 55 mm Hg) should be started on LTMV even if they are not experiencing symptoms. Often, these patients will experience symptomatic improvement even if they were unaware of symptoms initially.

D. Choosing Between Noninvasive and Invasive Ventilation

By virtue of its greater convenience, portability, lower cost of administration (24,28), and lower likelihood of contributing to infectious complications, noninvasive ventilation is widely considered to be the ventilator modality of first choice in patients meeting indications for LTMV. In most cases,this means nasal ventilation administered nocturnally. However, when deciding between noninvasive and invasive ventilation, the clinician should consider certain relative contraindications to noninvasive ventilation (Table 7). First, because noninvasive ventilation provides no direct access to the lower airways, patients must be able to protect their airway and mobilize airway secretions. Deciding when these functions are too compromised to justify a trial of nonivasive ventilation requires clinical judgment. Patients with bulbar muscle impairment can be managed noninvasively, and the available evidence suggests that their survival may be prolonged (29).

On the other hand, problems with oral air leaks are more common with noninvasive ventilation, and if severe impairment of the cough mechanism is combined with moderate to severe bulbar dysfunction (as occurs eventually in ALS patients), survival is likely to be brief unless invasive ventilation is promptly

Table 7 Contraindications to Noninvasive and Indications for Invasive Ventilation

Contraindications to noninvasive ventilation
Significant swallowing disorders
Severe cough impairment with chronic aspiration
Inability to clear secretions
Vocal cord paralysis
Inability to cooperate
Indications for invasive ventilation
Failure to tolerate noninvasive ventilation
Failure to adequately ventilate with noninvasive ventilation
Uncontrollable oral air leaks during noninvasive ventilation
High level of dependence on assisted ventilation (>20 hrs/day)

initiated. Likewise, excessive airway secretions or inspiratory stridor caused by vocal cord paralysis can be managed effectively only by resorting promptly to tracheostomy. In addition, noninvasive ventilation requires a cooperative patient who will not be continually removing the mask, so uncooperative, agitated patients will require invasive ventilation.

Because of the increasing use of noninvasive ventilation, patients using tracheostomy positive pressure ventilation are diminishing as a proportion of those using LTMV (30), but there are still important indications for invasive LTMV (see Table 7). The decision to proceed with tracheostomy should consider multiple factors. Clearly, if noninvasive ventilation is contraindicated and the patient desires continued ventilatory support, there is no alternative to tracheostomy. Also, if the patient fails a trial of noninvasive ventilation, tracheostomy is indicated. On the other hand, noninvasive ventilation should not be considered a failure unless every reasonable attempt to achieve compliance has been made. Reasons for failure vary, but most often it is related to difficulty in tolerating the mask. Multiple different mask types and styles are now available and, often, an acceptable commercial mask can be found. Newer face masks with soft silicone seals have become available, as have nasal masks with gel seals, and so-called "mini-masks" that can assuage feelings of claustrophobia. Custom-made masks may occasionally solve intolerance problems if skilled individuals are available for fabrication.

Sometimes, failure is related to inadequate support of ventilation. Here, consideration should be given to the adequacy of pressure settings, the possibility that rebreathing is contributing, or that excessive oral leaks are compromising efficacy. Obese patients and those with chest wall deformities have high respiratory impedances and may fail unless ventilators that are capable of generating high inflation pressures are used. Rebreathing may interfere with ventilatory assistance if expiratory pressures <4 cm H_2O are used during "bilevel" ventilation (31). Oral leaks are very common and although most patients tolerate them well, they compromise ventilation in some (32), who may improve after switching to a full-face mask. These possible manipulations must be considered and, if indicated, tried before noninvasive ventilation is declared a failure. In addition, some patients who are intolerant of NPPV may still respond favorably to other types of noninvasive ventilation that have enjoyed popularity in the past. Negative pressure ventilators, rocking beds, and "pneumobelts" may all be successfully applied, although induction of obstructive sleep apneas is a concern (39). The application of these devices is discussed in more detail in Chapter 10.

Some patients have initial success with noninvasive ventilation but eventually fail related to the natural progression of their disease. Increasing inflation pressure and/or the duration of ventilator use can sometimes reverse the failure. Many clinicians believe that beyond a certain level of dependency, switching to noninvasive ventilation is sensible for convenience and continued stability.

Arbitrarily, some authors have suggested that >16 hr/day of ventilator use justifies switching (35) whereas others argue that no level of support necessitates a switch to invasive ventilation as long as airway protection is adequate (36). However, the noninvasive management of patients who are entirely dependent on mechanical ventilation should be undertaken only at centers with experience and skill in managing such patients.

Placement of a tracheostomy increases the complexity of care because of the need for frequent suctioning, daily care of the stoma and tube, and periodic tube changes. Thus, the decision should be made only in consultation with the patient and caregivers. Bach (35) have surveyed long-term ventilator users and have found that noninvasive ventilation is preferred by most because of greater comfort and convenience. However, invasive ventilation is preferred by some because of greater security and better sleep. Age and physical dependency of the patient as well as skills and capabilities of the caregivers are considerations. Tracheostomies should be performed on patients with higher levels of dependency who have adequate caregiver support. Placement of a tracheostomy in a patient who lacks adequate caregiver support could necessitate transfer from home to a chronic care facility, and this may be unacceptable to some patients. Contrariwise, transfer from invasive to noninvasive ventilation can allow previously institution-bound patients to return home. This transfer is discussed in Chapter 11.

When indicated in appropriate and well-informed patients, tracheostomy ventilation remains a very efficient and safe mode of ventilation. Quality of life may actually improve compared with noninvasive ventilation because of the added security, improved sleep, and elimination of appliances from the face. Tracheostomy management is discussed in more detail in Chapter 9, but every effort must be made to optimize the rehabilitation of the patient. Whenever possible, tracheostomy tube cuffs should be deflated or eliminated to facilitate speech, and patients with adequate swallowing function should be encouraged to eat by mouth. Patients with limited oral intake due to swallowing dysfunction should have G or J tubes placed to maintain caloric balance. A brief stay in a rehabilitation hospital may be helpful before discharge home. When managed by clinicians knowledgeable about airway management and the needs of restrictive patients, tracheostomy ventilation can be safely and successfully administered to LTMV patients at home or in chronic care facilities for many years.

VI. Ethical Considerations Regarding Long-Term Mechanical Ventilation

The decision to proceed with LTMV can be very complex. Numerous considerations come into play, including the patient's and caregivers' wishes, the nature and natural history of the underlying process, the patient's age and comorbidity, the severity and distribution of physiologic impairment, and practical realities, such as the capabilities of the patient and caregivers and financial limitations. Although these considerations differ from patient to patient and decisions must always be individualized, certain general principles relating to the decision-making process can be elaborated.

First, patients and their caregivers should be educated and informed about the nature and probable consequences of their disease as soon as they come to medical attention. Particularly in patients with progressive neuromuscular diseases, such as Duchenne muscular dystrophy or ALS, patients should be prepared for the eventual respiratory deterioration and the decisions they must face. Clinicians must anticipate respiratory needs before crises occur whenever possible. In this way, noninvasive ventilation can be started at the optimal time, allowing time for adaptation. If patients deteriorate so that noninvasive support is no longer sufficient (due to swallowing or cough impairment, for example), then a tracheostomy can be placed in a timely fashion in patients who desire one, or hospice services can be provided at home for patients who don't. In this way, patients are informed and managed in a proactive rather than reactive fashion, crises and inappropriate use of medical resources are averted, and psychological stress to the patient and family is greatly reduced.

Second, patients should be given autonomy in making their medical decisions. The clinician should provide information in a gentle but frank manner and attempt to ascertain that the patient has a clear understanding of the consequences of different decisions. The decision to proceed with or forego tracheostomy in patients with progressive neuromuscular disorders may be particularly difficult, and having the patient speak to others who have had the procedure may be helpful. The clinician should try to be objective in administering advice, although, admittedly, biases are difficult to exclude entirely from these discussions. Also, although our ethical constructs prioritize patient autonomy, these decisions have implications for the family and should not be made in a vacuum. For example, a patient with ALS who has developed severe bulbar dysfunction may wish to return home with tracheostomy ventilation. However, unless family members are willing and able to make the time and emotional commitment necessary, the patient's wishes are unlikely to be met. Armed with this information, some patients may forego further efforts at ventilatory support rather than live with a tracheostomy in a chronic care facility.

The concept of medical futility has sometimes been used to argue against the use of invasive therapeutic interventions in diseases that will ultimately prove fatal. Medical futility is usually defined as a situation in which a therapy has little or no chance of bringing about a desired effect (36). However, the application of this concept to clinical decisions depends on how "little chance" and "desired effect" are defined. If the chance can be as low as one in a million, then fewer interventions will be considered futile than if the chances are one in ten. Likewise, if the desired outcome is reversal of a discrete physiologic dysfunction such as respiratory failure, then fewer therapies will be considered futile than if the desired outcome is restoration of a fully functional life. In this context, placement of a tracheostomy in a patient with ALS is not necessarily futile in that the physiologic defect, respiratory failure, can be reversed. On the other hand, some patients may consider it futile, because it does nothing to reverse the relentless progression of the underlying terminal illness.

Surveys of patients facing end-of-life decisions, mainly those with ALS, have provided some important insights. First, patient decisions may change over time. Patients who desire invasive ventilation when first informed of their illness may decide against it when asked again several months later, and others who decline invasive ventilation initially may opt for it when faced later with the reality of terminal respiratory failure. Second, patients vary markedly in their perceptions of life satisfaction, and may be more adaptable than they initially think. In one survey, only 10% of ALS patients decided to have a tracheostomy, but 90% of tracheostomized patients were happy with the decision (37). These observations highlight the fact that prospective decisions about end of life are not binding and should be reassessed periodically. Also, although most patients with ALS elect to forego tracheostomy, the decision to have one placed may be quite acceptable for a minority of patients, at least as determined by their satisfaction with life.

VII. Practical Application of Long-Term Mechanical Ventilation in Patients with Restrictive Thoracic Disorders

The practical application of LTMV is discussed in detail in Chapters 9 and 10 and will be considered only briefly here as regards restrictive thoracic disorders. Once an appropriate candidate has been selected based on the guidelines discussed above, ventilation must be initiated. Most often, noninvasive ventilation will be the first modality tried. If the patient is recovering from a bout of respiratory failure, then ventilation is initiated in the hospital, and the patient discharged home after comfort on initial settings has been established. Elective ventilatory assistance can be initiated on an outpatient basis, as long as the equipment supplier can provide skilled, experienced home respiratory therapists.

In either case, patient comfort with the initial setup is critically important. A nasal mask is most often tried initially, with the aim of optimizing fit and comfort and minimizing air leaks. The ventilator choice is based on convenience, economy, and any special patient needs. Most often, simple, lightweight, quiet, and inexpensive "bilevel" devices are chosen, unless the patient requires high inflation pressures, or needs more sophisticated monitoring because of the need for continuous ventilation. If started electively at the appropriate time, most patients require only nocturnal ventilation and sophisticated alarms or monitors are unnecessary. These patients should also be started with relatively low inflation pressures that can be tolerated without discomfort (inspiratory pressure roughly 8 cm H_2O). Once the patient becomes accustomed to the ventilator system, then pressures can be increased gradually as tolerated to achieve desired improvements in gas exchange. However, if excessive pressures are used initially, successful adaptation may be impossible. Eventually, inspiratory pressures in patients with neuromuscular disease are increased to between 14 and 20 cm H_2O, depending on patient tolerance, symptomatic response, and daytime and nocturnal gas exchange targets. For patients with chest wall restriction, inspiratory pressures are often higher, sometimes exceeding 30 cm H_2O in morbidly obese patients.

Minimal expiratory pressure can be used in patients with restrictive thoracic disorders because autoPEEP is rarely a concern unless patients have mixed obstructive and restrictive disease. The advantage of using lower expiratory pressure is that inspiratory pressure can be minimized at a given level of pressure support (inspiratory minus expiratory pressure). If rebreathing is a concern, as may be the case with "bilevel" ventilators, exhalation valves designed to minimize rebreathing, even at low expiratory pressures, can be used (31). Using a backup rate is advisable for patients with neuromuscular disease or the obesity hypoventilation syndrome, set slightly below the spontaneous breathing rate. This allows controlled breathing during sleep as the spontaneous rate slows slightly, permitting maximal rest of respiratory muscles. Typical backup rates are 15 to 20/min. The need for a backup rate is not as clear for patients with chest wall deformities, who tend to breathe at higher spontaneous rates and are less apt to allow the ventilator to control nocturnal breathing (38).

The noninvasive management of chronic respiratory failure in patients with restrictive thoracic disorders requires a long-term approach from knowledgeable and attentive clinicians. Unless there is urgency because of the severity of the patient's respiratory insufficiency, adaptation can take place gradually, with pressures gradually adjusted upward over several weeks to months. The expected rate of progression then determines the frequency of follow-up visits. Patients with postpolio syndrome or kyphoscoliosis who are likely to be stable for years may require minimal attention after successful adaptation. Patients with ALS or more rapidly progressive muscular dystrophies, on the other hand, may require follow-up every month or two when inspiratory pressure and/or duration of ventilator use per day can be gradually adjusted upward to maintain desired daytime arterial blood gas values.

When patients are poor candidates for or have failed noninvasive ventilation and desire invasive ventilatory support, tracheostomy ventilation should be initiated. Once the tracheostomy is placed, the focus should be on rehabilitation to help the patient attain the highest possible level of functioning. Acute medical problems should be stabilized and chronic conditions optimally treated. Nutritional balance should be restored, with a G or J tube placed in patients with swallowing impairment. Speech should be preserved in patients capable of speaking. If the patient is a candidate for home discharge, then the patient and family should be educated in the management of the tracheostomy and ventilator, including suctioning and preparation for emergencies. With a holistic approach that is detailed in Chapter 9, many patients with end-stage neuromuscular disease or chest wall deformity who would not otherwise be alive can be satisfactorily managed for years with home tracheostomy ventilation.

VIII. Outcomes of Long-Term Mechanical Ventilation in Patients with Restrictive Thoracic Disorders

Numerous studies have reported beneficial effects of LTMV on both early and long-term outcomes in large patient groups over extended periods of time. Early responses include the capacity for LTMV to correct hypoventilation associated with a prompt improvement in symptoms. Long-term studies report the maintenance of improvements in blood gases and symptoms, as well as less need for hospitalization, an enhanced quality of life, and good compliance with therapy. There is no question today that the therapy of choice for chronic hypoventilation in restrictive thoracic disorders is assisted ventilation. In contrast with COPD, the results published on restrictive patients are not controversial and show consistently favorable outcomes.

A. Early Benefits of Mechanical Ventilatory Assistance

In restrictive thoracic disorders, the beneficial effects of assisted ventilation are usually apparent soon after initiation. Symptoms related to hypoventilation improve (morning headaches, fatigue, daytime hypersomnolence) (40,41). In addition, signs of cor pulmonale usually resolve. Gas exchange is improved during wakefulness as well as during sleep as demonstrated by daytime blood gases and nocturnal recordings of Spo_2 and transcutaneous Pco_2 (42–44). Improvements during sleep include fewer respiratory disturbances, increased total sleep time, and enhanced sleep efficiency (27). Nevertheless, even during assisted ventilation, significant episodes of transient hypoventilation that contribute to sleep arousals may persist and appear to be related to mouth leaks (45,46). Because of the reduced tendency for air leaks, sleep quality may be better when ventilation is assisted using a mouthpiece interface or a tracheostomy than during nasal ventilation (34).

When symptoms respond promptly to assisted ventilation, success is virtually guaranteed, because of the strong motivating effect of symptomatic relief.

In addition, a large percentage of patients with restrictive thoracic disorders characteristically have a very strong will to improve and survive, even when their quality of life seems limited in the eyes of others without physical challenges. Often, these individuals (with postpolio syndrome, sequelae of TB, or slowly progressive neuromuscular diseases) have been adjusting to gradually increasing limitations throughout their lives, and the adjustment to assisted ventilation is another hurdle after many previous ones. A possible exception is patients with ALS, who tend to be afflicted later in life and often have more difficulty adapting to their illness. In addition, ALS progresses more rapidly than the others and is more apt to impair speech and swallowing functions, so although many are willing to try noninvasive ventilation, most forego invasive LTMV.

B. Sustained Benefits of Long-Term Mechanical Ventilation

Gas Exchange

The early improvement in arterial blood gases is sustained with the continuation of assisted ventilation. With noninvasive ventilation, the improvement is usually gradual as patients increase the number of hours per day of ventilator use. After a few weeks, stabilization occurs, often with $Paco_2$s remaining above normal limits, and varying considerably from patient to patient, depending on ventilatory limitations and the patient's tolerance for ventilator use. Daytime $Paco_2$ during spontaneous breathing varies from normal to 60 mm Hg (and sometimes even higher), but is still associated with symptom relief as long as sleep quality has improved. With tracheostomy ventilation, the $Paco_2$ is usually lowered more rapidly. Normal daytime $Paco_2$s are more often achieved, again depending on duration of use. During either NPPV or tracheostomy ventilation, the improvement in blood gases is usually sufficient to allow the patient to be completely free from supplemental oxygen or assisted ventilation during the day, even during exertion, and may be sustained for many years depending on the progression of the underlying illness (47).

Sleep

The reduction of respiratory disturbances during sleep and increases in sleep duration and efficiency found after the initiation of assisted ventilation are sustained for at least 3 yr and often much longer depending on the underlying illness (41). Several studies have evaluated the beneficial effects of noninvasive ventilation on sleep by temporarily withdrawing nocturnal ventilation from previously stabilized patients. In these studies, the patients presented with symptomatic chronic respiratory failure and had responded favorably to nocturnal ventilatory assistance (27,41,48). All of the studies observed a prompt recurrence of nocturnal hypoventilation, even during the first night without ventilatory assistance, especially during REM sleep. Sleep quality deteriorated, with less total sleep time, and a diminished proportion of slow wave and REM sleep. Symptoms reappeared progressively during the week or two of ventilator withdrawal and promptly resolved when assisted ventilation was resumed.

One of the studies (48) also observed a decrease in ventilatory responsiveness to CO_2 during the period of withdrawal, consistent with the idea that intermittent assisted ventilation works by reversing the blunting of respiratory drive that occurs with chronic CO_2 retention. Schoenhofer et al. (49) have shown that the period of assisted ventilation need not be during sleep. These investigators showed that the improvement in gas exchange following a month of NPPV was equivalent whether the patients used the ventilator nocturnally during sleep or during the daytime while awake.

Pulmonary Function and Exercise Capacity

Maximal inspiratory and expiratory pressures and vital capacity during wakefulness have shown some improvement after initiation of noninvasive ventilation in patients with restrictive disorders, but the changes have not been consistent (50–52). Measures of muscle endurance, such as the maximum sustainable minute ventilation may be more sensitive in detecting the improvements than the maximal inspiratory pressure, which is more a test of inspiratory muscle strength (52). The improvements in respiratory muscle function are thought to be related to muscle resting during assisted ventilation (53). However, resolution of hypercarbia has been associated with improved inspiratory muscle strength, so the improvement in blood gases may also be responsible (54). In addition, patients capable of exercising have improvements in cycle endurance or walking distances associated with smaller oxygen desaturations than before initiation of noninvasive ventilation (55).

Cardiac Function

Similar to long-term oxygen therapy (56), correction of hypoxemia associated with nocturnal ventilation allows stabilization or improvement in pulmonary hypertension and chronic cor pulmonale that is sustained for years. Recently, Schönhofer et al. (57) provided hemodynamic confirmation of these clinical observations by observing a significant improvement in pulmonary hypertension in kyphoscoliosis patients after 6 mo of NPPV.

Whether ventilatory assistance affects the progression of the cardiomyopathy in muscular dystrophies that impair cardiac function (such as Duchenne muscular dystrophy) is unknown. Some DMD patients have very long survivals on LTMV (living into their mid-40s), but whether these patients had less cardiac involvement to begin with or have been protected by LTMV is unclear.

Quality of Life

The quality of life with noninvasive ventilation has been evaluated using questionnaires. Patients with restrictive thoracic disorders consistently have an improvement in symptoms of chronic hypoventilation and better quality of sleep after starting ventilatory assistance. In a survey by Simonds et al. (58), 73% of the patients had less fatigue, 44% less breathlessness, and 48% decreased frequency of respiratory infections. The majority of patients were able to return to work at home and some returned to professional work. As assessed by SF-36 questionnaires that evaluate general health status (59), patients using noninvasive ventilation had comparable results to other patient groups with nonprogressive disorders despite a lower level of physical activity. In another study by Simonds et al. (60), quality of life measured in Duchenne muscular dystrophy patients using assisted ventilation did not differ significantly from age-matched male controls in domains such as mental health, role limitation related to physical and emotional factors, and social function. Bach has emphasized the observation that caregivers often underestimate patient quality of life in comparison to the patient's own ratings (61). Quality of life has not been as well studied in patients using invasive ventilation.

Effects on Hospitalization

The improved health status of restrictive thoracic disease patients using LTMV is exemplified by the drop in the number of days of hospitalization after initiation of assisted ventilation as compared with before. The reimbursement system in France allows precise tabulation of the days that patients spend in the hospital. A large follow-up series from France (62) showed that hospital days per patient per year dropped from 34 for the year before initiation of nocturnal NPPV to 6 and 5 for the first and second years afterward, respectively, for scoliosis, 31 days to 10 and 9 for the sequelae of tuberculosis, and 18 to 7 and 2 for DMD patients (all $p < 0.05$). Simonds et al. (58) reported similar results among DMD patients treated in England. In an earlier study from France, Robert et al. (63) also showed similar results among tracheostomized patients treated at home. These studies emphasize the medical stability of these patients after assisted ventilation is initiated and the potential benefits to the health care system in terms of reduced resource utilization if LTMV is begun at an appropriate time.

Survival Rate

In general, the natural history of patients with restrictive thoracic disorders leads to a significantly reduced life expectancy because of progressive respiratory insufficiency. Once respiratory impairment has advanced to a severe stage, or after the first episode of acute respiratory failure, it is likely that acute decompensations will recur and survival will be brief unless LTMV is implemented. Although LTMV has undoubtedly prolonged survival in most of the restrictive thoracic disorders, the differences in prognoses and responses to therapy among the various restrictive processes are so large that it is difficult to make any but the most sweeping generalizations without discussing each entity separately. Accordingly, the next section discusses the natural history and responses to therapy of the major restrictive thoracic disorders, not only with regard to survival but also other outcome variables, as well.

IX. Natural History and Response to Therapy of Patients with Main Restrictive Thoracic Disorders Treated with Long-Term Mechanical Ventilation

A. Thoracovertebral Deformities

Natural History

Idiopathic kyphoscoliosis (KS) and the mutilating sequelae of TB are the two main categories of disease that cause thoracovertebral deformities. Rarer etiologies that also have significant respiratory consequences include kyphosis secondary to spinal TB and abnormal spine development, such as spina bifida. Ankylosing spondylitis or other thoracic deformities, such as pectus excavatum, are rarely responsible for severe chronic respiratory insufficiency unless associated with other diseases.

For patients with idiopathic scoliosis, criteria are available that define the risk of developing chronic respiratory insufficiency (8,17). These include the age at onset, length and location of the scoliosis, and the degree of curvature. Scoliosis that appears before age 5 has the worst respiratory prognosis. For cervical/thoracic scoliosis and high thoracic scoliosis, the respiratory consequences are worse if the curve is long and extends to the upper spine. In addition, an angulation of more than 100 to 120° is considered very severe and induces chronic respiratory insufficiency. Further, a vital capacity of less than 45% at the time of bone maturity has an equally poor prognosis.

The angulation of scoliosis increases drastically during puberty and continues to worsen with aging and the development of osteoporosis, further contributing to the decline of respiratory function (3,5,8). Better prevention of thoracovertebral deformity with orthopedic treatment and early surgery to correct and stabilize spinal deformities have already drastically decreased the morbidity of congenital scolioses (64,65). Not all patients with thoracovertebral deformities, however, are candidates for surgery, and some come to medical attention after puberty when the scoliosis has already become advanced. Thus, there will continue to be scoliotic patients with some form of respiratory handicap (66).

The life expectancy of patients with thoracic deformities is usually reduced. In a group of 102 patients with idiopathic scoliosis and no surgical procedures, average age at death was reported to be 46 years (67), with chronic cor pulmonale cited as the cause of death in one third of the cases. The development of cor pulmonale is a grave development in these patients if untreated, with 50% dying within 1 yr and 80% after 2 yr (3). In addition, after an acute bout of cardiorespiratory failure without the implementation of LTMV, episodes of decompensation will recur. During a mean follow-up period of 6 yr after the first acute episode, there were 2.4 recurrences in one series, the extremes being 1 and 6 (3).

The second major group of patients with thoracic deformity has mutilating sequelae of TB. During the 1940s and 1950s before the wide availability of effective antibiotic regimens, deforming surgical procedures and other techniques such as phrenectomies and repeated iatrogenic pneumothoraces were performed in an attempt to control the disease within the lungs. These procedures, although very mutilating, prevented patient deaths. The mutilating sequelae of TB are diverse and several can be present in the same patient. Thoracoplasty, fibrothorax due to severe pleural thickening, pulmonary resection, and phrenectomy all cause restrictive ventilatory defects similar to those of scoliosis. In addition, these patients often have an obstructive component that may or may not respond to bronchodilators, and some have diffuse bronchiectasis. Hypoventilation generally occurs 30 to 40 yr after the mutilating procedures (66–68). The introduction of effective chemotherapy for TB during the 1950s virtually eliminated the use of surgical procedures to treat TB, and as a consequence, the number of patients suffering from late sequelae of TB is gradually dropping. Patients referred for hypoventilation are now usually older than 70.

Response to Long-Term Mechanical Ventilation

After polio patients, those with thoracic deformities were the next group to be treated with long-term assisted ventilation. Consequently, there is a large experience treating these patients over a long period of time. Initially, long-term oxygen therapy (LTOT) was proposed as a possible treatment for chronic respiratory failure in thoracic disorders because it was thought to be less cumbersome than assisted ventilation. However, although long-term oxygen therapy increases survival of these patients when compared with medical treatment and physiotherapy alone, the survival rate is much less than that of patients treated with assisted mechanical ventilation (69). For patients with sequelae of TB, the greater the thoracic deformity, the more significant the favorable impact of mechanical ventilation on prognosis. For kyphoscoliosis patients using LTOT, the age of the patient and the severity of hypoxemia without hypercarbia are the gravest prognostic factors. These studies stressed the observation that some patients survived because they added assisted ventilation during the evolution of their disease (70).

Other studies have reported favorable results with these patients using LTMV. Robert et al. (65) reported a 77% 5-yr survival for scoliosis patients using tracheostomy ventilation at home, with a good quality of life and no recurrent hospitalizations. More recently, however, NPPV has virtually replaced tracheostomy ventilation for restrictive thoracic patients. Table 8 lists the probabilities of continuing ventilator therapy and/or surviving over the first 5 yr of therapy as reported in several long-term studies in patients with kyphoscoliosis and sequelae of TB. All of the studies examined effects of NPPV or tracheostomy ventilation, except that by Jackson et al. (70), which reported survival rates of 70% at five years for a group of 25 patients with sequelae of TB treated by negative pressure ventilation via chest cuirass. In a subsequent study on patients who had undergone thoracoplasties, these authors (71) observed a 5-yr survival rate of 64% among 32 patients who were treated mainly with negative pressure ventilators but some with NPPV. Although the findings suggest that these patients may not fare as well as others with thoracic deformity, it is difficult to interpret these results in the absence of controls. Further, negative pressure ventilation is now usually avoided in patients with severe thoracic deformities, partly because of concerns about induction of sleep-disordered breathing (72).

Two studies have provided information on the outcomes of very large groups of patients with restrictive thoracic disorders who were treated with NPPV: 47 with kyphoscoliosis and 20 with sequelae of TB in the English report by Simonds and Elliott (58); and 105 with kyphoscoliosis and 80 with sequelae of TB in the French report by Leger et al. (62) (see Table 9). In these studies, continuation of NPPV is used as a surrogate of survival. However, it is likely to underestimate survival, because some patients discontinued due to intolerance and may have survived and others went on to tracheostomy. Simonds and Elliott reported the highest level of continuation after 5 yr on NPPV for both groups: 79% for kyphoscoliosis and 94% for sequelae of TB. In the French study, the probability of continuing NPPV was greater than that for surviving while using oxygen therapy alone. The major difference was found in the scoliosis patients at 5 yr: 73% continued nasal ventilation compared with 60% alive with oxygen therapy. For the sequelae of TB, the results at 5 yr were 60% and 53%, respectively. The survival of these patients is similar to that obtained in the past for patients with thoracovertebral abnormalities treated with tracheostomy (63).

In summary, NPPV improves survival for patients with thoracovertebral deformities compared with long-term oxygen therapy alone, appears to be superior to negative pressure ventilation in a number of respects, and compares favorably with tracheostomy ventilation with regard to prolongation of survival. Based on these observations and the fact that it has cost and convenience advantages over tracheostomy ventilation, NPPV is now considered the ventilator modality of first choice in patients with thoracic deformities.

Table 8 Invasive Versus Noninvasive Ventilation: Choosing Between Methods of LTMV

Method	Advantages	Disadvantages	Indication
Noninvasive Positive Pressure Ventilation	More physiologic Swallowing and phonation are maintained Patient autonomy	Leaks Efficacy of ventilation can be reduced by upper airway obstruction and mask or mouth leaks	First option for LTMV
Noninvasive Negative Pressure Ventilation	Swallowing and phonation are maintained	Cumbersome Risk of upper airway Obstruction Availability of equipment	Alternative to NIVPPV
Tracheostomy Ventilation	Ventilation Tracheal suction Reduce aspiration	Increased tracheal secretions Potential tracheal complications Additional equipment needed (humidification, suction machine . . .) Labor intensive—needs suctioning, trade maintenance (NM or severely handicapped)	Unweanable from invasive Contraindications of NIV Swallowing disorders Inability to clear secretion Failure of NIV High dependency of NIV

Table 9 Clinical Responses to Long-Term Mechanical Ventilation

Clinical responses	Results by etiology	
Initial PaO_2 and change after 1 year of NIPPV (PaO_2 and change are in mm Hg)	Scoliosis:	54; +10
	Sequels of TB:	52; +8
	Duchenne dystrophy:	75; +12
	Neuromuscular:	56; +14
Initial $PaCO_2$ and change after 1 year of NIPPV ($PaCO_2$ and change are in mm Hg)	Scoliosis:	53; −10
	Sequels of TB:	54; −7
	Duchenne dystrophy:	52; −8
	Neuromuscular:	61; −11
SLEEP		
Subjective sleepiness	improved	
Total sleep time	improved	
Efficiency	improved	
Nocturnal oxygenation	improved	
Pulmonary function test	unchanged	
Inspiratory muscle force	improved	
Inspiratory muscle endurance	improved	
Quality of life	improved	
Intolerance: % of patients who voluntarily interrupt NIPPV	Scoliosis	7%
	Sequels of TB	1%
	DMD	0%
Reduction in the number of days of hospitalization comparing before and after initiation of NIPPV	Significant for all restrictive patients during the first two years	

Source: Ref. 62.

B. Neuromuscular Disorders

In contrast to the situation with chest wall deformities, patients with neuromuscular disease receiving LTMV are increasing in number. This is due not only to advances in home health care (although the Budget Balancing Act of 1997 in the United States has reversed some of these gains) but also to the greater use of NPPV in this population of patients (73), who previously were often offered no ventilator options (74). In addition, the expanding knowledge of genetics and the potential for future novel and effective therapies have encouraged more interest in supporting these patients.

Neuromuscular diseases are not homogeneous and major differences exist among the various syndromes (75). Some are inherited and others are acquired. Some become manifest during infancy and others not until the senior years. The pattern of respiratory muscle involvement also varies considerably, sometimes even within the same disease category. For example, patients with amyotrophic lateral sclerosis (ALS, also referred to as motor neuron disease) may present with bulbar involvement, weakness of the inspiratory or expiratory muscles, any combination of these defects, or no respiratory muscle involvement whatsoever. In some cases, even the cardiac muscle may be affected (76).

Only some patients with neuromuscular disease develop severe respiratory insufficiency and need long-term mechanical ventilation. The proportion depends on the underlying disease, the pattern of respiratory muscle involvement and the rate of progression. The following discusses the natural history and response to LTMV of the more common neuromuscular syndromes.

Postpolio Syndrome

The victims of the polio epidemics were the pioneers of LTMV. Many used various forms of chronic ventilatory assistance, both invasive and noninvasive, for years after developing respiratory paralysis. Considering that the last polio epidemic occurred during the middle 1950s, many early survivors of acute respiratory paralysis who used LTMV have since expired. However, patients with the postpolio syndrome continue to come to medical attention, sometimes developing respiratory insufficiency late in life. This syndrome is thought to arise from the gradual dropout of neurons in areas of previous involvement by acute poliomyelitis. Some of these patients, whether ventilated or not during the acute phase of their disease, will progressively develop severe chronic respiratory failure and need ventilatory support.

The presence of thoracic deformity and respiratory muscle paralysis/weakness further aggravates the respiratory impairment of postpolio patients and can predispose to sleep-disordered breathing disorders. Patients with scoliosis have lower vital capacities and more severe disturbances in blood gas tensions than those without scoliosis. Hypercarbia is likely when patients have FVC <50% predicted, except for patients with the sequelae of bulbar poliomyelitis, including dysphagia or dysarthria, who may have hypercarbia even if FVC exceeds 50%. Not surprisingly, severe restriction and hypercarbia are associated with a poor prognosis (69).

The outcomes of postpolio patients receiving long-term ventilatory assistance, whether noninvasive or invasive, have been excellent. These patients have very slowly progressive conditions and may remain stable for many years. In their series of tracheostomized patients living at home, Robert et al. (63) reported a 5 year survival of 95% among their postpolio patients (see Table 8). In Simonds' survey of long-term NPPV (58), the continuation rate for postpolio patients was 100%. Considering that the last large polio epidemic was over 40 yr ago, surviving postpolio patients are among the longest users of LTMV. As was the case with thoracic deformities, NPPV is the ventilator modality of first choice for postpolio patients, unless they have severe bulbar involvement.

Spinal Cord Injury

Patients with spinal cord injury are increasing in number as therapeutic and rehabilitative options expand (77). Patients are divided into several categories depending on the level of spinal cord involvement. The diaphragm is innervated by C3 through C5 via the phrenic nerve. Accessory muscles of breathing are innervated by C5 through C8, and the thoracic nerves innervate the expiratory muscles (internal intercostals and abdominals). Thus, patients with C1 through C3 lesions have paralysis of both inspiratory and expiratory muscles and require acute and long-term ventilator support (78). Those with C4 or C5 lesions usually require ventilatory assistance acutely, but may have sufficient diaphragm function so that 50 to 80% wean eventually (79). Among those patients unable to wean from mechanical ventilation, if there is no concomitant head injury and upper airway muscles are intact, many are candidates for long-term mechanical ventilation in the home using noninvasive techniques (80).

Patients with C5 or C6 injuries sometimes require ventilatory support acutely, but diaphragm function should be intact. Thus, many of these patients are weaned and, as long as cough assistance is provided when needed, only a small percentage will require prolonged mechanical ventilation. Like the postpolio patients, some spinal cord injury patients may need ventilatory assistance when they become older. Both diseases usually progress very slowly, patients have time to adapt to the additional constraints related to the chronic respiratory insufficiency and the need for ventilatory support, and long-term survival rates are favorable (81).

Patients with high (C1 or C2) spinal cord lesions are usually left with intact bulbar function and, unless there was premorbid lung disease, should have structurally normal lungs. Accordingly, there are numerous options for ventilatory support (77,80). Endotracheal intubation with an early tracheostomy is the standard initial approach. Respiratory complications, including atelectasis, pneumonia, and pulmonary embolism, are common during this period and direct airway access is advantageous. Once stabilization has occurred, attempts to wean the patient from mechanical ventilation are indicated. If the patient has an inadequate vital capacity or fatigues easily during weaning trials, aggressive further weaning attempts may be counterproductive. Positive pressure ventilation via a tracheostomy is usually continued in this setting, although switching to noninvasive ventilation can also be considered (81) (see Chapter 11).

If noninvasive ventilation is desired, NPPV, either via a nose mask or mouthpiece, is the noninvasive method of first choice for nocturnal ventilatory assistance in quadriplegics (77,80). For daytime ventilatory assistance, abdominal insufflation belts can be used by some patients because they permit unimpeded speech (82). Mouthpiece positive pressure ventilation can be used for daytime use if the patient can turn the head enough to use a gooseneck apparatus attached to a wheelchair (77). Success with negative pressure ventilation has also been reported (81), but sleep should be monitored in these patients to assess the frequency and severity of obstructive apneas.

If noninvasive ventilation is selected, the patient should be taught glossopharyngeal breathing before decannulation. This technique permits up to several hours of ventilator-free time, and patients can be taught to "stack" breaths to enhance cough effectiveness (83). Some patients may be interested in having diaphragm pacers implanted as a means of freeing themselves from other mechanical ventilators, but the tracheostomy usually cannot be removed because of induction of apneas during sleep. Diaphragm pacers are expensive, at least initially, but advances in technology have facilitated placement and they are reliable means of providing ventilator support in high quadriplegics (84). Unfortunately, few comparative data are available to help in weighing the various options, so it is difficult to advise patients on the possible choices, other than to make suggestions based on personal preferences and biases.

Regardless of the ventilatory mode chosen, however, a severely weakened cough mechanism is universal in patients with high spinal cord lesions, so secretion removal must be a top priority. Close attention to assisting cough has decreased the incidence of pulmonary complications and need for ventilatory support after acute quadriplegia (85). Few long-term outcome studies have been done on high quadriplegics, but 5-yr mortality rates as high as 67% have been reported (78), reflecting the high complication rates (pneumonias, tracheal trauma, barotrauma) of long-term invasive ventilation.

Muscular Dystrophies

Duchenne muscular dystrophy has an X-linked recessive inheritance pattern and is the most common of the muscular dystrophies. It has a predictable rate of progression, with deterioration in functional abilities occurring between ages 8 and 12 leading to the inability to walk at approximately age 12 (86). Progressive respiratory muscle weakness leads to death at around age 20, although severe myocardiopathy also contributes to death in roughly 20% of cases (87). The FVC increases normally during infancy and early childhood, followed by a plateau during adolescence and a decline during late adolescence. During the decline phase, the average drop in FVC is 8.5% per year; the decline becomes more pronounced when the FVC falls below 1.7 L reaching a rate of 25% per year at the age 20 (88).

Respiratory function is worse for patients whose neuromuscular disease is complicated by spinal deformity, which compounds the ventilatory restriction. Patients whose neuromuscular impairment is manifest during infancy are at higher risk of developing spinal deformity, and should be closely monitored so that orthopedic intervention or surgery can be performed at the appropriate time to limit the deformity. Spinal fusion surgery should be considered when the angle of curvature progresses to 35 to 45° (89). Surgery improves patient comfort and appearance during sitting but does not seem to significantly slow the decline in respiratory function in the short term or at 5-yr follow-up (90). Also in DMD patients, if surgery is to be done, it must be performed before the occurrence of major cardiac involvement.

Ninety percent of patients require ventilatory assistance by age 20 if prolongation of survival is desired (50,75). During the late 1970s and early 1980s, DMD patients who were given assisted ventilation received either tracheostomy or negative pressure ventilation (74). DMD patients treated with negative pressure ventilation have survival extended an average of 6.3 yr, but have an increased need for ventilatory assistance of approximately 1 hr/24 hr/yr, and may eventually require tracheostomy (50,90). In addition, a large proportion of DMD patients have obstructive apneas while using negative pressure ventilation during sleep (91) that are eliminated by switching to NPPV (92). For this and for reasons of comfort and convenience, NPPV has replaced negative pressure ventilation as the ventilator modality of choice.

Tracheostomy and NPPV are estimated to increase survival in DMD by 7.9 and 4.5 yr, respectively (64,91). In an uncontrolled study, Vianello et al. (93) reported that 4 of 5 DMD patients treated with NPPV were alive after 2 yr, whereas only 1 of 5 similar patients who refused NPPV survived. However, outcomes of NPPV in DMD patients differ in the two large long-term surveys of NPPV users. Simonds et al. (58) found that 1- and 5-yr survival rates were 85% and 73%, respectively. Leger et al. (62), on the other hand, found that only 47% of the patients were still using NPPV after 3 yr, with some patients having switched to tracheostomies because of adverse effects or inadequate support during nasal ventilation. The differences between the two studies may be related to differences in the patient populations or in other therapeutic strategies, such as the aggressiveness of application of techniques to assist coughing. Nonetheless, it appears that survival of DMD patients using NPPV is not as good as that of patients with thoracic deformities or polio, mainly because of the more progressive nature of the disease and the contribution of cardiomyopathy. It also appears that although studies have not directly compared the two modalities, NPPV patients wishing to maximize survival should eventually switch to tracheostomy ventilation for better airway protection.

Becker muscular dystrophy is a more slowly progressive variant of DMD that shares a similar genetic defect and inheritance pattern (94). By definition, these patients remain ambulatory until after age 15, have a slow deterioration in pulmonary function thereafter, and usually survive into their fourth or fifth decades. Many require ventilatory assistance during adulthood, but generally not before their late 20s or 30s. No large series have evaluated outcomes in these patients specifically, but anecdotal reports suggest that outcomes with NPPV are as favorable as with other neuromuscular diseases (94).

A variety of other muscular dystrophies have different patterns of involvement and inheritance than DMD, but may also require ventilatory assistance. The *spinal muscular atrophies (SMA)* are a group of inherited neuromuscular disorders characterized by degeneration of the anterior horn cells of the spinal column (93). Infants with these disorders have reduced muscle tone and difficulty with motor tasks such as sitting (94). As the name implies, spinal muscles are involved early on, leading to spinal deformation. However, limb and other muscles are also involved, and individuals with advanced disease become quadriplegic. Four variants of SMA have been described, with types 1 and 2 having a rapid progression leading to early paralysis and death, often within a few years of birth. Types 3 and 4 have slower progression and permit life into adulthood, although muscle weakness leads to difficulty with ambulating. Severe ventilatory restriction characterizes the more advanced forms of this disease, and death is usually caused by progressive respiratory failure (93,94).

Limb girdle muscular dystrophy and *fascio-scapulo-humeral dystrophy* also cause restrictive ventilatory defects that lead to respiratory insufficiency during the third or fourth decades of life and sometimes later (95). Diaphragm dysfunction may contribute to the ventilatory insufficiency and accelerate the progression to chronic hypoventilation. Based on case reports and small series (96,97), these entities also respond favorably to NPPV, although no large series of patients has been reported.

Myotonic dystrophy is an inherited disorder that is characterized by a distinct pattern of temporal wasting and frontal balding and leads to a restrictive ventilatory impairment during middle age, sometimes with diaphragm paralysis (98). The restriction is frequently accompanied by breathing disorders during sleep, such as obstructive or central apnea, and central hypoventilation may contribute to the ventilatory defect (98). Cardiac involvement may also occur, often leading to arrhythmias and cardiac conduction disturbances. Even when their pulmonary function is relatively well preserved, these patients should be followed vigilantly for symptoms of hypoventilation because of the possible contribution of central hypoventilation. They respond well to NPPV, other noninvasive ventilators, or, sometimes, if obstructive sleep apnea has been excluded, oral progesterone supplementation (authors' personal observations).

Metabolic myopathies such as *acid maltase deficiency* can affect respiratory muscles predominantly. Symptoms of weakness or hypoventilation can be minimal and the disease may not become apparent until the patient experiences a stress, such as general anesthesia for surgery (99). Under other circumstances, the discovery of hypercarbia in a symptomatic patient suggests the diagnosis of acid maltase deficiency when the hypercarbia is out of proportion to the degree of respiratory muscle weakness.

Amyotrophic Lateral Sclerosis

Amyotrophic lateral sclerosis, also called motor neuron disease or Lou Gehrig's disease, is a degenerative neuropathy of unknown etiology that affects adults beginning in their 30s and has a peak incidence in their 50s to 60s (100). Although familial occurrence has been reported and a genetic predisposition has been suspected, no inheritance pattern has been established. The disease has an estimated incidence of 5/1,000,000 and is a common indication for chronic mechanical ventilatory assistance (102).

The disease often has an insidious onset, presenting with weakness of almost any part of the body. Often the diagnosis is made many months or even a year or two after the initial manifestation, awaiting the development of a more characteristic clinical pattern. The respiratory muscles may be spared initially, but eventually become involved in all cases, and most deaths are caused by respiratory failure (101). The three main groups of respiratory muscles, upper airway (bulbar), inspiratory, and expiratory, are affected, but the pattern of involvement and subsequent evolution of the disease varies considerably among individual patients. Approximately 30% of patients present with bulbar muscle involvement (slurred speech or dysphagia), and these muscles eventually become involved in all patients who survive long enough. This leads to swallowing disturbances and chronic aspiration that are often tolerated as long as the expiratory muscles are sufficient to generate an adequate cough. Some patients also present with isolated diaphragm dysfunction, and often respond favorably to noninvasive ventilation (101).

Although recent advances in pharmacotherapy (riluzole) have prolonged survival slightly (3 mo in the average case), functional capacity and quality of life have not yet been improved. Amyotrophic lateral sclerosis remains a devastating illness. It is characterized by a relentless loss of muscular function, eventually involving all skeletal muscles, and survival after diagnosis in untreated patients averages only a year or two. Noninvasive ventilation is being used increasingly for these patients, with an apparent increase in survival (102). Gay et al. (99) reported success in 7 of 9 patients with amyotrophic lateral sclerosis as part of a larger series of patients using nasal ventilation. These 7 patients had improvements in gas exchange and symptoms, and one patient remained stable after 26 mo. However, 3 of the 7 died within 6 mo, and most of the survivors had been ventilated for a year or less.

In a prospective, but nonrandomized trial of 20 consecutive ALS patients with bulbar features, Pinto et al. (29) treated the first 10 patients with oxygen, bronchodilators, and other palliative measures, and the following 10 patients with medical therapy plus NPPV. After 2 yr, 55% of the patients using NPPV were still alive compared with none of those receiving medical therapy alone. More recently, Aboussouan et al. (104) found that nasal NPPV was tolerated in 18 of 39 (46%) patients with respiratory insufficiency due to ALS. Risk of death was reduced by a factor of 3.1 if patients tolerated NPPV, and even though swallowing dysfunction is ordinarily considered a relative contraindication to the use of noninvasive ventilation, patients with bulbar involvement who tolerated NPPV also had improved survival. Bulbar involvement halved the likelihood of tolerating the device, however.

Despite the apparent success of NPPV in prolonging life for these unfortunate patients, they eventually become so weakened that they are unable to protect their airway. If they desire continued survival, tracheostomy ventilation becomes the only option. There is some question about how effective invasive ventilation is in prolonging survival. Bach et al. (105) found no difference in survival between 31 ALS patients institutionalized and tracheotomized and 21 patients who remained in the community mainly using NPPV (78%). However, this study was not controlled, and the institutionalized patients may have been sicker. When ALS progresses to the point at which patients cannot protect their airway, tracheostomy ventilation almost certainly prolongs survival, at least for awhile. However, considering that the disease eventually progresses to a "locked-in" state and may place a large burden on caregivers, it is arguable whether this prolongation merely amounts to an increase in quantity and not quality of life. As discussed above, this determination can only be made by the individual patient, but with the exception of ambulatory patients who have severe disproportinate bulbar involvement leading to chronic aspiration or vocal cord paralysis, tracheostomy is not an attractive option for most patients with this devastating disease.

Multiple Sclerosis

Like ALS, multiple sclerosis is a neuropathy of unknown cause that can involve all respiratory muscle groups including bulbar. Unlike ALS though, the disease progresses in fits and starts, and respiratory failure is a late and not inevitable manifestation, sometimes occurring decades after the initial diagnosis. Multiple sclerosis patients who develop respiratory failure usually experience an insidious onset. Nasal or mouth NPPV is the ventilator modality of choice (106), but tracheostomy ventilation may be necessary if bulbar involvement is severe. Negative pressure ventilation has also been used successfully in patients with intact bulbar function (107).

The decision to initiate mechanical ventilation raises ethical issues in patients with multiple sclerosis, just as it does in ALS patients. Most patients are still ambulatory when they develop chronic respiratory failure and elect to receive noninvasive ventilation (108). However, if significant bulbar involvement develops, tracheostomy ventilation may be necessary for adequate ventilatory support. This decision should be discussed with patients and their families well in advance of the need, so that emotional turmoil can be minimized. If invasive PPV is declined, referral to a home-based hospice program is advisable as patients approach the end stages of their disease.

Bilateral Diaphragm Paralysis

Bilateral diaphragm paralysis causes chronic respiratory failure that is characterized by sleep-disordered breathing, nocturnal hypoventilation, and orthopnea. It may occur as an isolated idiopathic entity, in association with other neuromuscular conditions such as ALS or multiple sclerosis, or as a consequence of surgery or trauma (109). Success with several different modes of noninvasive ventilation has been reported in the therapy of bilateral diaphragmatic paralysis. Negative pressure ventilation has been used and rocking beds have particular appeal because they assist diaphragm motion during sleep. In one series of patients with bilateral diaphragmatic paralysis occurring after cardiac surgery, the rocking bed was used to assist nocturnal ventilation until diaphragm function returned after 4 to 27 mo (110). Among noninvasive positive pressure modes, continuous positive airway pressure (CPAP) may be useful by shifting the active phase of the respiratory cycle to the expiratory muscles. However, more recently, nasal NPPV has been the main modality used (111).

C. Central Hypoventilatory Disorders

Central Alveolar Hypoventilation

This refers to hypoventilation that develops in the absence of underlying chest wall deformity or neuromuscular or lung disease. The problem occurs most often in infants, children, or young adults. The most common symptoms are fatigue, hypersomnolence, and morning headaches. Often, respiratory complaints are entirely absent, making the diagnosis difficult and placing the patient at risk of sudden respiratory compromise. The astute clinician may recognize the symptom complex as that of hypoventilation and obtain an arterial blood gas, but often the problem is discovered accidentally at the time of surgical anesthesia or when patients are given a hypnotic for sleep-related symptoms that precipitates a bout of acute respiratory failure (112).

The diagnosis of central alveolar hypoventilation is made when pulmonary function studies reveal no obstructive or restrictive defect to explain the hypoventilation, thyroid function tests are normal, and there is no evidence of a neuromuscular process (such as diaphragm paralysis or acid maltase deficiency). Despite these findings, the arterial blood gas shows CO_2 retention that is often aggravated by sleep. A sleep study should be obtained to rule out obstructive sleep apnea and demonstrate the characteristic sustained oxygen desaturation that occurs in association with increased hypoventilation during stages 3 and 4 sleep. In general, ventilation during REM sleep is preserved or less affected than during slow wave sleep. Once the above studies have ruled out alternative explanations for the hypoventilation, the definitive test is to show that the response to hypercarbia or hypoxia is severely attenuated. When hypoventilation is markedly exaggerated by sleep, as occurs in some individuals, the condition has been referred to as Ondine's curse (113).

The cause of central hypoventilation is thought to be a lack of central drive, either because of a failure to receive or respond to chemoreceptor feedback, or an inherent defect in the respiratory center. Central hypoventilation can be congenital or acquired as part of a number of neurologic syndromes, including cerebrovascular accidents involving the brain stem, myotonic dystrophy, as mentioned above, and Shy-Drager syndrome, among others (113). Some of these patients respond to pharmacologic respiratory stimulants such as progesterone (114). In the past, patients with central hypoventilation have also been treated successfully with diaphragm pacers (115) or negative pressure ventilators (116). However, NPPV is now considered the ventilatory modality of first choice, and most patients respond favorably to it.

Obesity Hypoventilation Syndrome

The obesity hypoventilation syndrome (OHS) occurs in the morbidly obese (>30% overweight), but relatively few such individuals actually have the syndrome. Other factors besides obesity alone seem to be responsible for hypoventilation, including decreased chest wall compliance and smaller lung volumes (TLC 20% smaller and MVV 40% lower) compared with similarly obese eucapnic subjects (117). In addition, compared with eucapnic obese individuals, OHS patients have a 40% reduction in maximal inspiratory pressure, a higher work of breathing (250% higher), and a greater CO_2 production. The breathing pattern also differs, as patients with OHS breathe more rapidly and shallowly.

A defect in the central respiratory controller appears to be the most important contributing factor, as the ventilatory response to CO_2 rebreathing and/or hypoxia is markedly attenuated (117). Many obese patients with hypoventilation also have obstructive sleep apnea, and it is important to obtain a polysomnogram to evaluate this possibility.

Like patients with other central hypoventilatory syndromes, patients with OHS may respond to pharmacologic respiratory stimulants. Noninvasive ventilation is also commonly effective, although high inspiratory pressures may be necessary because of the high respiratory impedance related to the large chest wall mass. Patients with OHS who fail to tolerate NPPV are poor candidates for alternative so-called "body" noninvasive ventilators because of difficulty with application (118), and usually require tracheostomies.

X. Summary and Conclusions

The restrictive thoracic disorders are a disparate group of illnesses that are characterized by low lung volumes. They fall into two main pathophysiologic categories: restriction due to chest wall stiffness (thoracic deformities) and restriction due to muscle weakness (neuromuscular processes). Central hypoventilatory disorders are sometimes lumped together with the others, because the net effect of all is to limit the capacity to generate an adequate minute volume, predisposing to hypoventilation. The various disorders differ markedly with regard to natural history, patterns of muscle involvement, and prognosis.

Although advances are rapidly being made concerning the genetic and biochemical defects that give rise to the disorders, very few effective pharmacologic therapies are currently available, and respiratory failure remains an inevitable consequence of most of them. Thus, assisted ventilation remains the main therapeutic intervention when ventilatory insufficiency occurs. The single most important development during the past 15 years has been the increasing use of NPPV to treat these diseases. NPPV has greatly extended survival and improved quality of life for many patients with restrictive thoracic diseases, obviating the need for tracheostomy and its attendant risks of complications. In general, NPPV is reserved for patients who have developed symptomatic hypoventilation, whether continuous or nocturnal only.

When implemented successfully, NPPV can be expected to improve gas exchange, symptoms, sleep quality, quality of life, and sometimes, pulmonary function and exercise capacity. However, NPPV is most effective when bulbar function is intact and may be ineffective in the face of severe bulbar involvement. Also, occasional patients fail to tolerate NPPV or are inadequately ventilated by it. Thus, some patients continue to receive tracheostomies, although this should only be done after the patient and family are fully informed about the consequences of living with a tracheostomy.

References

1. Kearon C, Viviani GR, Kirkley A, Killian KJ. Factors determining pulmonary function in adolescent idiopathic thoracic scoliosis. Am Rev Respir Dis 1993; 148:288–294.
2. Strumpf DA, Millman RP, Hill NS. The management of chronic hypoventilation. Chest 1990; 948:474–480.
3. Pehrsson K, Bake B, Larsson S, Nachemson A. Lung function in adult idiopathic scoliosis: A 20 year follow up. Thorax 1991; 46:474–478.
4. Kafer E. Idiopathic scoliosis. Gas exchange and the age dependence of arterial blood gases. J Clin Invest 1976; 58:825–833.
5. Kafer E. Idiopathic scoliosis. Mechanical properties of the respiratory system and the ventilatory response to carbon dioxide. J Clin Invest 1975; 55:1153–1163.
6. Black LF, Hyatt RE. Maximal respiratory pressures: Normal values and relationship to age and sex. Am Rev Respir Dis 1969; 99:696–702.
7. Bach JR, Ishikawa Y, Kim H. Prevention of pulmonary morbidity for patients with Duchenne muscular dystrophy. Chest 1997; 112:1024–1028.
8. Bergofsky EH. Respiratory insufficiency in mechanical and neuromuscular disorders of the thorax. In Roussos C, ed. The Thorax. New York: Marcel Dekker, 1995; 1556–1566.

9. McNicholas WT. Impact of sleep in respiratory failure. Eur Respir J 1997; 10:920–933.
10. Smith PEM, Calverly PMA, Edwards RHT. Hypoxemia during sleep in Duchenne muscular dystrophy. Am Rev Respir Dis 1988; 137:884–888.
11. George CF, Kryger MH. Sleep in restrictive lung disease. Sleep 1987; 10(5):409–418.
12. Sawicka EH, Branthwaite MA. Respiration during sleep in kyphoscoliosis. Thorax 1987; 42:801–808.
13. Piper AJ, Sullivan CE. Sleep-disordered breathing in neuromuscular disease. In Saunders NA, Sullivan CE, eds. Sleep and Breathing. 2nd ed. New York: Marcel Dekker, 1994; 761–786.
14. Bye PTP, Ellis ER, Issa FG, Donnelly PM, Sullivan CE. Respiratory failure and sleep in neuromuscular disease. Thorax 1990; 45:241–247.
15. Roussos CH. Respiratory muscle fatigue in the hypercapnic patient. Bull Eur Physiopathol Respir 1979; 15:117–123.
15. Roussos C. Function and fatigue of respiratory muscles. Chest 1985; 88:24S–132S.
16. White J, Bullock RE, Hudgson P, Gibson GJ. Neuromuscular disease, respiratory failure and cor pulmonale. Postgrad Med J 1992; 68,804:820–3.
17. Bergofsky EH. Respiratory failure in disorders of the thoracic cage. Am Rev Respir Dis 1979; 119:643–669.
18. Brooke MH, Fenichel GM, Griggs RC, et al. Clinical investigation of Duchenne muscular dystrophy. Arch Neurol 1987; 44:812–817.
19. Ferguson KA, Strong MJ, Ahmad D, George CF. Sleep disordered breathing in amyotrophic lateral sclerosis. Chest 1996; 110:664–669.
20. Gibson GJ. Diaphragmatic paresis: Pathophysiology, clinical features and investigation. Thorax; 1989, 44:960–964.
21. Braun NMT, Arora NS, Rochester DF. Respiratory muscle and pulmonary function in polymyositis and other proximal myopathies. Thorax 1983; 38:616–623.
22. Bach JR, Saporito LR. Indications and criteria for decannulation and transition from invasive to noninvasive long-term ventilatory support. Respir Care 1994; 39:515–531.
23. Sanders MH, Kern NB, Costantino JP, et al. Accuracy of end-tidal and transcutaneous PCO_2 monitoring during sleep. Chest 1994; 106:472–483.
24. Bach JR, Intintola P, Alba AS, Holland I. The ventilator-assisted individual: Cost analysis of institutionalization versus rehabilitation and in-home management. Chest 1992; 101:26–30.
25. Rideau Y, Gatin G, Bach J, Gines G. Prolongation of life in Duchenne's muscular dystrophy. Acta Neurol 1983; 5:118–124.
26. Raphael JC, Chevret S, Chastang C, et al. French multicenter trial of prophylactic nasal ventilation in Duchenne muscular dystrophy. Lancet 1994; 343:1600–1604.
27. Masa Jimenez JF, De cos Escuin JS, Vicente CD, Valle MH, Otero FF. Nasal intermittent positive pressure ventilation: Analysis of its withdrawal. Chest 1995; 107:382–388.
28. Strumpf DA, Carlisle CC, Millman RP, et al. An evaluation of the Respironics BiPAP bi-level CPAP device for delivery of assisted ventilation. Respir Care 1990; 35:415–422.

29. Pinto AC, Evangelista T, Carvalho M, Alves MA, Sales Luis ML. Respiratory assistance with a non-invasive ventilator (BiPAP) in MND/ALS patients: Survival rates in a controlled trial. J Neurol Sci 1995; 129(suppl):19–26.
30. Adams AB, Shapiro R, and Marini JJ. Changing prevalence of chronically ventilator-assisted individuals in Minnesota: Increases, characteristics, and the use of noninvasive ventilation. Respir Care 1998; 43:643–649.
31. Ferguson GT and Gilmartin M. CO_2 rebreathing during BiPAP ventilatory assistance. Am J Respir Crit Care Med 1995; 151:1126–1135.
32. Meyer TJ, Pressman MR, Benditt J, McCool FD, Millman RP, Natarajan R, Hill NS. Air leaking through the mouth during nocturnal nasal ventilation: Effect on sleep quality. Sleep 1997; 20:561–569.
33. Branthwaite MA. Noninvasive and domiciliary ventilation: Positive pressure techniques. Thorax 1991; 46:208–212.
34. Bach JR, Alba AS, Saporito LR. Intermittent positive pressure ventilation via the mouth as an alternative to tracheostomy for 257 ventilator users. Chest 1993; 103: 174–182.
35. Bach JR. A comparison of long-term ventilatory support alternatives from the perspective of the patient and care giver. Chest 1993; 104:1702–1706.
36. Schneiderman LJ, Jecker NS, et al. Medical futility: Its meaning and ethical implications. Ann Intern Med 1990; 112:949–954.
37. Moss AH, Casey P. Home ventilation for amyotrophic lateral sclerosis patients: Outcomes, costs and patient, family and physician attitudes. Neurology 1993; 43: 438–443.
38. Hill NS, Eveloff SE, Carlisle CC, et al. Efficacy of nocturnal nasal ventilation in patients with restrictive thoracic disease. Am Rev Respir Dis 1992; 101:516–521.
39. Hill NS, Redline S, Carskadon MA, Curran FJ, Millman RP. Sleep-disordered breathing in patients with Duchenne muscular dystrophy using negative pressure ventilators. Chest 1992; 102:1656–1662.
40. Kinnear WJM, Johnston IDA. Does Harrington instrumentation improve pulmonary function in adolescents with idiopathic scoliosis? A meta-analysis. Spine 1993; 8:1556–1559.
41. Hill NS, Eveloff SE, Carlisle CC, Goff SG. Efficacy of nocturnal nasal ventilation in patients with restrictive thoracic disease. Am Rev Respir Dis 1992; 145:365–371.
42. Barbé F, Quera-Salva MA, de Lattre J, Gajdos P, Agusti A. Long-term effects of nasal intermittent positive-pressure ventilation on pulmonary function and sleep architecture in patients with neuromuscular diseases. Chest 1996; 110:1179–1183.
43. Goldstein RS, Molotiu N, Skrastins R, Lone S, De Rosie J, Contrera M, et al. Reversal of sleep induced hypoventilation and chronic respiratory failure by nocturnal negative ventilation in patients with restrictive ventilatory impairment. Am Rev Respir Dis 1987; 135:1049–55.
44. Gay PC, Patel AM, Viggiano RW, Hubmayr RD. Nocturnal nasal ventilation for treatment of patients with hypercapnic respiratory failure. Mayo Clin Proc 1991; 66:695–703.
45. Bach JR, Robert D, Leger P, Langevin B. Sleep fragmentation in kyphoscoliotic individuals with alveolar hypoventilation treated by NIPPV. Chest 1995; 107: 1552–1558.

46. Meyer TJ, Pressman MR, Benditt J, McCool FD, Millman RP, Natarajan R, Hill NS. Air leaking through the mouth during nocturnal nasal ventilation: Effect on sleep quality. Sleep 1997; 20:561–569.
47. Piper AJ, Sullivan CE. Sleep-disordered breathing in neuromuscular disease. In: Saunders NA, Sullivan CE, eds. Sleep and Breathing. 2nd ed. New York: Marcel Dekker, 1994; 761–786.
48. Annane D, Quera-Salva MA, Lofaso F, Vercken JB, Lesieur O, Fromageot C, Clair B, Gajdos P, Raphael JC. Mechanisms underlying effects of nocturnal ventilation on daytime blood gases in neuromuscular diseases. Eur Respir J 1999; 13:157–162.
49. Schonhofer B, Geibel M, Sonneborn M, Haidl P, Kohler D. Daytime mechanical ventilation in chronic respiratory insufficiency. Eur Respir J 1997; 10:2840–2846.
50. Mohr CH, Hill NS. Long-term follow-up of nocturnal ventilatory assistance in patients with respiratory failure due to Duchenne-type muscular dystrophy. Chest 1990; 97:91–96.
51. Heckmatt JZ, Loh L, Dubowitz V. Night-time nasal ventilation in neuromuscular disease. Lancet 1990; 335:579–582.
52. Goldstein RS, De Rosie JA, Avendano MA, et al. Influence of noninvasive positive pressure ventilation on inspiratory muscles. Chest 1991; 99:408–415.
53. Braun NMT, Arora NS, Rochester DF. Respiratory muscle and pulmonary function in polymyositis and other proximal myopathies. Thorax 1983; 38:616–623.
54. Diaz Neg. $PaCO_2$.
55. Schoenhoffer ERJ. 99 Exercise.
56. Long Term O_2.
57. Schonhofer BM, Wenzel T, Barchfeld, Kohler D. Long-term effects of noninvasive mechanical ventilation of pulmonary hemodynamics in patients with chronic respiratory failure. Eur Respir J (in press).
58. Simonds AK, Elliott MW. Outcome of domiciliary nasal positive pressure ventilation in restrictive and obstructive disorders. Thorax 1995; 50:604–609.
59. Guyatt GH, Berman LB, Townsend M, Pugsley SO, Chambers LW. The measure of quality of life for clinical trials in chronic lung disease. Thorax 1987; 42:773–778.
60. Simonds AK, Muntoni F, Heather S, Fielding S. Impact of nasal ventilation on survival in hypercapnic Duchenne muscular dystrophy. Thorax 1998; 53:949–952.
61. Bach JR, Campagnolo DI, Hoeman S. Life satisfaction of individuals with Duchenne muscular dystrophy using long term mechanical ventilatory support. Am J Phys Med Rehabil 1991 70; 3:129–135.
62. Leger P, Bedicam JM, Cornette A, Reybet-Degat O, Langevin B, Polu JM, Jeannin L, Robert D. Nasal IPPV: Long term follow up in patients with severe chronic respiratory insufficiency. Chest 1994; 105:100–105.
63. Robert D, Gerard M, Leger P, et al. La ventilation mechanique a domicile definitive par tracheostomie de l'insuffisant respiratoir chronique. Rev Fr Mal Resp 1983; 11:923–936.
64. Kinear WJM, Johnston IDA. Does Harrington instrumentation improve pulmonary function in adolescents with idiopathic scoliosis? A meta-analysis. Spine 1993; 8: 1556–1559.

65. Wong CA, Cole AA, Watson L, Webb JK, Johnston IDA, Kinnear WJM. Pulmonary function before and after anterior spinal surgery in adult idiopathic scoliosis. Thorax 1996; 51:534–536.
66. Bredin CP. Pulmonary function in long-term survivors of thoracoplasty. Chest 1989; 85:18–20.
67. Philips MS, Kinnear WJM, Shneerson J. Late sequelae of pulmonary tuberculosis treated by thoracoplasty. Thorax 1987; 42:445–51.
68. Ricou B, Junod AF. Hypoventilation alvéolaire isolée dans les séquelles tuberculeuses. Rev Mal Resp 1990; 7:147–151.
69. Midgren B. Lung function and clinical outcome in postpolio patients: A prospective cohort study during 11 years. Eur Respir J 1997: 10:146–149.
70. Jackson M, Kinnear W, King M, Hockley S, Shneerson J. The effects of five years of nocturnal cuirass assisted ventilation in chest wall disease. Eur Respir J 1993; 6:630–635.
71. Jackson M, Smith I, King M, Shneerson J. Long term non-invasive domiciliary assisted ventilation for respiratory failure following thoracoplasty. Thorax 1994; 49:915–919.
72. Levy RD, Bradley TD, Newman SL, et al. Negative pressure ventilation: Effects on ventilation during sleep in normal subjects. Chest 1989; 5:95–99.
73. Adams AB, Whitman J, Marcy T. Surveys of long-term ventilatory support in Minnesota: 1986 and 1992. Chest 1993; 103:1463–1469.
74. Colbert AP, Schock NC. Respirator use in progressive neuromuscular diseases. Arch Phys Med Rehabil 1985; 66:760–762.
75. Rideau Y. Management of wheelchair muscular dystrophy patient death prevention. Fourth International Congress on Neuromuscular Disease, Los Angeles. Muscle Nerve 1986; 9:55.
76. Haverkamp LJ, Appel V, Appel SH. Natural history of amyotrophic lateral sclerosis in a database population. Validation of a scoring system, and a model for survival prediction. Brain 1995; 118:707–719.
77. Bach JR, Alba AS. Noninvasive options for ventilatory support of the traumatic high level quadriplegic. Chest 1990; 98:613–619.
78. Wicks AB, Menter RR. Long-term outlook in quadriplegic patients with initial ventilator dependency. Chest 1986; 90:406–410.
79. Mansel JK, Norman JR. Respiratory complications and management of spinal cord injuries. Chest 1990; 86:358–365.
80. Bach JR, O'Connor K. Electrophrenic ventilation: A different perspective. J Am Paraplegia Soc 1991; 14:9–17.
81. Viroslav J, Rosenblatt R, Tomazevic SM. Respiratory management, survival, and quality of life for high-level traumatic tetraplegics. In Noninvasive mechanical ventilation. Respir Care Clin North Am 1996; 2:313–322.
82. Bach JR, Alba AS. Total ventilatory support by the intermittent abdominal pressure ventilator. Chest 1991; 99:630–636.
83. Bach JR, Alba AS, Bodofsky E, et al. Glossopharyngeal breathing and noninvasive aids in the management of post-polio respiratory insufficiency. Birth Defects 1987; 23:99–113.
84. Glenn WWL, Broullette RT, Dentz B, et al. Fundamental considerations in pacing

of the diaphragm for chronic ventilatory insufficiency: A multicenter study. PACE 1988; 11:2121–2127.

85. McMichan JAMA 1980.
86. Brooke MH, Fenichel GM, Griggs RC. Duchenne muscular dystrophy: Pattern of clinical progression and effects of supportive therapy. Neurology 1989; 39:475–480.
87. Smith PEM, Calverley MB, Edwards RHT, et al. Practical problems in the respiratory care of patients with muscular dystrophy. N Engl J Med 1987; 316(19):1197–1205.
88. Miller RG, Chalmers AC, Dao H, et al. The effect of spine fusion on respiratory function in Duchenne muscular dystrophy. Neurology 1991; 41:38–40.
89. Robert D, Willig TN, Paulus J, Leger P. Long-term nasal ventilation in neuromuscular disorders: Report of a consensus conference. Eur Respir J 1993; 6:599–606.
90. Curran FJ, Colbert AP. Ventilatory management in Duchenne muscular dystrophy and post poliomyelitis syndrome: Twelve years' experience. Arch Phys Med Rehabil 1989; 70:180–185.
91. Hill NS, Redline S, Carskadon MA, Curran FJ, Millman RP. Sleep-disordered breathing in patients with Duchenne muscular dystrophy using negative pressure ventilators. Chest 1992; 102:1656–1662.
92. Ellis ER, McCauley VB, Mellis C, Sullivan CE. Treatment of alveolar hypoventilation in a six-year-old girl with intermittent positive pressure ventilation through a nose mask. Am Rev Respir Dis 1987; 136:188–191.
93. Vianello A, Bevilacqua M, Salvador V, Cardaioli C, Vincenti E. Long-term nasal intermittent positive pressure ventilation in advanced Duchenne's muscular dystrophy. Chest 1994; 105:445–448.
94. McDonald CM, Abresch RT, Carter GT, Fowler WM. Jr, Johnson ER, Kilmer DD. Profiles of neuromuscular diseases: Becker's muscular dystrophy. Am J Phys Med Rehabil 1995; 74(suppl 5):S93–S103.
95. Iannacone ST. Spinal muscular atrophy. Semin Neurol 1998; 18:19–26.
96. Carter GT, Abresch RT, Fowler WMJr, Johnson ER, Kilmer DD, McDonald CM. Profiles of neuromuscular diseases: Spinal muscular atrophy. Am J Phys Med Rehabil 1995; 74(Suppl 5):S150–S159.
97. McDonald CM, Johnson ER, Abresch RT, Carter GT, Fowler WMJr, Kilmer DD. Profiles of neuromuscular diseases: Limb-girdle syndromes. Am J Phys Med Rehabil 1995; 74(Suppl 5):S117–S130.
98. Leger P, Jennequin J, Gerard M, et al. Home positive pressure ventilation via nasal mask for patients with neuromuscular weakness or restrictive lung or chest wall deformities. Respiratory Care 1989; 34:73–77.
99. Gay PC, Patel AM, Viggiano RW, et al. Nocturnal nasal ventilation for treatment of patients with hypercapnic respiratory failure. Mayo Clin Proc 1991; 66:695–703.
100. Begin P, Mathieu J, Almirall J, Grassino A. Relationship between chronic hypercapnia and inspiratory muscle weakness in myotonic dystrophy. Am J Resp Crit Care Med 1997; 156:133–139.
101. Trend PSJ, Wiles CM, Spencer GT, Morgan Hughes J, Lake BD, Patrick AD. Acid maltase deficiency in adults. Brain 1992; 108:845–860.

102. Haverkamp LJ, Appel V, Appel SH. Natural history of amyotrophic lateral sclerosis in a database population: Validation of a scoring system, and a model for survival prediction. Brain 1995; 118:707–719.
103. Schiffman PL, Belsh JM. Pulmonary function at diagnosis of amyotrophic lateral sclerosis: Rate of deterioration. Chest 1993; 103:508–513.
104. Aboussouan LS, Khan SU, Meeker DP, Stelmach K, Mitsumoto H. Effect of noninvasive positive pressure ventilation on survival in amyotrophic lateral sclerosis. Ann Intern Med 1997; 127:450–453.
105. Bach JR. ALS: Communication status and survival with ventilatory support. Am J Phys Med Rehab 72:343–349.
106. Bach JR, Ishikawa Y, Kim H. Prevention of pulmonary morbidity for patients with Duchenne muscular dystrophy. Chest 1997; 112:1024–1028.
107. Splaingard ML, Frates RC Jr, Harrison GM, et al. Home-positive-pressure ventilation: Twenty years' experience. Chest 1983; 84:376–384.
108. Kelly B, Luce JM. The diagnosis and management of neuromuscular disease causing respiratory failure. Chest 1991; 99:1485–1494.
109. Gibson GJ. Diaphragmatic paresis: Pathophysiology, clinical features and investigation. Thorax 1989; 44:960–964.
110. Abd AG, Braun NMT, Baskin MI, et al. Diaphragmatic dysfunction after open heart surgery: Treatment with a rocking bed. Ann Intern Med 1991; 111:881–886.
111. Lin MC, Liaw MY, Huang CC, Chuang ML, Tsai YH. Bilateral diaphragmatic paralysis—a rare cause of acute respiratory failure managed with nasal mask bilevel positive airway pressure (BiPAP) ventilation. Eur Respir J 1997; 10:1922–1924.
112. Idiopathic congenital central hypoventilation syndrome: Diagnosis and management. Am J Resp Crit Care Med 1999; 160:368–373.
113. Central Hypovent
114. Progest
115. Moxham J, Shneerson JM. Diaphragmatic pacing. Am Rev Respir Dis 1993; 148: 533–536.
116. Celli B, Lee H, Criner G, et al. Diaphragm paralysis.
117. Rapoport DM, Garay SM, Goldring RM. Chronic hypercapnia in obstructive sleep apnea syndrome: A re-evaluation of the pickwickian syndrome. Chest 1986; 89: 627–635.
118. Hill NS. Clinical applications of body ventilators. Chest 1986; 90:897–905.

7

Long-Term Mechanical Ventilation in Severe COPD

MARK W. ELLIOTT

St. James's University Hospital
Leeds, England

I. Introduction

Chronic obstructive pulmonary disease (COPD) is the most common cause of respiratory failure worldwide and is associated with considerable morbidity and mortality (1,2). The aim of pharmacologic therapy is to alleviate symptoms by reversing correctable abnormalities, but in many patients the changes are largely irreversible. In time, patients develop respiratory failure, pulmonary hypertension, and cor pulmonale. Once peripheral edema supervenes, the prognosis is very poor with a 5-yr mortality of between 70 and 100% (3). Therefore various therapeutic strategies have been developed to treat the consequences of chronic airway obstruction in an attempt to improve survival and reduce symptoms. These include long-term oxygen therapy (LTOT), respiratory stimulant drugs, and mechanically assisted ventilation.

Following a number of preliminary, uncontrolled studies suggesting benefit, two large randomized controlled trials of domiciliary oxygen therapy were organized in the United States (Nocturnal Oxygen Therapy Trial, NOTT) and the United Kingdom (Medical Research Council, MRC) (4,5). Although the protocols were different, both showed a significant reduction in mortality. Accordingly, domiciliary oxygen therapy remains the gold standard for the treatment of chronic respiratory failure due to COPD. Nonetheless, there are a number of reasons for considering alternative therapies. In the MRC trial, there was no survival advantage from oxygen until 500 days of treatment had elapsed. The best predictor of death, and therefore a lack of benefit from oxygen, was a combination of polycythemia and hypercapnia. In contrast, the NOTT study showed that a change in hematocrit was unrelated to survival. Thus, hypercapnia alone may be responsible for the worse prognosis and lack of response to oxygen therapy. Further evidence for this hypothesis comes from the study of Cooper et al. (6) in which, although the benefit from oxygen was apparent immediately, 29 of the 57 patients who were hypercapnic at entry died during the course of the study compared with only 3 of 15 normocapnic patients. On the other hand, a study of 4552 patients with COPD in Japan did not show any difference in outcome between patients with hypercapnia and those who were normocapnic (7). Connors et al. (8) found that patients with COPD with $Paco_2$ >50 mm Hg at or just before admission to hospital had a 50% mortality at 2 yr.

The reason why hypercapnia should be associated with a worse prognosis is not clear. Although compliance with LTOT has been very good in experimental trials, this is not always the case in routine clinical practice. The main reason for noncompliance is the restriction placed upon lifestyle by the need for 16 hr of oxygen per day. Symptomatic patients are more likely to comply with therapy, whereas asymptomatic patients tend to use oxygen for insufficient time to gain a survival benefit (9,10). A further problem with LTOT is the failure to control hypercapnia, which appears to be associated with a worse prognosis (1,2,4). These limitations of LTOT suggest that a therapy such as noninvasive ventilation, which does not interfere with daily activity and reduces CO_2 tension in COPD patients, may be better tolerated and improve survival, compared with LTOT.

Early experience of noninvasive ventilation in COPD was with negative pressure devices. These were usually used for short periods in hospital with the aim of resting the respiratory muscles (11–14). However, the use of negative pressure devices at home and during sleep in patients with COPD has been largely unsuccessful (13,15); in two controlled trials patients were generally unable to sleep during negative pressure ventilation and most either failed to complete the protocol, because of lack of improvement or discomfort associated with the use of the equipment (15), or did not wish to continue treatment after the study was completed (13). Negative pressure devices are relatively inefficient, particularly when the impedance to inflation is high, and may not be able to provide adequate ventilation during sleep. All negative pressure devices predispose to the development or accentuation of upper airway collapse (16) and this may be a particular problem during sleep in the obese patient with COPD. However, these studies did suggest that it is the hypercapnic patient who is most likely to benefit from assisted ventilation. Negative pressure ventilation has largely been superseded by noninvasive positive pressure ventilation (NPPV) and, following the success of the technique in the management of patients with extrapulmonary restrictive disorders (17,18), the spotlight has switched to its use in the numerically much more common group of patients with COPD.

II. Pathophysiology of Ventilatory Failure and Symptoms in Chronic COPD

The effectiveness of assisted ventilation in restrictive chest wall disease is not surprising, given that there is a primary abnormality of the respiratory muscle pump, the patient's own ventilator. The situation is very different in COPD in that the primary abnormality lies in the patient's lungs. However, a logical case can also be made for the extension of the technique to this patient group.

To understand why assisted ventilation should be effective in improving gas exchange, even during spontaneous breathing, requires a basic understanding of the pathophysiology of ventilatory failure. For breathing to be effective, the respiratory muscles must have the capacity to sustain ventilation against a given load. It also requires neural drive from the respiratory center in the brain stem. In other words, there needs to be a balance between load and capacity with the system receiving adequate neural drive. In the patient with COPD all three of these components may be abnormal (Table 1). Changes in load, drive and capacity are neither an "all or nothing" phenomenon nor are they static. Airway obstruction has a direct effect upon load by increasing the impedance to inflation. It also leads to hyperinflation and may cause the development of intrinsic positive end-expiratory pressure (PEEPi) because alveolar emptying is incomplete by the

Table 1 Pathophysiology of Ventilatory Failure and Symptoms in Patients with Chronic COPD

Increased load
Airway obstruction
Inspiratory threshold load because of PEEPi
Pulmonary hypertension
Reduced capacity
Mechanical disadvantage due to hyperinflation
Effects of hypoxia, hypercapnia and acidosis upon muscle function
Drive
Reduced chemosensitivity because of bicarbonate retention during sleep
Sleep
Quality impaired, ?contribution of hypoxia and hypercapnia
Nocturnal desaturation, ?important in genesis of pulmonary hypertension

end of expiration. Gas flow into the alveoli occurs only when the pressure within them falls below the pressure at the mouth and nose. In the presence of PEEPi, there is an inspiratory threshold load; the first part of each inspiratory effort is wasted because gas decompression occurs without airflow. This increases the work of breathing and decreases ventilatory efficiency. Hyperinflation also reduces capacity by causing the intercostal muscles and diaphragm to be working at a mechanical disadvantage (19), which has led to the proposal that ventilatory failure occurs because of fatigue of the respiratory muscles (20). Abnormalities of the pulmonary vasculature may place a secondary load on the respiratory muscles by increasing the need for ventilation to maintain gas exchange. Ventilation is reduced during sleep in normal individuals because of a sleep-induced reduction in drive to breathe (21). A rise in carbon dioxide (CO_2) of up to 1 kPa is normal, but if the rise is excessive, a transient acidosis results that leads to a compensatory renal retention of bicarbonate. Consequently, chemosensitivity to CO_2, which is mediated by changes in pH, is reduced.

Polysomnographic studies show that oxygen desaturation may occur in patients with COPD, particularly marked during rapid eye movement (REM) sleep (22,23), and alveolar hypoventilation is the predominant mechanism. Patients with COPD have a higher physiologic dead space than normal subjects and the rapid shallow breathing that normally occurs during REM sleep produces an even greater decrease in alveolar ventilation. In addition, hyperinflated patients with COPD are more dependent on intercostal and accessory muscle activity than normal subjects. During REM sleep, the diaphragm alone is unable to maintain ventilation. However, the effect of these derangements during sleep upon survival and daytime function is not well known.

Nocturnal hypoxemia is thought to be important in the genesis of pulmonary hypertension in COPD patients (24). The REM-related falls in oxygen saturation may be associated with rises in pulmonary artery pressure (PAP) of up to 20 mm Hg (25). However the effect of transient rises in PAP during sleep is not clear. Higher mean PAP and red cell masses were found in 36 patients with COPD and mild to moderate oxygen desaturation (desaturation to at least 85% and at least 5 min spent with oxygen saturation [Sao_2] less than 90%) than in 30 patients who did not desaturate (26). However, there were also significant differences in awake oxygenation.

The effect of the interaction between hypoxia and hypercapnia upon the human pulmonary circulation is not well known. In isolated lung preparations, hypercapnia leads to a variety of different responses in the pulmonary circulation: vasoconstriction (dogs), vasodilatation (rats), or a biphasic response (cats) (27). In man, acidosis is a potent vasoconstrictor and therefore transient rises in CO_2 during sleep may exacerbate the vasoconstrictor response to hypoxia. Therefore, improvement of hypercapnia in addition to hypoxia could be advantageous to pulmonary hemodynamics.

Impaired sleep quality is also well recognized in COPD patients compared with age-matched controls (28). Experience from obstructive sleep apnea (OSA) suggests that sleep disruption is associated with impaired neuropsychiatric functioning and reduced quality of life. White et al. (29) showed that normals who were sleep deprived had abnormal ventilatory responses to both hypoxia and hypercapnia by day and this may further contribute to a reduction in chemosensitivity in these patients. The effect of supplemental oxygen on sleep quality is controversial, with some investigators showing an improvement (30) and others no benefit (31). In neither study was CO_2 tension measured. Although severe hypoxia (Sao_2 <70%) may not cause arousal in humans (32), acute hypercapnia, with a rise in $Paco_2$ of 6 to 15 mm Hg, is a powerful arousal stimulus (33). A reduction in carbon dioxide during sleep may therefore improve sleep quality. In patients with OSA, arousal is related to the magnitude of esophageal pressure change (34), and it is possible that large negative esophageal pressure swings in patients with COPD may further disrupt sleep. The complex interactions in the

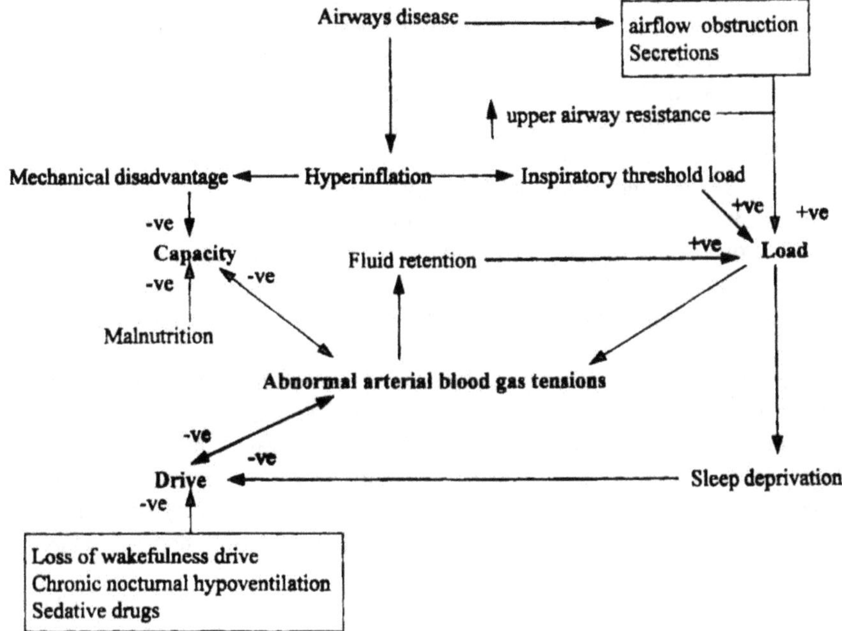

Figure 1 The complex interactions leading to the development of diurnal ventilatory failure. In COPD, the primary abnormality is of an increase in load, but this may have secondary effects upon the respiratory muscles and the central drive to breathe as well as upon sleep quality. Abbreviations: −ve, reduces; +ve, increases.

pathogenesis of diurnal ventilatory failure and daytime symptoms are shown in Figure 1. Although the effect of nocturnal abnormalities of gas exchange in COPD upon the genesis of daytime symptoms and signs is not clear, the experience in patients with chest wall deformity and neuromuscular disorders in whom correction of the nocturnal abnormality results in improved daytime function suggests that similar benefit might be achieved in COPD.

III. Evidence Base for Use of NPPV in COPD

A number of studies have looked at the feasibility of using NPPV during sleep in patients with COPD. Early experience with negative pressure devices in this condition were disappointing, with most patients unable to use the equipment satisfactorily at home or during sleep (15,35). A number of workers have reported successful nasal positive pressure ventilation in uncontrolled studies showing improved daytime blood gas tensions and sleep quality, suggesting that it is feasible (17,18,36–40). Sivasothy et al. (41) retrospectively studied the effect of domiciliary NPPV in 26 consecutive patients with hypercapnic ventilatory failure due to COPD in whom oxygen therapy caused worsening hypercapnia. Patients were ventilated with a variety of different ventilators, both volume- and pressure-cycled machines, used for a median of 7.81 hr/day during sleep and daytime naps. Supplemental oxygen was added if it was not possible to increase Sao_2 >90% with NPPV despite a reduction in $Paco_2$. After 1 yr, Pao_2 had increased by a median of 2.4 kPa and $Paco_2$ had fallen by a median of 1.4 kPa. Daytime $Paco_2$ correlated with overnight transcutaneous carbon dioxide tension ($Ptcco_2$). Hematocrit improved and there was an improvement in the "role limitation physical" domain of the short form 36 health status questionnaire. Survival was comparable to oxygen-treated patients in other studies and better than that in historical controls.

Jones et al. (42) followed 11 patients with severe stable COPD and hypercapnic ventilatory failure for 2 yr. In addition to sustained improvements in arterial blood gas tensions, they also found that hospitalization rates and General Practitioner consultation rates were halved in the year after starting NPPV compared with the previous year. These data suggest that there may be economic advantages to home ventilation, but these findings need to be confirmed in larger prospective studies.

There have been few controlled trials and most of these had small numbers of patients followed over a short period of time. Strumpf et al. (43) performed a randomized controlled crossover study in 19 patients with COPD and found that 7 of 19 were unable to tolerate the nasal mask and a further five withdrew because of intercurrent illness. In the seven who did complete the study, there were significant differences only in the neuropsychologic testing. Acclimatization was performed as an outpatient, but with regular visits from a respiratory therapist. Adequacy of ventilation was confirmed during wakefulness by measurement of end-tidal CO_2 tensions, though this measure may be unreliable in patients with severe COPD, and the adequacy of control of nocturnal hypoventilation was not confirmed. In addition, the patients were not particularly hypercapnic (mean $Paco_2$ 46 mm Hg). Meecham Jones et al. (44) performed a similarly designed crossover study of the use of nasal pressure support ventilation and oxygen with oxygen alone and showed improved daytime arterial blood gas tensions, better quality sleep and improved quality of life during the pressure support limb of the study. The improvement in daytime $Paco_2$ correlated with a reduction in overnight transcutaneous CO_2.

Lin (45) studied 12 patients in a prospective randomized crossover study of oxygen alone, NPPV alone, and oxygen plus NPPV, each for 2 wk. There were no differences in tidal volume, minute volume, spirometry, diurnal arterial blood gas tensions, mouth pressures or ventilatory drive. Sleep efficiency was worse during NPPV than with oxygen alone. However, the maximum tolerated inspiratory pressure ranged from only 8 cm H_2O to a maximum of 15 cm H_2O. No data were given about the effect of NPPV on blood gas tensions during ventilation and there was no statistically significant improvement in sleep hypoventilation with NPPV. Since a primary aim of noninvasive ventilation delivered during sleep is to control nocturnal hypoventilation, it can be argued that this was not achieved, and therefore, it is not surprising that there was no evidence of any therapeutic effect with NPPV. Also, low levels of pressure support are less likely to unload the respiratory muscles. The fact that no patient could tolerate an inspiratory positive airway pressure (IPAP) of more than 15 cm H_2O in the Lin study is surprising since in the study of Meecham Jones et al. (44) the mean IPAP for the group was 18 cm H_2O. Further, in the study of Ambrosino et al. (46), the mean IPAP was 22 cm H_2O, and in the study of Elliott et al. (37), in which volume-cycled flow generators were used, most patients tolerated peak inflation pressures of 35 to 40 cm H_2O. Practical experience with both NPPV and continuous positive airway pressure (CPAP) demonstrates that most patients require several weeks of acclimatization before they are comfortable, and confident, with the delivery of ventilatory support during sleep. Therefore, the short time period of the Lin study may not have been sufficient. It may also be significant that acceptance of NPPV in this patient group is more likely when it is initiated as an inpatient (37,44). The two unfavorable studies clearly show that there may be problematic application of NPPV in patients with severe COPD, but the absence of therapeutic benefit cannot be taken as definitive evidence that NPPV in this patient group has no therapeutic effect compared with conventional treatment. The possible explanations for the lack of benefit seen in these studies are

Table 2 Possible Explanations for Failure of NPPV in COPD in Controlled Studies

Patients not sufficiently hypercapnic
Insufficient inflation pressures to achieve adequate ventilation
Effectiveness of control of nocturnal hypoventilation not confirmed
Patients not sufficiently acclimatized to the technique
NPPV unable to achieve therapeutic benefit in some patients

summarized in Table 2. In the one controlled study in which a beneficial effect was seen, this related to the effectiveness of the control of nocturnal hypoventilation as evidenced by the reduction in transcutaneous CO_2 during sleep.

These data from short-term studies certainly do not justify the routine use of noninvasive ventilation in COPD. Two more long-term uncontrolled studies (17,18) have shown 5-yr survival rates comparable to the oxygen-treated patients in the NOTT and MRC studies. It should be acknowledged that most of the patients recruited to these studies were hypercapnic and thus, on the basis of the MRC study, less likely to benefit from LTOT. Also, and at the time when NPPV was started, the patients were deemed to have failed oxygen therapy. The results in a group of "oxygen failures" were therefore encouraging. However, what constituted "oxygen failure" was not defined and it is inappropriate to make comparisons with historical controls from over 20 yr ago. The results of two multicenter European trials comparing NPPV with LTOT in COPD are awaited. Until further data are available, a trial of NPPV can only be justified in patients who have failed with or cannot tolerate the gold standard treatment, namely LTOT.

These studies do show, however, that patients with COPD have difficulty acclimatizing to NPPV, and there is some evidence to suggest that if nocturnal hypoventilation is controlled, there is a therapeutic effect. In light of this, if NPPV is to be tried in COPD patients, the effective control of nocturnal hypoventilation should be targeted.

More recently, the use of noninvasive ventilation as a means of unloading the respiratory muscles during exercise has been investigated. During exhaustive exercise in patients with COPD, Kyroussis et al. (47) showed slowing of the maximum relaxation rate of the sniff esophageal pressure waveform, which is thought to indicate the presence of respiratory muscle fatigue (48). The same group (49) showed that this could be reduced by the use of inspiratory pressure support during exercise. Bianchi et al. (50) showed that CPAP, pressure support ventilation, and proportional assist ventilation (PAV) all increased exercise time and reduced dyspnea, but with the greatest changes seen with PAV. These findings suggest that noninvasive ventilation may have a role in improving exercise capacity in COPD patients if an easily portable ventilator with an acceptable interface, perhaps a mouthpiece, can be developed. An alternative strategy is to use a fixed noninvasive ventilator during exercise training, on a treadmill or static cycle, as part of a rehabilitation program. The offloading of the respiratory muscles could allow more exercise, increasing the training effect on the cardiac and peripheral muscles.

IV. Mechanism of Benefit

An understanding of the pathophysiology of ventilatory failure and of the effects of sleep disordered breathing is important both in selecting patients who are likely to benefit from noninvasive ventilation and also in targeting the appropriate therapeutic outcome. In the early studies of noninvasive ventilation in COPD, benefit was seen in hypercapnic but not in eucapnic patients. This is perhaps not surprising given that one is augmenting the individual's own ventilator (i.e., the respiratory muscle pump and its controller). If reversal of hypoventilation is important in the therapeutic response to noninvasive ventilation, then it is not surprising that little apparent benefit derives from assisted ventilation when the function of the patient's own ventilator is adequate and able to maintain a normal or near-normal carbon dioxide tension.

It has been suggested that assisted ventilation improves blood gas tensions by the relief of chronic respiratory muscle fatigue (20). Early studies to test this hypothesis used negative pressure devices during the day (12–15,51). The period of ventilation ranged from 3 to 6 hr for 3 days to 8 hr once weekly for several months. Improvements were seen in arterial blood gas tensions during spontaneous breathing, maximal inspiratory and expiratory mouth pressures, transdiaphragmatic pressures, quality of life, and exercise capacity. The improvements, particularly in mouth pressures, were cited as evidence for the effectiveness of respiratory muscle rest and the existence of chronic fatigue. However, this analysis is flawed for three reasons. First, although accessory muscle and diaphragmatic electromyogram (EMG) activity can be reduced by both negative (52) and positive pressure devices (53), in most cases this has not been documented during the study. Rodenstein et al. (54) have shown that accessory muscle and diaphragmatic EMG activity may not be reduced at all in naive patients, and Ambrosino et al. (14), who measured integrated EMG activity during negative pressure ventilation, stated that activity was reduced by 50% only *temporarily*. The assumption that abolition of EMG activity occurring under ideal conditions, when ventilator controls have been adjusted to achieve this goal, also occurs during routine use may not be valid and it is therefore possible that the respiratory muscles were not rested at all in these studies. Second, patients were often recruited during recovery from an acute exacerbation (55,56); the changes seen may reflect the natural history of recovery, rather than any beneficial effect of assisted ventilation per se. Third, individual patients have shown large improvements in arterial blood gas tensions despite decreases in mouth pressures suggesting that, at least in these patients, other factors may be important (12).

Studies using NPPV are similarly flawed. Most have had small numbers of patients, have been uncontrolled, and have not considered other possible explanations for improvement, such as changes in load and respiratory drive. Small increases in maximal inspiratory pressures have been cited as evidence of improved capacity though in the absence of a control group these may have been due to learning effects and/or better motivation. In addition, it is not clear whether the improvements in mouth pressures are the cause or the consequence of the fact that the patients have improved arterial blood gas tensions. However, others (57,58) have reported improved daytime arterial blood gas tensions in the absence of changes in the indices of respiratory muscle strength.

In an attempt to answer definitively whether respiratory muscle fatigue exists in stable chronic COPD, Shapiro et al. (59) studied 184 patients randomized to active or sham negative pressure ventilation at home using a poncho wrap ventilator. They did not show any significant difference between the two groups, but compliance with treatment was much less than anticipated. They found no relationship between their primary end point, a 6-min. walking test, with the total duration of ventilation (to serve as an index of the "dose" of respiratory muscle rest actually delivered). They also found that there was no relationship between these variables or baseline characteristics such as hypercapnia, forced expiratory volume in 1 sec (FEV_1), etc., and benefit. They concluded that respiratory muscle fatigue did not exist and little was to be gained by resting the respiratory muscles. However 6-min walking distance is an unconventional measure of respiratory muscle fatigue and is affected by other factors. In addition, subgroup analysis lacks the necessary power to ascertain that there was no relationship. It also is noteworthy that the mean $Paco_2$ of the patients studied was only 44 mm Hg and a review of the literature suggests that it is hypercapnic patients who are most likely to benefit from noninvasive ventilation.

Because of the poor compliance with negative pressure ventilation and the use of a crude measure of respiratory muscle fatigue, it is difficult to draw any meaningful conclusions from this study. Other studies, as outlined above, have made the control of sleep-related hypoventilation the primary therapeutic aim. If the nocturnal rise in CO_2 can be prevented, bicarbonate retention will not occur and indeed, if the CO_2 is lowered and a mild alkalosis induced, there will be excretion of bicarbonate and restoration of chemosensitivity to CO_2. Berthon-Jones and Sullivan (60) showed a left shift of the ventilatory response curve to progressive hypercapnia in patients with severe obstructive sleep apnea after 90 days of treatment with continuous positive airway pressure. In eight patients with severe COPD ventilated noninvasively during sleep for 6 mo, Elliott et al. (57)

showed a reduction in bicarbonate and base excess and a leftward shift of the ventilatory response to CO_2.

Individuals with sleep-disordered breathing have poor-quality sleep that leads to daytime symptoms such as fatigue and hypersomnolence. This can be extreme, as with severe obstructive sleep apnea, even when overall ventilation is unchanged, as evidenced by the maintenance of a normal carbon dioxide tension. In patients with severe COPD, symptomatic benefit has been seen when nocturnal hypoventilation is controlled and sleep quality improved (37,44). However, this does not mean that this is the mechanism by which NPPV works. It is also likely that the reduction in CO_2 during ventilation was accompanied by unloading, and therefore "rest," of the respiratory muscles. Petrof et al. (61) found no improvement in daytime pulmonary function when the respiratory muscles of patients with COPD were unloaded during sleep by CPAP. Schonhofer et al. (62) have attempted to elucidate possible mechanisms of the improvement in physiologic parameters. Patients with neuromuscular disease or skeletal deformity were allocated to receive NPPV either during sleep or during the day for a 1-mo period. In the latter group, patients were prevented from sleeping by having to respond to intermittent prompts by pressing a button when a light came on. They were thus able to compare the effects of NPPV during sleep and wakefulness. There were no differences between the two groups, with each showing improved diurnal blood gas tensions, increased respiratory muscle strength, and a slight reduction in the pressure generated during the first 100 msec of an inspiratory effort (P0.1), a measure of central drive. Overnight oxygen saturation and transcutaneous CO_2 tensions were also improved in both groups at the end of the study during spontaneous breathing overnight. Sleep quality also improved in a small subgroup who underwent full polysomnography. They concluded that nocturnal derangements of gas exchange were not important in the development of ventilatory failure.

On the other hand, the observation that ventilation during wakefulness was as effective as that during sleep does not necessarily mean that abnormalities developing during sleep are unimportant. Respiratory muscles can be rested and bicarbonate can be excreted just as well by daytime as by nighttime NPPV. Also, because of the resetting of the central respiratory controller and improved capacity of the respiratory muscle pump, spontaneous ventilation during sleep can be improved even by daytime assisted ventilation. This was, in fact, what was seen in this study. In addition, the withdrawal of NPPV from patients with restrictive chest wall disease is associated with little change in sleep quality or daytime gas exchange over 2 wk, though symptoms returned (63). Thus, there is little doubt that nocturnal assisted ventilation is effective and is clearly more convenient for the patient. There are, however, some individuals who are unable to tolerate NPPV during sleep and in these assisted ventilation by day may be an alternative.

It seems unlikely that NPPV exerts its effect exclusively through one mechanism. Therefore, the ventilator should be adjusted to reduce respiratory muscle activity, to lower arterial CO_2, and to improve sleep quality. Fortunately, these are not mutually exclusive and, indeed, it is difficult to achieve one without a significant effect on the others.

V. Practical Issues

For NPPV to be effective, the right patient must be selected, an appropriate ventilator must be chosen that is effective and tolerated by the patient, and the correct interface between the ventilator and the patient must be used (Table 3). In addition, ventilator settings must be optimized and, if used in the assist mode, the ventilator trigger must be responsive to the patient. Finally it is important to confirm by appropriate monitoring that effective ventilation is delivered both during wakefulness and sleep. The current literature suggests that NPPV of patients with COPD is more challenging than in patients with neuromuscular disease and chest wall disease. There are a number of theoretical reasons why this should be. The impedance to inflation is high in patients with COPD. High pres-

Table 3 Choices in Noninvasive Ventilation

Patient selection
On maximum effective treatment for COPD
Intolerant of oxygen because of symptomatic hypercapnia
Deteriorating despite LTOT—intractable edema, frequent hospitalization
Motivated
Ventilator selection
Volume or pressure cycled
Local expertise
Patient preference
Cost
Interface/headgear selection
Patient preference
Best fit
Preferably nasal
Full-face mask if incorrigible mouth breather or poor fit with nasal mask
To minimize dead space
Ventilator settings selection
To achieve adequate control of nocturnal hypoventilation (confirmed by overnight monitoring)
To minimize respiratory muscle activity (confirmed by observation)
To optimize patient tolerance (may be at odds with other goals)

sures may be needed to achieve effective ventilation but may be uncomfortable. Lower pressures, while better tolerated, may not be effective. In addition, PEEPi may predispose to patient/ventilator asynchrony, and finally, COPD patients often have a cough, with or without secretions, which may interfere with ventilation.

A. Patient Selection

Indications for NPPV in patients with severe stable COPD have not been established. Until further data are available, NPPV should be reserved for those patients who remain symptomatic despite maximal conventional therapy, including LTOT. Only when these measures fail should domiciliary NPPV be considered. The use of a noninvasive ventilator requires a considerable amount of patient cooperation during the early stages and should only be considered in patients who are motivated. The patient who is intolerant of an oxygen mask or who cannot be bothered to use it is unlikely to persist with NPPV. According to the literature, it is the patients with COPD who are hypercapnic who are most likely to benefit from NPPV. In general, the more hypercapnic the patient the more likely the technique is to succeed. Finally, anecdotally, the patient with symptomatic sleep-disordered breathing is more likely to benefit.

B. Choice of Ventilator

Many different ventilators are available of widely varying complexity and cost. The clinician must choose between pressure-cycled and volume-cycled machines. Both have been shown to be effective in improving arterial blood gas tensions (64–66). In large measure, the choice comes down to clinician preference and patient comfort (Fig. 2). Pressure-cycled machines deliver a predetermined pressure and the volume delivered will depend upon the impedance to inflation. If there is a leak in the circuit, flow will increase to compensate, but if there is airway obstruction, tidal volume will be reduced. Volume-cycled machines deliver a fixed tidal or minute volume and will generate a pressure sufficient to achieve this. If the impedance to inflation is high, pressure will be increased and the targeted tidal volume will be delivered. However, if there is a leak, a lower pressure will be generated, there will be no increase in flow rate to compensate, and the delivered tidal volume will fall. Restrick et al. (64) found no difference in overnight oxygenation between pressure-support and volume-cycled ventilators. Each type of ventilator was used for only one night, but the effect upon overnight CO_2 was not determined.

Schonhofer et al. (66) compared 1 mo each of pressure-cycled ventilation with volume-cycled ventilation in 30 consecutive patients requiring home mechanical ventilation, including 3 with COPD. Most patients could be satisfactorily

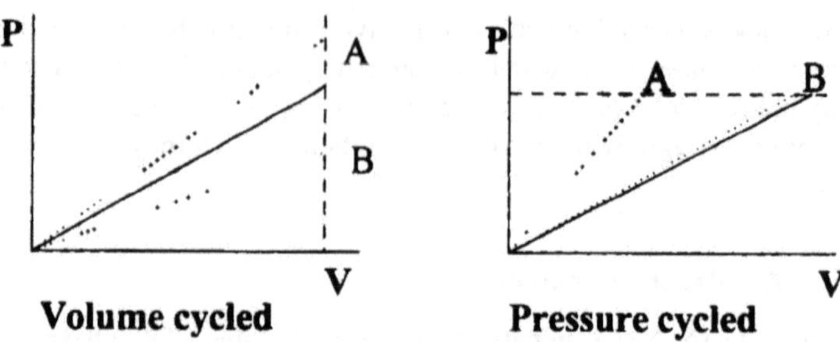

A = Increased impedance - i.e. increased airway obstruction, sputum retention, coughing

	Volume cycled	Pressure cycled
Effects:	Increased airway pressure VT maintained Discomfort	Pressure constant VT falls No discomfort

B = Increased leak - mouth breathing, leak under mask

	Volume cycled	Pressure cycled
Effects:	Pressure falls VT falls	Pressure maintained VT maintained

Figure 2 Volume-cycled generators vs. pressure-cycled generators: the effects upon ventilation and inflation pressure of changes in impedance and leak.

ventilated using either device, but 10 were deemed to be nonresponders to pressure-controlled ventilation either because of immediate symptomatic deterioration ($n = 3$) or because of a deterioration in symptom score or Pa_{O_2} ($n = 7$) after 1 mo. These patients were subsequently satisfactorily ventilated with volume-cycled machines. It was interesting that the nonresponders to pressure-cycled ventilation reported significantly more dyspnea, less mobility, and worse sleep quality than with volume-cycled machines, suggesting that in these patients, overnight ventilation was not adequate with pressure-cycled machines. Conversely, Smith and Shneerson (67) reported an improvement in diurnal blood gas tensions in 10 patients switched from a volume-cycled machine to a pressure-cycled machine. Theoretically, pressure-cycled machines are more comfortable for the patient since sudden increases in pressure are avoided. These may occur during use of volume-cycled ventilation, caused for instance by coughing or swallowing during the inspiratory phase, and may be uncomfortable for the patient. The ability to add PEEP (or EPAP) is an important consideration if patients with COPD are going to be expected to trigger some or all breaths (see below).

C. Choice of Interface

The variety of commercially available masks is ever increasing and it is usually possible to find something to suit most face shapes. Occasionally, a custom-built mask is required, but these may be expensive and the expertise is confined to a few centers. The major choice lies between a nasal mask or a full-face mask. A nasal mask is usually more comfortable, but patients with COPD are often mouth breathers and may find it difficult to breathe exclusively through the nose, in which case, a full-face mask is preferable. However, full-face masks have a bigger dead space that could interfere with CO_2 clearance and are more apt to induce claustrophobic reactions. It is important to choose the correct headgear to assure that the mask is retained comfortably in place. Rebreathing of carbon dioxide is also affected by the type of expiratory valve in the circuit; the standard vent used for various "bi-level" devices may allow significant rebreathing. This can be reduced either by using a nonrebreathing valve, which may slightly reduce tidal volume, or by increasing the level of expiratory airway pressure (EPAP), which effectively lavages the mask and circuit (68,69).

D. Choice of Ventilator Settings

This depends on the type of ventilator used. The more complex machines allow selection of a wide variety of different parameters, including inspiratory and expiratory time, inspiratory and expiratory trigger sensitivities, and the pattern of delivery of gas flow (rise time), whereas others allow only the inspiratory and expiratory pressures to be set by the operator. Most allow a choice among timed modes, in which ventilation is delivered independently of the patient's own inspiratory efforts, spontaneous mode, in which each machine-delivered breath is triggered in response to the patient's inspiratory effort, or a combination of the two.

There are no clear data about which mode is preferable, but the inclusion of the facility to trigger breaths (i.e., a spontaneous mode) is probably preferable. This is because patients, particularly those with COPD, may have quite irregular patterns of breathing during the transition from wakefulness to sleep and during rapid eye movement sleep. In this context it is noteworthy that Meecham Jones et al. (44) and Elliott et al. (37) used such ventilators, whereas Strumpf et al. (43) used the timed mode.

Where there is more flexibility in the choice of ventilator parameters, the first aim should be to match the machine to the patient's own pattern of breathing. This can be done by a combination of asking the patient which settings they prefer and by operator observation. Minor further adjustments can then be made in response to measurements of arterial blood gas tensions and monitoring of oxygenation and breathing pattern.

The choice of the correct level of PEEP or EPAP is particularly important in patients with COPD. The presence of intrinsic PEEP may cause significant patient/ventilator asynchrony because initial inspiratory efforts are not accompanied by airflow sufficient to trigger the ventilator (70,71). This may be uncomfortable for the patient and significantly increases the work of breathing. The addition of extrinsic PEEP (PEEPe) significantly reduces the work of breathing compared with pressure support alone (72). It is impractical to measure intrinsic PEEP in these patients, but the level of extrinsic PEEP can be titrated against patient comfort and to reduce the degree of ventilator/patient asynchrony. In addition, EPAP may improve gas exchange during sleep; in a small study, the addition of 5 cm H_2O of EPAP significantly improved overnight gas exchange in patients with extrapulmonary restrictive disease. Although there was a trend toward improvement in the patients with COPD, this did not reach statistical significance (73). Also, EPAP may have a lavaging effect preventing carbon dioxide rebreathing (69) and stabilizes the upper airway in patients with coexisting OSA. As a rough rule of thumb, EPAP should not be increased above 7 to 8 cm H_2O, at least initially, although this recommendation is not based on any published data.

E. Monitoring

As already stated, effective ventilation must be confirmed by measurement of arterial blood gas tensions during wakefulness once the patient is comfortable and acclimatized to the ventilator. Depending on these results, ventilator settings can then be adjusted. It is also important to observe the patient during this stage to ensure that inspiratory effort is minimized. This is best done by observing the degree of activation of accessory muscles—effective ventilation is accompanied by reduction or abolition of accessory muscle use. If the patient continues to make vigorous inspiratory efforts, improved blood gas tensions may be achieved despite insufficient ventilatory assist, resulting in inappropriate ventilator settings. Once satisfactory gas exchange has been achieved during wakefulness, and the patient is sleeping with the ventilator, adequacy of ventilation must be confirmed by overnight monitoring. If supplemental oxygen is not being used (and this should be the aim whenever possible), oxygen saturation is a simple and reliable measure of the adequacy of overnight ventilation. If supplemental oxygen is administered the transcutaneous P_{CO_2} should be measured. However transcutaneous CO_2 measurements are difficult in adults with COPD and at best can only be used to monitor trends. Arterial blood gas sampling remains the only way to be certain about the effectiveness of ventilation, but it is really impractical during sleep even with an arterial line in place. End-tidal P_{CO_2} is not a reliable measure in patients with severe airway disease.

VI. Initiation of NPPV in Patients with COPD

During the initiation phase, most patients require time and support from the nursing and/or technical staff while they acclimatize to the ventilator. Investment of time at this stage is usually well spent. If the process is hurried, the confidence of the patient may be lost and a much greater investment of time and effort will be required subsequently. There should be discussion of the implications and practical aspects of ventilation allowing time for questions to be answered. Most patients are apprehensive about the mask, headgear, and the ventilator, and the sensation of air pressure is often initially uncomfortable. The patient should be reassured that most individuals find this initial stage difficult and that they are not unusual if their first thought is that they will never get to tolerate ventilation. It is better to be pleasantly surprised that it was not as bad as they expected than to enter the process with high hopes that are rapidly dashed. It is important during these early stages that patients feel in control and not that they have been taken over by a machine. Although there are no firm data, inpatient acclimatization is probably preferable. Acclimatization to NPPV in the negative study of Strumpf et al. (43) was performed as an outpatient, whereas in the positive study of Meecham Jones et al. (44) patients started NPPV in hospital. In the study of Elliott et al. (37), the first three patients were acclimatized as outpatients; all struggled, with two of the three discontinuing NPPV before the trial was completed. Subsequent patients remained in hospital until they were confident in the use of the equipment during sleep. However, the reasons for some patients failing to acclimatize in these studies, and in routine practice, are multifactorial and no hard and fast rules can be made, with practice best determined by local circumstances and experience.

Acclimatization is aided by the patient first having the mask and headgear on without the ventilator connected and this also allows early identification of mask fitting problems. Good mask fit is very important and manufacturers' sizing gauges are a useful aid to correct selection. Patients should be allowed to experiment with different masks so that they are aware of the choices available. They should be shown how to put the mask on, how to take it off, and how to disconnect the tubing. Attention must also be paid to the headgear, which allows the mask to sit correctly and comfortably; poorly fitting headgear can lead to an ill-fitting mask.

When ventilation is tried for the first time the headgear should be removed and the mask held in place by the patient. Once they are comfortable with the sensation of positive pressure ventilation, the head straps can be used to hold the mask in place. If the patient is apprehensive, the initial use of a mouthpiece may help to build confidence until they get used to the sensation of being ventilated. The ventilator is set to match the patient's inspiratory and expiratory pattern by asking if they have enough time to breathe in and out and whether the breaths are coming too quickly. It is not uncommon for patients to complain that the machine is going too fast, when in fact all breaths are triggered! Coaching is usually sufficient, but if not, to encourage slower breathing, the trigger sensitivity can be reduced. Because there is no need for ventilation to be improved immediately, the ventilator should initially be set at a low pressure or flow, even if this is unlikely to be sufficient for adequate ventilation. Starting with high pressures will be uncomfortable and it is much easier to gain the patient's confidence if they are comfortable. Ventilation can then be increased over time to the clinically desired pressure or flow.

Someone should stay with the patient until a measure of confidence is gained. When left alone for the first time it is important that the patient should know what to do if they start to panic and how to summon help. The patient should practice disconnecting the ventilator tubing from the mask. This will usually cause alarms to sound, but they should be reassured that this is no cause for concern. Although it is seldom necessary, practice of this "emergency" drill helps to instill the feeling that the patient, and not the machine, is still in control.

Arterial blood gas tensions should be checked after about 1 hr of continuous ventilation and ventilator settings adjusted as necessary. Initially the patient may only manage a few minutes on the ventilator, but with practice and encouragement this is usually soon increased to several hours. When the patient is reasonably happy with daytime use, ventilation during sleep should be encouraged. This is usually possible the first night, but if the patient has had great difficulty it is best to give them a break and try again the next day. Once the patient is comfortable and confident, they should be encouraged to use the ventilator while sleeping through the night. They will feel the benefit of reversal of ventilatory failure more rapidly and the practice will increase their confidence. Although this schedule sounds daunting, patients often achieve between 10 and 16 hr a day. However, they should be encouraged for whatever progress they make, even if it is only a few minutes on the first day. It should be made clear that if they do subsequently require a ventilator at home, then this will only be needed at night—most would find the idea of 16 hr of ventilation per day for the rest of their lives unacceptable! It is important that the adequacy of ventilation be checked not only with arterial blood gas analysis by day, but also by overnight pulse oximetry and, if available, transcutaneous carbon dioxide measurement. Oxygen saturation should be above 90% for most of the night and an excessive rise in $Ptcco_2$ should be avoided. Ideally, $Ptcco_2$ should be lower overnight during NPPV than during spontaneous breathing by day. However, what can be achieved will depend upon the severity of ventilatory failure and nocturnal hypoventilation at presentation. Inadequate ventilation during sleep may occur because of mouth leaks and can be minimized by the use of a chin strap, a full-face mask, or by increasing ventilator settings.

VII. Home Ventilation via Tracheostomy

Tracheostomy ventilation has been largely superseded by NPPV, but a small number of patients, usually those who have proved unweanable following invasive mechanical ventilation, may require home ventilation via tracheostomy (tPPV). Robert et al. (74) reported their experience in 222 patients ventilated at home with tPPV some of whom were followed for up to 25 yr. This group included 50 patients with COPD. Survival in patients with polio, kyphoscoliosis, other neuromuscular disorders, and previous tuberculosis was much better than that reported with other therapies, but that in the COPD patients was similar to the oxygen-treated patients in the MRC study. However, importantly, survival was no worse, despite the presence of a tracheostomy, which may be associated with significant morbidity and mortality (75). The patients with chest wall deformity and neuromuscular disease had better arterial blood gas tensions during unassisted ventilation, more trips outside the house, and fewer days hospitalized or confined to the house because of illness than the COPD patients. A small group ($n = 10$) with bronchiectasis had the worst survival and required the most intensive ventilatory support (average 20 hr per day) and the most frequent bronchial suctioning (average 50 times per day).

Muir et al. (76), in a multicenter study in France, reported survival and long term follow-up data on 259 tracheostomized patients treated by home mechanical ventilation (HMV). Twenty-four percent of patients did not require assisted ventilation and 67% required oxygen in addition to MV. Patients ventilated without added oxygen required ventilatory support for 14.4 ± 4.4 hr/day compared with 11.8 ± 4.7 hr for those receiving additional oxygen. Some patients were ventilated only during the night and some only during the day. The 5-yr survival rate of 44% was similar to oxygen-treated patients in the LTOT studies. Patients had severe airflow limitation with a mean FEV_1 of 0.73l and hypercapnic ventilatory failure with a mean Pa_{O_2} 50.4 mm Hg and Pa_{CO_2} 56 mm Hg. Improvements in diurnal blood gas tensions were similar to those reported in patients receiving domiciliary NPPV. The tracheostomies were performed during episodes of acute respiratory failure in 230 of the 259 patients (89%).

Thirty-seven patients had complications from the tracheostomy: tracheal stenosis (14 of 37), granulomas (11 of 37), and tracheal hemorrhage or ulceration (6 of 37). The risk of complications was lower in those with uncuffed tubes (9 vs. 18%). Almost 50% of patients had a further episode of acute respiratory failure, usually because of bronchopulmonary infection. Estimated costs in the year before tracheostomy were $43,062 falling to $28,255 in the first year, with further small falls in years two and three. After year eight, however, hospitalization rates, and presumably therefore also costs, increased. Survival was better with age <65, use of an uncuffed tube, and $Pa_{O_2} > 56$ mm Hg breathing room air at 3 mo after tracheostomy.

Ventilation via tracheostomy is an option for HMV in patients with COPD. Muir et al. (77) have suggested increasingly aggressive treatment for ventilatory failure as COPD progresses. Initial oxygen therapy is followed by NPPV and, when this is no longer sufficient, tPPV substituted. It is probable, however, that in most cases tPPV will follow a bout of acute respiratory failure treated with invasive mechanical ventilation, when weaning proves difficult. Since NPPV has now been shown to be effective in promoting weaning (78–80), it is likely that most patients can be managed using noninvasive techniques, which are preferable because of their lower complication rates.

VIII. Conclusion

NPPV may be successfully used in severe stable COPD. However, careful patient selection, intensive acclimatization, and adequate monitoring of therapeutic effect are vital to a successful outcome. At present, NPPV should be reserved for hypercapnic patients who have failed conventional treatment. It remains to be seen whether the use of NPPV has advantages over long-term oxygen therapy in terms of survival or quality of life. However, it seems reasonable to offer such patients a trial of noninvasive ventilation since a few studies suggest that benefit may be achieved. Furthermore, given the complexities and associated discomfort of using NPPV, they are unlikely to continue treatment in the absence of any perceived beneficial effect. There is no doubt that large-scale prospective randomized controlled trials are sorely needed, powered to measure quality of life as well as survival, and incorporating a health economic analysis.

References

1. Burrows B, Earle RH. Course and prognosis of chronic obstructive lung disease. N Engl J Med 1969; 280:397–404.
2. Boushy SF, Thompson HK, North LB, Beale AR, Snow TR. Prognosis in chronic obstructive pulmonary disease. Am Rev Respir Dis 1973; 108:1373–1383.
3. Sahn SA, Nett LM, Petty TL. Ten year follow-up of a comprehensive rehabilitation program for severe COPD. Chest 1980; 77(suppl):311–314.
4. Nocturnal Oxygen Therapy Trial Group. Continuous or nocturnal oxygen therapy in hypoxemic chronic obstructive lung disease: A clinical trial. Ann Intern Med 1980; 93:391–398.
5. Medical Research Council Working Party Report. Long term domiciliary oxygen therapy in chronic hypoxic cor pulmonale complicating chronic bronchitis and emphysema. Lancet 1981; 1:681–685.
6. Cooper CB, Waterhouse J, Howard P. Twelve year clinical study of patients with hypoxic cor pulmonale given long term domiciliary oxygen therapy. Thorax 1987; 42:105–110.
7. Aida A, Miyamoto K, Nishimura M, et al. Prognostic value of hypercapnia in patients with chronic respiratory failure during long term oxygen therapy. Am J Respir Crit Care Med 1998; 158:188–193.
8. Connors AF Jr, Dawson NV, Thomas C, et al. Outcomes following acute exacerba-

tion of severe chronic obstructive lung disease. The SUPPORT investigators (Study to Understand Prognoses and Preferences for Outcomes and Risks of Treatments). Am J Respir Crit Care Med 1996; 154:959–967.
9. Baudouin SV, Waterhouse JC, Tahtamouni T, Smith JA, Baxter J, Howard P. Long term domiciliary oxygen treatment for chronic respiratory failure reviewed. Thorax 1990; 45:195–198.
10. Walshaw MJ, Lim R, Evans CC, Hind CRK. Factors influencing compliance of patients using oxygen concentrators for long-term home oxygen therapy. Respir Med 1990; 84:331–333.
11. Cropp A, Dimarco AF. Effects of intermittent negative pressure ventilation on respiratory muscle function in patients with severe chronic obstructive pulmonary disease. Am Rev Respir Dis 1987; 135:1056–1061.
12. Gutierrez M, Beroiza T, Contreras G, et al. Weekly cuirass ventilation improves blood gases and inspiratory muscle strength in patients with chronic airflow limitation and hypercarbia. Am Rev Respir Dis 1988; 138:617–623.
13. Celli B, Lee H, Criner G, et al. Controlled trial of external negative pressure ventilation in patients with severe chronic airflow limitation. Am Rev Respir Dis 1989; 140:1251–1256.
14. Ambrosino N, Montagna T, Nava S, et al. Short term effect of intermittent negative pressure ventilation in COPD patients with respiratory failure. Eur Respir J 1990; 3:502–508.
15. Zibrak JD, Hill NS, Federman EC, Kwa SL, O'Donnell C. Evaluation of intermittent long term negative-pressure ventilation in patients with severe COPD. Am Rev Respir Dis 1988; 138:1515–1518.
16. Schiavina M, Fabiani A, Gunella G. External negative pressure ventilation techniques. Monaldi Arch Chest Dis 1994; 49:516–521.
17. Simonds AK, Elliott MW. Outcome of domiciliary nasal intermittent positive pressure ventilation in restrictive and obstructive disorders. Thorax 1995; 50:604–609.
18. Leger P, Bedicam JM, Cornette A, et al. Nasal intermittent positive pressure ventilation: Long-term follow-up in patients with severe chronic respiratory insufficiency. Chest 1994; 105:100–105.
19. Rochester DF, Braun NMT. Determinants of maximal inspiratory pressure in chronic obstructive pulmonary disease. Am Rev Respir Dis 1985; 132:42–47.
20. Macklem PT. The clinical relevance of respiratory muscle research: J Burns Aberson Lecture. Am Rev Respir Dis 1986; 134:812–815.
21. Douglas NJ, White DP, Pickett CK, Weil J, Zwillich CW. Respiration during sleep in normal man. Thorax 1982; 37:840–844.
22. Douglas NJ, Calverley PMA, Leggett RJE, Brash HM, Flenley DC, Brezinova V. Transient hypoxaemia during sleep in chronic bronchitis and emphysema. Lancet 1979; 1:1–4.
23. Fletcher EC, Gray BA, Levin DC. Nonapneic mechanisms of arterial oxygen desaturation during rapid-eye-movement sleep. J Appl Physiol 1983; 54:632–639.
24. Boysen PG, Block AJ, Wynne JW, Hunt LA, Flick MR. Nocturnal pulmonary hypertension in patients with chronic obstructive pulmonary disease. Chest 1979; 76:536–542.
25. Coccagna G, Lugaresi E. Arterial blood gases and pulmonary and systemic arterial

pressure during sleep in chronic obstructive pulmonary disease. Sleep 1978; 1:117–124.

26. Fletcher EC, Luckett RA, Miller T, Costarangos C, Kutka N, Fletcher JG. Pulmonary vascular hemodynamics in chronic lung disease patients with and without oxyhemoglobin desaturation during sleep. Chest 1989; 95:757–764.
27. Emery CJ, Sloan PJ, Mohammed FH, Barer GR. The action of hypercapnia during hypoxia on pulmonary vessels. Bull Eur Physiopathol Respir 1977; 13:763–776.
28. Arand DL, McGinty DJ, Littner MR. Respiratory patterns associated with hemoglobin desaturation during sleep in chronic obstructive pulmonary disease. Chest 1981; 80:183–190.
29. White DP, Douglas NJ, Pickett CK, Zwillich CW, Weil JV. Sleep deprivation and control of ventilation. Am Rev Respir Dis 1983; 128:984–986.
30. Calverley PMA, Brezinova V, Douglas NJ, Catterall JR, Flenley DC. The effect of oxygenation on sleep quality in chronic bronchitis and emphysema. Am Rev Respir Dis 1982; 126:206–210.
31. Fleetham JA, West P, Mezon B, Conway W, Roth T, Kryger M. Sleep, arousals, and oxygen desaturation in COPD. Am Rev Respir Dis 1982; 126:429–433.
32. Berthon-Jones M, Sullivan CE. Ventilatory and arousal responses to hypoxia in sleeping humans. Am Rev Respir Dis 1982; 125:632–639.
33. Hedemark L, Kronenberg R. Ventilatory responses to hypoxia and CO_2 during natural and flurazepam induced sleep in normal adults (abstr). Am Rev Respir Dis 1981; 123:190.
34. Rees K, Spence DP, Earis JE, Calverley PM. Arousal responses from apneic events during non-rapid-eye-movement sleep. Am J Respir Crit Care Med 1995; 152:1016–1021.
35. Shapiro SH, Ernst P, Gray-Donald K, et al. Effect of negative pressure ventilation in severe chronic obstructive pulmonary disease. The Lancet 1992; 340:1425–1429.
36. Carroll N, Branthwaite MA. Control of nocturnal hypoventilation by nasal intermittent positive pressure ventilation. Thorax 1988; 43:349–353.
37. Elliott MW, Simonds AK, Carroll MP, Wedzicha JA, Branthwaite MA. Domiciliary nocturnal nasal intermittent positive pressure ventilation in hypercapnic respiratory failure due to chronic obstructive lung disease: Effects on sleep and quality of life. Thorax 1992; 47:342–348.
38. Marino W. Intermittent volume cycled mechanical ventilation via nasal mask in patients with respiratory failure due to COPD. Chest 1991; 99:681–684.
39. Perrin C, El Far Y, Vandenbos F, et al. Domiciliary nasal intermittent positive pressure ventilation in severe COPD: effects on lung function and quality of life. Eur Respir J 1997; 10:2835–2839.
40. Alfaro V, Torras R, Palacios L, Ibanez J. Long-term domiciliary treatment with nasal intermittent positive-pressure ventilation plus supplemental oxygen in COPD with severe hypercapnia. Respiration 1997; 64:118–120.
41. Sivasothy P, Smith IE, Shneerson JM. Mask intermittent positive pressure ventilation in chronic hypercapnic respiratory failure due to chronic obstructive pulmonary disease. Eur Respir J 1998; 11:34–40.
42. Jones SE, Packham S, Hebden M, Smith AP. Domiciliary nocturnal intermittent

positive pressure ventilation in patients with respiratory failure due to severe COPD; long term follow up and effect on survival. Thorax 1998; 53:495-498.

43. Strumpf DA, Millman RP, Carlisle CC, et al. Nocturnal positive-pressure ventilation via nasal mask in patients with severe chronic obstructive pulmonary disease. Am Rev Respir Dis 1991; 144:1234-1239.
44. Meecham Jones DJ, Paul EA, Jones PW, Wedzicha JA. Nasal pressure support ventilation plus oxygen compared with oxygen therapy alone in hypercapnic COPD. Am J Respir Crit Care Med 1995; 152:538–544.
45. Lin CC. Comparison between nocturnal nasal positive pressure ventilation combined with oxygen therapy and oxygen monotherapy in patients with severe COPD. Am J Respir Crit Care Med 1996; 154:353–358.
46. Ambrosino N, Nava S, Bertone P, Fracchia C, Rampulla C. Physiologic evaluation of pressure support ventilation by nasal mask in patients with stable COPD. Chest 1992; 101:385–391.
47. Kyroussis D, Polkey MI, Keilty SE, et al. Exhaustive exercise slows inspiratory muscle relaxation rate in chronic obstructive pulmonary disease. Am J Respir Crit Care Med 1996; 153:787–793.
48. Mulvey DA, Koulouris NG, Elliott MW, Laroche CM, Moxham J, Green M. Inspiratory muscle relaxation rate after voluntary maximal isocapnic hyperventilation in humans. J Appl Physiol 1991; 70:2173–2180.
49. Polkey MI, Kyroussis D, Mills GH, et al. Inspiratory pressure support reduces slowing of inspiratory muscle relaxation rate during exhaustive treadmill walking in severe COPD. Am J Respir Crit Care Med 1996; 154:1146–1150.
50. Bianchi L, Foglio K, Pagani M, Vitacca M, Rossi A, Ambrosino N. Effects of proportional assist ventilation on exercise tolerance in COPD patients with chronic hypercapnia. Eur Respir J 1998; 11:422–427.
51. Nava S, Ambrosino N, Zocchi L, Rampulla C. Diaphragmatic rest during negative pressure ventilation by pneumowrap assessment in normal and COPD patients. Chest 1990; 98:857–865.
52. Rochester DF, Braun NM, Laine S. Diaphragmatic energy expenditure in chronic respiratory failure. Am J Med 1977; 63:223–231.
53. Carrey Z, Gottfried SB, Levy RD. Ventilatory muscle support in respiratory failure with nasal positive pressure ventilation. Chest 1990; 97:150–158.
54. Rodenstein DO, Stanescu DC, Cuttita G, Liistro G, Veriter C. Ventilatory and diaphragmatic EMG responses to negative-pressure ventilation in airflow obstruction. J Appl Physiol 1988; 65(4):1621–1626.
55. Scano G, Gigliotti F, Duranti R, Spinelli A, Gorini M, Schiavina M. Changes in ventilatory muscle function with negative pressure ventilation in COPD. Chest 1990; 97:322–327.
56. Corrado A, Bruscoli G, De Paola E, Ciardi-Dupre GF, Baccini A, Taddel M. Respiratory muscle insufficiency in acute respiratory failure of subjects with severe COPD: Treatment with intermittent negative pressure ventilation. Eur Respir J 1990; 3:644–648.
57. Elliott MW, Mulvey DA, Moxham J, Green M, Branthwaite MA. Domiciliary nocturnal nasal intermittent positive pressure ventilation in COPD: Mechanisms underlying changes in arterial blood gas tensions. Eur Respir J 1991; 4:1044–1052.

58. Barbe F, Quera-Salva MA, de Lattre J, Gajdos P, Agusti A. Long-term effects of nasal intermittent positive pressure ventilation on pulmonary function and sleep architecture in patients with neuromuscular diseases. Chest 1996; 110:1179–1183.
59. Shapiro SH, Ernst P, Gray-Donald K, et al. Effect of negative pressure ventilation in severe chronic obstructive pulmonary disease. Lancet 1992; 340:1425–1429.
60. Berthon-Jones M, Sullivan CE. Time course of change in ventilatory response to CO_2 with long-term CPAP therapy for obstructive sleep apnea. Am Rev Respir Dis 1987; 135:144–147.
61. Petrof BJ, Kimoff RJ, Levy RD, Cosio MG, Gottfried SB. Nasal continuous positive airway pressure facilitates respiratory muscle function during sleep in severe chronic obstructive pulmonary disease. Am Rev Respir Dis 1991; 143:928–935.
62. Schonhofer B, Geibel M, Sonnerborn M, Kohler D. Daytime mechanical ventilation in chronic respiratory insufficiency. Eur Respir J 1997; 10:2840–2846.
63. Jiminez JFM, Sanchez de Cos Escuin J, Vicente CD, Valle MH, Otero FF. Nasal intermittent positive pressure ventilation: Analysis of its withdrawal. Chest 1995; 107:382–388.
64. Restrick LJ, Fox NC, Braid G, Ward EM, Paul EA, Wedzicha JA. Comparison of nasal pressure support ventilation with nasal intermittent positive pressure ventilation in patients with nocturnal hypoventilation. Eur Respir J 1993; 6:364–370.
65. Meecham Jones DJ, Wedzicha JA. Comparison of pressure and volume preset nasal ventilator systems in stable chronic respiratory failure. Eur Respir J 1993; 6:1060–1064.
66. Schonhofer B, Sonnerborn M, Haidl P, Bohrer H, Kohler D. Comparison of two different modes for noninvasive mechanical ventilation in chronic respiratory failure: Volume versus pressure controlled device. Eur Respir J 1997; 10:184–191.
67. Smith IE, Shneerson JM. Secondary failure of nasal intermittent positive pressure ventilation using the Monnal D: Effects of changing ventilator. Thorax 1997; 52: 89–91.
68. Lofaso F, Brochard L, Touchard D, Hang T, Harf A, Isabey D. Evaluation of carbon dioxide rebreathing during pressure support ventilation with airway management system (BiPAP) devices. Chest 1995; 108:772–778.
69. Ferguson GT, Gilmartin M. CO_2 rebreathing during BiPAP ventilatory assistance. Am J Respir Crit Care Med 1995; 151:1126–1135.
70. Elliott MW, Mulvey DA, Moxham J, Green M, Branthwaite MA. Inspiratory muscle effort during nasal intermittent positive pressure ventilation in patients with chronic obstructive airways disease. Anaesthesia 1993; 48:8–13.
71. Nava S, Bruschi C, Fracchia C, Braschi A, Rubini F. Patient-ventilator interaction and inspiratory effort during pressure support ventilation in patients with different pathologies. Eur Respir J 1997; 10:177–183.
72. Appendini L, Patessio A, Zanaboni S, et al. Physiologic effects of positive end-expiratory pressure and mask pressure support during exacerbations of chronic obstructive pulmonary disease. Am J Respir Crit Care Med 1994; 149:1069–1076.
73. Elliott MW, Simonds AK. Nocturnal assisted ventilation using bilevel positive airway pressure: The effect of expiratory positive airway pressure. Eur Respir J 1995; 8:436–440.

74. Robert D, Gerard M, Leger P, et al. Domiciliary ventilation by tracheostomy for chronic respiratory failure. Rev Fr Mal Resp 1983; 11:923–936.
75. Stauffer JL, Olson DE, Petty TL. Complications and consequences of endotracheal intubation and tracheostomy. Am J Med 1981; 70:65–75.
76. Muir JF, Girault C, Cardinaud JP, Polu JM, and the French Co-operative Group. Survival and long-term follow-up of tracheostomized patients with COPD treated by home mechanical ventilation: A multicenter French study in 259 patients. Chest 1994; 106:201–209.
77. Muir J. Intermittent positive pressure ventilation (IPPV) in patients with chronic obstructive pulmonary disease (COPD). Eur Respir Rev 1992; 2(10):335–345.
78. Udwadia ZF, Santis GK, Steven MH, Simonds AK. Nasal ventilation to facilitate weaning in patients with chronic respiratory insufficiency. Thorax 1992; 47:715–718.
79. Restrick LJ, Scott AD, Ward EM, Feneck RO, Cornwell WE, Wedzicha JA. Nasal intermittent positive-pressure ventilation in weaning intubated patients with chronic respiratory disease from assisted positive-pressure ventilation. Respir Med 1993; 87: 199–204.
80. Nava S, Ambrosino N, Clini E, et al. Noninvasive mechanical ventilation in the weaning of patients with respiratory failure due to chronic obstructive pulmonary disease. A randomized, controlled trial. Ann Intern Med 1998; 128:721–728.

74. Robert D, Gerard M, Leger P, et al. [illegible] ventilation by tracheostomy for [illegible] respiratory failure. Rev Fr Mal Resp 1983; 11:923–[illegible].
75. [illegible] complications and consequences of endotracheal [illegible] and tracheostomy. [illegible]
76. [illegible] and the French Language Group. Survival and long-term follow-up [illegible] patients with COPD treated by [illegible] ventilation. A multicentric French study in [illegible] patients. Chest [illegible]
77. [illegible] positive pressure ventilation (NPPV) in patients with chronic [illegible] pulmonary disease (COPD). Eur Respir Rev 1992; 2(10):[illegible]
78. [illegible] Nasal ventilation in [illegible] chronic [illegible] insufficiency. [illegible]
79. [illegible]
80. [illegible]

8

Long-Term Mechanical Ventilation in Infants and Children

W. GERALD TEAGUE

Emory University School of Medicine
Atlanta, Georgia

I. Introduction

Fewer than two decades have elapsed since the first articles describing long-term home mechanical ventilation for children were published (1,2). During this era, long-term mechanical ventilation for the pediatric patient with chronic respiratory failure has evolved from an extraordinary measure to routine care for many disorders. This chapter is a comprehensive review of the current knowledge and challenges associated with long-term mechanical ventilation in the pediatric patient. The reader interested in further information may refer to an early position statement by the American Thoracic Society in 1990 (3), and recent consensus reports published by the American College of Chest Physicians (4) and the American Association of Respiratory Care (5) pertaining to long-term mechanical ventilation and noninvasive positive pressure ventilation (NPPV) of pediatric patients, respectively.

Three trends in modern medicine sustained over the past two decades have resulted in a significant increase in the number of infants and children treated at home with mechanical ventilators (6). One has been improved survival in pediatric patients with both acute lung injury and disorders known to progress to chronic respiratory failure. In infants born in the United States, low birth weight is the most important variable determining the risk of acute respiratory failure and postnatal mortality (7). The percentage of low birth weight infants born in the United States reached its highest level in over two decades in 1996. As a result, occurrences of chronic lung disease of infancy or bronchopulmonary dysplasia (BPD) have increased in centers with neonatal intensive care nurseries across the country (8). In addition, new rescue therapies, such as extracorporeal membrane oxygenation (ECMO) and high-frequency ventilation, appear to have increased survival for older children with acute lung injury who fail standard positive pressure ventilation. Survivors of acute lung injury often develop structural abnormalities and chronic respiratory insufficiency during the repair phase (9).

A second modern trend supporting the steady rise in the number of both adult and pediatric patients using long-term mechanical ventilation has been the development of new respiratory equipment for home care. Soft nasal masks and flow-triggered portable pressure ventilators are examples of technologies developed in the last decade. These and other devices have been rapidly introduced into the market by commercial vendors and, as a natural consequence, applied to patients of all ages. Most of this activity has been market-driven, well in advance of controlled trials critically examining the effectiveness and safety of specific methods.

Parental expectation of long-term survival of their child is a third factor supporting the growth of home mechanical ventilation in pediatric patients with respiratory disorders. Although pediatricians in training clearly opposed long-term mechanical ventilation for children with severe CNS injury, one survey found that parental requests for prolonged care altered treatment plans significantly (10). Physicians themselves differ widely in how they counsel parents of children with incurable disorders of the respiratory system. Such patients are typically followed in the hospital by a number of medical and surgical specialists and conflicts related to such care decisions are frequent. Often the caregivers of children with irreversible respiratory failure are not informed of the broad financial and lifestyle implications of a decision to attempt home mechanical ventilation.

As a result of these trends, the number of infants and older children at risk for prolonged dependence on assisted ventilatory devices continues to grow in the United States. Expenditures for U.S. children with chronic respiratory failure enrolled in government-sponsored financial assistance programs contribute substantially to total health care expenditures (11). In 1983, this challenge to the health care system was recognized by the U.S. Surgeon General, who called for "longitudinal studies" to determine the results of caring for ventilator-dependent children at home (6). However, a variety of ventilator methods have been used in the past for long-term assisted ventilation in pediatric patients. Published reports of these therapeutic trials are limited to case series with small numbers of patients in countries with highly developed medical systems. Thus, the plea made by Surgeon General Koop in 1983 has not been completely addressed, and very little objective evidence is available to judge the success of long-term mechanical ventilation in pediatric patients.

II. Distinguishing Features of Chronic Respiratory Failure in Pediatric Patients

A. Functional Instability of the Developing Respiratory System

Development of Respiratory Muscle and Lung Mechanical Functions

The human respiratory system is relatively prone to dysfunction during early postnatal development as a result of the mechanical interdependence between the unstable rib cage and small lung (Table 1) (12). In young infants, the rib cage is highly compliant and its outward recoil tendency low. Due to the balance of static forces between the chest wall and lung at end-expiration, predicted functional residual capacity (FRC) should be nearly equal to total lung capacity (TLC). In fact, dynamic measurements of FRC in young infants are closer to 40% of estimated TLC (13). This dynamic elevation of FRC is likely due to expiratory flow limitation via the larynx, a compensatory response that is lost

Table 1 Functional Disadvantages of the Developing Respiratory System

High chest wall compliance in association with a relatively low elastic recoil pressure
Predicted FRC close to total lung capacity
FRC dependent on active expiratory braking mechanism
Dependent airways close at FRC during tidal breathing
Fraction of diaphragmatic force development is wasted on chest wall distortion
Increased risk of respiratory muscle fatigue
Relatively less fatigue-resistant diaphragm muscle fiber types
Shape of diaphragm at FRC not conducive to optimal force development
Limited zone of apposition between the diaphragm and chest wall
Unfavorable upper airways properties
Nasal resistance contributes significantly more to the total respiratory resistance
Airway tends to collapse in the hypopharyngeal region
Brisk laryngeal closure response to liquid stimulation
Disadvantages in conducting airways function
Airways hyperreactivity to methacholine greatest in the very young
Dysanapsis in the growth rates of the small and large conducting airways
Impaired sleep respiratory function
More time in REM sleep with hypotonia of the respiratory muscles
Diminished arousal responses to hypoxemia and hypercarbia
Ventilatory response to hypoxia not sustained compared to adults

following tracheostomy. A second disadvantage of the unstable chest wall in young infants is that increases in diaphragmatic force development are "wasted" on chest wall distortion and not coupled to effective increases in alveolar ventilation (14). These factors increase the load on the immature respiratory muscles, which may be at increased risk of fatigue due to the distribution of fiber types (15) and a relatively smaller zone of apposition between the diaphragm and rib cage (14).

In the immature human lung, alveolar maturation is incomplete. Due to the distribution of surface forces, the deflation static pressure-volume relationship in young infants is curvilinear. With increasing age up to young adulthood, it becomes more linear (16). The elastic recoil properties of the lungs determine the distribution of pleural pressure and in conjunction with the flow-resistive properties of the airways determine the distribution of alveolar ventilation. In infants and very young children during tidal breathing some of the dependent airways close at FRC (17). This results in intermittent inadequate ventilation of some of the terminal lung units and in infants with lung disease probably contributes significantly to impaired respiratory gas exchange.

Properties of the Upper and Lower Airways

In young infants the flow resistance of the nasal airway is great and makes up a significant portion of the total respiratory system resistance (18,19). Common childhood conditions blocking the nasopharyngeal airway, such as hypertrophy of the adenoids and tonsils, may be fatal if severe and untreated (20). A number of disorders leading to respiratory failure in children are associated with intermittent upper airway collapse and obstructive apnea (21). In the human infant, unlike the adult, the airway tends to collapse at the level of the oropharynx or even lower (22). Infants also demonstrate particularly strong glottic closure in response to liquid stimulation (23). Such airway responses may be triggered during episodes of gastroesophageal reflux, a common condition in pediatric patients with respiratory disorders.

In young infants, the number and size of the lower conducting airways are well developed relative to the alveolar structures. As a result, specific conductance normalized to lung volume is greater in young infants than it is in the adult (24). The peripheral airways, those distal to the tenth or twelfth generation, increase in size relative to the central airways after the fifth year of life (25). As a result, absolute airway conductance, relative to lung volume, progressively increases during childhood (12). In contrast to earlier observations, recent studies show that the immature human airways have sufficient surrounding smooth muscle to constrict and relax in response to various stimuli (26). Methacholine elicits bronchoconstriction at a relatively low dose in young infants, a response that tends to decrease during the first year of postnatal development (27).

Neural Respiratory Drive, Sleep Stages, and Lung Volume

Young infants normally spend 30 to 50% of their total sleep time in the rapid eye movement (REM) phase (28). In REM sleep, control of breathing is more automatic and less dependent on neural control pathways, and relaxation of the respiratory muscles can further decrease FRC (29). The low FRC promotes hypoxemia, accounting for the arterial oxygen desaturation that occurs in young infants during REM sleep. This pattern is enhanced in patients with lung disease. One striking difference between young infants and adults occurs during a phase of infant development when ventilatory control is heavily influenced by carotid chemoreceptor function. Infant lambs that undergo carotid chemo-denervation just after birth acutely hypoventilate but appear well for a period of 5 to 6 wk, and then approximately half die unexpectedly during sleep (30). Another difference between neonates and adults is the ventilatory response to hypoxia. Although hypoxia triggers a biphasic increase and then depression in minute ventilation in both adults and neonates, the neonate cannot sustain the increase in ventilation for as long (31). About two-thirds of otherwise normal infants do not arouse from quiet sleep in response to hypoxia (32).

B. Pathophysiology of Chronic Respiratory Failure in Pediatric Patients

Definition and Classification

Respiratory failure results when the pump function of the ventilatory muscles paced by the neural respiratory drive does not achieve a critical level of alveolar gas exchange to meet the metabolic demands of cellular respiration. A number of variables impact the respiratory "load" as defined by the magnitude of cellular oxygen (O_2) consumption and carbon dioxide (CO_2) production (Fig. 1). Dysfunction of any of the critical components of this system, including the respiratory muscles, neural drive, or the lung mechanical properties, can lead to respiratory failure at a point that is determined by the metabolic rate. Keens (33) was one of the first to point out that respiratory failure in children with progressive neuromuscular disease does not occur until the pubertal growth spurt, when the metabolic demands necessary to sustain a larger body mass overwhelm the gas exchange capacity of the respiratory system. In a second example of this principle, infants with BPD showed sustained elevation of resting oxygen consumption that could not be attributed to the expected increase in energy expenditure of the respiratory muscles necessary to overcome the mechanical work of breathing (34).

Respiratory failure in both pediatric patients and adults may be classified according to the presence or absence of alveolar hypoventilation (35,36). Type I respiratory failure is manifested by hypoxemia with a low arterial Pa_{O_2} and

- Abnormal lung function
- Respiratory muscle fatigue
- Decreased neural drive
- Increased resting energy expenditure
- High carbohydrate dietary load

- Increased neural drive
- Distribution of blood flow away from diseased lung units
- Diaphragm energy reserves
- Intermittent diaphragm rest?
- Renal HCO_3 reabsorption

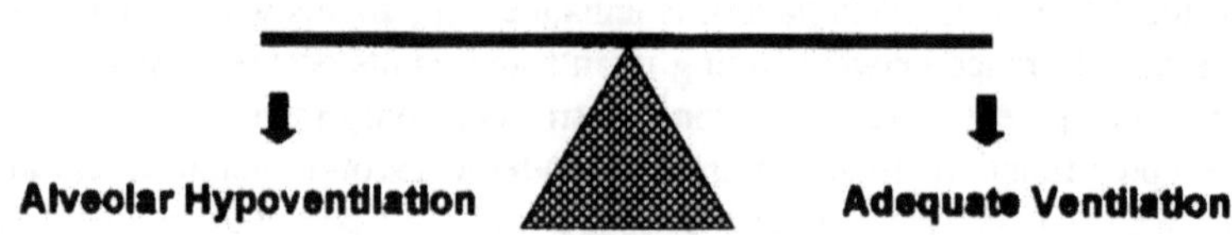

Figure 1 Variables promoting and impeding respiratory failure in pediatric patients. (Modified from Ref. 33.)

normal to low $Paco_2$. The predominant cause of type I failure is ventilation/perfusion mismatch. Type I failure typically occurs in acute conditions, such as status asthmaticus and acute respiratory distress syndrome (ARDS), in which poorly ventilated air spaces remain perfused despite regional hypoxia-induced vasoconstriction. Type II respiratory failure is caused by alveolar hypoventilation and manifested by an elevated arterial $Paco_2$ with or without hypoxemia. This type of respiratory failure is more likely to result from conditions impairing ventilation, such as depressed neural ventilatory drive, neuromuscular weakness, marked obesity, and rib cage abnormalities. In pediatric patients with significant upper airway obstruction, type II respiratory failure may occur during sleep despite sustained activity of the respiratory muscles (37).

Respiratory failure in children is typically classified as acute or chronic depending on the time course of presentation and underlying disorder. Children with chronic respiratory failure typically can lead a relatively normal life provided there is adequate renal compensation for the underlying acid-base disruption associated with hypercarbia. In a common clinical sequence, children with disorders complicated by compensated chronic respiratory failure present with acute or chronic respiratory acidosis brought on by an infection (38). A second common sequence occurs in pediatric patients with respiratory distress and type I respiratory failure. Such patients can develop respiratory muscle fatigue and progress to a mixed or a predominately type II pattern of respiratory failure (39). Another fundamental point to consider in children with disorders of neuromuscular weakness or impaired ventilatory control is that they may not exhibit classic physical signs of respiratory distress in the face of profound abnormalities in respiratory gas exchange. In such patients, an arterial or capillary blood gas analysis is essential to gauge the magnitude of respiratory system compromise.

Respiratory Mechanics in Children with Acute and Chronic Lung Disease

Young infants with the respiratory distress syndrome are at significant risk for alveolar hypoventilation as a result of a number of derangements in lung mechanical function. In the presence of a significant decrease in dynamic lung compliance, both the respiratory rate and dead space/tidal volume ratio nearly double (40). Because the chest wall is highly compliant, compensatory increases in diaphragmatic contraction manifest in young infants as asynchronous movements of the thorax and abdomen (termed retractions or in-drawing). The compliant chest wall also promotes a relatively low end-expiratory lung volume, so young infants with respiratory disease are particularly prone to hypoxemia (41). The decrease in respiratory muscle tone during REM sleep enhances the effect of the floppy chest wall in impairing diaphragmatic function (29). Rapid eye movement sleep is a time when infants with respiratory disease are particularly vulnerable to derangements in respiratory gas exchange.

Respiratory Control and Response to Treatment in Children with Chronic Lung Disease

Pediatric patients with chronic lung disease can develop abnormalities in respiratory control through the effects of hypoxemia, hypercarbia, and sleep stage (42). In children with cyanotic congenital heart disease, the ventilatory response to hypoxia is depressed but normalizes following surgical correction of the cause of cyanosis (43). Although chronic hypercarbia appears to promote a sustained increase in respiratory center output, it may blunt the ventilatory response to CO_2 in children with chronic lung disease (42). Long-term furosemide therapy associated with systemic chloride depletion can further blunt the ventilatory response to hypercarbia (44). Furosemide therapy complicated by hypochloremic metabolic alkalosis was an important risk factor for increased mortality in infants with BPD (45). During REM sleep, depressed ventilatory responses to both hypoxemia and hypercarbia in association with lung and chest wall mechanical factors can promote significant episodes of hypoxemia (46). In normal children, oxygen saturation (Sao_2) drops by a mean of 2.2% during sleep, with no decreases in oxygen saturation greater than 4% (42). Decreases in oxygen saturation greater than 4% are common during sleep in children with chronic respiratory disease.

Long-term assisted ventilation may also impact respiratory control in pediatric patients with chronic respiratory failure. Adults with chronic respiratory disorders associated with hypercarbia treated with intermittent noninvasive positive pressure ventilation (NPPV) demonstrated a significant reduction in daytime arterial $Paco_2$ (47). Increased elimination of CO_2 at night most likely restores the ventilatory response to hypercarbia, thereby resulting in an increase in daytime CO_2 elimination (48). In a preliminary report, similar improvement in daytime respiratory gas exchange was found in pediatric patients with chronic hypoventilation disorders treated with intermittent NPPV (38). Oxygen therapy may exacerbate the degree of hypoventilation in adults with chronic obstructive pulmonary disease. However, oxygen therapy in children with chronic lung disease may not worsen hypoventilation in specific conditions (8,49). Oxygen therapy alone in the absence of assisted ventilation can exacerbate hypercarbia and may be unsafe in older children with conditions associated with sustained impairment of the ventilatory response to hypercarbia such as spina bifida and obesity hypoventilation syndrome (50).

III. Historical Perspective

Although definitive documentation is lacking, probably the earliest attempts at assisted respiration of infants and children stem from the use of bellows in the late seventeenth century for victims of near-drowning (51). One of the first devices to incorporate the principle of negative pressure ventilation was designed by Braun in 1889 for infant resuscitation and used in 50 consecutive cases (52). In 1929, Charles F. McKhann, a pediatrician, along with Drinker and Shaw, developed the first "iron lung" device for resuscitation after industrial accidents (Table 2). In the same year, Drinker and McKhann (53) published an article describing its use in an 8-yr-old girl with poliomyelitis. The Emerson negative pressure ventilator, a modification of the Drinker device, was used extensively for long-term assisted ventilation of pediatric patients during the poliomyelitis epidemics of 1930s to 1950s in the United States and abroad. Dr. John Effeldt and colleagues at Ranchos Los Amigos in 1953 began to send respirator-dependent survivors of poliomyelitis home with trained attendants (54). A key legacy of this era was to affirm the concept that home care for children with chronic respiratory insufficiency was preferable to institutional care.

The modern era of prolonged mechanical ventilation with positive pressure ventilators in pediatric patients began in the early 1950s (55). The introduction of polyvinyl nasotracheal tubes in 1962 eliminated the need for tracheostomy and significantly advanced positive pressure mechanical ventilation in newborns (56). This was quickly followed by pioneering applications of positive pressure ventilators in newborns with hyaline membrane disease in the United States, Canada, and Europe (57).

Table 2 Historical Landmarks in Long-Term Mechanical Ventilation of Pediatric Patients

1929	Charles F. McKhann et al. treat a child with poliomyelitis with a tank ventilator.
1953	John Effeldt et al. pioneer the concept of home mechanical ventilation in children with poliomyelitis.
1971	Robert Kirby et al. design a volume-controlled ventilator for pediatric patients.
1978	Carl Hunt et al. treat three neonates with CCH with bilateral phrenic pacing.
1981	President Ronald Reagan waives existing regulations to permit supplemental income benefits beyond Medicaid to Katie Beckett, a ventilator-dependent child.
1983	Barbara Burr et al. publish an article in the New England Journal of Medicine reporting satisfactory outcomes in five children treated at home with mechanical ventilation.
1989	Nielson et al. transition a child with CCH from TPPV to NPPV successfully.

In early applications, adult ventilators with high flow rates and inspiratory pressures were adjusted to accommodate the rapid breathing patterns of infants with respiratory distress (58). This approach, while improving survival in larger infants, did not work with infants under 1500 g in body weight. However, in 1971, Gregory et al. (59) significantly improved survival in small neonates with respiratory distress syndrome through the introduction of continuous positive airway pressure. During the same year, Kirby et al. (60) designed the first safe and effective unit for intermittent mandatory volume-regulated ventilation for pediatric patients.

Further advances in medical technology and knowledge during the 1960s and 1970s applied to children with diverse causes of respiratory failure resulted in a large population of children unable to be weaned from mechanical ventilation. In 1978, Hunt et al. (61) reported the use of phrenic nerve electrical stimulation to artificially ventilate three neonates with congenital central alveolar hypoventilation syndrome. In the mid-1980s, the first reports of successful home care for ventilator-dependent children using either positive or negative pressure devices began to appear in the medical literature (1,54,62,63). By 1983, the Surgeon General of the United States, C. Everett Koop (6), called for longitudinal studies to analyze the results of caring for ventilator-dependent children at home.

One of the first descriptions of noninvasive ventilation was reported in 1969 in spinal injury patients treated with positive pressure ventilation via a mouthpiece (64). By the late 1980s long-term noninvasive positive pressure ventilation of pediatric patients became possible through the introduction of soft nasal masks and portable pressure-targeted ventilators (65–67). In one of the earliest reported applications, long-term NPPV via nasal mask was substituted for conventional invasive positive pressure home ventilation to facilitate tracheal decannulation in a 12-yr-old girl with central hypoventilation syndrome (68).

IV. Methods Available for Long-Term Mechanical Ventilation of Pediatric Patients

A. Overview

The most important disorders causing respiratory failure in 455 pediatric patients treated with long-term mechanical ventilation in 19 articles published from 1983 to 1998 included progressive and nonprogressive myopathies (26%), BPD (26%), congenital and acquired central hypoventilation syndromes (18%), assorted congenital anomalies including heart disease (16%), spinal injury (6%), and obstructive hypoventilation syndromes (4%) (Table 3). Positive pressure ventilation via tracheostomy (TPPV) was the predominant (71%) method used in these reports. Other methods less frequently applied included positive pressure ventilation via nasal mask (NPPV) (13%), electrophenic stimulation of the diaphragm (9%), negative pressure ventilation via a tank (5%) or chest cuirass (1%), tracheostomy with continuous positive airway pressure (CPAP) (1%), the rocking bed (<1%), and the pneumobelt (<1%). Treatment with negative pressure ventilators peaked in the decade following the polio epidemic, but utilization fell after the introduction of portable positive pressure units suitable for pediatric patients. Descriptions of long-term NPPV via nasal mask in pediatric patients appeared in the literature only recently, but this method appears to be the fastest growing based on early success and the number of recent publications in support of NPPV in pediatric patients (38,65,67–72).

The selection of a specific method of long-term mechanical ventilation for an infant or child with chronic respiratory failure should involve consideration of a number of factors (4). These include the age of the patient, pattern and degree of respiratory dysfunction, educational and financial characteristics of the caregivers, the anticipated site of care, and the need for portability. Young infants with incurable or progressive disorders are most likely to need an artificial airway and a positive pressure unit. Patients with neuromuscular disorders may compensate very well for a number of years but then need ventilatory assistance with the onset of puberty or in association with an acute respiratory infection (33). Intermittent nocturnal noninvasive ventilation may work well in these patients and delay the need for a tracheostomy.

B. Invasive Methods of Mechanical Ventilation

Invasive mechanical ventilation involves a permanent tracheostomy interfaced with a positive pressure ventilator or electrophrenic pacing apparatus. As a general principle, young infants with significant respiratory dysfunction have most

Table 3 Diagnoses and Methods in Pediatric Patients Treated with Long-Term Mechanical Ventilation 1983–1998

Diagnosis	n	TPPV	NPPV	Tank	Cuirass	CPAP	Phrenic pacing
Central hypoventilation syndromes (1,38,54,61,75,82,83,97,117,137)							
n = 82 (18%)							
Mean duration of follow-up 3.7 yr							
Mean Survival 79%							
CCH	72	32	2	0	1	0	41
Arnold-Chiari malformation	5	0	5	0	0	0	0
Metabolic/acquired	5	5	0	0	0	0	0
Neuromuscular disorders (1,54,63,69,75,107,108,115,117,128,129,137)							
n = 157 (34%)							
Myopathies	117	72	22	19	5	1	0
Spinal injury	27	23	0	4	0	0	0
Chest wall deformity	13	4	8	0	0	1	0
Parenchymal lung diseases (63,71,75,117,118)							
n = 127 (28%)							
BPD	117	178	0	0	0	0	0
CF	9	1	7	0	0	1	0
Interstitial lung disease	1	1	0	0	0	0	0
Congenital anomalies (54,63,75,117,137)							
n = 73 (16%)							
Heart diseases	30	27	0	0	0	3	0
Hypoplastic lungs	2	2	0	0	0	0	0
Assorted anomalies	41	40	0	0	0	1	0
Obstructive hypoventilation syndromes (38,117)							
n = 16 (4%)							
Obesity	10	0	10	0	0	0	0
Anatomic	6	0	6	0	0	0	0
Totals (%)	455	324 (71)	60 (13)	23 (5)	6 (1)	7 (1)	41 (9)

often been treated with invasive methods (4). A tracheostomy may also be necessary in patients treated with negative pressure units. Patients treated with negative pressure ventilators not uncommonly develop occlusive apnea and hypoxemia during sleep. Nasal CPAP may be used to stabilize the upper airways of such patients, thereby avoiding tracheostomy (73).

Positive Pressure Ventilation via Tracheostomy

Time-Cycled Constant Flow Ventilators

Time-cycled constant flow ventilators provide a high level of background flow and therefore are typically designed for medical transport of small infants. The Newport E100I® can function as either a volume-limited or pressure plateau ventilator in one of three modes: synchronized intermittent mandatory ventilation (SIMV), assist control, or spontaneous ventilation (74). In home use, the air–oxygen blender is not used because the blender consumes a large volume of oxygen to pneumatically drive the ventilator. To raise the fraction of inspired oxygen (FIO_2), oxygen is blended into the inspiratory circuit and the system is driven pneumatically by an air compressor. This ventilator has limited transport capabilities in that oxygen cylinders are required to provide a high-pressure gas source. Wheeler et al. (75) reported successful outcomes in young infants with chronic lung disease treated with this type of ventilator.

Microprocessor-Controlled Volume Ventilators

These ventilators are not driven by air compressors and therefore offer enhanced portability over time-cycled constant flow units (74). Most feature a wide range of volumes, inspiratory times, and breathing rates, and can be used in patients of all sizes. Modern units such as the Aequitron LP 10® feature a spring-loaded valve that operates independently of the microprocessor to limit inspiratory pressure in the assist control or SIMV mode. This function alters the normal pressure waveform by providing a plateau that may be especially effective in pediatric patients by reducing barotrauma and maintaining a more constant minute ventilation in the presence of a variable leak around the uncuffed tracheostomy (33,76). However, the concept of pressure plateau mechanical ventilation is difficult to teach caregivers in preparation for home care. A second major drawback to these ventilators when used in the SIMV or assist control mode is that significant ventilatory effort is necessary to trigger a spontaneous ventilator-assisted breath. Since these units do not provide a constant flow source, an external flow source is required for small infants to reduce the work of breathing (77).

Electrophrenic Pacing

This invasive method involves intermittent electrical stimulation of the phrenic nerve via an external radiofrequency transmitter and subcutaneous receiver-electrode system (78). Unlike adult patients in whom unilateral pacing has been used effectively, bilateral simultaneous pacing applied intermittently has been the most successful method in infants and children (61,79,80). Pediatric patients with electrophrenic pacers are typically treated with TPPV at night to avoid injury to the phrenic nerve through constant stimulation (61). Patients from infancy to adolescence require a tracheostomy for electrophrenic pacing to avoid obstructive apneas caused by dyssynchronous contractions of the diaphragm and laryngeal muscles. The tracheostomy maintains upper airway patency and provides an interface for positive pressure ventilation (81). The method has been most often used in infants and children with congenital central hypoventilation syndrome (CCH) (61,79,82,83).

C. Noninvasive Methods of Mechanical Ventilation

Positive Pressure Ventilation via Nasal Mask

Noninvasive positive pressure ventilation augments alveolar ventilation with a positive pressure ventilator connected to the patient through a nasal or full-face mask interface not requiring an invasive artificial airway (5). Although volume-controlled units may be used, in most domestic settings NPPV in pediatric patients is accomplished using portable pressure-targeted, flow-triggered ventilators and nasal masks (84). Full-face masks can be used in older children, but may be dangerous in young infants at risk of gastric perforation (85). Advantages of NPPV with pressure-targeted ventilators include avoidance of tracheostomy, portability, simplicity of operation, and improved patient comfort by coupling spontaneous respiratory efforts with an adjustable level of inspiratory positive airway pressure. Important drawbacks to most commercially available pressure-targeted ventilators include a pressure-dependent exhalation system with potential rebreathing of CO_2 (86) and lack of an integrated oxygen blender to raise the FIO_2 (87). Modern portable pressure-support ventilators include an FIO_2 control setting and improved expiratory ports to decrease the likelihood of rebreathing CO_2 (86).

In spite of early promising reports and growing use (88), NPPV is still considered by some to be an experimental mode of long-term ventilatory support for pediatric patients (4). In nearly all of the published case reports to date, nasal mask interfaces have been effective despite significant gas leaks via the mouth (38,39,65–68,72). When necessary, the FIO_2 may be raised by blending pure oxygen directly into a small mask port or into the inspiratory tubing (38,89). In clinical practice, low flow rates suffice when the first method is used, whereas high flow rates are necessary as a result of the high background flow rate when the oxygen is blended into the inspiratory tubing.

Negative Pressure Ventilators

Tank Ventilators

Negative pressure ventilators are based on the application of external intermittent subatmospheric pressure to expand the rib cage, lungs, and abdomen. Tank ventilators seal the trunk and extremities of a patient within a chamber, and adjustment of the rate and magnitude of subatmospheric pressure swings permits augmentation of tidal volume. Large tank ventilators termed "iron lungs" were used extensively in pediatric patients during the early 1950s polio epidemic with mixed efficacy and are still in use in patients with Duchenne's muscular dystrophy (54). Recently, continuous negative extrathoracic pressure applied via a custom incubator reduced the incidence of chronic lung disease in neonates with acute respiratory failure (90). Today, tank ventilators have been largely replaced by customized chest shells. The main advantage of both tank and shell ventilators is to avoid or delay tracheostomy in children with hypoventilation associated with neuromuscular weakness. Disadvantages of large tank ventilators include limited portability, agitation in young children, and obstructive apnea/hypopnea syndrome in small patients with inherently unstable upper airway function (4).

Chest Shell and Wrap Ventilators

The chest shell is a modification of the large tank ventilator in which subatmospheric pressure is applied intermittently to the external thorax via a tightly fitted mold or cuirass. Commercial molds are limited to children older than 4 yr, although custom fits are available for young infants and older children with chest wall deformities (91). As with the large tank ventilators, chest shells are most useful in patients with normal lung mechanics and hypoventilation due to neuromuscular weakness in an attempt to avoid tracheostomy (4). They are not reliable in patients with reduced lung compliance or high airway resistance in whom high airway pressures may be necessary.

Rocking Bed and the Pneumobelt

Both of these methods are infrequently used but isolated case reports of their success as a primary mode of therapy (54) or in combination with other techniques (92) have been published. A rocking bed involves tilting the abdominal contents back and forth, thereby decreasing and expanding the intrathoracic volume. It is limited by lack of portability and can require a tracheostomy to be effective. The pneumobelt consists of a bladder held within an abdominal corset that is inflated intermittently by a positive pressure generator to raise intra-abdominal pressure and displace the abdominal contents cephalad. Alveolar ventilation results from expansion of the intrathoracic volume during the gravity-driven descent phase of the cycle. This method has very limited utilization in young patients and is restricted to older children and adolescents.

D. Electronic Monitoring

Appropriate electronic monitoring of the ventilator circuit and the child's cardiorespiratory status is essential for young patients treated at home with mechanical ventilation. The incidence of death and severe hypoxia-induced encephalopathy secondary to airway accidents in patients treated at home is 2.3 per 10,000 patient days, nine times higher than the expected incidence in an intensive care unit (93). Positive pressure ventilators when used with a tracheostomy should be equipped with disconnect alarms that sound in response to a minimally acceptable pressure in the ventilator circuit (4). Airway pressure monitoring is also indicated in patients treated at home with NPPV whose disease status is such that sudden disconnection from the external interface would result in cardiorespiratory instability (5). Impedance electronic monitors for apnea and bradycardia are indicated for all tracheostomy-dependent infants and children and ventilator-dependent patients with decreased central respiratory drive (4). It is a common practice to use pulse oximeters as a backup to thoracic impedance monitors in technology-dependent children. A recent review in home ventilator-dependent patients suggests that this practice may decrease the incidence of serious airway-related accidents (93). Pulse oximeters may also be used to guide the level of home oxygen therapy.

V. Long-Term Mechanical Ventilation for Pediatric Disorders Complicated by Chronic Respiratory Failure

A. Congenital and Acquired Central Alveolar Hypoventilation Syndromes

Congenital Central Hypoventilation Syndrome

Congenital central hypoventilation syndrome is often referred to as Ondine's curse. This term is both a literary and scientific misnomer, in that according to the original story, Ondine cursed no one and her lover was not rendered breathless (94). Congenital central hypoventilation syndrome is part of a spectrum of congenital autonomic nervous system abnormalities, termed the neurocristopathy syndrome, that likely result from defects in the migration and differentiation of neural crest tissues during embryogenesis (95). Infants with CCH hypoventilate during quiet (non-REM) sleep as a result of failure of the central chemoreceptors to respond to elevations in CO_2 (76). The ventilatory response to CO_2 during REM and wakefulness remains impaired in CCH patients; however, they do not appear to hypoventilate as much in these states since environmental cues stimulate respiratory efforts via higher cortical pathways (96). CCH is a lifelong disorder with significant co-morbidity as a result of colonic dysfunction, cardiac dysrhythmias, and neuroendocrine cell malignancies (76,95).

The primary mode of therapy for patients with CCH is long-term support with TPPV alone (1,54,82,97) or TPPV in association with bilateral phrenic nerve pacing of the diaphragm (Table 4) (61,80,92). Whereas long-term continuous electrophrenic pacing may lead to structural phrenic nerve injury (61), in most

Table 4 Selected Published Case Series of Long-Term Mechanical Ventilation in Pediatric Patients with Acquired and Congenital Central Hypoventilation Syndromes

First author	Year	n	Primary and co-morbid conditions	Modes of assisted ventilation	Survival and outcomes
Invasive methods					
Hunt (61)	1978	3	CCH, cor pulmonale	Diaphragm pacing	2 yr 33% 1 death from phrenic injury
Hyland (92)	1978	1	CCH, cor pulmonale, polycythemia	Diaphragm pacing/rocking bed	Not listed
Burr (1)	1983	4	CCH, asphyxia, recurrent pneumonia, seizures	TPPV 3 TPPV/diaphragm pacing 1	4 yr 100%
Goldberg (137)	1984	3	CCH	TPPV	Not listed
Frates (54)	1985	5	Acquired hypoventilation with encephalitis	TPPV	1.5 yr 40%
Oren (97)	1987	6	CCH, cor pulmonale, seizures	TPPV	8 yr 100%
Marcus (82)	1991	13	CCH, cor pulmonale, poor growth, seizures	TPPV 10 Cuirass 1 Diaphragm pacing 6	7 yr 92%
Weese-Mayer (83)	1992	32	CCH, cor pulmonale, heart block, Hirschsprung's	Diaphragm pacing/TPPV	6 yr 69%
Noninvasive methods					
Ellis (67)	1987	1	CCH	NPPV via nasal mask	3 mo 100%
Nielson (68)	1990	1	CCH, tracheitis	NPPV via nasal mask	3 yr 100%
Teague (38)	In review	5	Spina bifida, pneumonia	NPPV via nasal mask	2 yr 80%

case series diaphragm pacing is alternated with TPPV. Both methods require a tracheostomy early in life (81). Pharmacologic respiratory stimulants are generally not effective, but have not been studied in combination with other therapies (4,98). Only recently, a few older children with CCH have been weaned from tracheostomy and treated with intermittent NPPV (67,68). This approach remains experimental and likely will not be effective in small infants and toddlers without further advances in nasal mask design and pressure-targeted ventilators that will cycle reliably in a timed mode.

The Arnold-Chiari Malformation

The Arnold-Chiari malformation is a congenital anatomic abnormality that involves elongation of the hindbrain. The most common variant, type II, is defined by downward displacement of the medulla and cerebellum and is associated with myelomeningocele. Although patients with Arnold-Chiari malformation can present with a wide spectrum of respiratory abnormalities including vocal cord paresis secondary to brain stem dysfunction (99), hypoventilation usually results from central impairment of respiratory control and is likely to be lifelong (50). Infants with Arnold-Chiari malformation who undergo polysomnographic study have prolonged episodes of central apnea (100) and impaired arousal responses to both hypoxia and hypercarbia (101). Rarely, the magnitude of central alveolar hypoventilation is severe enough to require long-term assisted ventilation (4,38).

Inborn Errors of Metabolism and Acquired Forms of Central Hypoventilation

Central hypoventilation associated with chronic respiratory failure may be caused by a number of rare inborn errors of metabolism, including pyruvate dehydrogenase complex deficiency (102), Leigh disease (103), carnitine deficiency, and congenital abnormalities of the brain stem nuclei as in Mobius syndrome. Infants with these disorders may present with clinical signs and symptoms indistinguishable from CCH. In addition, pediatric patients may present with acquired central hypoventilation following brain stem injury from asphyxia (104), encephalitis caused by *Listeria monocytogenes* (105), or in association with Reye's syndrome (106). In general, the overall prognosis for many of these conditions is poor even with long-term mechanical ventilatory support.

Summary of Evidence in the Management of Central Hypoventilation Disorders

Although there have been no controlled clinical trials, available evidence via case series suggests that TPPV with or without supplemental diaphragmatic pacing prolongs survival and permits a reasonable quality of life in children with CCH.

The main advantage of supplemental diaphragmatic pacing is to permit independence from TPPV during the day, but may be complicated by phrenic nerve injury, infection, and technical failure of the implanted electronic components. It is not at all established whether supplemental diaphragmatic pacing with TPPV prolongs survival in children with CCH compared with TPPV alone. Respiratory pharmacologic stimulants may decrease the magnitude of hypoventilation in selected patients; however, they do not appear to be efficacious in the primary management of CCH. Noninvasive methods such as negative pressure devices or NPPV may permit removal of the tracheostomy in selected cases of CCH. However, at present, experience with this mode of treatment is limited to a few isolated case reports and is not validated at all in small patients.

B. Restrictive Pulmonary Disorders

Neuromuscular Weakness

Pediatric patients with progressive and nonprogressive disorders associated with neuromuscular weakness present with respiratory failure when the respiratory muscles are too weak to sustain adequate alveolar ventilation (107). Respiratory failure is inevitable over time in progressive neuromuscular disorders such as spinal muscular atrophy or muscular dystrophy. Children with both progressive and nonprogressive neuromuscular disorders often compensate until adolescence or late school-age when the weak respiratory muscles cannot keep pace with the metabolic demands of an increased body mass (4). In an all too common scenario, previously stable pediatric patients with neuromuscular disorders require mechanical ventilation as a complication of an acute lower respiratory tract infection. Once intubated, these patients may be very difficult to wean as a result of impaired cough clearance, atelectasis, and respiratory muscle weakness (38).

Current published evidence suggests that these patients may be ideal candidates for long-term mechanical ventilation in specific circumstances (4). In one notable exception, Rutherford et al. (108) found that long-term survival was nil in very young infants with congenital myotonic dystrophy who required mechanical ventilation for longer than thirty days. In contrast, Gilgoff et al. (107) reported survival rates of 87% over a mean follow-up period of 8 yr in 15 pediatric-age patients with spinal muscular atrophy treated with long-term mechanical ventilation. Although studies analyzing specific outcomes by treatment mode have not been published in pediatric patients, some trends are apparent from review of several published case series (Table 5). As has been found in adult patients with neuromuscular diseases, pediatric patients with neuromuscular diseases appear to progress through an initial phase of nocturnal hypoventilation that is associated with episodic obstructive apnea (21). If recognized, treatment with intermittent NPPV at this early phase may significantly improve daytime respiratory gas exchange and functional status (38). However, in a large randomized clinical trial

Table 5 Selected Published Case Series Abstracted for Results of Long-Term Mechanical Ventilation in Pediatric Patients with Neuromuscular Disorders

First author	Year	n	Primary and co-morbid conditions	Modes of assisted ventilation	Follow-up and survival
Invasive assisted ventilation					
Goldberg (137)	1984	5		TPPV	Not listed
Frates (54)	1985	41	Neuromuscular 24 Spinal injury 17	TPPV	5 yr 67% 3 yr 65%
Schreiner (63)	1987	14	Neuromuscular 9 Spinal 5	TPPV	3 yr 71%
Rutherford (108)	1989	4	Congenital myotonic dystrophy	TPPV	9 mo 0%
Gilgoff (107)	1989	15	Spinal muscular atrophy	TPPV	8 yr 87%
Heckmatt (128)	1989	7	Nonprogressive neuromuscular disease	TPPV 2 Cuirass 5	3 yr 86%
Canlas-Yamsuan (117)	1993	12	Neuromuscular 6 Spinal injury 6	TPPV 10	2.6 yr 75%
Noninvasive assisted ventilation					
Heckmatt (69)	1990	14	Assorted neuromuscular disorders 12 Rigid spine 2	NPPV	1.5 yr 100% 4/14 did not tolerate NPPV
Khan (129)	1996	8	Congenital myopathy 4 Duchenne's 2 Rigid spine 2	NPPV	4 yr 100%

in patients with muscular dystrophy and normocapnia, "early" intermittent use of NPPV did not delay the onset of hypercapnia or interrupt the expected decline in FVC (109).

The optimal method of ventilatory assistance for children with advanced neuromuscular disease is not clear based on the current evidence. Once the degree of respiratory muscle weakness and hypoventilation reach a critical stage, continuous mechanical ventilation is necessary and long-term survival declines (21,54). The goals of management should be identified and a method selected based on criteria presented earlier. Controlled trials comparing various methods are needed. In an interesting review of home care in adults, Leger reported that the probability of continuing with NPPV long-term was lower in patients with muscular dystrophy than with other causes of hypoventilation (110,111). Treatment with continuous NPPV at this stage may be impractical, and as a result TPPV or tracheostomy with negative pressure ventilation are suitable alternatives.

Chest Wall Dysfunction

Idiopathic scoliosis in the absence of respiratory muscle weakness can reduce lung volume when the spinal angle exceeds 70° (112). Advanced uncorrected scoliosis can lead to hypoventilation and compromise respiratory muscle function (113). Hypoventilation has also been described in infants with congenital disorders affecting the development of the chest wall, including asphyxiating thoracic dystrophy, short-limbed dwarfism, and giant omphalocele (114). Before the advent of NPPV, patients with hypoventilation associated with chest wall dysfunction were treated commonly with negative pressure ventilation and other ventilatory adjuncts. Common reasons for failure of negative pressure ventilation include young age and advanced scoliosis (115). For pediatric patients with advanced scoliosis, a custom mold is often necessary to achieve a tight seal for effective mechanical ventilation with the cuirass (4). Considering that NPPV is effective for adult patients with restrictive impairment from chest wall dysfunction (47), its use should be contemplated early on in the management of pediatric patients with similar conditions.

C. Disorders Involving Lung Parenchyma and Airways

Bronchopulmonary Dysplasia

Bronchopulmonary dysplasia is a highly variable disorder that is associated with premature birth and exposure to both hyperoxia and positive pressure mechanical ventilation during the neonatal period (8,9). When severe, BPD can result in chronic respiratory failure due to a combination of obstructive airways dysfunction with loss of alveolar units and fibrosis. The pattern of BPD has changed over the years, probably because of the introduction of artificial surfactant to treat the neonatal respiratory distress syndrome and advances in respiratory management (90). Unlike the previous two decades, it is less common today to find infants with BPD who require long-term mechanical ventilation at home. With appropriate management, the prognosis for significant improvement in pulmonary function over time is very good although functional impairment with exercise does persist well into school age and adolescence (116).

Long-term mechanical ventilation in infants with BPD is typically initiated in the hospital and continued after discharge in the patient's home (Table 6). Tracheostomies were necessary in all patients reported to date interfaced with a range of positive pressure devices, including CPAP units (117), volume- and pressure-cycled ventilators (63,75,118), and portable flow-triggered bilevel pressure ventilators (70). In all of the published reports except one (118), short-term survival was greater than 90% and eventual weaning and tracheal decannulation were the norm (63,75,117). In the study with low survival, the patient population included primarily hospital-based infants observed over a relatively short span starting from birth (118). This is a time when mortality would be expected to be highest. In contrast, the case mix in three long-term studies with good survival rates includes older infants stable enough to go home on a ventilator (63,75,117). However, the hospital readmission rate for these infants was high with significant morbidity associated with respiratory infections during the first year of life (117).

Cystic Fibrosis and Other Chronic Lung Diseases

Cystic fibrosis (CF) is a genetic disease with a pervasive reduction in chloride transport across epithelial apical membranes due to impaired function of a transmembrane regulatory protein. Children with advanced cystic fibrosis typically have severe obstructive pulmonary dysfunction and bronchiectasis associated with endobronchial colonization with various bacteria, including *P. aeruginosa*. Although survival rates in recent years have significantly improved, most patients die in young adulthood from respiratory failure. There is a general consensus among clinicians that mechanical ventilation is rarely justified for cystic fibrosis patients with advanced pulmonary involvement since weaning is typically prolonged and survival post-extubation is only for a few weeks (119). The possibility of immediate improvement through lung transplantation may change this paradigm. Despite growing use of long-term mechanical ventilation in adults with chronic obstructive pulmonary disease, experience with long-term home mechanical ventilation is very limited for CF patients, with poor outcomes generally reported (117).

Early reports of intermittent NPPV treatment in patients with cystic fibrosis are encouraging (65,72,120). In young adult patients with advanced disease, nocturnal NPPV eliminated the increase in Pa_{CO_2} associated with supplemental oxygen therapy (72). In a case series of patients with severe gas exchange abnormali-

Table 6 Published Case Reviews of Long-Term Mechanical Ventilation in Pediatric Patients with Bronchopulmonary Dysplasia

Author	Year	n	Method	Survival	Comments
Schreiner (63)	1987	35	TPPV	1 yr 97%	19/35 discharged from the hospital on TPPV, only 1/32 with primary pulmonary disease treated with TPPV died
Canlas-Yamsuan (117)	1983	3	Trach-CPAP	2.6 yr 100%	All discharged from the hospital, 2/3 underwent tracheal decannulation, high hospital readmission rate
Overstreet (118)	1991	58	TPPV	4 mo 10%	Primarily a hospital-based cohort, mortality associated with level of respiratory support
Wheeler (75)	1994	20	TPPV	31 mo 90%	16/20 discharged from the hospital on TPPV, 15/20 ultimately weaned, 19/20 had tracheomalacia

ties, intermittent NPPV was well tolerated, improved the quality of life, and was viewed as a successful bridge therapy to lung transplantation (65). Further studies are needed to examine the role of intermittent NPPV in cystic fibrosis patients with regard to specific outcomes. Similar to adults with COPD, the role of NPPV may well be to reduce hospitalization and improve functional but not physiologic outcomes.

Pediatric patients can acquire chronic respiratory failure as a result of a number of disorders damaging the airways and lung parenchyma. Unusual but serious conditions in this category include the repair phase of severe ARDS, interstitial lung diseases, and bronchiolitis obliterans. Experience with long-term mechanical ventilation in these disorders is lacking and, to date, generally unsuccessful with regard to long-term survival (117). However, most of the experience predates lung transplantation as an option for these patients. Home mechanical ventilation could be considered as a bridge therapy to transplantation in individual patients.

D. Syndromes Complicated by Obstructive Hypoventilation

This is a heterogeneous group of disorders characterized by hypoventilation from upper airway obstruction and typically exacerbated by sleep. Patients with obstructive hypoventilation syndrome (OHS) often have primary disorders associated with restrictive changes in lung function. Included within this category are infants and children with morbid obesity, cerebral palsy, and craniofacial syndromes characterized by fixed upper airway obstruction (Table 7). Obstructive hypoventilation syndrome is diagnosed best by overnight polysomnography with prolonged episodes of hypopnea accompanied by thoracoabdominal asynchrony and hypercarbia (37). Periods of complete airflow obstruction are not typical due to sustained activity of the diaphragm but at the price of a significant increase in work of breathing. These patients may also hypoventilate during the day. Fatigue of the respiratory muscles in association with a decrease in central respiratory drive are thought to play a role in the pathogenesis of OHS.

Patients with OHS often have co-morbid conditions, such as cardiac anomalies, gastroesophageal reflux disease, scoliosis, and recurrent pneumonia, that may contribute significantly to the total pattern of respiratory impairment. Obstructive hypoventilation syndrome is frequently termed an "overlap" syndrome due to the combination of upper and lower respiratory tract dysfunction. For example, children with obesity hypoventilation syndrome have severe nocturnal obstructive apnea/hypopnea (121) in association with restrictive changes in lung function. The degree of respiratory dysfunction may require mechanical ventilation (122). Infants and toddlers with Down syndrome have functional upper airway obstruction from hypotonia and macroglossia that is further complicated by lower respiratory tract dysfunction, typically due to cardiac anomalies and a high

Table 7 Disorders Associated with Obstructive Hypoventilation Syndrome in Pediatric Patients

Morbid obesity
Prader-Willi syndrome
Obesity hypoventilation syndrome
Cerebral palsy
Associated with upper airway obstruction from laryngeal dysfunction and/or malposition of the tongue
Frequently exacerbated by scoliosis and parenchymal dysfunction from recurrent infection
Myelomeningocele with bulbar dysfunction and vocal cord paresis
Frequently accompanied by chronic aspiration lung injury
Craniofacial syndromes with maxillary hypoplasia
Apert's syndrome
Crouzon's syndrome
Treacher-Collins syndrome
Carpenter's syndrome
Rubinstein-Taybi syndrome
Fetal alcohol syndrome
Choanal atresia/stenosis
Subglottic stenosis with or without GERD
Vocal cord paresis
Down syndrome
Complicated by sleep obstructive apnea
Often associated with variable lower respiratory tract obstruction (tracheomalacia)
Severe primary laryngo- and tracheomalacia
Often associated with gastroesophageal reflux disease
Complicated obstructive sleep apnea syndrome
Associated with massive adenotonsillar hypertrophy and cor pulmonale
Associated with pharyngeal flap repair of cleft palate

incidence of tracheomalacia. During sleep there may be significant hypoxemia in these patients, of sufficient magnitude to increase the pulmonary vascular resistance (123).

Treatment with supplemental oxygen alone while improving oxygenation does not relieve the severity or frequency of obstructive episodes (49). Tracheostomy is the primary mode of treatment for pediatric patients with severe hypoventilation due to upper airway obstruction. Due to its invasive nature and the social disadvantages of tracheostomy, older patients with obstructive hypoventilation syndrome may be treated with nasal mask CPAP (124) or NPPV (38). Nasal CPAP therapy in patients with long-standing obstructive hypoventilation may be complicated by central hypoventilation, especially in the obese (125). For this reason NPPV should be considered as an alternate and possibly preferred treatment to CPAP in children with morbid obesity and obstructive hypoventilation (125). In five toddlers with OHS from anatomic upper airway obstruction, NPPV was an effective "bridge" therapy to corrective airway surgery (38). There is also an important role for NPPV in patients with upper airway obstruction from adenotonsillar hypertrophy at risk for perioperative decompensation (126). Long-term survival and quality of life in patients with OHS depend in part on successful surgical management (127) and the prognosis of the underlying disorder.

VI. Survival, Complications, and Family Issues

A. Survival

Long-term survival for pediatric patients treated with mechanical ventilation is influenced significantly by the prognosis of the underlying disorder (75,117). As a general principle, patients with reversible disorders of the lung parenchyma, such as BPD, fare better than those with nonreversible parenchymal disorders, such as CF and progressive neurologic conditions. The average 5-yr cumulative survival abstracted from 14 case reports for 265 pediatric patients with a variety of disorders treated with home mechanical ventilation was approximately 85% (1,38,54,69,75,82,83,97,107,108,117,128,129) (Fig. 2). The average duration of follow-up in these reports was 3.3 yr and survival estimates beyond 5 yr are relatively less accurate.

In pediatric patients with central hypoventilation syndromes, average cumulative survival from discharge over a mean 5-yr period of follow-up exceeded 90% in 70 infants treated with both TPPV alone and TPPV with daytime electrophrenic pacing (Fig. 3) (1,54,82,83,97). It is not at all clear whether supplemental electrophrenic pacing prolongs survival in infants with CCH. Patients do appear to benefit in respect to quality of life by not being dependent on the ventilator during the day. The role of NPPV in the treatment of pediatric patients with CCH deserves further study since preliminary reports suggest that it might be an effective alternate to TPPV in older patients.

Cumulative 5-yr survival estimates in 137 pediatric patients treated with long-term mechanical ventilation at home for assorted neuromuscular diseases were slightly lower (75%) than those reported for chest wall or central hypoventilation syndromes (Fig. 4). This high-risk cohort includes patients with spinal injury and progressive neuromuscular disorders who typically are dependent on continuous mechanical ventilation. Unlike infants with CCH and BPD, many are older when treated with mechanical ventilation. Cumulative survival from 2 to 5 yr postdischarge in patients treated with negative pressure devices (54,115) was similar to if not higher than it was in those treated with TPPV (54,63,107,117).

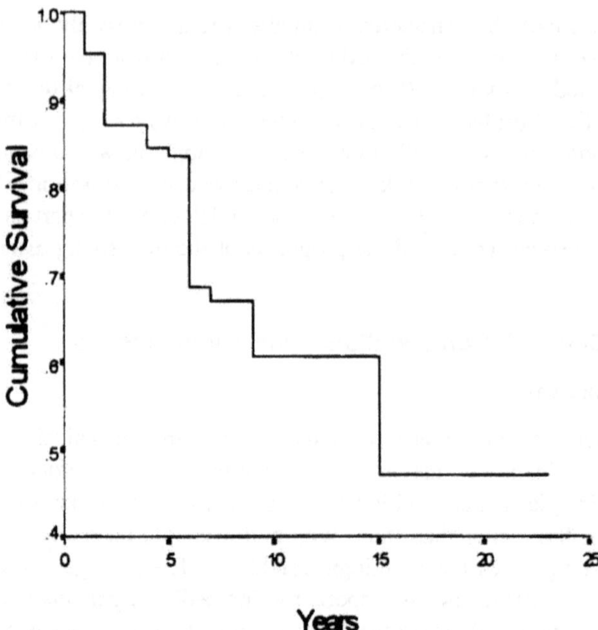

Figure 2 Cumulative survival from discharge to home in pediatric patients with chronic respiratory failure associated with several disorders treated with long-term mechanical ventilation. The data were abstracted from case reports published from 1983 to 1998 including 265 patients with central hypoventilation syndromes, neuromuscular diseases, congenital anomalies, and parenchymal disorders. The mean duration of follow-up in these reports was 3.3 yr.

With regard to parenchymal disorders, most of the published experience relates to outcomes in infants with BPD. In this diagnostic group, overall mean cumulative survival was 93% over an average 1.5 yr of follow-up (63,75). The likelihood of weaning and tracheal decannulation in these reports was high. However, these publications report the outcomes of infants who were stable enough to be discharged for home care and not all infants with BPD. Mortality was much higher in the report by Overstreet et al. (118) wherein survival of infants who required mechanical ventilation for BPD followed from birth was much lower. With respect to severe parenchymal disorders, such as CF, in older children, survival with home mechanical ventilation was poor in the few patients reported in previous case series (117). Although there is no evidence at present that it will prolong survival, NPPV appears to be an exceptionally promising mode of therapy in these patients.

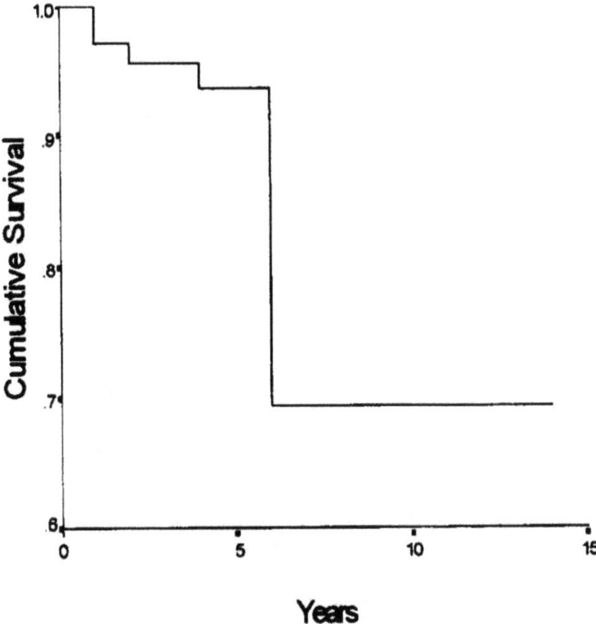

Figure 3 Cumulative survival from discharge in 70 pediatric patients with congenital central hypoventilation syndrome treated at home with TPPV or nocturnal TPPV and daytime electrophrenic pacing. The mean duration of follow-up in these reports was 5 yr.

B. Complications of Long-Term Mechanical Ventilation

Tracheostomy both in the hospital and at home is an exceptionally high-risk method of maintaining the pediatric airway. In one pediatric case series, tracheostomy was associated with a complication rate of 26% 130. Complications related to tracheostomy include death from accidental decannulation, obstruction with a mucus plug, and infection (Table 8) (130–132). In 22 children transferred from endotracheal intubation to tracheostomy for the purposes of long-term mechanical ventilation, colonization of the airway with bacteria occurred in 95%, although the infection rate was no higher following tracheostomy than it was following transtracheal intubation (133). Traumatic injury to the trachea and stoma is common with a high rate of granuloma formation, suprastomal tracheomalacia, and acquired tracheal stenosis. Significant bleeding may occur in association with episodes of tracheobronchitis and mucosal injury or erosion through the tracheal wall into the thyrocervical artery. The presence of a tracheostomy per se diminishes the protective function of the larynx against aspiration of salivary and gastric contents. Social complications include difficulty in attending school, impaired

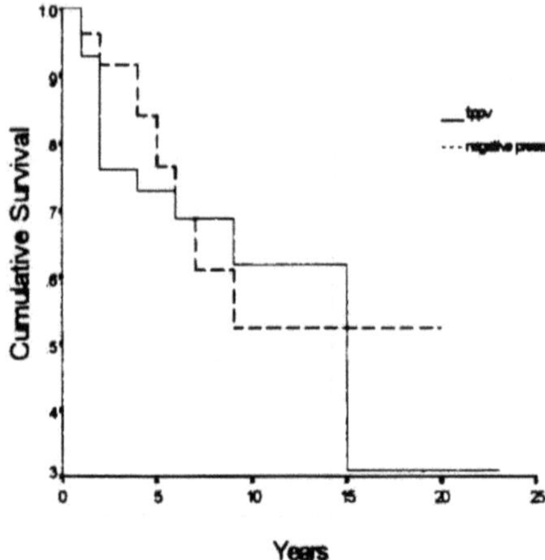

Figure 4 Cumulative survival after discharge from the hospital in 137 pediatric patients with neuromuscular disorders treated at home with long-term mechanical ventilation. The solid line indicates patients treated with positive-pressure ventilation via tracheostomy and the interrupted line indicates patients treated with negative pressure ventilation via a tank device. The mean duration of follow-up in these case reports was 3.3 yr.

speech, and potential water aspiration with swimming or baths. The risk of significant complications from the tracheostomy is related in part to the age of the patient, with adverse outcomes being more uncommon in the very young (131).

Recurrent pneumonia is cited most often as a complication of long-term mechanical ventilation in pediatric patients and is an important cause of hospital readmission (see Table 8). The second most cited complication of TPPV relates to accidents involving the tracheostomy and ventilator circuit. In one case series, tracheostomy complications were as common in children who required a tracheostomy for mechanical ventilation as they were in children with tracheal stenosis (134). Medical cardiovascular complications include congestive heart failure in patients with congenital neuromuscular disorders and as a complication of pulmonary artery hypertension in patients with chronic hypoxemia. Feeding problems with a reduction in growth velocity are an important complication of TPPV in pediatric patients due to swallow and laryngeal dysfunction as a consequence of the tracheostomy. Many patients ultimately require a permanent feeding gastrostomy.

C. Impact on the Family

Families with ventilator-dependent children in the home often experience significant levels of stress, both social and financial. Most report inadequate finances

Table 8 Complications of Long-Term Invasive Mechanical Ventilation via Tracheostomy in Pediatric Patients

Infection
Recurrent pneumonia (0.6)[a]
Fatal bacterial tracheobronchitis (0.05)
Medical
Recurrent hospital admissions (0.35)
Pulmonary artery hypertension (0.25)
Congestive heart failure (0.20)
Occult hypoxemia and hypercarbia (0.15)
Pulmonary embolism (0.05)
Atelectasis (0.05)
Tracheostomy and ventilator circuit dysfunction
Accidental ventilator disconnect (0.20)
Acquired supra-stomal tracheomalacia (0.15)
Bleeding (0.15)
Granulation tissue (0.05)
Power failure (0.05)
Accidental decannulation (0.05)
Mechanical obstruction with mucus (0.05)
Intracranial bleed following an accidental fall (0.05)
Feeding problems/aspiration
Failure to thrive (0.15)
Aspiration pneumonia (0.10)
Oral aversion (0.10)

[a] Figures in parenthesis indicates fractional proportion of articles listing the complication.

as the most frustrating aspect of providing the child's care. In nearly every case, the direct costs of home care for a ventilator-dependent child are less than hospital-based care (4). Whereas governmental assistance and commercial insurance may compensate for most of the direct costs, families frequently report large out of pocket expenses and reduced income as a result of providing the child's care. The net economic impact of family caregiver's efforts may be considerable (135), to the extent that in unusual cases hospital care may cost less than home care when all costs are considered (136).

In 1981, President Reagan waived the eligibility rules for Supplemental Security Income and allowed Katie Beckett, a ventilator-dependent child, to return home without losing Medicaid benefits (1). Families who qualify through reduced income may receive home nursing assistance for a ventilator-dependent child through the federal Model Waiver program. This program was actually designed for oxygen-dependent children to provide a limited amount of home nursing for the purposes of educating the family in providing the child's long-term care. Caregivers who receive benefits via this program frequently get into conflicts with the home health care company regarding allocation of nursing hours and limits on various supplies such as the number of suction catheters that may be used each day.

VII. Summary and Conclusions

Published case reports support the use of long-term mechanical ventilation as a safe and life-sustaining therapy for pediatric patients with a wide spectrum of chronic respiratory disorders, but no randomized, controlled trials have been done. In the future, the number of children who will need long-term mechanical ventilation is expected to increase as improvements in critical care pediatrics increase survival of children with previously fatal types of acute lung injury. Important unanswered questions remain regarding the optimum method of support for children with specific disorders. Whereas positive pressure ventilation via tracheostomy is the predominant method currently utilized, noninvasive positive pressure ventilation is being increasingly used in conditions amenable to intermittent treatment. As new and improved modes of ventilatory assistance suitable for children evolve, it will be necessary to test these in controlled trials so as to better guide clinical decision making.

References

1. Burr BH, Guyer B, Todres ID, Abrahams B, Chiodo T. Home care for children on respirators. N Engl J Med 1983; 309:1319–1323.
2. Splaingard ML, Frates RC, Harrison GM, Carter RE, Jefferson LS. Home positive-pressure ventilation: 20 years experience. Chest 1983; 84:376–382.
3. American Thoracic Society, Board of Directors. Home mechanical ventilation of pediatric patients. Am Rev Respir Dis 1990; 141:258–259.
4. Make BJ, Hill NS, Goldberg AI, Bach JR, Criner GJ, Dunne PE, et al. Management of pediatric patients requiring long-term ventilation. Chest 1998; 113:289S–344S.
5. Bach JR, Brougher P, Hess DR, Hill NS, Kacmarek RM, Kreimer D, et al. Consensus statement: Noninvasive positive pressure ventilation. Respir Care 1997; 42: 364–369.
6. Koop CE. Excerpts from keynote address. In: Report of the Surgeon General's Workshop. DHHS Publ PHS-83-50194. Washington, DC: U.S. Government Printing Office, 1983; 9.
7. Guyer B, Martin JA, MacDorman MF, Anderson RN, Strobino DM. Annual summary of vital statistics—1996. Pediatrics 1997; 100:905–918.
8. Hazinski TA. Bronchopulmonary dysplasia. In: Chernick V, Kendig EL, eds. Disor-

ders of the Respiratory Tract in Children. 5th ed. Philadelphia: Saunders, 1990; 300–320.
9. O'Brodovich HM, Mellins RB. Bronchopulmonary dysplasia: Unresolved neonatal acute lung injury. Am Rev Respir Dis 1985; 132:694–709.
10. Rubenstein JS, Unti SM, Winter RJ. Pediatric resident attitudes about technologic support of vegetative patients and the effects of parental input: A longitudinal study. Pediatr 1994; 94:8–12.
11. Ireys HT, Anderson GF, Shaffer TJ, Neff JM. Expenditures for care of children with chronic illnesses enrolled in the Washington state medicaid program, fiscal year 1993. Pediatr 1997; 100:197–204.
12. Bryan AC, Wohl MB. Respiratory mechanics in children. In: Macklem PT, Mead J, eds. Handbook of Physiology. Bethesda, MD. American Physiological Society, 1986; 179–191.
13. Nelson NM, Prod'Hom LS, Cherry RB, Lipsitz PJ, Smith CA. Pulmonary function in the newborn infant. V. Trapped gas in the normal infant's lung. J Clin Invest 1963; 42:1850–1857.
14. Hershenson MB. The respiratory muscles and chest wall. In: Beckerman RC, Brouillette RT, Hunt CE, eds. Respiratory Control Disorders in Infants and Children. Baltimore: Williams & Wilkins, 1992; 28–46.
15. Keens TG, Bryan AC, Levison H. Developmental patterns of muscle fiber types in human ventilatory muscle. J Apply Physiol 1978; 44:909–913.
16. Wohl MB, Mead J. Age as a factor in respiratory disease. In: Chernick V, Kendig EL, eds. Disorders of the Respiratory Tract in Children. 5th ed. Philadelphia: Saunders, 1990; 175–182.
17. Mansell AL, Bryan AC, Levison H. Airway closure in children. J Appl Physiol 1972; 33:711–718.
18. Lacourt G, Polgar G. Interaction between nasal and pulmonary resistance in newborn infants. J Appl Physiol 1971; 30:870–873.
19. Stocks J, Godrey S. Nasal resistance during infancy. Respir Physiol 1978; 34:233–246.
20. Levy AM, Tabakin BS, Hanson JS. Hypertrophied adenoids causing pulmonary hypertension and severe congestive heart failure. N Engl J Med 1967; 277:506–511.
21. Khan Y, Heckmatt JZ. Obstructive apnoeas in Duchenne muscular dystrophy. Thorax 1994; 49:157–161.
22. Roberts JL, Reed WR, Thach BT. Factors influencing regional patency and configuration of the upper airway in human infants. J Apply Physiol 1985; 58:635–644.
23. Davies AM, Koenig JS, Thach BT. Upper airway chemoreflex responses to saline and water in preterm infants. J Appl Physiol 1988; 64:1412–1420.
24. Stocks J, Godfrey S. Specific airway conductance in relation to post-conceptual age during infancy. J Appl Physiol 1977; 43:144–150.
25. Hogg JC, Williams J, Richardson JB. Age as a factor in the distribution of lower-airway conductance and in the pathologic anatomy of obstructive lung disease. N Engl J Med 1970; 282:1283–1290.
26. Tepper RS. Airway reactivity in infants: A positive response to methacholine and metaproterenol. J Appl Physiol 1987; 62:1028–1034.

27. Montgomery GL, Tepper RS. Changes in airway reactivity with age in infants and young children. Am Rev Respir Dis 1990; 142:1372–1376.
28. Dittrichova J. Development of sleep in infancy. J Appl Physiol 1966; 21:1243–1246.
29. Muller N, Gulston C, Cade D, Whitton J, Froese AB, Bryan MH, et al. Diaphragmatic muscle fatigue in the newborn. J Appl Physiol 1979; 46:688–695.
30. Bureau MA, Lamarche J, Foulon P, Dalle D. Postnatal maturation of respiration in intact and carotid body-chemodenervated lambs. J Apply Physiol 1985; 59:869–874.
31. Rosen CL, McColley SA, eds. Development of respiratory control: An overview. Chicago: Proceedings of the American Thoracic Society, 1998; 1–7.
32. Davidson-Ward SL, Bautista DB, Keens TG. Hypoxic arousal responses in normal infants. Pediatr Pulmonol 1989; 7:276A.
33. Keens TG, Jansen MT, DeWitt PK. Home care for children with chronic respiratory failure. Semin Respir Med 1990; 11:269–281.
34. Kurzner SI, Garg M, Bautista DB. Growth failure in bronchopulmonary dysplasia: Elevated metabolic rates and pulmonary mechanics. J Pediatr 1988; 112:73–80.
35. Newth CJL. Recognition and management of respiratory failure. Pediatr Clin North Am 1979; 26:617–643.
36. Pagtakhan RD, Pasterkamp H. Intensive care for respiratory disorders. In: Chernick V, Kendig DL, eds. Disorders of the Respiratory Tract in Children. 5th ed. Philadelphia: Saunders, 1990;205–224.
37. Rosen CL, D'Andrea L, Haddad GG. Adult criteria for obstructive sleep apnea do not identify children with serious obstruction. Am Rev Respir Dis 1992; 146:1231–1234.
38. Teague WG, Harsch A, Lesnick B. Non-invasive positive pressure ventilation as a long-term treatment for pediatric patients with chronic hypoventilation disorders. Am J Respir Crit Care Med 1999; 159:A297.
39. Fortenberry JD, Del Toro J, Jefferson LS, Evey L, Haase D. Management of pediatric acute hypoxemic respiratory insufficiency with bilevel positive pressure (BiPAP) nasal mask ventilation. Chest 1995; 108:1059–1064.
40. Avery ME, Fletcher BD, Williams RG. Methods of study of pulmonary function in infants. In: The Lung and Its Disorders in the Newborn Infant. 4th ed. Philadelphia: Saunders, 1981; 63–84.
41. Henderson-Smart DJ, Read DJ. Reduced lung volume during behavioral active sleep in the newborn. J Apply Physiol 1979; 46:1081–1085.
42. Loughlin GM, McColley SA. Respiratory control disorders in children with chronic lung disease. In: Beckerman RC, Brouillette RT, Hunt CE, eds. Respiratory Control Disorders in Infants and Children. Baltimore: Williams & Wilkins, 1992; 306–321.
43. Edelman NH, Lahiri S, Braudo L, Cherniack NS, Fishman AP. The blunted ventilatory response to hypoxia in cyanotic congenital heart disease. N Engl J Med 1970; 282:405–411.
44. Hazinski TA. Furosemide decreases ventilation in young rabbits. J Pediatr 1985; 106:81–86.
45. Perlman JM, Moore V, Siegel MJ, Dawson J. Is chloride depletion an important

contributing cause of death in infants with bronchopulmonary dysplasia? Pediatrics 1986; 77:212–216.

46. Garg M, Kurzner SI, Bautista DB, Keens TG. Clinically unsuspected hypoxia during sleep and feeding in infants with bronchopulmonary dysplasia. Pediatrics 1988; 81:635–642.
47. Hill NS, Eveloff SE, Carlisle CC, Goff SG. Efficacy of nocturnal nasal ventilation in patients with restrictive thoracic disease. Am Rev Respir Dis 1992; 145:365–371.
48. Hill NS. Noninvasive ventilation: Does it work, for whom, and how? Am Rev Respir Dis 1993; 147:1050–1055.
49. Marcus CL, Carroll JL, Bamford O, Pyzik P, Loughlin GM. Supplemental oxygen during sleep in children with sleep-disordered breathing. Am J Respir Crit Care Med 1995; 152:1297–1301.
50. Swaminathan S, Paton JY, Davidson-Ward SL, Jacobs RA, Sargent CW, Keens TG. Abnormal control of ventilation in adolescents with myelodysplasia. J Pediatr 1989; 115:898–903.
51. Baker AB. Artificial respiration: The history of an idea. Med Hist 1971; 15:336–345.
52. Smith RA, Rasanen JO, Downs JB. Evolution of mechanical ventilation. In: Grenvik A, Downs JB, Rasanen J, Smith R, eds. Mechanical Ventilation and Assisted Respiration: Past, Present, and Future. New York: Churchill Livingston, 1991; 1–14.
53. Drinker P, McKhann CF. The use of a new apparatus for the prolonged administration of artificial respiration. I. A fatal case of poliomyelitis. JAMA 1929; 92:1658–1667.
54. Frates RC, Splaingard ML, Smith EO, Harrison GM. Outcome of home mechanical ventilation in children. J Pediatr 1985; 106:850–856.
55. Bloxsom A. Asphyxia neonatorium: New method of resuscitation. JAMA 1951; 146:1120–1125.
56. Brandstater B. Prolonged intubation: An alternative to tracheostomy in infants. Vienna: Proceedings of the First European Conference on Anesthesia, 1962; 106A.
57. Delivoira-Papadopoulos M, Levison H, Swyer P. Intermittent positive pressure respiration as a treatment in severe respiratory distress syndrome. Arch Dis Child 1965; 40:474–480.
58. Mushin WW, Mapleson WM, Lunn JN. Problems of automatic ventilation in infants and children. Br J Anaesth 1962; 34:574–578.
59. Gregory GA, Kitterman JA, Phibbs RH, Tooley W. Treatment of the idiopathic respiratory distress syndrome with continuous positive airway pressure. N Engl J Med 1971; 284:1333–1340.
60. Kirby RR, Robison EJ, Schulz J, de Lemos R. A new pediatric volume ventilator. Anesth Analg 1971; 50:533–538.
61. Hunt CE, Matalon SV, Thompson TR, Demuth S, Loew JM, Liu HM, et al. Central hypoventilation syndrome: Experience with bilateral phrenic nerve pacing in three neonates. Am Rev Respir Dis 1978; 118:23–28.
62. Frates RC, Harrison GM, Splaingard ML. Home care for children on respirators. N Engl J Med 1984; 310:1126–1127.

63. Schreiner M, Donar ME, Kettrick RG. Pediatric home mechanical ventilation. Pediatr Clin North Am 1987; 34:47–60.
64. Alba A, Solomon M, Trainor FS. Management of respiratory insufficiency in spinal cord lesions. Proceedings of the 17th Veterans Administration Spinal Cord Injury Conference. Washington, D.C.: US Government Printing Office, 1971; 436:200–213.
65. Padman R, Lawless S, Von Nessen S. Use of BiPAP by nasal mask in the treatment of respiratory insufficiency in pediatric patients: Preliminary investigation. Pediatr Pulmonol 1994; 17:119–123.
66. Teague WG, Fortenberry JD. Noninvasive ventilatory support in pediatric respiratory failure. Respir Care 1995; 40:86–96.
67. Ellis ER, McCauley VB, Mellis C, Sullivan CE. Treatment of alveolar hypoventilation in a six year old girl with intermittent positive pressure ventilation through a nose mask. Am Rev Respir Dis 1987; 136:188–191.
68. Nielson DW, Black PG. Mask ventilation in congenital central alveolar hypoventilation syndrome. Pediatr Pulm 1990; 9:44–46.
69. Heckmatt JZ, Loh L, Dubowitz V. Night-time nasal ventilation in neuromuscular disease. Lancet 1990; 335:579–582.
70. Brown RW, Grady EA, Van Laanen CJ, Dean JM, Hurvitz EA, Nelson VS, et al. Home use of bi-level positive airway pressure (BLPAP) ventilation for chronic respiratory failure in children (abstr). Am J Respir Crit Care Med 1994; 149:A376.
71. Padman R, Nadkarni VN, Von Nessen S, Goodill J. Noninvasive positive pressure ventilation in end-stage cystic fibrosis: A report of seven cases. Respir Care 1994; 39:736–739.
72. Gozal D. Nocturnal ventilatory support in patients with cystic fibrosis: Comparison with supplemental oxygen. Eur Respir J 1997; 10:1999–2003.
73. Samuels MP, Southall DP. Negative extrathoracic pressure in the treatment of respiratory failure in infants and young children. Br Med J 1989; 299:1253–1257.
74. Burstein L. Home care. In: Barnhart SL, Czervinske MP, eds. Perinatal and Pediatric Respiratory Care. Philadelphia: Saunders, 1995; 658–679.
75. Wheeler WB, Maguire EL, Kurachek SC, Lobas JG, Fugate JH, McNamara JJ. Chronic respiratory failure of infancy and childhood: Clinical outcomes based on underlying etiology. Pediatr Pulmonol 1994; 17:1–5.
76. Gilgoff IS, Peng RC, Keens TG. Hypoventilation and apnea in children during mechanically-assisted ventilation. Chest 1992; 101:1500–1506.
77. Kacmarek RM. Home mechanical ventilatory assistance for infants. Respir Care 1994; 39:550–561.
78. Ilbawi MN, Idriss FS, Hunt CE, Brouillette R, DeLeon SY. Diaphragmatic pacing in infants: Techniques and results. Ann Thorac Surg 1985; 40:323–329.
79. Weese-Mayer DE, Morrow AS, Brouillette RT, Ilbawi MN, Hunt CE. Diaphragm pacing in infants and children. A life-table analysis of implanted components. Am Rev Respir Dis 1989; 139:974–979.
80. Ilbawi MN, Hunt CE, DeLeon SY, Idriss FS. Diaphragm pacing in infants and children: Report of a simplified technique and review of experience. Ann Thorac Surg 1981; 31:61–65.
81. Hyland RH, Hutcheon MA, Perl A, Bowes G, Anthonisen NR, Zamel N, et al. Upper airway occlusion induced by diaphragm pacing for primary alveolar hypo-

ventilation: Implications for the pathogenesis of obstructive sleep apnea. Am Rev Respir Dis 1981; 124:180–185.

82. Marcus CL, Jansen MT, Poulsen MK, Keens SE, Nield TA, Lipkser LE, et al. Medical and psychosocial outcome of children with congenital central hypoventilation syndrome. J Pediatr 1991; 119:888–895.
83. Weese-Mayer DE, Silvestri JM, Menzies LJ, Morrow-Kenny AS, Hunt CE, Hauptman SA. Congenital central hypoventilation syndrome: diagnosis, management, and long-term outcome in 32 children. J Pediatr 1992; 120:381–387.
84. Strumpf DA, Carlisle CC, Millman RP, Smith KW, Hill NS. An evaluation of the Respironics BiPAP bi-level CPAP device for delivery of assisted ventilation. Respir Care 1990; 35:415–422.
85. Garland JS, Nelson DB, Rice T, Neu J. Increased risk of gastrointestinal perforations in neonates mechanically ventilated with either face mask or nasal prongs. Pediatr 1985; 76:406–410.
86. Ferguson GT, Gilmartin M. CO_2 rebreathing during BiPAP ventilatory assistance. Am J Respir Crit Care Med 1995; 151:1126–1135.
87. Kacmarek RM. Characteristics of pressure-targeted ventilators used for noninvasive positive pressure ventilation. Respir Care 1997; 42:380–388.
88. Marcus CL, Gozal D, Teague WG. Efficacy of non-invasive positive pressure ventilation in children (letter to the editor). Chest 1998; 114(6):1794–1795.
89. Teague WG. Pediatric application of non-invasive ventilation (NPPV). Respir Care 1997; 42:414–423.
90. Samuels MP, Raine J, Wright T, Alexander JA, Lockyer K, Spencer SA, et al. Continuous negative extrathoracic pressure in neonatal respiratory failure. Pediatrics 1996; 98:1154–1160.
91. O'Leary J, King R, Leblanc M. Cuirass ventilation in childhood neuromuscular disease. J Pediatr 1979; 94:419–421.
92. Hyland RH, Jones NL, Powles ACP, Lenkie SCM, Vanderlinden RJ, Epstein SW. Primary alveolar hypoventilation treated with nocturnal electrophrenic respiration. Am Rev Respir Dis 1978; 117:165–172.
93. Downes JJ, Pilmer SL. Chronic respiratory failure: Controversies in management. Crit Care Med 1993; 21:S363–S364.
94. Comroe JH. Frankenstein, Pickwick, and Ondine. In: Retrospectroscope. 4th ed. Menlo Park: Von Gehr Press, 1983:136–139.
95. Stovroff MC, Dykes F, Teague WG. The complete spectrum of neurocristopathy. J Pediatr Surg 1995; 30:1218–1221.
96. Fleming PJ, Cade D, Bryan MH, Bryan AC. Congenital central hypoventilation and sleep state. Pediatr 1980; 66:425–428.
97. Oren J, Kelly DH, Shannon DC. Long-term follow-up of children with congenital central hypoventilation syndrome. Pediatr 1987; 80:375–380.
98. Oren J, Newth CJL, Hunt CE, Brouillette RT, Bachand RT, Shannon DC. Ventilatory effects of almitrine bismesylate in congenital central hypoventilation syndrome. Am Rev Respir Dis 1986; 134:917–919.
99. Krieger AJ, Detwiler JS, Trooskin SZ. Respiratory function in infants with Arnold-Chiari malformation. Laryngoscope 1976; 86:718–723.
100. Davidson-Ward SL, Jacobs RA, Gates EP, Hart LD, Keens TG. Abnormal ventila-

tory patterns during sleep in infants with myelomeningocele. J Pediatr 1986; 109: 631–634.

101. Davidson-Ward SL, Nickerson BG, van Der Hal A, Rodriguez AM, Jacobs RA, Keens TG. Absent hypoxic and arousal responses in children with myelomeningocele and apnea. Pediatr 1986; 78:44–50.
102. Johnston K, Newth CJL, Sheu KF, Patel MS, Heldt GP, Schmidt KA, et al. Central hypoventilation syndrome in pyruvate dehydrogenase complex deficiency. Pediatr 1984; 74:1034–1040.
103. Lonsdale D, Mercer RD. Primary hypoventilation syndrome. Lancet 1972; 2:487.
104. Brazy JE, Kinney HC, Oakes WJ. Central nervous system structural lesions causing apnea at birth. J Pediatr 1987; 111:163–175.
105. Jensen TH, Hansen PB, Broderson P. Ondine's curse in listeria monocytogenes brain stem encephalitis. Acta Neurol Scand 1988; 77:505–506.
106. Liebhaber M, Robin ED, Lynn-Davies P, Sachs DPL, Sinatra F, Theodore J, et al. Reye's syndrome complicated by Ondine's curse. West J Med 1977; 126:110–118.
107. Gilgoff IS, Kahlstrom E, MacLaughlin E, Keens TG. Long-term ventilatory support in spinal muscular atrophy. J Pediatr 1989; 115:904–909.
108. Rutherford MA, Heckmatt JZ, Dubowitz V. Congenital myotonic dystrophy: Respiratory function at birth determines survival. Arch Dis Child 1989; 64:191–195.
109. Raphael JC, Chevret S, Chastang C. Randomized trial of preventive nasal ventilation in Duchenne muscular dystrophy. Lancet 1994; 343:1600–1604.
110. Leger P. Noninvasive positive pressure ventilation at home. Respir Care 1994; 39: 501–513.
111. Leger P, Bedicam JM, Cornette A, Reybet-Degat O, Langevin B, Polu JM. Nasal intermittent positive pressure ventilation: Long-term follow-up in patients with severe chronic respiratory insufficiency. Chest 1994; 105:100–105.
112. Kafer E. Idiopathic scoliosis: Gas exchange and age dependence of arterial blood gases. J Clin Invest 1976; 58:825–833.
113. Lisboa C, Moreno R, Fava M, Ferretti R, Cruz E. Inspiratory muscle function in patients with severe scoliosis. Am Rev Respir Dis 1985; 132:48–52.
114. Hershenson MB, Brouillette RT, Klemka L, Raffensperger JD, Poznaski AS, Hunt CE. Respiratory insufficiency in newborns with abdominal wall defects. J Pediatr Surg 1985; 20:348–353.
115. Splaingard ML, Frates RC, Jefferson LS, Rosen CL, Harrison GM. Home negative pressure ventilation: Report of 20 years experience in patients with neuromuscular disease. Arch Phys Med Rehabil 1985; 66:239–241.
116. Mitchell SH, Teague WG. Reduced gas transfer at rest and during exercise in school-age survivors of bronchopulmonary dysplasia. Am J Respir Crit Care Med 1998; 157:1406–1412.
117. Canlas-Yamsuan M, Sachez I, Kesselman M, Chernick V. Morbidity and mortality patterns of ventilator-dependent children in a home care program. Clin Pediatr 1993; 32:706–713.
118. Overstreet DW, Jackson JC, van Belle G, Truog WE. Estimation of mortality risk in chronically ventilated infants with bronchopulmonary dysplasia. Pediatr 1991; 88:1153–1160.

119. Davis PB, di Sant'Agnese PA. Assisted ventilation for patients with cystic fibrosis. JAMA 1978; 239:1851–1855.
120. Piper AJ, Parker S, Torzillo PJ, Sullivan CE, Bye PT. Nocturnal nasal IPPV stabilizes patients with cystic fibrosis and hypercapnic respiratory failure. Chest 1992; 102:846–850.
121. Mallory GB, Fiser DH, Jackson R. Sleep-associated breathing disorders in morbidly obese children and adolescents. J Pediatr 1989; 115:892–897.
122. Bourne RA, Maltby CC, Donaldson JD. Obese hypoventilation syndrome of early childhood requiring ventilatory support. Int J Pediatr Otorhinolaryngol 1988; 16: 61–68.
123. Loughlin GM, Wynne JW, Victoria BE. Sleep apnea as a possible cause of pulmonary hypertension in Down syndrome. J Pediatr 1981; 98:435–437.
124. Guilleminault C, Nino-Murcia G, Heldt G, Baldwin R, Hutchinson D. Alternative treatment to tracheostomy in obstructive sleep apnea syndrome: Nasal continuous positive airway pressure in young children. Pediatrics 1986; 78:797–802.
125. Piper AJ, Sullivan CE. Effects of short-term NIPPV in the treatment of patients with severe obstructive sleep apnea and hypercapnia. Chest 1994; 105:434–440.
126. Rosen GM, Muckle RP, Mahowald MW, Goding GS, Ullevig C. Postoperative respiratory compromise in children with obstructive sleep apnea syndrome: Can it be anticipated? Pediatrics 1994; 93:784–788.
127. Burstein F, Cohen S, Scott P, Teague W, Montgomery G, Kattos A. Surgical therapy for severe refractory sleep apnea in infants and children: application of the airway zone concept. Plast Reconstr Surg 1995; 96:34–41.
128. Heckmatt JZ, Loh L, Dubowitz V. Nocturnal hypoventilation in children with nonprogressive neuromuscular disease. Pediatrics 1989; 83:250–255.
129. Khan Y, Heckmatt JZ, Dubowitz V. Sleep studies and supportive ventilatory treatment in patients with congenital muscle disorders. Arch Dis Child 1996; 74:195–200.
130. Orlowski JP, Ellis NG, Amin NP, Crumrine RS. Complications of airway intrusion in 100 consecutive cases in a pediatric ICU. Crit Care Med 1980; 8:324–331.
131. Schreiner MS, Downes JJ, Kettrick RG. Chronic respiratory failure in infants with prolonged ventilator dependency. JAMA 1987; 258:3398–3404.
132. Downes JJ, Schreiner MS. Tracheostomy tubes and attachments in infants and children. Inter Anesthesiol Clin 1985; 23:37–60.
133. Morar P, Singh V, Jones AS, Hughes J, Van Saene R. Impact of tracheotomy on colonization and infection of lower airways in children requiring long-term ventilation. Chest 1998; 113:77–85.
134. Sheikh AA, Schreiner MS, Wetmore RF. Tracheal complications of airway managment in chronic respiratory failure of infancy. Crit Care Med 1986; 14:423
135. Leonard B, Brust JD, Sapienza JJ. Financial and time costs to parents of severely disabled children. Public Health Rep 1992; 107:302–312.
136. Sevick MA, Bradham DD. Economic value of caregiver effort in maintaining long-term ventilator-assisted individuals at home. Heart Lung 1997; 26:148–157.
137. Goldberg AI, Faure EA, Vaugh CJ, Snarski R, Seleny FL. Home care for life-supported persons: an approach to program development. J Pediatr 1984; 104:785–795.

9

Management and Monitoring of Long-Term Invasive Mechanical Ventilation

JOHN M. TRAVALINE and GERARD J. CRINER

Temple University School of Medicine
Philadelphia, Pennsylvania

I. Introduction

Long-term invasive mechanical ventilation in patients unable to support spontaneous breathing demands special attention from a variety of health care professionals. The needs of such patients frequently are complex, and in addition to the usual needs common to other groups of chronically ill patients, these patients require specific care to address the particular needs encountered during long-term mechanical ventilation. Typically, a multidisciplinary team approach (Table 1) is employed to provide effective comprehensive care in patients requiring this form of therapy.

This chapter focuses on the management of patients requiring long-term invasive mechanical ventilation. Special needs in these patients, such as assistance with communication and eating, evaluation and treatment of psychological dysfunction, and solving problems in patient–ventilator interactions are addressed. In addition, aspects of monitoring and preventing complications in patients receiving chronic invasive ventilation are discussed. First, however, we discuss the selection of patients for long-term invasive mechanical ventilation, the goals of their management, and the appropriate means of providing this form of therapy.

Table 1 Team Members Involved in Management of Long-Term Mechanically Ventilated Patients

Nurses
Respiratory therapists
Pulmonary and critical care physicians
Respiratory trained nurses
Physical therapists
Occupational therapists
Psychologist
Nutritionist
Speech therapist
Social worker
Home care vendor
Home health nurse

II. Determination of Unweanability

When spontaneous efforts are unable to sustain adequate alveolar ventilation, mechanical ventilation is required. The most obvious group of patients to identify as candidates for long-term invasive mechanical ventilation are those with absent or severely impaired spontaneous breathing efforts (Table 2). Examples of patients in this category are those with severe hypoventilation secondary to inadequate central respiratory drive (i.e., intracranial hemorrhage, cerebrovascular accidents, central alveolar hypoventilation) or severe respiratory muscle weakness (i.e., high spinal cord injury). Patients in this group are unable to sustain any spontaneous breathing effort and are dependent upon mechanical ventilation continuously for life support. Patients who require continuous mechanical ventilation

Table 2 General Characteristics of Patients Requiring Prolonged Invasive Ventilation

Absent or severely impaired spontaneous, breathing efforts
Central disorders (i.e., major strokes)
Major insults to the respiratory system secondary to catastrophic medical or surgical illnesses
S/P ARDS
Cardiomyopathy
Chronic disorder that precipitates recurrent bouts of respiratory failure
Severe COPD
Severe kyphoscoliosis

usually require more support personnel and respiratory equipment (i.e., backup ventilators) and are at a much greater risk for catastrophic complications.

Patients who fail repeated attempts at weaning from mechanical ventilation represent another group of patients who may require long-term mechanical ventilation. These patients typically have suffered some disorder that precipitates an acute bout of respiratory failure, and despite reversal of the acute problem, fail repeated attempts at weaning from mechanical ventilation and require prolonged ventilation. These patients may have suffered a major insult to the respiratory system as a result of a severe medical illness or postoperative catastrophe, or developed an acute illness superimposed on a chronic disorder that further impairs an already compromised respiratory pump (i.e., malnutrition, advanced age, cardiac disease, systemic infections). Some patients in this category may be able to breathe spontaneously for several hours, however, longer periods of spontaneous breathing result in worsened respiratory failure and require reinstitution of mechanical ventilation. Because some patients in this group are not totally dependent upon mechanical ventilation, in the event of ventilator malfunction, these patients are less likely to suffer adverse sequelae. Overall, patients who can maintain spontaneous ventilation for significant periods of time (i.e., ≥4 hr) are easier to monitor and require less support personnel and respiratory equipment (i.e., monitoring equipment, backup ventilators).

The third, and potentially largest group of patients who may require long-term ventilation are patients with chronic disorders that precipitate recurrent bouts of respiratory failure. Each episode of respiratory failure necessitates intensive care unit (ICU) hospitalization and repeated treatment with mechanical ventilation. Examples of diseases in this group of patients include severe chronic obstructive pulmonary disease (COPD), kyphoscoliosis, and severe or slowly progressive neuromuscular disorders.

Determining whether a patient can live independent of the ventilator is sometimes difficult. In some situations, such as a high spinal cord injury, the need for continued invasive mechanical ventilation for the long-term is usually obvious. Other situations, however, are less clear. For example, in the patient with severe underlying cardiopulmonary disease who has suffered an acute insult, such as a severe bout of sepsis, the prognosis for ventilator independence is less certain, and the inability to successfully wean the patient from the ventilator only becomes evident over time.

In patients requiring augmentation of ventilation, the choice between noninvasive or invasive forms of mechanical ventilation should be considered. Noninvasive forms of ventilation (e.g., noninvasive positive pressure ventilation with a nasal or nasal–oral mask, external negative pressure ventilation via cuirass, tank, or "pulmowrap" ventilators) have been reported to be successful in patients with underlying neuromuscular diseases, central alveolar hypoventilation, obesity-hypoventilatory syndromes, chest wall deformities, and those with stable or slowly progressive neuromuscular syndromes who have intact upper airway function (1). In addition, noninvasive ventilation has been shown in several studies to be beneficial in avoiding the need for tracheostomy and prolonged ventilatory support or in enhancing the ability of the patient to be extubated and avoid tracheostomy in those who initially receive invasive ventilation via endotracheal intubation (2–4). Its role, however, in patients with chronic respiratory failure secondary to COPD is currently unclear, and additional studies must be performed demonstrating its efficacy before it can be recommended as standard therapy (5–7).

In general, invasive ventilation is most frequently employed in patients who have suffered an acute bout of respiratory failure and failed to respond to repeated weaning attempts, or have difficulty with recurrent pulmonary aspiration, upper airway obstruction, or severe debilitation (1). In select cases, patients may be converted from long-term invasive ventilation to noninvasive ventilation based on the experience of the practitioner when the underlying disease mandates less intensive augmentation of nocturnal hypoventilation, or when long-term cannulation of the airways for upper airway support or secretion clearance is no longer needed.

III. Goals for Long-Term Mechanical Ventilation

A. Patient Goals

Restoring the patient to the maximum level of functioning possible is the foremost goal in the management of patients receiving long-term mechanical ventilation. Working toward maximizing a patient's physical condition to allow the patient to be mobile and perform usual daily activities is the basis for all therapy provided. More specific goals include respiratory and whole body muscle reconditioning, decreased dependence on mechanical ventilation, improved mobility, stabilization of cardiopulmonary function, secretion clearance, optimization of communication, restoration of eating, patient and family education about chronic illness, psychological support, skin care, discharge planning, and successful transition of the patient to the home or to an institutional chronic care facility. Although specific data showing each of these rehabilitative strategies in patients receiving invasive ventilation have not been extensively reported, data demonstrating the efficacy of these maneuvers in other patient groups illustrate their potential role in rehabilitating ventilator-dependent patients.

B. Institutional Goals

Recently, limited ICU resources and cost containment policies have fostered the development of multiple sites (e.g., skilled nursing facility, nursing home, acute hospital, noninvasive respirator care units) to care for patients requiring long-term invasive mechanical ventilation. The duration of time a patient spends at a given location is now influenced by the institution's goals and policies in caring for long-term invasive mechanical ventilation patients. For example, once patients achieve a chronic state of stability but still require invasive ventilation, some institutions transfer them to an off-site skilled nursing facility or nursing home where weaning attempts, rehabilitation, and other medical care are assumed by other practitioners and support staff. In other institutions, such as ours, patients who require chronic invasive ventilation are transferred to a ventilator rehabilitation unit (VRU), which is located within our tertiary care facility. In the VRU, patients are aggressively rehabilitated and weaned from mechanical ventilation, treated with invasive or noninvasive forms of ventilation, and in some cases treated pre- or postoperatively for lung, heart, and heart–lung transplantation.

Dependent upon the institutional policies, therefore, patient goals may be totally achieved at different locations within that institution or some may be addressed outside the institution. Regardless of the location of care, however, patients receiving invasive mechanical ventilation have complex problems and are prone to develop new or worsening conditions that require ongoing medical evaluation, and at times, specialized care, to ensure optimum outcome. The subgroup of patients that requires the greatest scrutiny are those who have an acute medical or surgical illness that precipitates respiratory failure, superimposed on a chronic disorder.

To illustrate this point, we recently evaluated 25 consecutive patients (58 ± 13 yr) who were transferred out of the intensive care unit to our VRU for new or changing medical conditions that affected their weaning outcome (8). Causes of respiratory failure in these patients included pneumonia, postoperative conditions, congestive heart failure, acute respiratory distress syndrome, sepsis, renal failure, diaphragm dysfunction, and obesity; the majority of patients (n = 23) had more than one of the above causes contributing to their respiratory failure. Patients were intubated and received invasive ventilation for approximately 17 ± 7 days in the intensive care unit and required another 16 ± 14 days of mechanical ventilation until totally weaned in the VRU. Nine patients (36%) were able to wean within 7 days of presenting to the VRU, but 64% of patients (n = 16) required 21 ± 15 days to wean from mechanical ventilation. In the group that took a longer time to wean, new problems that affected weaning duration and outcome included sepsis, volume overload, worsening bronchospasm, ileus, renal failure, cardiac arrhythmias, changes in blood pressure, seizure disorder, and tracheal bleeding. Despite the development of newer or worsening medical problems, 81% of patients in the latter group also successfully weaned from medical ventilation with 10 of 13 discharged directly to home, 1 of 13 requiring home mechanical ventilation, and 2 of 13 dying from multiple organ failure after ICU transfer.

We conclude from this preliminary information that new or worsening medical problems must be identified since they can complicate weaning outcome in patients receiving chronic invasive ventilation. Despite their development, however, close attention to medical problems ensured successful weaning outcome in the majority of patients. These data also substantiate that despite the location where patients receive chronic invasive ventilation, special attention must be given to detecting and correcting new medical problems to ensure optimal outcome.

IV. Rehabilitative Strategies in Invasive Ventilator-Dependent Patients

A. Need for Rehabilitation in Ventilator-Dependent Patients

Chronic ventilator-dependent patients are deconditioned due to the underlying disease precipitating respiratory failure, the immobility associated with mechanical ventilation, and the indirect effects of concomitant therapy (high-dose corticosteroids and neuromuscular blocking agents). However, data demonstrating the degree of deconditioning and the impact of physical therapy on outcome are extremely limited.

We recently evaluated 25 consecutive patients (12 females, 58 ± 14 yrs) admitted to our VRU for weaning from invasive ventilation (9). Prior to transfer to the VRU, patients were intubated and ventilated for 17 ± 7 days and in the intensive care unit and then for an additional 29 ± 17 days in the VRU. No patient had an underlying neuromuscular disorder, 23 patients had more than one cause for respiratory failure, including sepsis, congestive heart failure, COPD, pneumonia, postoperative conditions, and renal failure. Overall, 40% of these patients were exposed to neuromuscular blocking agents during their intensive care unit stay to facilitate mechanical ventilation.

On admission to the VRU, physical therapy was started on all patients. On initial presentation, deconditioning was assessed with a 5-point motor score that considered resistance and range of motion in all muscle groups and the use of a 7-point previously validated dependence functional score to measure the degree of independent function. Evaluations were performed on VRU admission, during daily physical therapy sessions, and at VRU discharge by a skilled physical therapist. Table 3 shows the impact of whole-body rehabilitation on functional status and motor score in patients admitted to our ventilator rehabilitation unit. On initial presentation, patients exhibited marked weakness in shoulder, elbow, hip, knee, and foot flexion, which showed substantial improvements after daily physical therapy. Moreover, compared with admission, ventilator-dependent patients receiving invasive ventilation were more likely to sit and stand at VRU discharge after daily whole-body physical therapy. These preliminary data confirm that in-

Table 3 Impact of Whole Body Rehabilitation on Functional Status in Chronic Invasive Ventilator-Dependent Patients

	Motor strength	
	VRU admission	VRU discharge[a]
Shoulder flexion	1.6 ± 0.6	2.8 ± 0.6
Elbow flexion	2.1 ± 0.8	3.4 ± 0.7
Hip flexion	1.9 ± 0.8	2.8 ± 0.7
Knee flexion	1.8 ± 0.8	2.7 ± 0.7
Dorsiflexion	1.5 ± 0.6	2.7 ± 0.6

Functional score VRU admission vs. discharge	
Supine to sit	$p < 0.001$
Sit to stand	$p < 0.001$

[a]$p < 0.001$

vasive ventilator-dependent patients are deconditioned and suggest that daily physical therapy helps to improve whole body function.

B. Respiratory and Nonrespiratory Muscle Reconditioning

Many studies on COPD patients have demonstrated the effectiveness of multidisciplinary rehabilitation programs that involve some form of arm and leg exercise (10–12). At the completion of these programs, patients have increased maximal oxygen uptake, enhanced muscle strength and endurance, improved muscle coordination, more desirable body composition with increased muscle mass and less body fat, diminished breathlessness, and an improved overall sense of well-being (10–12). It has even been suggested in some studies that patients who participate in rehabilitation programs have a lower rate of hospitalization when compared with historical controls. Whether it is participation in a rehabilitation program per se, or the performance of whole body exercise that is responsible for the improvements, however, is unclear.

Keens et al. (13) demonstrated in seven children with cystic fibrosis that strenuous training of the upper extremities achieved by 4 wk of daily 1.5-hr periods of rowing, swimming, or canoeing was associated with hyperventilation, increased maximum voluntary ventilation (MVV), and maximal sustainable ventilatory capacity. Belman and Mittman (14) in a small number of patients with stable COPD showed that 15-min daily sessions of isocapnic hyperventilation increased MVV, sustainable ventilatory capacity, and the maximum oxygen uptake of the respiratory muscles over a 6-wk period. In another study, Belman and Kendregan (15) found that daily performance of arm or leg exercise on a bicycle ergometer in COPD patients for 6 wk did not increase sustainable ventilatory capacity or respiratory muscle maximum oxygen uptake. Although some of the results are conflicting, these studies have stimulated interest in the role of arm exercise and the pectoral girdle muscles in the respiratory muscle function of patients with severe obstructive lung disease. These muscles may apply considerable forces to the upper rib cage, which may affect intrathoracic pressure, the shape of the rib cage, and even the mechanical performance of the conventional chest wall respiratory muscles. Studies by ourselves (16,17) and others (18) suggest that arm posture and/or contraction of the pectoral girdle muscles affect lung volume, rib cage dimensions, diaphragm and abdominal inspiratory muscle activity, and overall ventilatory capacity.

Three studies that have incorporated extensive upper extremity training into rehabilitation programs have shown an improvement in respiratory muscle strength and ventilatory muscle endurance (13,18,19). The previously mentioned Keens study (13) on cystic fibrosis patients observed a 57% increase in ventilatory muscle endurance at the end of the training program. Clanton et al. (19) studied the effect of swim training on lung volume, inspiratory muscle strength, and endurance in 16 women varsity swimmers between the ages of 17 and 21, and compared them to an age-matched nontraining control group. Swim training including running for 40 to 60 min and isometric conditioning of upper extremity muscle groups using Nautilus machines each session for three sessions per week and swimming a distance of at least 2200 m/day over a 4-wk period. Women who underwent swim training showed a 25% increase in maximum inspiratory pressure and a greater than 100% increase in endurance time compared with the nontrained age-matched control group. Finally, Estenne et al. (18) studied the effect of isometric exercises on pectoralis muscle function in six C5-C6 tetraplegia subjects. They found an increase in expiratory reserve volume after 6 wk of training.

In COPD patients, upper extremity exercise also appears to have a benefit. Lake et al. (20) randomized 28 COPD patients with severe airflow obstruction to upper limb training, lower limb training, or both as part of an outpatient rehabilitation program. Twenty-six patients completed the 8-wk training program and, as expected, improvements in muscle group–specific tasks were demonstrated. In addition, when upper limb exercise was combined with lower limb exercise, not only was exercise performance enhanced but an improvement in self-efficacy score, an assessment of quality of life, self-confidence, and self-esteem, was also found. All of these above studies demonstrate that extensive upper extremity exercise may enhance ventilatory muscle function and ventilatory capacity in normal subjects and patients with a variety of obstructive and restrictive chest wall disorders. Although these studies have not evaluated ventilator-dependent subjects, it is reasonable to expect that such patients who can cooperate with an exercise program stand to realize similar benefits.

Because ventilator-dependent patients differ so much, the prescription for exercise training must be individualized. In our VRU, an initial evaluation by a physiatrist and physical therapist is performed upon admission. Specific goals for increasing muscle strength, endurance, and mobility are then established for each patient. Physical therapy may involve as little as passive range of motion, to active strengthening exercises, weight bearing, upper extremity exercise, pedaling, stair climbing, and ambulation. Depending on the patient's condition, therapy should occur at least daily. Frequently, however, as a patient becomes less dependent on the ventilator and acute medical issues are treated, the patient will attend two physical therapy sessions per day, one in the morning and one in the afternoon, separated by a period of rest. In all patients, when possible, upper extremity strength and endurance training is incorporated into the program of whole body retraining in order to maximize the recovery of ventilatory function.

C. Respiratory Muscle Training and Breathing Techniques

Respiratory muscle strength estimated by a maximal inspiratory pressure maneuver along with other variables, such as minute ventilation and underlying diagnosis, are important components in a model predictive of weaning outcome in long-term ventilated patients (21). In managing long-term ventilator patients, therefore, attention specifically to respiratory muscle weakness is important. In fact, there is some evidence that inspiratory muscle resistive training may facilitate weaning from mechanical ventilation (22).

In nearly all of our long-term ventilated patients, we suspect some degree of respiratory muscle weakness. This is particularly so in COPD patients, in whom chronic hyperinflation, undernutrition, increased airway resistance, and increased physiologic dead space all lead to a greater amount of energy expended for breathing and impose an added stress on the respiratory muscles. In our VRU, we generally initiate inspiratory muscle training using a threshold device set at approximately one-third the maximal inspiratory pressure measured with a unidirectional valve connected to the tracheotomy tube. Training sessions are performed for 10 to 15 min 2 to 3 times per day. The threshold is then adjusted weekly based on reassessment of maximal inspiratory pressure.

Many studies over the past two decades have examined the effects of training on ventilatory endurance and strength of the respiratory muscles (23–25). These studies for the most part were conducted either on normal subjects (13,24), or stable COPD patients (5–30). Patients requiring long-term mechanical ventilation, however, commonly have underlying severe lung disease, whether related to chronic obstruction or some other process that similarly impairs respiratory muscle function. These studies, therefore, can provide some insight into the utility of respiratory muscle training.

In a controlled prospective study, Levine et al. (25) showed that isocapnic hyperventilation produced significant increases in maximum sustainable ventilation, increases in endurance time during lower extremity cycling and treadmill exercise, and increased peak oxygen uptake during progressive incremental work. They also found a significant improvement in psychological testing and the ability of patients to perform the activities of daily living.

Pardy et al. (26) demonstrated that inspiring against an inspiratory resistance for two 15-min periods daily increases the ability to sustain ventilation against high levels of external resistance, associated with an increased lower extremity ergometry endurance time, maximum power output, and maximum oxygen uptake. Others (27,28) also demonstrated increases in inspiratory muscle strength and endurance achieved by daily inspiratory resistive breathing exercises, although improvement in whole body exercise measured by treadmill or bicycle performance was not consistently demonstrated (27).

After having 10 COPD patients perform two 15-min sessions of resistive breathing daily for 6 wk, Belman et al. (29) showed no significant increases in maximum respiratory pressure or the ability to sustain breathing through a higher resistive load. When these investigators coached the subjects to breathe with a longer inspiratory time, lower peak mouth pressure, and a lower frequency, however, they were able to show an increase in the resistive load that the subjects could endure for 15 min. In addition, the pressure time index of the inspiratory muscles (i.e., the area under the pressure time curve) was significantly greater during coaching. In another study on 10 patients with moderately severe COPD, Larson et al. (30) showed that 7 wk of daily 30-min training sessions of inspiring against a threshold load that was one-third of the maximum inspiratory pressure increased maximum inspiratory pressure, endurance to breathe against an inspiratory pressure load, and performance on a 12-min walk test.

In patients with chronic congestive heart failure, respiratory muscle training has also been suggested to be of benefit. Mancini et al. (31) evaluated eight patients with congestive heart failure (CHF) who underwent 3 mo of supervised respiratory muscle training that involved isocapnic hyperpnea, resistive inspiratory muscle training, inspiratory and expiratory strength training, and breathing calisthenics to strengthen the abdominal muscles. This group was compared with six patients with CHF who did not undergo the training protocol. They found that there was a significant increase in ventilatory muscle endurance, increased inspiratory and expiratory muscle strength, increased 6-min walk distance, increased peak oxygen uptake during exercise, and reduced sensation of dyspnea during isocapnic hyperpnea.

Inspiratory muscle training in chronic cervical spinal cord–injured patients has also recently been evaluated (32). Ten patients with chronic spinal cord injury (level C4-C7) and no history of lung disease prior to spinal injury underwent resistive inspiratory muscle training for two 15-min session daily for 8 wk. Compliance with the training session was good (48 to 100%) with no patient missing more than eight consecutive sessions. After 8 wk, there was a significant improvement in maximum inspiratory pressure ranging from 6 to 78 cm H_2O), and forced vital capacity (2.8 to 3.07 L). There was no statistically significant difference in dyspnea score as assessed with the modified Borg scale, although subjects generally reported reduced levels of perceived difficulty in breathing.

While respiratory muscle function may be improved with specific inspiratory training and exercise performance may also be enhanced through structured training protocols, it appears important that the training involve a controlled pattern of breathing (33). This need to control breathing pattern certainly limits the application of respiratory muscle training in the clinical setting. Moreover, at present, there are no studies that have examined the effect of inspiratory muscle strength training or isocapnic hyperventilation on the incidence of respiratory failure, the need for hospitalization, functional status, or the mortality of patients with moderate to severe underlying lung disease.

D. Breathing Techniques

In addition to respiratory muscle training, breathing techniques to facilitate weaning from mechanical ventilation have been assessed. For example, deep diaphragmatic breathing in patients with severe COPD and chronic hypercapnia was recently evaluated (34). In this study, 25 patients with severe COPD recovering from a recent exacerbation, 15 of whom had required mechanical ventilation (4 to 15 days) during their exacerbation (6 invasive, 9 noninvasive), were evaluated. Five of the patients had tracheostomy, but breathed spontaneously during the study. Maximum inspiratory pressures in both groups were similarly reduced. Diaphragmatic breathing was supervised in all subjects by the same certified respiratory therapist. Measurements were made during 15 min of deep diaphragmatic breathing and compared with the final 5 min of a 15-min period of the patient's naturally adopted breathing pattern. Diaphragmatic breathing was associated with a lower transcutaneous carbon dioxide (CO_2), higher transcutaneous oxygen (O_2), and a higher minute ventilation; however, it was also associated with an increase in inspiratory muscle effort (greater swings in esophageal pressure, increased pressure time product, and pressure time index) and worsened dyspnea score. Other breathing exercises have also been utilized in patients on long-term mechanical ventilation (35).

E. Weaning from Mechanical Ventilation

Even though total liberation from mechanical ventilation is not always the optimum goal, at least partial independence from mechanical ventilation should be attempted in all patients receiving long-term invasive ventilation. Independence from the ventilator allows reconditioning and physical therapy to occur more easily. The process of weaning from mechanical ventilation is facilitated by progress in restoring physical function, and often coincides with improvement in nonrespiratory areas. In reconditioning the ventilator patient, however, one must be careful not to overwork the patient and impede the weaning process. Further, overzealous attempts at total withdrawal from mechanical ventilation should be avoided so as not to leave the patient so drained that whole body rehabilitation cannot be considered. Overall, frequent assessment of the patient by the various members of the multidisciplinary team (physical therapists, nurses, physicians) should detect when the reconditioning or weaning programs are too intense or need to be modified so that both programs can be conducted concurrently to maximize patient gain.

F. Early Mobilization

Early mobilization of the ventilator-dependent patient has long been recognized as an important component of the rehabilitation process (36). Such mobilization may simply involve repositioning the patient in the bed, first sitting them upright in bed, then in a chair, increasing the duration of time out bed, standing, and ambulating. Early mobilization may reduce muscle and skeletal wasting, risk of thromboembolism, decubitus ulcers, and despair (36). Ventilator dependence should not impede the process of early mobilization. If the patient is able to sustain spontaneous respiration, the process is made easier. In patients requiring continuous mechanical ventilation, while there may be more effort involved with mobilization of the patient, it remains a critical component to recovery of the patient. Typically, we use portable ventilators to facilitate patient mobility, alternatively, in many patients, we employ manual ventilation with a bag system using 100% oxygen connected to the tracheotomy tube (Fig. 1).

Working to restore a patient's level of functioning to perform activities of daily living and other common tasks occurs throughout the rehabilitation process. Nurses, physical therapists, occupational therapists, and respiratory therapists all work in concert to restore independent patient function.

G. Renutrition

The high metabolic demands imposed on the critically ill patient over time inevitably lead to an undernourished state despite aggressive nutrition support (Table 4). The role of malnutrition is particularly important in the chronic respiratory failure patient. We know that malnutrition is associated with decreased muscle mass of the diaphragm, reduced maximum voluntary ventilation, and reduced respiratory muscle strength (37). In addition to adversely affecting muscle func-

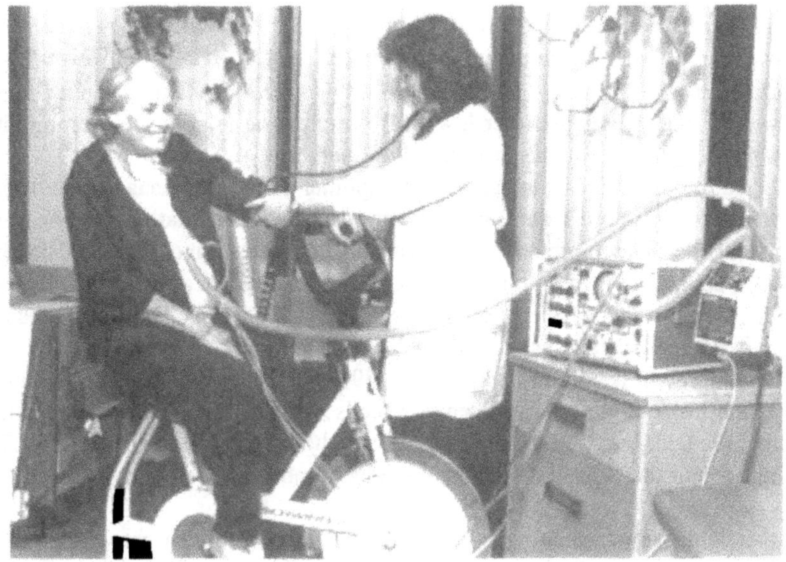

Figure 1 Whole body exercise performed in a patient requiring chronic invasive ventilation via portable volume ventilator. (From Ref. 43.)

tion, undernutrition impairs ventilatory drive, weakens host defense mechanisms placing patients at risk for infections, and impedes wound healing. In patients with COPD, reduced body weight is associated with higher mortality. However, whether malnutrition is an independent factor contributing to a higher mortality, or simply a marker of disease severity is unclear. In an attempt to evaluate this question, Gray-Donald et al. (38) analyzed a cohort of 348 patients with severe COPD. They separated this cohort into those patients who were hospitalized (n = 184) and those not hospitalized (n = 164). They found that body mass index (BMI) for the group was an independent factor on survival with heavier patients

Table 4 Consequences of Malnutrition in Patients Receiving Long-Term Invasive Ventilation

Decreased diaphragm muscle mass
Reduced maximum voluntary ventilation
Decreased ventilatory drive
Weakened host defenses
Impaired normal healing

living longer. For the hospitalized subgroup, BMI was not independently predictive of mortality, but in the nonhospitalized group it was the only significant predictor of total mortality. Like the others, however, this study was not able to answer the question of whether low BMI has a causal relationship to mortality in severe COPD, or whether it is simply a marker of severe disease.

An important factor in determining optimal nutritional management of patients, especially those requiring long-term mechanical ventilation, is a measure of patient energy requirements. Most typically, a predication of nutritional needs is based upon patient weight. In the patient who survives an acute critical illness, patient weight as a measure of predicting nutritional needs is inaccurate because of body edema. In such cases, adjusted weight may be more accurate for predicting energy expenditure. Cutts et al. (39) evaluated critically ill ventilator-dependent patients and estimated energy needs with the Harris-Benedict equation using both actual weight and an adjusted weight to reflect lean body mass. The authors found that adjusted weights provided a more accurate prediction of energy needs.

In addition to refeeding patients, the use of recombinant growth hormone has been touted as producing a positive nitrogen balance, promoting skeletal muscle anabolism, and improving peripheral muscle function. To evaluate this claim, Pichard et al. (40) studied 20 mechanically ventilated patients requiring prolonged mechanical ventilation (i.e., greater than 7 days) randomly assigned to receive recombinant growth hormone or placebo for 12 days. When compared with the control group, those patients receiving growth hormone had a significant increase in body cell mass and nitrogen retention; however, muscle function assessed using a computer-controlled electrical stimulation technique applied to the adductor pollicis was no different between the treated and untreated groups. Similarly, there was no difference between the two groups with respect to weaning from mechanical ventilation, gas exchange variables, or duration of mechanical ventilation.

Strategies for facilitating the weaning of mechanical ventilation by altering the fat or carbohydrate composition in refeeding patients weaning from mechanical ventilation has also been examined and found not to affect the weaning process. Van den Berg et al. (41) provided high fat nutrition to 15 patients and standard feeding (isocaloric) to 17 patients weaning from mechanical ventilation. They found that while CO_2 excretion and respiratory quotient values were lower in the high-fat feeding group, there was no effect on the duration of weaning from mechanical ventilation.

Protein–calorie malnutrition is a major factor contributing to the pathogenesis of chronic ventilator dependency. It remains important, therefore, to address this issue early on in the care of critically ill patients, and to continue nutritional evaluation in patients as they transition to more active weaning from the ventilator or become ventilator independent.

V. Selection of Tracheostomy Tubes and Ventilator

A. Tracheostomy Tube Selection

Long-term invasive mechanical ventilation requires chronic airway access that is tolerated by the patient, minimizes impairment of swallowing function, and, as much as possible, facilitates speech. Most often, tracheostomy tubes that optimize comfort, facilitate speech and swallowing, and meet the goals of mechanical ventilation are relatively small (4 to 6 mm, internal diameter), cuffless, plastic or metal tubes. In patients who are able to sustain spontaneous ventilation for periods of time, a fenestrated tracheostomy tube may permit a greater volume of air to flow through the larynx for better voice quality and intensity.

In long-term mechanically ventilated patients who are unable to tolerate periods of spontaneous breathing, a cuffless tracheostomy tube that allows for phonation may be appropriate. The tidal volume delivered by the ventilator can be increased by 150 to 200 cc in order to compensate for the leak that occurs when a cuffless tube is used. Another option for the patient unable to tolerate periods of independent ventilation is a tracheostomy tube designed to have the cuff inflated only with each cycle of inspiration. On expiration, the cuff is allowed to deflate and phonation is possible.

The increased tidal volume used to compensate for the leak that occurs when a cuffless tracheostomy tube is used to facilitate speech in a ventilated patient may cause hypocapnia. Unfavorable effects of hypocapnia (e.g., shifting oxygen-hemoglobin dissociation curve, decreasing oxygen availability at the tissue level, decreasing cerebral blood flow) may be avoided by inserting dead space into the circuit. Such a strategy has been evaluated and shown to be effective (42). Cuffed tracheostomy tubes are necessary in patients with severe swallowing impairment to minimize the risk of aspiration. They also are appropriate for patients who have had strokes or bulbar dysfunction that has rendered them speechless. Some patients are not adequately ventilated with cuffless tubes and for them, a partially inflated cuff may provide a sufficient tidal volume as well as enough air leak to permit phonation. Other patients may deflate the cuff during the daytime for speech and then inflate it at night when the continued air leak can interfere with sleep.

If cuffs are used, patients must be cautioned about over-inflating them. They should be instructed in the minimal leak inflation technique, and should be told never to exceed a maximal inflation volume, such as 6 to 8 cc. Contrary to a commonly held belief, it is not necessary to inflate the cuff for meals unless gross aspiration has been documented.

B. Ventilator Selection

Several important changes occur with respect to the need for mechanical ventilation as a patient moves from an acute condition to a more chronic stable state

(43). For one, the demands placed upon the mechanical ventilator are generally less. High levels of minute ventilation are not typically required, nor are complex mechanisms to ensure maintenance of end-expiratory lung volume by requiring positive end-expiratory pressure (PEEP). Ventilator modes, such as pressure support and flow-by, which are options on some ventilators, are not needed for the patient requiring chronic stable invasive ventilation. Also, in this phase, patients are generally more mobile, and a smaller, lighter ventilator with a battery source

Table 5 Criteria for Admission of Invasive Ventilator-Dependent Patients to Our Ventilator Rehabilitation Unit

Respiratory stability
Airway: Tracheostomy for invasive ventilation, minimal aspiration
Secretions: Manageable with infrequent suctioning
Oxygen: $Fio_2 \leq 40\%$, PEEP ≤ 5 cm, $Spo_2 \geq 90\%$
Ventilator settings: Stable, no sophisticated mode, no change in settings for 1–2 wk prior to discharge
PEEP: ≤ 5 cm H_2O
Patient assessment: Comfortable on ventilator, prefer at least 1–2 hr of spontaneous breathing time per day
Weaning technique: Tracheal collar
Nonrespiratory medical stability
Sepsis identified and controlled: Continuation of antibiotic therapy to complete course
No uncontrolled hemorrhage: No active bleeding
No uncontrolled cardiac arrhythmia, heart failure, or angina: No unstable cardiac condition
No coma, awake, cooperative: Awake, alert, responsive to verbal command
Secure intravenous access: Only permanent intravenous access if required
Secure alimentation route: Gastrostomy or jejunostomy tubes only
Socioeconomic status
Insurance coverage for institutional and professional care: Involvement of 3rd party payor
Insurance coverage for disposable and nondisposable supplies: Disposable supplies and home care coverage secured
Psychological stability: Participates in care plan
Significant other for support: Support system requisite for sophisticated respiratory care at home
Comprehensive discharge plan[a]: All aspects of home medical, nursing, respiratory, rehabilitative, and follow-up care organized and in place

[a]Medical, respiratory, rehabilitative, and emergent care coordinated with active family support and financial coverage of all aspects of care.

of power is preferred to a larger, "critical care" ventilator to facilitate patient mobility. Portable ventilators are also significantly less expensive than the "critical care" ventilators.

Patients who are candidates for portable mechanical ventilation require less extensive monitoring and alarm capabilities and are manageable with less sophisticated modes or types of ventilators. Table 5 shows selection criteria for admission of ventilator-dependent patients to our ventilator rehabilitation unit and the requirements for clinical stability, ventilatory support, and financial resources in these patients. Overall, these patients are stable despite the need for mechanical ventilation and easily accommodate the use of smaller, portable ventilators with internal batteries.

VI. Special Management Issues in Patients Receiving Prolonged Invasive Ventilation

A. Swallowing Dysfunction

Swallowing dysfunction and aspiration occur commonly in patients receiving ventilatory support via a cuffed tracheostomy tube following translaryngeal intubation (44,45). Although several case reports and small series of patients describe swallowing abnormalities and aspiration in patients receiving mechanical ventilation via a cuffed tracheotomy tube, the overall incidence is unknown. In an early study that used dysphagia as a marker of swallowing dysfunction in patients with tracheostomies, the incidence of swallowing abnormalities was low (7%) (46). In more recent studies, when aspiration is used to indicate the presence of swallowing dysfunction, the incidence is reported to be 40 to 50% (44,45,47). We examined the effects of prolonged mechanical ventilation on swallowing (47), and found that long-term positive pressure mechanical ventilation in patients requiring prolonged intubation (translaryngeal followed by tracheostomy) produced a high incidence of swallowing abnormalities (Table 6). These abnormalities, moreover, were independent of the presence or absence of significant underlying neuromuscular illnesses. We also found that the abnormalities were complex and frequently multiple in any given patient.

Tracheostomy impairs upper airway/laryngeal reflexes, and chronic aspiration represents a major complication associated with this procedure. Because a tracheostomy involves fixation of the trachea, there is reduced elevation and anterior displacement of the larynx during deglutition (47). This impairment in laryngeal movement allows for the incomplete protection of the airway during swallowing. In addition, tracheal cuff inflation may exert extrinsic compression on the esophagus and further impair swallowing. Chronic upper airway bypass by the tracheostomy also produces desensitization of the larynx and diminunition of protective laryngeal reflexes, further diminishing swallowing function.

Table 6 Findings on Initial Modified Barium Swallow with Videofluoroscopy in Invasive Ventilator-Dependent Patients (n = 19)

	NMD present (n = 11)				NMD absent (n = 8)			
		Abnormal				Abnormal		
Parameters	Normal	Mild	Moderate	Severe	Normal	Mild	Moderate	Severe
Lingual propulsion	5	2	3	1	4	2	2	0
Premature spillage[a]	3	4	3	1	1	3	2	2
Swallowing reflex	4	5	2	0	1	4	2	1
Tracheal aspiration[a]	7	1	3	0	2	2	0	4
Vallecular stasis[a]	3	2	2	4	3	1	0	4
Pyriform sinus stasis[a]	3	2	2	4	3	1	0	4
Pharyngeal coating[a]	4	2	2	3	2	1	1	4
Laryngeal elevation	5	0	4	2	5	2	0	1
Cricopharyngeal spasm[a]	7	0	2	2	8	0	0	0

[a]"Normal" indicates that this finding was absent on the study.
Modified from Ref. 47.

Other factors thought to contribute to swallowing dysfunction include an underlying neuromuscular disorder (48–50), acute medical or surgical illness, prolonged inactivity of swallowing muscles, use of corticosteroids, anesthetics, neuromuscular blocking agents, and prior translaryngeal intubation causing vocal cord dysfunction.

Evaluation of Swallowing Dysfunction

All of our VRU patients receiving long-term mechanical ventilation are evaluated at the bedside by an experienced speech pathologist. This evaluation includes a review of the patient's medical history and an examination of the oral anatomy. The patients are then closely observed while they swallow materials of different textures (thin and thick liquids, and semisolid paste) to which food dye is added to help evaluate for aspiration as suggested by "tinting" of the tracheal secretions. A modified barium swallow (MBS) with videofluoroscopy is then performed on all patients in whom the bedside evaluation is found to be abnormal.

In addition to the initial bedside evaluation and MBS, our evaluation includes direct laryngoscopy to more fully assess hypopharyngeal sensation, detect vallecula and pyriform sinus pooling, observe hypopharyngeal muscle contraction, and observe the integrity of epiglottic and vocal cord function. We have found that examination of the unanesthetized upper airway via fiberoptic laryngoscopy provides important information and is well tolerated by the patient (47,51). We position the flexible pediatric bronchoscope above the glottis and observe swallowing after the oral administration of color-tinted water-ice (to assess the response to thermal stimulation) and other textured material. This allows us to assess the coordinated action of the hypopharyngeal muscles, epiglottis, and vocal cords directly.

Treatment of Swallowing Dysfunction

The initial goal in the patient with swallowing dysfunction is to prevent aspiration. The early establishment of alternative routes of enteral nutrition, therefore, is advised (47). Gastrostomy or jejunostomy feeding tubes are the routes most commonly employed for long-term enteral nutrition, and are associated with relatively low morbidity. We look for concomitant neurologic processes because if they exist, they may represent one of the more treatable causes of swallowing dysfunction. Inspection of the tracheostomy tube is also performed to ensure that its size is appropriate and that the cuff is not overinflated. Tracheostomy tube strings or Velcro collars should be secured to decrease excessive movement of the tube and prevent the weight of the ventilator tubing from applying torque and rotating the tube.

In addition to the above evaluation and establishing alternate routes of nourishment, proper positioning of the patient is important to minimize the risk of aspiration (Table 7), particularly in patients with poor head and upper body control. Patients who are able to take nutrition by mouth should be carefully evaluated and instructed by a trained speech therapist to ensure proper upper airway function and decrease the risk for aspiration. Various techniques are available for training the patient to compensate for the swallowing abnormality. The response to therapy and prognosis for recovery of swallowing dysfunction in mechanically ventilated patients are uncertain. While some have suggested that swallowing dysfunction is transient (44), others (47) suggest that swallowing abnormalities do not quickly resolve. Nonetheless, ongoing evaluation and therapy by a speech therapist trained in swallowing dysfunction are recommended so as to maximize a patient's chance for resumption of oral feeding.

B. Psychological Dysfunction

The incidence of psychological dysfunction in critically ill ICU patients has been reported to range from 14 to 72% (52). In our study of 28 long-term ventilated patients, the prevalence of cognitive deficits was high (53) (Fig. 2). At least one of five cognitive deficits examined (orientation, long-term memory, short-term memory, language, and reasoning) was found by a clinical psychologist after neuropsychologic testing in 93% of the patients, and most of the patients had three or more deficits (Fig. 3). Severity of illness, patient immobility, the inability to speak, and the use of sedating agents while on mechanical ventilation may have all contributed to psychological problems. Such problems include agitation,

Table 7 Therapeutic and Compensatory Techniques for Managing Dysphagia

Technique	Desired effect
Flex neck	Reduce aspiration
Turn head to one side	Direct bolus to the ipsilateral side (away from side of weakness)
Hold breath before swallowing	Seal larynx, reduce aspiration
Thicken liquids (avoid thin)	Reduce aspiration, improve bolus control
Thin liquids (avoid thick)	Reduce pharyngeal retention
Slow rate of eating	Improve oral bolus control, avoid overloading pharynx
Mendelsohn maneuver	Prolong pharyngoesophageal sphincter opening, improve pharyngeal clearance
Glottic adduction exercises	Improve airway protection, reduce aspiration
Use glossectomy spoon	Bypass anterior mouth, place food directly into posterior oral cavity
Stimulate soft palate with cold	Increase sensitivity for eliciting swallow
Feeding gastrostomy	Bypass oral cavity and pharynx

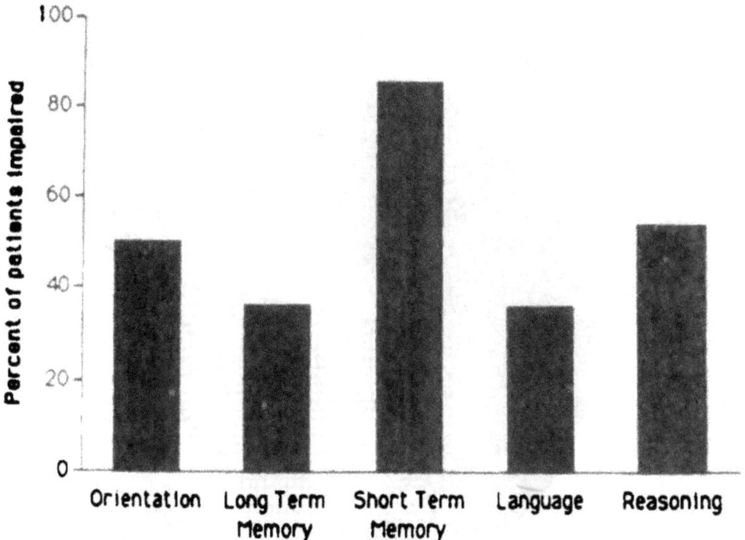

Figure 2 Cognitive deficits present in 28 patients receiving chronic invasive mechanical ventilation. Memory was most commonly impaired with the majority of patients showing deficits in short-term memory. Disorientation and impaired reasoning were observed in 50 and 56% of patients, respectively, while 36% of patients showed impairment in long-term memory and language function. (From Ref. 54.)

anxiety, confusion, depression, fear and delirium (54). Severity of illness, sleep and sensory deprivation, altered underlying physiology secondary to the disease process, medications, and the process of mechanical ventilation itself are among the major causes for these psychological abnormalities (55) (Table 8).

Severity of Illness

The severity of illness is an important factor that contributes to psychological disturbance. In one study on patients with congestive heart failure (CHF), Class IV patients had a 100% incidence of postoperative delirium compared with a 29% incidence in patients with class I CHF (56). Moreover, the investigators found that the duration of cardiopulmonary bypass time, and the complexity of operative procedure further increased the risk for development of postoperative delirium. It was speculated that subclinical infection, anoxia, and a greater incidence of electrolyte disturbances may have been present in the patients with more severe disease.

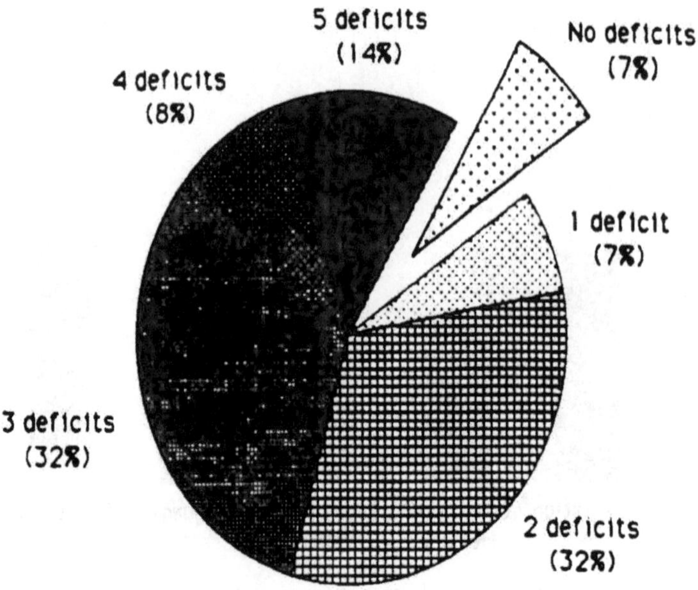

Figure 3 Breakdown of cognitive deficits in all chronically invasively ventilated patients. Only 7% of patients showed normal cognitive function testing. The majority of patients showed several cognitive deficits. (From Ref. 54.)

Sleep Deprivation

Several studies have shown that sleep deprivation may be an important factor contributing to the development of psychological disturbances (57,58). Restless sleep, nightmares, and the total absence of dreaming are commonly reported in ICU patients who develop delirium or other psychological disturbances. Multiple

Table 8 Contributing Factors to Psychological Dysfunction in Chronic Invasively Ventilated Patients

Severity of illness
Patient immobility
Inability to speak
Use of sedative agents
Sleep and sensory deprivation
Physiologic derangements (i.e., gas exchange abnormalities)
Process of mechanical ventilation

factors present in the ICU setting contribute to sleep deprivation (59). Nursing interventions, nocturnal medical care and treatments, and noise generated by the ventilator, monitors, and oxygen outlets on the wall are among such factors producing a state of sleep deprivation. Studies confirm that noise levels measured at the heads of beds in the ICU are high (60,61). The noise generated by ventilators, alarms, and oxygen outlets was equivalent to that of a radio playing at full volume 90% of the time (60). In another study (61), noise levels were shown to far exceed a recommended level set by the U.S. Environmental Protection Agency. Table 9 shows the major sources of noise in the ICU and the mean sound levels.

Sensory Deprivation

Besides sleep deprivation, sensory deprivation may contribute to psychological dysfunction. Whether the patient's room has a window or not has been shown to affect mental status (62). Wilson compared the incidence of delirium in 50 surgical patients treated for three or more days in ICU rooms without windows with 50 surgical patients treated in ICU rooms with windows. The patients were similar with respect to age, operative procedure, and nursing care; however, the patients treated in the windowless rooms had a threefold greater incidence of postoperative delirium.

Acoustic stimulation provided by the harsh sounds of the ventilator, oxygen outlets, and monitors in chronically ventilated patients may also have a detrimen-

Table 9 Major Causes of Noise in the Intensive Care Unit Setting

Noise	% of time[a]	Mean peak sound ± SEM, dBA
Air conditioner	2	74.8 ± 1.2
IV alarm	0.9	77.3 ± 2.0
Ventilator	8	78.0 ± 1.1
Monitor alarm	20	79.0 ± 0.7
Television	23	79.1 ± 0.5
Ventilator alarm	5	79.7 ± 1.3
Telephone	0.8	79.9 ± 2.5
Nebulizer	0.6	80.6 ± 0.6
Oximeter alarm	5	81.1 ± 1.6
Intercom	0.5	83.7 ± 2.1
Miscellaneous	7	84.0 ± 1.1
Beeper	0.9	84.3 ± 5.5
Talking	26	84.6 ± 0.7

[a]Total observation time, 160 min.

tal effect on psychological function. Intermittent auditory stimulation may produce visual and auditory hallucinations in normal subjects (63). Egerton and Kay (57) also speculated that hallucinations and thought disorders in their open heart surgery patients were provoked by exposing patients to auditory driving by 1 to 6 clicks of sound per second for several days. These data suggest that a variety of abnormal auditory stimuli coupled with sleep and sensory deprivation routinely encountered in long-term ventilated patients contribute to psychological dysfunction.

Underlying Lung Disease

Patients requiring long-term mechanical ventilation almost by definition have some impairment of their respiratory system either as a primary process (e.g., severe emphysema), a secondary process (e.g., postoperative acute respiratory distress syndrome [ARDS]), or both. Features common to these groups that may contribute to psychological dysfunction include gas exchange abnormalities and chronic dyspnea.

Abnormalities in Gas Exchange

Hypoxemia and hypercapnia have been associated with a variety of cognitive impairments, such as inappropriate behavior, impaired short-term memory, short attention span, apathetic attitude, perceptual distortions, and impaired judgment (64). In one study (65) evaluating the use of nocturnal versus continuous supplemental oxygen in hypoxemic COPD patients, the investigators found that moderate to severe cognitive impairments were three times more common in ambulatory hypoxemic COPD patients (mean Pa_{O_2} 51 mm Hg) compared with a nonhypoxemic control group. In the hypoxemic COPD patients, higher cognitive functions (abstract reasoning, complex perceptual motor integration) were more severely affected, and 50% of these patients also showed impairments in coordination, strength, and motor speed. In a subsequent study, Heaton et al. (66) found that COPD patients had higher scores on neuropsychological testing after 12 months of continuous oxygen administration compared with patients treated with only nocturnal oxygen supplementation. These data suggest that cognitive impairment is commonly present in patients with severe COPD and may be exacerbated by the presence of hypoxemia.

Chronic Dyspnea

The experience of dyspnea may precipitate anxiety in patients, which may further increase the sensation of dyspnea, independent of actual physiologic changes (67,68). In many patients with chronic lung disease, the fear of dyspnea leads to a decreased expression of any emotion, which has resulted in this group of patients being described as living in an emotional "straightjacket" (69). Many patients with severe lung problems have developed a systematically decreased tolerance for dyspnea, and often exhibit anxiety or avoidance in the anticipation of any physical exertion. In patients on mechanical ventilation, the implementation of weaning trials or initiation of any exercise program may provoke displays of fearfulness and apprehension that are more related to the anticipation of dyspnea, rather than to the stress of the activity itself.

Medication Effects

Medications commonly used in the treatment long-term mechanically ventilated patients may contribute to the psychologic disturbance. Sympathomimetic agents, for example, may produce agitation and excitation. Corticosteroids may produce bizarre, inappropriate behavior and affective disturbances (70,71). Aminophylline has been reported to affect patient mood, behavior, and performance on neuropsychological testing (72), although contrary evidence is also present regarding the last effect (73). Benzodiazepines may contribute to short-term memory deficits, and narcotics or their withdrawal may cause disorientation or even hallucinations.

Mechanical Ventilation

A number of emotional stressors that are specific to the process of mechanical ventilation have been recognized as contributing to psychological dysfunction. Mechanical ventilation necessitates a loss of independence and control over breathing. A tracheostomy tube impairs not only speech but also other expressions of emotion, such as a sigh or gasp. This ''communicator isolation'' (64) further exacerbates feelings of isolation and abandonment. Riggio et al. (74) described the perceptions of ventilated patients regarding sources of psychological stress and found that the inability to communicate, memory loss, disorientation, and pain were all perceived as major problems.

Other aspects of long-term ventilation have also been described as additional stresses. Most patients describe endotracheal suctioning as extremely unpleasant and compare suctioning to suffocating or gagging. As discussed above, noise from the ventilator, and other adjunctive apparatus contribute to aberrant sensory input and sleep disturbances. Limited physical activity because of being tethered to the ventilator may produce a sense of isolation and helplessness. Realization that mechanical malfunction or failure of the ventilator may result in a worsened condition or even death produces added anxiety, apprehension, and fear.

In contrast to patients who require only brief mechanical ventilatory support, those who require long-term ventilation have additional psychological and emotional problems. The incidence of patients' perceptions of fatigue while receiving long-term mechanical ventilation is high (75). Higgins (75) evaluated 20 patients receiving long-term mechanical ventilation (mean ICU length of stay

20.5 days), and found that all of the patients rated themselves as fatigued on a visual analogue scale. Whereas 20% of the patients considered themselves mildly fatigued, 45% considered themselves severely fatigued. This study also found that associated factors such as nutritional status as determined by serum albumin and hemoglobin did not correlate with the perception of fatigue. The presence of a depressed mood state, however, strongly correlated with perception of fatigue. In addition, the perception of sleep effectiveness was inversely related to the perception of fatigue.

Bergbom-Engberg and Haljamae (76) retrospectively assessed patients' recall of their reactions to mechanical ventilation after discharge from the hospital. These patients required mechanical ventilation for acute medical and/or surgical problems including trauma. The mean duration of mechanical ventilation was approximately six days. They found that 47% of the patients felt fearful or anxious during the period of mechanical ventilation and that 90% of the patients recalled the experience of mechanical ventilation as unpleasant and stressful up to 4 yr posttreatment.

While data suggest that chronic ventilation is associated with depression and hopelessness, an evaluation of the psychological status of patients with amyotrophic lateral sclerosis (ALS) receiving chronic ventilatory support came to a different conclusion. McDonald et al. (77) administered a battery of standardized tests to assess psychological status to 18 patients with ALS on chronic mechanical ventilation and another 126 ALS patients not requiring ventilatory support. The authors found that there was no significant difference between the two groups with respect to psychological status. In fact, many of the ventilated patients experienced a high quality of life and psychological well-being despite their limitations. It should be recalled, however, that patients with ALS receiving long-term invasive mechanical ventilation are a highly selected subgroup.

Treatment of Psychological Dysfunction

A general approach to treatment of psychological problems in the long-term ventilated patient involves a systematic plan for reversing the factors contributing to the psychological dysfunction (e.g., limited mobility, sterile environment, impaired communication and swallowing). More specific interventions include altering the environment for the patient and pharmacotherapy.

Altering the Environment

To promote a more favorable environment for the patient, a setting should be established that minimizes patient seclusion and enhances interactions with the family and medical staff. In such a setting, the patient is in an individual room, interventions that disturb sleep are minimized, and monotonous sensory input is reduced by placing unnecessary monitoring equipment outside of the patient's room. Further, the room is equipped with orientation aids, such as clocks, calendars, and family artifacts. In addition, the room is spacious to foster patient mobility, and preferably, an outside window is present.

Pharmacotherapy

The selective use of psychotropic medications may be helpful in addition to behavioral techniques and supportive psychotherapy (69). Anxiolytics, such as the benzodiazepines, may be useful in patients who suffer from extreme anxiety. Moreover, small doses of neuroleptic agents may be helpful in controlling restless or agitated ventilated patients. In some instances, antidepressant agents may be needed to treat the extreme fatigue and apathy manifested in some chronically ill, ventilated patients.

C. Verbal Communication

Various devices are available to facilitate speech in patients receiving long-term mechanical ventilation. In general, the devices include the electrolarynx, self-activating pneumatic voicing systems, and speaking tracheostomy tubes (Fig. 4). The limitations of the electrolarynx include its cost, unnatural voice quality, and need for coordination in holding the device properly on the neck (78). The pneumatic voicing system is also limited in part because of articulation difficulty secondary to the intraoral catheter. Speaking tracheostomy tubes may produce better voice quality and may be simpler to use. However, they require specific instruction and training for optimal use (78).

Ventilator-dependent patients are unable to phonate without the use of some accessory device that allows airflow to occur on exhalation through the vocal cords. Other means of communication such as lipreading, writing, or communication boards are used but have limitations. The introduction of the Passy-Muir unidirectional flow valve applied to the tracheostomy tube directly or in line with the breathing circuit apparatus from the ventilator has greatly enhanced the ability of ventilator-dependent patients to communicate with others by speaking.

In one study, performed in ventilator-dependent patients with tracheostomy, use of the valve while on mechanical ventilation resulted in the facilitation of speech, improved sense of well-being, a reduction in airway secretions, improved cough and a return of the sense of smell after 1 wk of use (79). Important precautions when using this valve, however, must be taken. For one, if a cuffed tracheostomy tube is used, in order to achieve ventilation goals, the tidal volume may need to be increased to offset air leaking around the tracheostomy tube on inspiration. In addition, the cuff on the tracheostomy tube must be deflated, not only to allow for airflow to pass through the vocal cords, but also to avoid the hyperinflation and possible barotrauma that will occur with the cuff inflated and the one-way valve in place. Overall, in patients who have intact upper airway

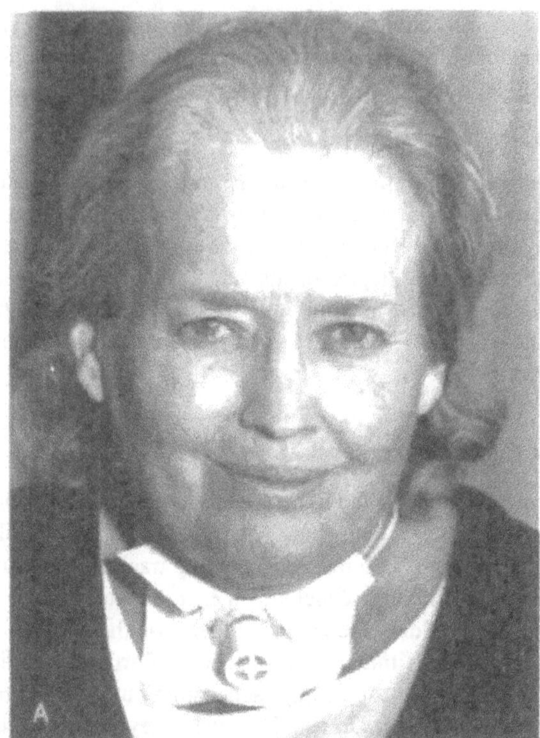

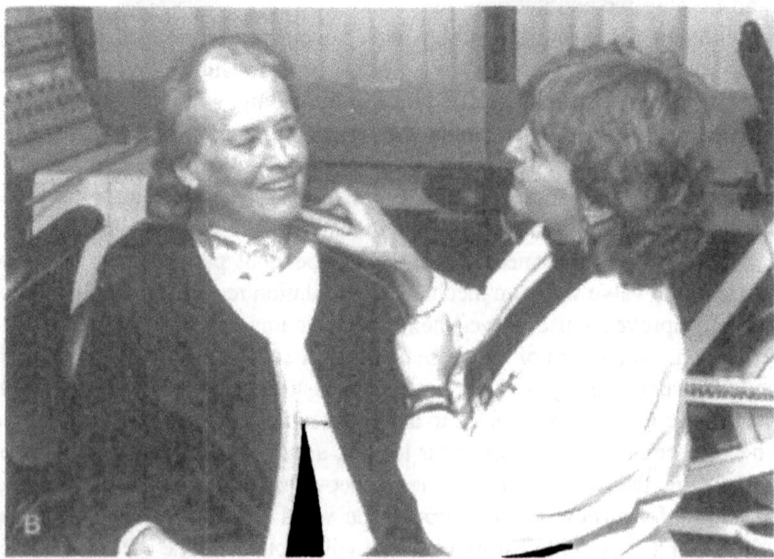

Figure 4 Communication skills illustrated with a Passy-Muir valve (A) and electrolarynx (B) in a chronically invasively ventilated patient. (From Ref. 43.)

control and a near-normal mental status, this valve can be of great value in facilitating communication with health care providers, family, and friends.

VII. Monitoring Long-Term Invasive Mechanical Ventilation

The essentials for monitoring patients receiving long-term invasive mechanical ventilation are identical to those tests and procedures used routinely in intensive care units. In those patients who achieve long-term clinical stability and are transferred to locations outside the intensive care unit, ensuring access to needed tests is usually what is required. The most crucial element of monitoring outcome in patients receiving long-term invasive ventilation is the acumen and experience of the medical personnel. Nurses, respiratory therapists, and physicians who are well versed in all aspects of respiratory care and ventilator management are prerequisites for the successful evaluation and treatment of such patients. All members of the multidisciplinary team that runs programs to rehabilitate patients receiving long-term invasive ventilation must be familiar with the patient's respiratory status and essential aspects of airway and ventilator management in order to maximize their contributions to patient care and minimize complications.

Oxygen saturation is monitored continuously in all patients receiving invasive long-term ventilation entering our ventilator rehabilitation unit. When patients reach a chronic state of stability, however, oxygen saturation need be monitored only intermittently. Easily heard low-pressure alarms that are monitored in a central nursing station are also required for patients who are dependent on continuous ventilation. Routine cardiac telemetry is not usually necessary, but occasionally may be helpful. Patients with uncontrolled cardiac arrhythmias are not admitted to our ventilator rehabilitation unit until the underlying arrhythmia is adequately treated.

Tests helpful in predicting weaning outcome and evaluating disorders contributing to respiratory failure include arterial blood gases (Pao_2, $Paco_2$, pH), maximum inspiratory and expiratory mouth pressures, and spontaneous ventilatory variables (i.e., minute ventilation and its components of tidal volume and respiratory rate). Indices such as the rapid shallow breathing index (f/V_T) are derived from these parameters and in addition to predicting weaning success or failure are used to determine when to initiate and end weaning trials (80). These tests have been used to predict weaning outcome in patients receiving mechanical ventilation for ≤ 7 days, but they may be less helpful in patients receiving prolonged ventilatory support. Additional studies are needed to establish the utility of these tests in predicting weaning outcome of long-term ventilator users.

Because patients requiring long-term invasive mechanical ventilation usually have complex underlying medical disorders that need ongoing assessment and treatment, measures of electrolytes, metabolic parameters, and specific blood levels of pharmaceutical agents must be available. The monitoring capabilities of units caring for patients requiring long-term invasive mechanical ventilation must be individually tailored to meet specific patient and institutional goals.

VIII. Preventing Complications

A. Management of Airway Secretions

Maintaining an airway clear of excessive secretions is a major component of care for patients receiving long-term mechanical ventilation. Airway secretions may impair ventilation, adversely affect gas exchange, and promote bacterial infection leading to pneumonia. Although many patients on long-term mechanical ventilation have an intact cough reflex, it is often weakened because of diminished flow rates secondary to the increased resistance from the endotracheal tube (81). Hence, adequate clearance of secretions from the airway necessitates intermittent suctioning to diminish the untoward effects of excessive airway secretions. Suction catheters and machines must therefore always be present at the patient's bed. Suggested suctioning techniques include preoxygenation and bagging to produce hyperinflation and/or hyperventilation prior to suctioning to minimize the risk of hypoxemia. However, these are unnecessary in long-term ventilation once the patient has stabilized unless chronic hypoxemia is known to be a problem. Instillation of saline "bullets" into the trachea prior to suctioning is sometimes performed to additionally stimulate cough and help loosen secretions. There is no minimal amount of suctioning or fixed frequency to suction a patient on mechanical ventilation. The frequency of suctioning depends on individual patient needs (82).

Chest physical therapy (CPT) may also aid the management of airway secretions. The benefit of bronchial drainage has long been recognized in patients with lung diseases (83,84). Positioning of the patient to promote drainage of an affected area of the lung is a key component to CPT. One needs to be careful, however, when positioning patients because of changes in V/Q matching that may occur. Also, positioning a patient may contribute to dyspnea by altering chest wall mechanics, and the therapist administering CPT must be aware of this.

Chest percussion is another technique employed to promote secretion clearance. When combined with vibration techniques, chest percussion has been shown to increase production of secretions in intubated, mechanically ventilated patients with respiratory failure (85). There is no agreement on the optimal force to apply, the frequency of percussion, and whether to percuss directly to the skin or through padding (86).

Mucolytic agents (e.g., pulmozyme or acetylcysteine) are also sometimes helpful in gaining control of airway secretions. These drugs, however, are not routinely employed, partly because of concerns about bronchospasm.

B. Bronchospasm

Frequently, patients receiving long-term mechanical ventilation have underlying chronic airway disease, and bronchospasm may be a manifestation of suboptimally controlled disease. Airway hyperreactivity may also be worsened by infection, trauma to the airway mucosa from frequent suctioning, or heart failure. Recognition of bronchospasm in patients receiving mechanical ventilation is important so that treatment is begun promptly and the sequelae of dynamic hyperinflation are avoided. The patient typically will be distressed, high pressure alarms will be triggered because of increased airways resistance, and the patient will be breathing out of synchrony with the ventilator. Wheezes may not be heard on examination of the chest, but the thorax will appear hyperinflated and hyperresonant to percussion. Treatment consists of the prompt administration of bronchodilators to the airways directly, either via a small-volume nebulizer or using multiple "puffs" from a metered-dose inhaler. Doses of beta agonists are titrated depending on the individual patient's response.

Mechanical ventilation may affect the amount of aerosolized bronchodilator actually delivered to the airways. Ventilator tubing and the tracheal tube may trap some of the droplet medication, reducing the amount deposited into the patient's airways. Humidification within the circuit can also affect the droplet size such that less deposition occurs. A high inspiratory flow or respiratory rate may also lessen the amount of delivered medication. Newer generation ventilators with a built-in nebulizer function allow for easier administration of aerosolized medication by using the ventilator as the source of compressed gas. Because of concerns about the unpredictable delivery of aerosolized medication during mechanical ventilation, however, we prefer to administer aerosolized bronchodilators during spontaneous unassisted breathing, if possible.

C. Tracheobronchitis

The presence of an artificial airway interferes with natural barrier defense mechanisms and increases the risk for infection in the lower respiratory tract. A patient's artificial airway is colonized by hospital flora within a few days of hospital admission. Further, by the time a patient is transferred to our long-term ventilator unit, airway flora frequently include antibiotic-resistant gram-negative bacilli and other potential pathogens that may pose a challenge for effective treatment.

Nurses, respiratory therapists, and physicians pay attention to the characteristics of secretions suctioned from the airway. This information is noted in the patient's medical chart. A change in secretion characteristics, such as increased volume, altered consistency, or change in color suggests the presence of an infection in the lower respiratory tract. These should prompt further investigation, including a sputum gram stain and culture, as well as a chest x-ray if fever or leukocytosis is present. Antibiotics are used judiciously with specific end points in mind. Typically, a course of antibiotic therapy may last 1 to 2 wk. The regular use of aerosolized or prophylactic antibiotics is not advocated in our unit.

D. Venous Thromboembolism

Immobility that occurs as a result of prolonged critical illness is the major risk factor for venous thromboembolism encountered in long-term mechanically ventilated patients. In general, low-dose subcutaneous heparin, low-molecular-weight heparin, or intermittent pneumatic compression devices are appropriate for prophylaxis against venous thromboembolism. The need for prophylaxis is tailored to the individual patient and, for the most part, as a patient becomes reconditioned through physical therapy, spends more time out of bed, ambulates, and exercises, prophylaxis becomes unnecessary.

E. Skin Care

In one study, investigators prospectively evaluated 60 medical ICU patients and found that 40% developed pressure ulcers within 2 wk of admission (87). Since pressure is the most important risk factor for the development of pressure sores, the key intervention is to relieve pressure. This is most commonly achieved by repositioning the patient frequently and mobilizing the patient as early as possible. Other interventions, such as special mattresses, cushions, or specialty beds, are also sometimes employed. Optimization of nutritional status is also an important component in management of the patient at risk for skin breakdown (88).

IX. Nutritional Management

Malnutrition is common in hospitalized patients, and is associated with increased morbidity and mortality (89). Moreover, malnutrition contributes to respiratory muscle weakness (e.g., expiratory muscle weakness impairs cough and limits airway secretion clearance, inspiratory muscle weakness contributes to ventilatory pump failure). Undernutrition also reduces metabolic rate and minute ventilation (90) and diminishes ventilatory response to hypoxia (91). To minimize the ill effects of malnutrition in patients receiving long-term mechanical ventilation, all patients in our VRU receive formal nutritional evaluation by a dedicated nutritionist. A history, examination, and selected laboratory studies, which include an evaluation of nitrogen balance and serum proteins, form the basis of an assessment of each patient's nutritional status. Recommendations are provided based upon this assessment in order to achieve the goals of preventing undernutrition and improving overall outcome. In general, renutrition goals include the provision of 2000 to 2500 kcal/day with approximately 20% of total calories as protein.

Thrice weekly follow-up visits by the nutritionist help ensure maintenance of nutritional therapy.

The use of high-fat, low-carbohydrate formulations has been recommended for patients with pulmonary disease to decrease carbon dioxide production; however, studies evaluating these diets have yielded conflicting results. In one study, a high-fat, low-carbohydrate diet resulted in a lower $Paco_2$ and less time on mechanical ventilation (92). Van den Berg et al. (41), however, showed no difference in ventilator time in patients receiving a high-fat, low-carbohydrate diet, even though there was a reduction in carbon dioxide production.

The route of feeding is probably also important (93). In our VRU, the route of renourishing patients is almost entirely via the gastrointestinal tract, and commonly this is achieved via surgically or percutaneously placed gastrostomy tubes or jejunostomy tubes. A number of patients, however, are able to take nutrition by mouth after formal evaluation, including modified barium swallow with videofluoroscopy and bedside flexible laryngoscopy demonstrates an intact swallowing mechanism. Many patients also receive tube feedings nocturnally and eat during the day. On occasion, total parenteral nutrition is employed when bowel rest is mandatory; however, enteral feeding remains the primary route of feeding.

X. Summary

Advances in critical care medicine and mechanical ventilation have improved the survival of critically ill patients, some of whom require long-term invasive ventilation for life support. Patients who require long-term invasive ventilation usually suffer from a complex blend of medical, physiologic, and psychological disturbances. Careful evaluation and treatment of these complex medical, physiologic, and psychological disorders by members of a multidisciplinary team may improve the patients' ability to tolerate spontaneous ventilation and maximize functional capacity thereby resulting in improvement in their quality of life.

References

1. Make BJ, Hill NS, Goldberg AI, Bach JA, Criner GJ, Dunne PE, Gilmartin ME, Heffner JE, Kacmacek R, Keens TG, McInturff S, O'Donohue WJ, Oppenhiemer EA, Robert D. Mechanical ventilation beyond the Intensive Care Unit. Report of a concensus conference by the American College of Chest Physicians. Chest 1998; 113(5):289–344.
2. Bach JR, Saporito LR. Criteria for extubation and tracheostomy tube removal for patients with ventilatory failure: A different approach to weaning. Chest 1996; 11: 1566–1571.

3. Meduri GU, Abou-Shala N, Fox RC, et al. Noninvasive face mask ventilation in patients with acute hypercapneic respiratory failure. Chest 1991; 100:445–454.
4. Nava S, Ambrosino N, Clini E, Prato M, Orlando G, Vitacca M, Brigada P, Racchia C, Rubin F. Noninvasive mechanical ventilation in the weaning of patients with respiratory failure due to chronic obstructive pulmonary disease: A randomized controlled trial. Ann Intern Med 1998; 128:721–728.
5. Gay PC, Hubmayr RD, Stroetz RW. Efficacy of nocturnal nasal ventilation in stable, chronic obstructive pulmonary disease during a 3-month controlled trial. Mayo Clin Proc 1996; 71:533–542.
6. Strumpf DA, Millman RP, Carlisle CC, Grattan LM, Ryan SM, Erickson AD, et al. Nocturnal positive pressure ventilation via nasal mask in patients with severe chronic obstructive pulmonary disease. Am Rev Respir Dis 1991; 144:1234–1239.
7. Meecham Jones DP, Paul EA, Jones PW, Wedzicha JA. Nasal pressure support ventilation plus oxygen compared with oxygen therapy alone in hypercapnic COPD. Am J Resp Crit Care Med 1995; 152:538–544.
8. Martin UJ, Hincapie L, Gilmartin ME, Kreimer D, Criner GJ. Impact of whole body rehabilitation on functional status in chronic ventilator-dependent patients. Am J Resp Crit Care Med 1999; 159:A374.
9. Gilmartin ME, Martin UJ, Kreimer DT, Criner GJ. Impact of new or worsening medical disorders on weaning progress in patients receiving long-term mechanical ventilation. Am J Resp Crit Care Med 1999; 159:A374.
10. Celli B. Arm and leg exercise training in pulmonary rehabilitation. In: Hodgkin JE, Connors GI, Bell CW, eds. Pulmonary Rehabilitation. Philadelphia: Lippincott, 1993.
11. Nicholas JJ, Gilbert R, Gabe R, Auchincloss JH Jr. Evaluation of an exercise therapy program for patients with chronic obstructive pulmonary disease. Am Rev Respir Dis 1970; 102:1–9.
12. Paez PN, Phillipson EA, Masangkay M, Sproule BJ. The physiologic basis of training patients with emphysema. Am Rev Respir Dis 1967; 95:944–953.
13. Keens TG, Krastins IRB, Wanamaker EM, et al. Ventilatory muscle endurance training in normal subjects and patients with cystic fibrosis. Am Rev Respir Dis 1977; 116:853–860.
14. Belman MJ, Mittman C. Ventilatory muscle training program improves exercise capacity in chronic obstructive disease patients. Am Rev Respir Dis 1980; 121:273–280.
15. Belman MJ, Kendregan BA. Physical training fails to improve ventilatory muscle endurance in patients with chronic obstructive pulmonary disease. Chest 1982; 81:440–443.
16. Criner GJ, Celli BR. Effect of unsupported arm exercise on ventilatory muscle recruitment in patients with severe chronic airflow obstruction. Am Rev Respir Dis 1988; 138:856–861.
17. Criner GJ, Muza SR, Kelsen SG. Respiratory action of the canine deep pectoral muscles. Resp Physiol 1994; 98:43–51.
18. Estenne M, Kroop C, VanVaerenbergh J, Heilporn A, DeTroyer A. The effect of pectoralis muscle training in tetraplegia subjects. Am Rev Respir Dis 1989; 139:1218–1222.

19. Clanton T, Dixon G, Drake J, Gadek J. Effects of swim training on lung volumes and inspiratory muscle condition. J Appl Physiol 1987; 62:39–46.
20. Lake FR, Henderson K, Briffa T, Openshaw J, Musk AW. Upper-limb and lower-limb exercise training in patients with chronic airflow obstruction. Chest 1990; 97: 1077–1082.
21. Tobin MJ, Laghi F, Walsh JM. Monitoring of respiratory neuromuscular function. In: Tobin MJ, ed. Principles and Practice of Mechanical Ventilation. New York: McGraw-Hill, 1994.
22. Aldrich TK, Karpel JP, Uhrlass RM, Sparapani MA, Eramo D, Ferranti R. Weaning from mechanical ventilation: Adjunctive use of inspiratory muscle resistive training. Crit Care Med 1989; 17:143–147.
23. Leith DE, Bradley M. Ventilatory muscle strength and endurance training. J Appl Physiol 1976; 41:508–516.
24. Belman MJ, Gaesser GA. Ventilatory muscle training in the elderly. J Appl Physiol 1988; 64:899–905.
25. Levine S, Weiser P, Gillen J. Evaluation of a ventilatory muscle endurance training program in the rehabilitation of patients with chronic obstructive pulmonary disease. Am Rev Respir Dis 1986; 133:400–406.
26. Pardy RL, Rivington RN, Despas PJ, et al. The effects of inspiratory muscle training on exercise performance in chronic airflow limitation. Am Rev Respir Dis 1981; 123:426–433.
27. Chen H, Dukes R, Martin BJ. Inspiratory muscle training in patients with chronic obstructive pulmonary disease. Am Rev Respir Dis 1985; 131:251–255.
28. Sonne LJ, Davis JA. Increased exercise performance in patients with severe COPD following inspiratory resistive training. Chest 1982; 81:436–439.
29. Belman MJ, Thomas SF, Lewis MI. Resistive breathing training in patients with chronic obstructive pulmonary disease. Chest 1986; 90:663–670.
30. Larson J, Kim M, Sharp J, Larson D. Inspiratory muscle training with a pressure threshold breathing device in patients with chronic obstructive pulmonary disease. Am Rev Respir Dis 1988; 138:689–696.
31. Mancini DM, Henson D, LaManca J, et al. Benefit of selective respiratory muscle training on exercise capacity in patients in chronic congestive heart failure. Circulation 1995; 91:320–329.
32. Ruchik A, Weissman AR, Almenoff PL, et al. Resistive inspiratory muscle training in subjects with chronic cervical spinal cord injury. Arch Phys Med Rehabil 1998; 79:293–297.
33. Smith K, Cook D, Guyatt G, Madhavan J, Oxman A. Respiratory muscle training in chronic airflow limitation: A meta-analysis. Am Rev Respir Dis 1992; 145:533–539.
34. Vitacca M, Clini E, Bianchi L, et al. Acute effects of deep diaphragmatic breathing in COPD patients with chronic respiratory insufficiency. Eur Respir J 1998; 11:408–415.
35. Holtackers TR. Physical rehabilitation of the ventilator-dependent patient. In: Irwin S, Tecklin JS, eds. Cardiopulmonary Physical Therapy. 3rd ed. St. Louis: Mosby, 1995; 471–485.
36. Burns JR, Jones Fl. Early ambulation in patients requiring ventilatory assistance. Chest 1975; 68:608.

37. Arora NS, Rochester DF. Respiratory muscle strength and maximal ventilation in undernourished patients. Am Rev Respir Dis 1982; 126:5–8.
38. Gray-Donald K, Gibbons L, Shapiro SH, et al. Nutritional status and mortality in chronic obstructive pulmonary disease. Am J Respir Crit Care Med 1996; 153:961–966.
39. Cutts ME, Dowdy RP, Ellersieck MR, et al. Predicting energy needs in ventilator-dependent critically ill patients: effect of adjusting weight for edema or adiposity. Am J Clin Nutr 1997; 66:1250–1256.
40. Pichard C, Kyle U, Chevrolet JC, et al. Lack of effects of recombinant growth hormone on muscle function in patients requiring prolonged mechanical ventilation: A prospective, randomized, controlled study. Crit Care Med 1996; 24:403–413.
41. Van den Berg B, Bogaard JM, Hop WCJ. High fat, low carbohydrate, enteral feeding in patients weaning from the ventilator. Intensive Care Med 1994; 20:470–475.
42. Watt JWH, Devine A. Does dead space ventilation always alleviate hypocapnia? Anaesthesia 1995; 50:688–691.
43. Criner GJ, Tzouanakis A, Kreimer DT. Overview of improving tolerance of long-term mechanical ventilation. Crit Care Clin 1994; 10(4):845–866.
44. Devita MA, Spierer-Rundback MS. Swallowing disorders in patients with prolonged intubation or tracheostomy tubes. Crit Care Med 1990; 18:1328–32.
45. Elpern EH, Scott MG, Petro L, Ries MH. Pulmonary aspiration in mechanically ventilated patients with tracheostomies. Chest 1994; 105:563–66.
46. Bonanno PC. Swallowing dysfunction after tracheostomy. Ann Surg 1971; 174:29–33.
47. Tolep K, Getch KL, Criner GJ. Swallowing dysfunction in patients requiring prolonged mechanical ventilation. Chest 1996; 109:167–172.
48. Horner J, Massey MD, Riski JE, Lathrop MA, Chase KN. Aspiration following stroke: Clinical correlates and outcome. Neurology 1988; 38:1359–62.
49. Sonies BC, Dalakas MC. Dysphagia in patients with the post-polio syndrome. N Engl J Med 1991; 324:1162–1167.
50. Walton J, ed. The parkinsonian syndrome. In: Walton J. Brain's Diseases of the Nervous System. London: Oxford University Press, 1985; 325–328.
51. Rossini G, McGowan E, Criner GJ. Correlation between modified barium swallow and fiberoptic endoscopic evaluation of swallowing in chronic ventilated patients (abstr). Am J Respir Crit Care Med 1999; 159:A374.
52. Wilson M. Intensive care delirium. Arch Intern Med 1972; 130:225–226.
53. Isaac L, Hungerpillar J, Criner G. Neuropsychologic deficits in chronic ventilator-dependent patients. Chest 1989; 96:255S.
54. Criner GJ, Isaac L. Psychological problems in the ventilator-dependent patient. In: Tobin MJ, ed. Principles and Practice of Mechanical Ventilation. New York: McGraw-Hill, 1994.
55. Criner GJ, Isaac L. Psychological problems in the ventilator-dependent patient. Clin Pulm Med 1994; 1:47–57.
56. Blachy PH, Starr A. Post-cardiotomy delirium. Am J Psychiat 1964; 121:371–375.
57. Egerton N, Kay JH. Psychological disturbances associated with open heart surgery. Brit J Psychiat 1964; 110:443–439.
58. Parker MM, Schubert W, Shelhamer JH, Parrillo JE. Perceptions of a critically ill

patient experiencing therapeutic paralysis in an ICU. Crit Care Med 1984; 70:69–71.

59. Krachman SL, D'Alonzo GE, Criner GJ. Sleep in the intensive care unit. Chest 1995; 107:1713–1720.
60. Woods N, Falk S. Noise stimuli in the acute care area. Nurs Res 1974; 23:144.
61. Kahn DM, Cook TE, Carlisle CC, Nelson DL, Kramer NR, Millman RP. Identification and modification of environmental noise in an ICU setting. Chest 1998; 114: 535–540.
62. Wilson M. Intensive care delirium. Arch Intern Med 1972; 130:225–226.
63. Neher A. Auditory driving observed with scalp electrodes in normal subjects. Electroencephalogr Clin Neurophysiol 1961; 13:449–451.
64. Gale J, O'Shannick GJ. Psychiatric aspects of respirator treatment and pulmonary intensive care. Adv Psychosom Med 1985; 14:93–108.
65. Grant I, Heaton RK, McSweeney J, Adams K, Timms R, et al. Neuropsychologic findings in hypoxemic chronic obstructive pulmonary disease. Arch Intern Med 1982; 142:1470–1476.
66. Heaton RK, Grant I, McSweeny AJ, Adams KM, Petty TL. Psychologic effects of continuous and nocturnal oxygen therapy in hypoxemic chronic obstructive pulmonary disease. Arch Intern Med 1983; 143:1941–1947.
67. Dudley DL, Glaser EM, Jorgenson BN, Logan DL. Psychosocial concomitants to rehabilitation in chronic obstructive pulmonary disease. Part I. Psychosocial and psychological considerations. Chest 1980; 77:413–420.
68. LaFont L, Horner J. Psychosocial issues related to long-term ventilatory support. Probl Resp Care 1988; 1(2):241–256.
69. Sandhu HS. Psychosocial issues in chronic obstructive pulmonary disease. Clin Chest Med 1986; 7:629–642.
70. Boston Collaborative Drug Surveillance Program. Acute adverse reactions to prednisone in relation to dosage. Clin Pharmacol 1972; 13:694–698.
71. Smyllie H, Connolly C. Incidence of serious complications of corticosteroid therapy in respiratory disease. Thorax 1968; 23:571–581.
72. Young LD, Bouton D, Alford P, et al. Do medications reduce cerebral blood flow in COPD patients? Psychosomatics 1986; 27:240.
73. Lindgren S, Lokshin B, Stromquist A, Weinberger M, Massif E, McCubbin M, Frasher R. Does asthma or treatment with theophylline limit children's academic performance? N Engl J Med 1992; 327:926–930.
74. Riggio RE, Singer RD, Hartaran K, Sneider R. Psychological issues in the care of critically ill respirator patients: Differential perceptions of patient's relatives and staff. Psychol Rep 1982; 51:363–369.
75. Higgins PA. Patient perception of fatigue while undergoing long-term mechanical ventilation: Incidence and associated factors. Heart Lung 1998; 27:177–183.
76. Bergbom-Engberg I, Haljamae H. Assessment of patient's experience of discomforts during respirator therapy. Crit Care Med 1989; 17:1068–1072.
77. McDonald ER. Evaluation of the psychological status of ventilatory-supported patients with ALS/MND. Palliative Med 1996; 10:35–41.
78. Leder SB. Importance of verbal communication for the ventilator-dependent patient. Chest 1990; 98:792–793.

79. Manzano JL, Lubillo S, Henriquez D, et al. Verbal communication of ventilator-dependent patients. Crit Care Med 1993; 21:512–517.
80. Yang KL, Tobin WJ. A prospective study of indexes predicting the outcome of trials of weaning from mechanical ventilation. N Engl J Med 1991; 324:1445–1450.
81. Gal TJ. Effects of endotracheal intubation on normal cough performance. Anesthesiology 1980; 52:324–329.
82. Hess D, Kacmarek RM. Technical aspects of the patient-ventilator interface. In: Tobin MJ, ed. Principles and Practice of Mechanical Ventilation. New York: McGraw-Hill, 1994.
83. Ewart W. Treatment of bronchiectasis and chronic bronchial afflictions by posture and respiratory exercises. Lancet 1901; 2:70–72.
84. Stewart HE. Diathermy in pneumonia. Physiother News Bull 1925; 3(5):7–12.
85. Mackenzie CF, Ciesla N, Imle C, et al. Chest physiotherapy in the intensive care unit. Baltimore, MD: Williams & Wilkins, 1981.
86. Zadai CC. Physical therapy for the acutely ill medical patient. Phys Ther 1981; 61(12):1746–1754.
87. Bergstrom N, Demuth PJ, Braden BJ. A clinical trial of the Braden scale for predicting pressure sore risk. Nurs Clin North Am 1987; 22(2):417.
88. Bergstrom N. Pressure Ulcers. In: Hall JB, Schmidt GA, Wood LDH, eds. Principles of Critical Care. New York: McGraw-Hill, 1992.
89. Souba WW. Nutritional support. N Engl J Med 1997; 336:41–48.
90. Angelillo VA, Bedi S, Durfee D, et al. Effect of low and high carbohydrate feedings in ambulatory patients with chronic pulmonary disease and chronic hypercapnia. Ann Intern Med 1985; 103:883–885.
91. Doekel RC, Zwillich CW, Scoggin CH, et al. Clinical semi-starvation: Depression of hypoxic ventilatory response. N Engl J Med 1979; 295:358–365.
92. Al-Saady NM, Blackmore CM, Bennett ED. High fat, low carbohydrate, enteral feeding lowers PaCO2 and reduces the period of ventilation in artificially ventilated patients. Intensive Care Med 1989; 15:290-295.
93. Kudsk KA, Croce MA, Fabian TC, et al. Enteral versus parenteral feeding: effects on septic morbidity following blunt and penetrating abdominal trauma. Ann Surg 1992; 215:503–513.

10

Management of Long-Term Noninvasive Ventilation

NICHOLAS S. HILL

Brown University School of Medicine
Rhode Island Hospital
Providence, Rhode Island

I. Introduction

Noninvasive ventilation has been used for the long-term therapy of respiratory failure dating back to the polio epidemics of the 1920s and 1930s (1). Negative pressure ventilation was the main ventilatory mode used until the 1960s, when positive pressure techniques gained favor. Although noninvasive positive pressure ventilation (NPPV) was used for long-term ventilation at some centers dating back to the 1960s (2), use of invasive techniques predominated at most centers. During the late 1970s and early 1980s, several reports described the successful long-term application of intermittent nocturnal negative pressure ventilation for patients with restrictive thoracic diseases (3–5), but these techniques were not used at most centers (6).

The rising popularity of noninvasive positive pressure techniques to administer long-term mechanical ventilation awaited the introduction during the mid-1980s of nasal continuous positive airway pressure (CPAP) to treat obstructive sleep apnea (OSA) (7). Investigators learned that nasal masks interfaced with standard portable positive pressure ventilators could be used nocturnally to assist ventilation in patients with chronic respiratory failure due to restrictive thoracic diseases (8–10). Stimulated by the demand to treat OSA, manufacturers developed a variety of commercially available nasal masks that proved to be useful for noninvasive ventilation as well. By virtue of its convenience and efficacy advantages compared with negative pressure ventilation, and its safety compared with invasive ventilation, NPPV rapidly gained acceptance among clinicians and patients alike as the preferred ventilator mode for patients with chronic respiratory failure requiring intermittent ventilatory assistance (11,12). This chapter discusses the general approach to the patient requiring long-term noninvasive ventilation, including patient evaluation, selection, initiation, adaptation, monitoring, and management of complications. Other chapters examine the evidence supporting the use of NPPV for specific causes of respiratory failure, and discuss specific indications and applications.

II. Evaluation of Patients

Patients being considered for noninvasive ventilation should undergo a thorough evaluation to determine that they are appropriate candidates. This should consist of a clinical examination and battery of tests to assess the severity of symptoms, the specific respiratory impairment, and the gas exchange defect.

A. Symptoms of Chronic Respiratory Failure

Patients undergoing consideration for long-term noninvasive ventilation usually present with symptoms of chronic hypoventilation or are recovering from a bout of acute respiratory failure. The typical symptoms are those associated with sleep deprivation: fatigue, hypersomnolence, difficulty concentrating, or nightmares (Table 1). Presumably, these are caused by sleep fragmentation that occurs when gas exchange deteriorates at night. Worsening hypercapnia and hypoxemia are thought to contribute to arousals, disrupting sleep (13). Enuresis may occur if the gas exchange derangement is severe, and hypercarbia also gives rise to the common symptom of morning headache that is ascribed to hypercapnia-induced cerebrovascular dilation and increased intracranial pressure.

Dyspnea is an unreliable symptom of chronic respiratory failure. Patients with severe neuromuscular weakness may be unaware of any symptoms directly attributable to the respiratory system despite severe hypercarbia. This is most likely due to the insidious onset of respiratory failure that allows them to compensate for the increasing respiratory acidosis, and the severe limitation that neuromuscular disease may place on their ability to exercise. On the other hand, some patients have orthopnea that should lead to an evaluation of possible diaphragm or cardiac dysfunction. Clinicians must be aware that when patients with severe respiratory impairment present with fatigue or difficulty sleeping, hypnotics should never be prescribed without a pulmonary evaluation and blood gases, since these symptoms may signal the onset of respiratory failure.

Table 1 Symptoms and Signs in Patients with Chronic Respiratory Failure

Symptoms
CO_2 retention
Morning headaches
Difficulty concentrating
Enuresis
Sleep disturbance
Excessive fatigue
Hypersomnolence
Pulmonary dysfunction
Dyspnea
Signs
Cor pulmonale
↑ Intensity of P_2
RV impulse
Tricuspid regurgitation murmur
Liver enlargement
Pedal edema

B. Signs of Chronic Respiratory Failure

Tachypnea and tachycardia may signal progressive respiratory deterioration, although patients with severe neuromuscular disease sometimes present with severe respiratory failure and only mild tachypnea. The physical examination may also reveal insights into the nature of the respiratory muscle impairment. Reduced excursion and paradoxical motion of the rib cage may be seen in patients with intercostal muscle paralysis. Contrariwise, paradoxical abdominal motion in the supine patient suggests severe diaphragm weakness or paralysis. Evaluation of cough effectiveness is useful in identifying patients at risk of secretion retention by virtue of expiratory muscle weakness or inability to close the glottis.

Progressive hypoventilation leads to worsening alveolar hypoxia, causing hypoxic pulmonary vasoconstriction and structural remodeling. These pathophysiologic responses lead to sustained pulmonary hypertension and cor pulmonale; structural or functional changes in the right ventricle attributable to respiratory disease (see Table 1). The earliest and most sensitive sign of pulmonary hypertension is an increase in the intensity of the pulmonic heart sound (P_2), as determined by a more prominent second heart sound at the left upper sternal border (or pulmonic area) compared with the right (or aortic area) (14). Normally, the second heart sound in the aortic area is more prominent, reflecting the higher pressures in the systemic circulation. With advanced cor pulmonale, a right ventricular (RV) impulse or heave may be palpable at the left sternal border. Other manifestations of cor pulmonale include distension of the jugular veins, pedal edema, hepatomegaly due to passive congestion, and ascites. Most patients develop symptoms associated with hypoventilation before signs of cor pulmonale appear, so these signs are usually indicators of advanced chronic respiratory failure. It is well to keep in mind, however, that severe emphysema with hyperinflation may obscure some of the signs of cor pulmonale (14).

C. Laboratory Evaluation

Patients being considered for noninvasive ventilation should undergo pulmonary function testing, including spirometry, lung volumes, and arterial blood gases on room air (Table 2). Maximal inspiratory and expiratory pressures serve as indexes of respiratory muscular strength that may be of prognostic value (15), but imprecision in the measurements limits the clinical value. For patients with neuromuscular disease, measurement of peak expiratory flow may be a useful indicator of cough effectiveness (16). Noninvasive end-tidal or transcutaneous measurements of gas exchange may be useful for trending or for nocturnal monitoring (17), but these measurements have not been shown to be sufficiently accurate to replace arterial blood gases (18).

In addition to routine studies such as electrocardiogram (ECG) and chest x-ray, other laboratory tests that should be obtained include a hemogram for evidence of polycythemia, blood chemistries to exclude electrolyte or other meta-

Table 2 Laboratory Evaluation of Patients with Chronic Respiratory Failure

Blood tests
Complete blood count
Thyroid function tests
Calcium, magnesium
Pulmonary functions
Spirogram
Lung volumes
Arterial blood gases
Maximal inspiratory and expiratory pressures
Sleep evaluation
? Nocturnal oximetry
? Multichannel recorder
? Full polysomnogram
Special studies
Transdiaphragmatic pressure measurements
Nerve conduction studies

bolic disorders. Hypophosphatemia, hypomagnesemia, and hypothyroidism may all depress respiratory drive and contribute to hypoventilation. When bilateral diaphragm paralysis is suspected, transdiaphragmatic pressure measurements may be useful in confirming the diagnosis.

D. Sleep Evaluation

Patients with chronic hypoventilation syndromes almost invariably hypoventilate more during sleep (13). Depending on the underlying condition, they may have hypoventilation without upper airway obstructions, sleep-disordered breathing with frequent hypopneas, or frank obstructive sleep apnea. Despite the frequency of these sleep abnormalities, the role of routine polysomnography in the evaluation of these patients has not been established. It might be argued that whether an initial polysomnogram shows persisting hypoventilation or frank sleep apnea, the therapeutic approach will be the same; patients with symptomatic daytime hypoventilation will be placed on NPPV regardless. Nonetheless, some investigators believe that full polysomnography should be routine in all patients considered for noninvasive ventilation (19). Polysomnography provides an accurate assessment of sleep-disordered breathing and permits initial titration of ventilator settings so that elimination of hypopneas and apneas can be assured. However, full polysomnography is expensive and not universally available, and even when it is available, scheduling delays are frequent. Ultimately, the need to do a full polysomnogram as part of the initial evaluation will depend on its effect on the outcome of NPPV therapy. If patients initiated on NPPV without an initial full polysomnogram have the same symptomatic, functional, and gas exchange responses as those evaluated with one, then full polysomnography may be deemed unnecessary.

In the absence of a definitive answer to the above debate, it is reasonable to perform some baseline sleep monitoring before initiating NPPV. At the least, home monitoring of pulse oximetry may be useful to serve as a baseline for later comparisons. In addition, the severity and duration of desaturations may serve as rough indicators of the severity of sleep-disordered breathing. Although few insurers will cover home oximetry, some vendors will perform the service at no charge if it is performed as part of the NPPV initiation process. Home multichannel recordings that include not only oximetry but also measures of airflow and chest wall motion are capable of more precisely characterizing sleep-disordered breathing. It should be recalled, however, that these studies may be insensitive and misleading, and should not be used to exclude sleep-disordered breathing abnormalities (20).

E. Optimization of Therapy

In addition to defining the patient's physiologic deficiencies, the initial evaluation should also identify reversible factors that are then optimally treated before NPPV is initiated. For example, airway obstruction should be minimized, fluid overload corrected, and hypothyroidism adequately treated. Often, the precipitating factor for a bout of worsened respiratory failure is an upper respiratory infection. This may increase airway secretions and airway resistance in patients with severe underlying airway obstruction or cough impairment. These infectious exacerbations should be treated aggressively with antibiotics, steroids, bronchodilators, and cough-enhancing techniques as indicated. Some of these patients may be treated with noninvasive ventilation during the acute exacerbation to avert the need for invasive ventilation (21). However, long-term noninvasive ventilation should be reserved for those patients whose reversible contributing factors have been treated and who remain candidates as determined by selection guidelines as discussed below.

III. Patient Selection

Guidelines for selection of patients to receive NPPV are discussed in detail elsewhere. Please refer to Chapters 6 and 7 dealing with restrictive thoracic and obstructive disorders for specific selection guidelines. This section discusses general considerations for selecting patients with the highest likelihood of success. A number of patient factors are important for optimizing rates of success (Table 3). Patients should be symptomatic; most clinicians find that unless motivated by the desire for symptom relief, patients tend to comply poorly. For this reason, prophylactic use of NPPV in patients with progressive neuromuscular diseases who are asymptomatic is unlikely to succeed, as was suggested in a controlled

Table 3 Factors to Consider in Optimizing Success of Long-Term Noninvasive Ventilation

Patient characteristics
Selected using appropriate guidelines
Motivated
Capable of comprehending the therapy
Adequate family (caregiver) support
Adequate financial resources
Mask selection
Patient desires; nasal mask usually preferred
Mask type; ? mini-mask or softseal
Optimal fit; use fitting gauge
Ventilator selection
Need for alarms, monitoring
Need for high inflation pressures

trial (22). Patients should also be motivated, cooperative, and able to comprehend the purpose and implementation of the therapy.

Success rates also depend on patient physical characteristics. For example, success rates are lower in morbidly obese patients (23) because of the increased impedance of the respiratory system. Occasionally, however, these patients may succeed with volume-limited ventilators that are able to generate high peak inspiratory pressure (up to 35 to 40 cm H_2O) when pressure-limited ventilators fail. Patients should also have adequate upper airway function. Some aspiration and difficulty with hypersecretion are tolerable if the cough mechanism is intact, but severe swallowing impairment combined with a severely weakened cough is a lethal combination that responds poorly to noninvasive ventilation. If patients with these defects value maximal prolongation of life, ventilation via a tracheostomy is preferred. Finally, anatomic abnormalities, including severe deviation of the nasal septum that interferes with nasal ventilation or facial abnormalities that interfere with mask fitting, may render futile the application of noninvasive ventilation. Some investigators have observed that intact dentition is important in fitting masks to minimize air leaking through the mouth (24).

Other important considerations include the availability of social supports. Noninvasive ventilation is much easier to implement in the home than invasive ventilation (25). However, patients with severe neuromuscular impairment may still require a high level of assistance in the home for monitoring and applying and removing the ventilator. The availability of family members and others caregivers for providing this assistance should be established before long-term NPPV is begun. Likewise, financial resources should be adequate. NPPV is much less costly than invasive ventilation (26), but coverage by insurers should be ascertained in advance.

Guidelines for the selection of patients to receive long-term noninvasive ventilation after hospitalization for a bout of acute respiratory failure have not been established. However, a substantial number of patients who receive long-term noninvasive ventilation start in this manner. Commonly used selection criteria include a severe underlying ventilatory defect, persisting respiratory distress, tachypnea during spontaneous breathing, sustained or increasing hypercarbia, and a history of repeated bouts of respiratory failure requiring hospitalization. Application of these criteria to patients with COPD is particularly difficult, however, considering the lack of evidence to support this approach. The decision in these patients is often arbitrary, depending on the beliefs of the treating practitioner and patient preferences.

IV. Initiation of Noninvasive Ventilation

After the evaluation is completed and an appropriate candidate is selected, noninvasive ventilation can be initiated. Initiation necessitates a number of choices, including a location for initiation, selection of an appropriate mask (or interface) and ventilator, and optimal adjustment of ventilator settings. The following sections discuss each of these choices, based on scientific evidence where possible, pointing out areas of controversy, and relying on personal experience and opinion where necessary.

A. Location

Noninvasive ventilation for long-term applications should be initiated in a quiet, relaxed setting. Of course, inpatient initiation is obligatory for patients who begin noninvasive ventilation during a bout of acute respiratory failure. Even for patients who are otherwise medically stable, however, a brief hospitalization is sometimes used to initiate noninvasive ventilation (17,27). This permits closer observation and monitoring over a period of days, so that mask and ventilator adjustments can be made promptly and frequently. However, hospitalization is expensive, has not been demonstrated to increase patient compliance rates, and may be impractical because of constraints on hospital bed usage in some countries such as the United States.

Alternatively, noninvasive ventilation may be initiated in a sleep laboratory. This can be done either during a daytime nap study or as part of a "split" nocturnal study, in which the first half is diagnostic, and the second used for initiation and titration of noninvasive ventilation. This type of initiation is preferred by some clinicians (19) because it affords an accurate assessment of sleep-disordered breathing and rapid optimization of ventilator settings. Some consider it desirable to optimize ventilator settings during sleep, when respiratory control and upper airway resistance differ from the awake state (13,28). On the other hand, use of a sleep laboratory may not be practical if none is available or long delays are necessitated by crowded sleep laboratory schedules. Further, patients with severe neuromuscular disease often have special needs that are poorly met in many sleep laboratories, and unless a caregiver can stay in the sleep laboratory with the patient, the experience may be unpleasant.

Other location options include the physician's office or the patient's home. If noninvasive ventilation is initiated in the physician's office, the home respiratory vendor should be contacted to provide equipment and a therapist for the office visit. The therapist assists in selecting and fitting the interface and adjusting the ventilator, while the physician makes certain that these are optimized and educates and motivates the patient. For initiation in the patient's home, a home respiratory vendor delivers equipment to the patient's home and a respiratory therapist provides education and training in noninvasive ventilation techniques. Because skill and experience with these techniques vary considerably among different home respiratory therapy companies and their therapists, home initiation is discouraged unless the therapist is highly skilled in the initiation of noninvasive ventilation.

B. Selection of an Interface

The interface (or mask) serves as the contact between the patient and the ventilator, serving as a conduit for pressurized gas to enter the patient's upper airway. Selection of a properly fit and comfortable interface is crucial to the success of noninvasive ventilation, and this point cannot be overemphasized. In order to achieve this, the clinician must have familiarity with the various types of interfaces available and an appreciation for their relative advantages and disadvantages (29). Interfaces commonly used for long-term noninvasive ventilation include nasal masks, oronasal masks, and mouthpieces, and these are considered separately below.

Nasal Masks

Because they leave the mouth free for speech and eating, nasal masks are the interfaces most commonly chosen for long-term applications of noninvasive ventilation. Partly because of the large demand for nasal interfaces created for therapy of obstructive sleep apnea, many sizes and varieties are commercially available. They consist of several different types, including standard nasal masks, nasal "pillows" or "seals," mini-masks, and custom-made masks.

Standard nasal masks are dome-shaped, clear plastic appliances, usually with triangular bases made of soft silicon or other rubber flanges that are applied to the skin to form an air seal (Fig. 1, top). They come in a wide variety of sizes and shapes, and most manufacturers supply "fitting gauges" to permit rapid sizing (Fig. 1, bottom). Consisting of plastic sheets with stamped contours corresponding to the various mask sizes, use of these gauges is encouraged. Commonly, inexperienced practitioners select masks that are too large, necessitating excessive mask pressure on the skin to achieve an adequate air seal. A mask that just clears the perimeter of the nose is usually the best fit, and fitting gauges facilitate this determination. In an effort to enhance comfort and minimize pressure on sensitive areas of the skin, some masks come with "forehead spacers," foam rubber cushions that are used to minimize pressure on the bridge of the nose where redness or frank ulceration is apt to occur. Others come with thin cellophane-like flanges that permit air sealing with minimal pressure on the skin. Standard nasal masks are attached to the ventilator tubing via a swivel device that permits position changes, and most have several nipples for attachments to oxygen tubing or manometers.

Nasal "pillows" or "seals" are used as alternatives to standard nasal masks (Fig. 2). They consist of soft cone-shaped rubber pledgets that are inserted into each nostril and connected to the ventilator via a plastic tubing assembly. They leave the nasal bridge free, and sometimes permit use of eyeglasses. They are used by patients who develop pressure sores on the bridge of the nose or

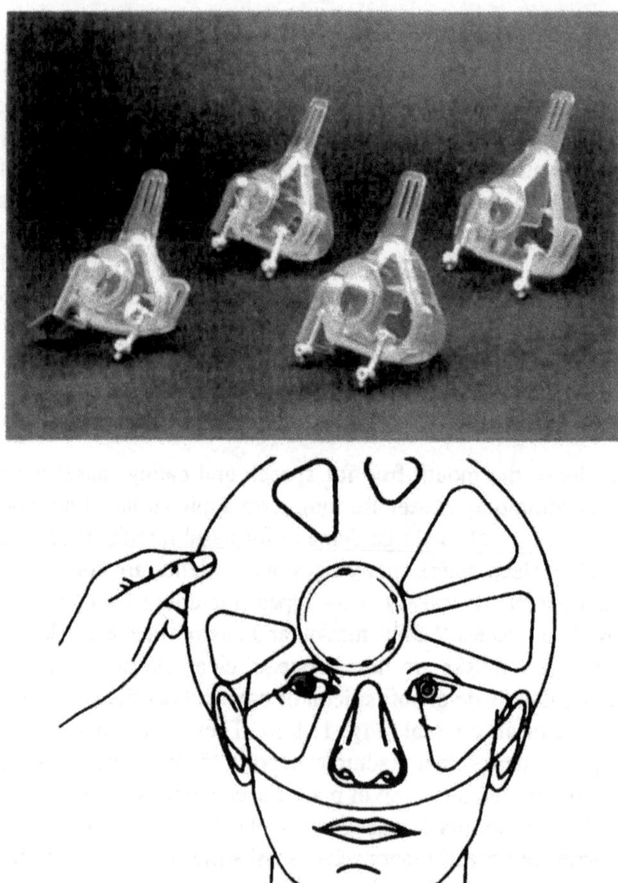

Figure 1 (Top) Standard nasal masks (Respironics, Inc., Pittsburgh, PA) are shown in a variety of sizes and shapes. (Bottom) A fitting gauge is used to select the appropriately sized nasal mask.

become claustrophobic during use of standard nasal masks, and some patients alternate use of one mask type with another.

Recent efforts have been directed at reducing the bulk of nasal masks and creating softer flanges for contact with the skin. Mini-masks, as the name implies, attempt to minimize mask size and contact with the face. One type uses a soft rubber membrane to cover the area over the nares, and is strapped with only two points of attachment. This mask is well tolerated by claustrophobic patients, but its attachment is less stable than with larger standard nasal masks, and air leakage

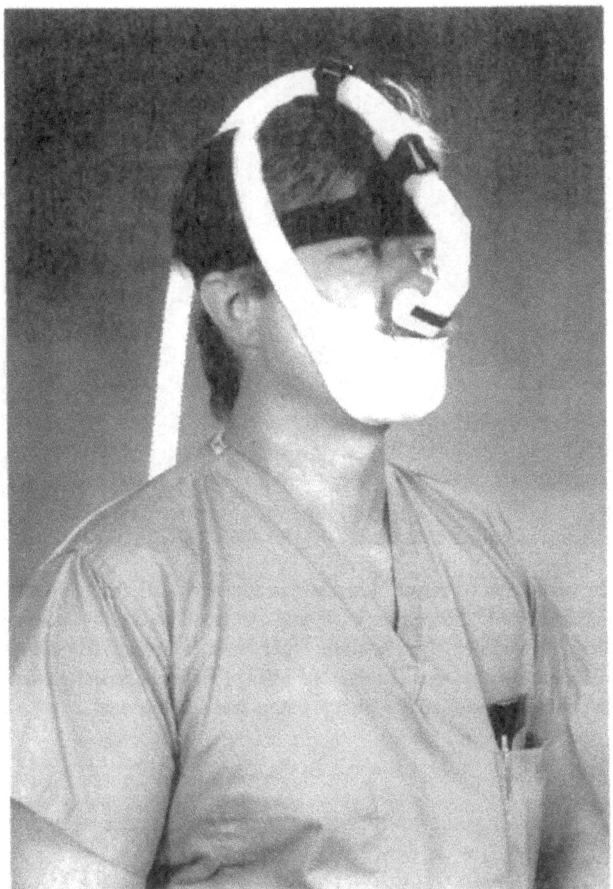

Figure 2 Nasal "pillows" (Mallinkrodt, Lenexa, KS) are shown with a chin strap that helps to reduce air leaking. (From Ref. 29.)

around the mask may be problematic during sleep. Other recently introduced masks that appear to enhance patient comfort include "gel masks" that use gel seals to reduce pressure on the skin, and more compact masks that use very soft silicone seals (Fig. 3).

Kits for custom-made masks are commercially available but not often used, at least in the United States, because of the wide variety of pre-formed masks available. These customizing kits consist of malleable rubber or plastic that is shaped to the patient's anatomy and hardened using a chemical substance or heating and cooling. These masks can be molded to fit any facial contour and

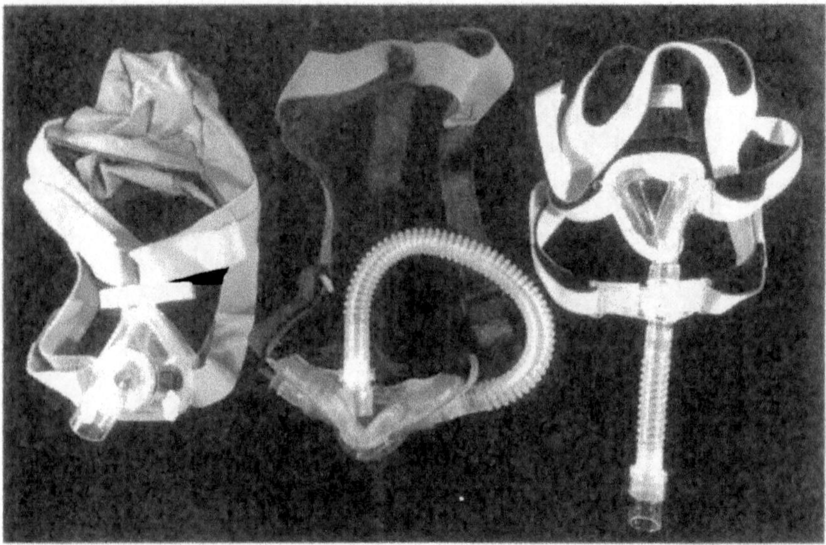

Figure 3 An assortment of newer masks and headgear. (Left) The Goldseal™ (Respironics, Inc., Pittsburgh, PA) incorporates a gel seal and is attached to a four-point Softcap™ headgear assembly. (Middle) The Phantom™ gel mask (Sleepnet, Manchester, NH) utilizes a two-point headgear system. (Right) The Mirage™ nasal mask (Resmed, San Diego, CA) utilizes a compact design and a highly compliant silicone seal.

are durable, but they may be time consuming to fit, expensive, and they require some skill for application. A few centers offer customized masks made on site by individuals with special skills and interests (29). However, considering the plethora of nasal masks commercially available, such customized masks are not often needed.

Oronasal Masks

Oronasal masks consist of clear plastic, dome-shaped appliances that are placed over the nose and mouth, similar in appearance to, but somewhat larger than, a standard nasal mask (Fig. 4). Traditionally, they have had air-filled cuffs to create an air seal, but more recently, foam-filled cuffs or soft silicone flanges similar to those used with nasal masks have gained in popularity. These masks are used less often in the long-term than in the acute setting because they cover the mouth and interfere with speech and eating. They may also intensify feelings of claustrophobia. In addition, they may interfere with coughing and airway clearance in patients who are prone to excessive airway secretions or vomiting. Further, as-

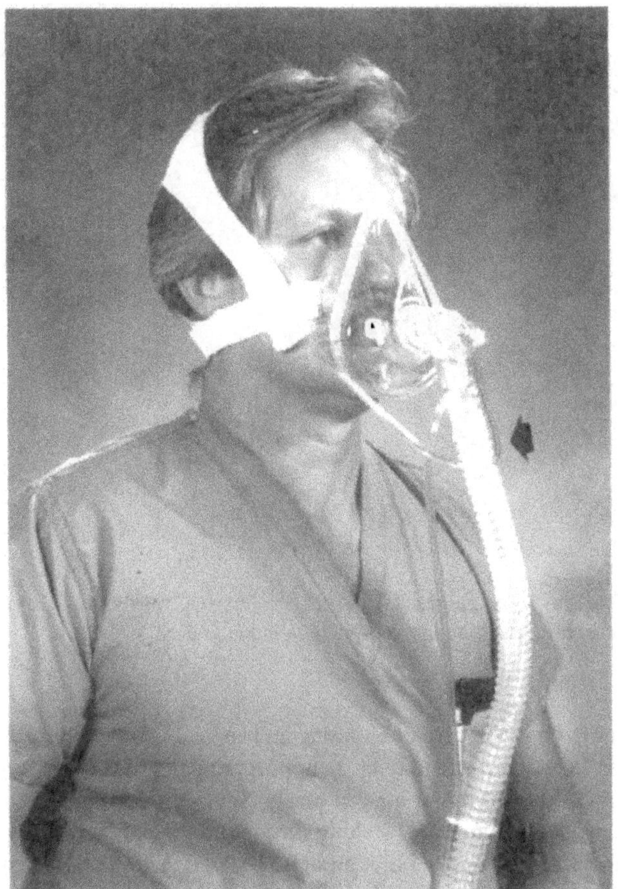

Figure 4 Spectrum™ oronasal mask (Respironics, Inc., Pittsburgh, PA) specifically designed for noninvasive ventilation. It incorporates an "anti-asphyxia" valve that prevents rebreathing in the event of machine failure, and a rapid release strap (arrow) to be used in the event of vomiting.

phyxiation due to rebreathing may be a concern in the event of ventilator failure in a quadriplegic patient using an oronasal mask.

On the other hand, oronasal masks are being used increasingly for patients with excessive air leaking through the mouth during use of nasal masks. Also, advances in nasal mask design are being applied to oronasal masks, so recently introduced versions have soft, comfortable silicone flanges (Fig. 5). In addition, oronasal masks designed specifically for noninvasive applications include quick

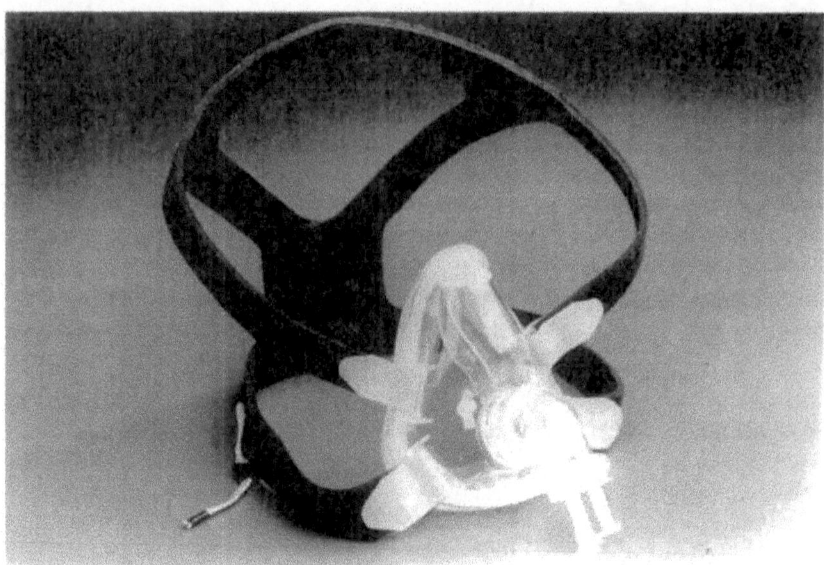

Figure 5 Mirage™ oronasal mask (Resmed, San Diego, CA) with headgear incorporates low dead space design and highly compliant silicone seal.

release straps to be use in case of vomiting and special valves to prevent rebreathing. Thus, an oronasal mask may be an appropriate choice for long-term NPPV, and the choice between it and a nasal mask should be determined by considerations such as the amount of air leaking through the mouth and patient comfort. Concerns about dead space ventilation have been raised with regard to oronasal masks, and some manufacturers have inserted foam rubber on the insides of masks to minimize this potential problem. However, data are unavailable to determine how much dead space ventilation actually occurs.

A larger version of the oronasal mask has been described and may help when large uncontrollable air leaks occur during use of other masks (30). Similar in appearance to a hockey goalie's mask, the "total" face mask seals around the perimeter of the face, thus minimizing air leakage. Perhaps because it is clear and does not affix directly over the nose or mouth, it is well tolerated even by patients with claustrophobia.

Mouthpieces

Dating back to the 1960s, mouthpieces have been used at certain rehabilitation centers to provide long-term noninvasive ventilation to patients with neuromuscular disease (2,31). Mouthpieces may be inserted through lip seals that are strapped in place or may be custom-fashioned by an orthodontist so that oral retention is possible without straps (Fig. 6). This latter manner of fixation is preferred in tetraplegic patients who can then expectorate the devices when they wish to remove the mask. Mouthpieces may also be suspended from a gooseneck clamp attached to a wheelchair for daytime use in patients with severe neuromuscular impairment. Use of mouthpiece ventilation has been reported to be highly effective, even for patients who have little or no vital capacity (31). Such patients may receive assisted ventilation around the clock using this method, or may use a nasal interface for sleep at night and switch back to mouthpiece ventilation during the daytime.

Initially, patients may complain of increased salivation and gagging when using mouthpieces, but these symptoms usually subside with continued use. Patients have been supported by mouthpiece ventilation for periods ranging up to decades, with dental deformity as the only significant adverse outcome reported (31). In occasional patients, efficacy may be limited by air leaking through the nose that may be controlled by inserting cotton plugs into the nose.

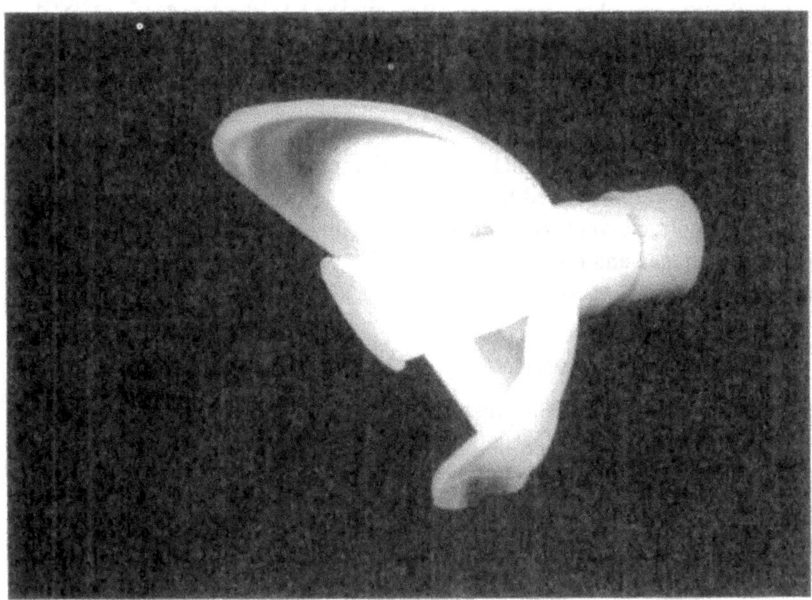

Figure 6 Lipseal (Mallinkrodt) with mouthpiece that is inserted between the teeth and strapped over lips to achieve air seal.

Headgear (or Straps)

The term "headgear" refers to the straps used to keep the interface in place. Individual masks are designed to work with particular strapping systems, but numerous variations are possible (Fig. 3). Headgear design is extremely important in the application of noninvasive ventilation, because comfort, safety, and efficacy depend partly on it. In general, the stability of the mask on the face is greater when more points of attachment are used, and the greater the stability, the less air leaking between the skin and mask. Accordingly, masks have been designed with up to five different attachment points. However, more points of attachment complicate the strap system, increasing the likelihood of entanglement or error and reducing comfort due to the bulk of the straps required. Thus, most systems use three or four points of attachment.

Soft straps that are durable and wide enough to minimize abrasion of the skin on the neck or ears are desirable, as are designs that avoid slipping of straps on the back of the head. In this regard, straps that are sewn into soft caps have achieved popularity (Fig. 3). Velcro is used with almost all straps as a fastener because it offers almost limitless options for adjusting strap tension. Some mask models also use clips for rapid fastening or detachment, once strap tension has been optimized. In an effort to stabilize the mandible and minimize air leakage through the mouth, chin straps are often attached to the headgear via Velcro fasteners (Fig. 2), but these are optional accessories.

C. Selection of a Ventilator

The original reports of nocturnal nasal ventilation used portable volume-limited ventilators that were designed for use with tracheostomies. More recently, pressure-limited portable ventilators have gained popularity. The following sections discuss advantages and disadvantages of these ventilator types, as well as other noninvasive options when NPPV fails.

Positive Pressure Ventilators

Pressure-Limited Portable Ventilators

These were created by the addition of a valve in blower devices that were originally designed to deliver nasal CPAP (32) (Fig. 7). The additional valve permitted delivery of higher inspiratory and lower expiratory positive airway pressure. This ability to provide two levels of airway pressure has given rise to the term "bilevel" ventilators for this group, although, in essence, most deliver typical pressure support and/or pressure control modes. Use of these ventilators has achieved wide popularity for long-term noninvasive ventilation, particularly for patients using nasal ventilation just at night. They are highly portable, weighing only 4 to 8 kg, and are relatively inexpensive. They generate high peak inspiratory flow

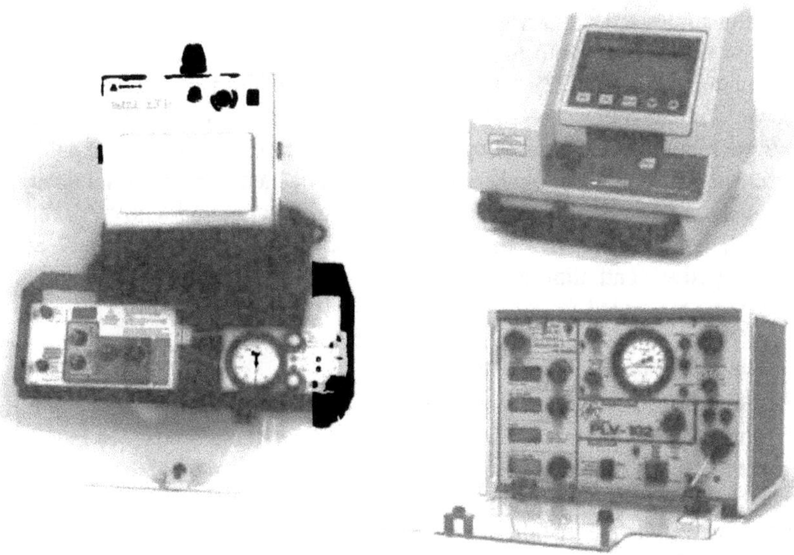

Figure 7 Examples of portable ventilators used for long-term noninvasive ventilation. (Left) BiPAP™ (Respironics, Inc., Pittsburgh, PA) is a prototype "bilevel" ventilator. (Top right) The 335 "bilevel" ventilator (Mallinkrodt, Lenexa, KS) incorporates digital screen and adjustable inspiratory and expiratory triggers. (Bottom right) The PLV-102 portable volume-limited ventilator (Respironics).

rates (120 to 180 L/min) that enable them to compensate quite effectively for air leaks. In addition, they are simple to operate with airflow patterns that are usually sensed as comfortable by patients. Their paucity of alarms may be advantageous in patients requiring only nocturnal ventilation because of fewer interruptions in patient or caregiver sleep. They also lack built-in battery backup systems, although external batteries may be added that can power the ventilators for up to 8 hr.

These features have created a large demand for these devices, and many different types are now commercially available. However, it should be borne in mind that some of the above-listed advantages are disadvantages in certain situations. The lack of alarms or an internal battery may be problematic in patients who are dependent on continuous mechanical ventilation, or if the devices are used during invasive ventilation. In addition, because these devices use a single tube for inhalation and exhalation, removal of carbon dioxide (CO_2) from the circuit depends on flow of gas through fixed exhalation valves. With the use of certain exhalation valves at low expiratory pressures, insufficient air may escape through the valve so that substantial rebreathing may occur. This can interfere with ventilator efficiency (33) but is usually not a problem during nasal ventilation in the chronic setting because much of the CO_2 is exhausted via air leaks through the mouth (34). Rebreathing can be life threatening, however, should it occur during ventilator failure when the device is attached to an oronasal device or endotracheal tube. For this reason, oronasal masks to be used with "bilevel" ventilators have incorporated "anti-asphyxia" valves, and use of "bilevel" devices for invasive ventilation is discouraged unless appropriate monitoring and alarm systems are added.

Volume-Limited Portable Ventilators

Designed for the delivery of long-term invasive mechanical ventilation, volume-limited portable ventilators have been available for several decades (see Fig. 7). They were the first ventilators used to deliver nocturnal nasal ventilation (8–10). However, because of greater weight and expense in comparison with "bilevel" ventilators as well as the inability to automatically compensate for air leaks and the inclusion of unnecessary alarm systems, they are less often used for this indication presently. Nonetheless, they are effective at delivering noninvasive ventilation, as long as delivered tidal volume is set slightly above that generally used for invasive ventilation to compensate for the inevitable air leaks (10 to 15 ml/kg). Considering that they contain a backup battery and more sophisticated alarms than most of the pressure-limited portable ventilators, some clinicians prefer them for use in patients with severe ventilatory impairment who require continuous noninvasive ventilation (35).

Because they are capable of delivering substantially higher inspiratory pressures than the pressure-limited ventilators, the volume-limited portable ventilators may be preferred in certain settings. They may be used successfully for patients with requirements for high inspiratory pressure, such as those with morbid obesity or severe restriction, when the "bilevel" ventilators are incapable of generating sufficient pressure. In addition, they can be used to "stack" breaths, with the patient retaining air for several consecutive breaths to achieve a large tidal volume and enhance cough efficacy (35). These ventilators offer volume control, assist/control, and synchronized intermittent mandatory ventilation (SIMV) modes, but for noninvasive ventilation, the assist/control mode is preferred. Use of the SIMV mode has been discouraged because of high resistance in some of the demand valves (36). Also, because there are separate inspiratory and expiratory circuits provided with these ventilators, rebreathing is not a problem.

Table 4 Features of Portable Pressure- Versus Volume-Limited Ventilators

	Pressure	Volume
Peak inspiratory pressure	20–35 cm H_2O	60–70 cm H_2O
Leak compensation	Excellent	Poor
Alarms	Low/high pressure disconnect	Multiple
Monitoring	Variable, estimated tidal volume	Greater, accurate tidal volume
Weight (kg)	4–8	12–16
Patient comfort	Greater	Less
Patient activated cycling[a]	Yes	No
Internal battery	No	Yes
Cost	Less	More

[a]Mechanism for cycling from inspiration to expiration.

Table 4 lists differences between the two types of ventilators, which have been compared in a number of studies in both acute and chronic settings. Vitacca et al. (37) and Girault et al. (38) both found that pressure-limited and volume-controlled ventilation performed similarly in avoiding intubation among COPD patients with acute exacerbations. In addition, although the latter group found that volume-controlled ventilation reduced work of breathing more effectively, both groups of investigators found that patient "compliance" or comfort with the therapy was better with pressure support ventilation. In other comparison studies, pressure-limited ventilation and volume-limited ventilation were found to be equally effective in supporting gas exchange after a few hours during the daytime in COPD patients (39), and overnight in a variety of patients with chronic respiratory failure (40).

More recently, Schonhofer et al. (41) treated 30 patients with chronic respiratory failure with volume-limited ventilation for a month, then switched them to pressure-limited ventilation. Only two patients failed with volume-limited ventilation and these subsequently succeeded with pressure-limited ventilation. Of the remaining 28 patients who were switched from volume- to pressure-limited ventilation, 10 failed (5 within the first week) and were returned to volume-limited ventilation. The authors inferred that either volume- or pressure-limited modes can effectively deliver NPPV and acknowledged that the uncontrolled design of their study prevented them from drawing conclusions about the relative effectiveness of the two modes. In summary, although findings vary among studies, it is fair to conclude that either pressure- or volume-limited modes can be used to successfully assist ventilation in the majority of patients requiring long-term ventilation. Therefore, the choice between them should be determined by considerations such as patient comfort or the perceived need for more sophisticated alarms or high inspiratory pressures.

Other Noninvasive Ventilators

For the past dozen years or so, NPPV has been the preferred method for providing noninvasive ventilation. Prior to that time, various ventilators were used to provide noninvasive ventilation, commonly referred to as ''body'' ventilators because they acted by applying pressure to various body surfaces. These ventilators are no longer in common use in most parts of the world, but because they may still be effective for patients who fail NPPV, they are described briefly here.

Negative Pressure Ventilators

Negative pressure ventilators were among the earliest mechanical ventilators described, dating back to the 1840s (42). They work by intermittently applying subatmospheric pressure to the surfaces of the thorax and abdomen, augmenting chest expansion and downward motion of the diaphragm, and thereby assisting inhalation. Exhalation is achieved by passive recoil, although some negative pressure ventilators are able to apply a positive pressure over the thorax and abdomen in an attempt to assist expiration. Negative pressure ventilators consist of three basic types (Fig. 8): (1) tank ventilators, which are rigid cylinders or chambers that encompass the entire body except the head, which protrudes through a neck seal; (2) ''poncho,'' ''wrap,'' or ''jacket'' ventilators, which consist of an impervious garment into which a rigid chestpiece is inserted and positioned over the thorax and abdomen to prevent the garment from collapsing on the skin during generation of negative pressure within; and (3) ''shell'' or cuirass ventilators, which use a rigid dome positioned over the anterior thorax and abdomen. Both the shell and wrap (and some tank) ventilators must be connected to an external negative pressure pump for generation of intermittent subatmospheric pressure.

The efficiency of negative pressure ventilators, i.e., the tidal volume generated for a given negative pressure, depends on the surface area of the thorax and abdomen over which the negative pressure is applied. Hence, the tank ventilator is most efficient and the cuirass the least. This efficiency makes tank ventilators suitable for therapy of acute respiratory failure (43,44), but the wrap and cuirass

Figure 8 Negative pressure ventilators include the tank-type ''iron lung'' (top), which was used widely during the polio epidemics, and the ''wrap'' (middle) and cuirass (bottom) ventilators. The curved perforated plastic device shown with the wrap is positioned over the chest to permit generation of negative pressure over the chest and abdomen. Both the wrap and cuirass ventilators are shown attached to negative pressure pumps.

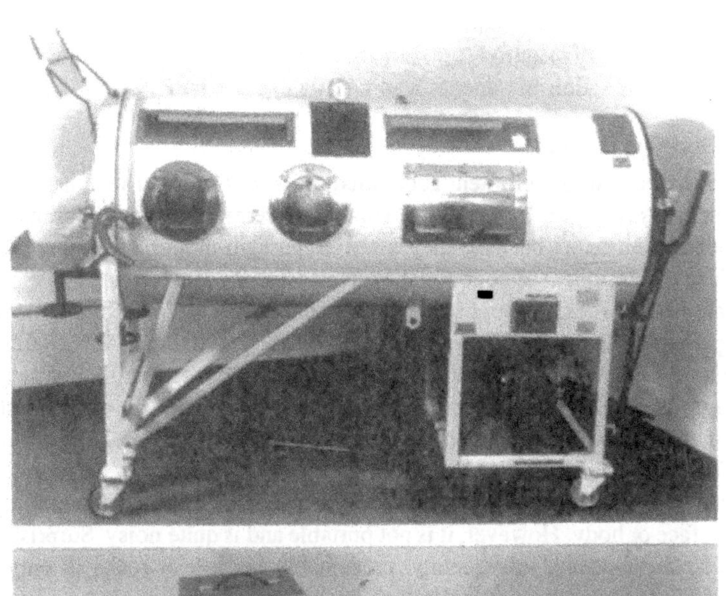

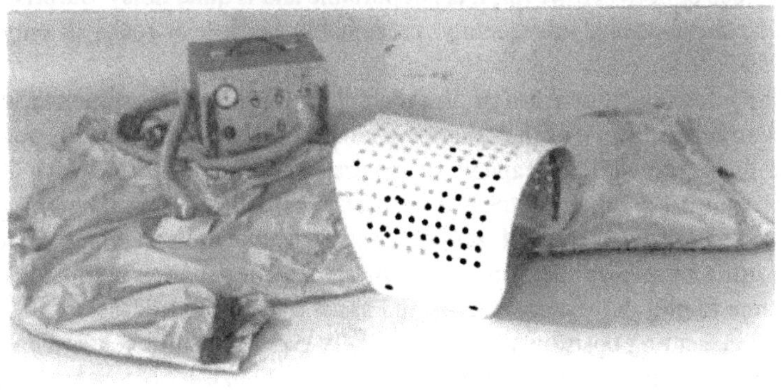

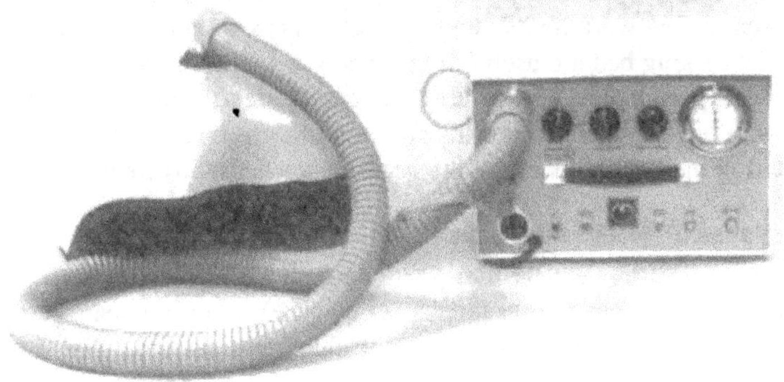

ventilators should be reserved for long-term applications. Currently, the main indication for use of negative pressure ventilation is as a second-line form of noninvasive ventilation in patients who cannot tolerate NPPV.

Other "Body" Ventilators

The rocking bed and intermittent abdominal pressure respirator (or pneumobelt) are other types of "body" ventilators, sometimes referred to as "abdominal displacement" ventilators because they assist diaphragm motion by taking advantage of the displacement of abdominal contents (Fig. 9). The rocking bed consists of a mattress that rocks through an arc of approximately 40° on a fulcrum placed at the patient's hip level. When the head is down, gravitational force pulls the abdominal viscera cephalad, assisting exhalation. When the feet rock down, the diaphragm is pulled caudad, assisting inhalation. By rocking in such a fashion at a rate of 12 to 20/min, the device effects diaphragm motion, assisting ventilation. The chief advantages of the rocking bed are simplicity of operation and enhanced patient comfort by eliminating the need for any attachments to the patient's face or body. However, it is not portable and is quite noisy. Surprisingly, motion sickness occurs infrequently, presumably because it rocks in only one plane.

The pneumobelt consists of an inflatable rubber bladder contained within a corset strapped firmly to the anterior abdomen. When attached to a portable positive pressure ventilator capable of generating pressures up to 60 or 70 cm H_2O, intermittent inflations of the bladder assist ventilation. These inflations force the abdominal viscera cephalad, actively assisting exhalation. As long as the patient is sitting in at least a 30° upright position, bladder deflation permits gravitational force to pull the viscera caudad and assist inhalation. Because of the need to remain in a sitting position, patients generally use the pneumobelt as a daytime aid. Nonetheless, patients occasionally have been able to use pneumobelts round-the-clock, once they have adapted to sleeping in a semi-upright position (45).

Because they work mainly by assisting diaphragm motion, both the pneumobelt and rocking bed are useful in patients with bilateral diaphragm paralysis (46,47). The pneumobelt is also used in some patients with high spinal cord lesions who have lost diaphragm function and desire freedom of the face and hands during the daytime without the need for tracheostomy ventilation (48).

Disadvantages of "Body" Ventilators

These ventilators were widely used for long-term ventilatory assistance in the past, but they have been largely supplanted by NPPV in recent years because of a number of disadvantages. First, they are much less portable. The iron lung weighs approximately 300 kg and is 3 m long, and even the more portable fiberglass tank ventilators weigh 30 to 50 kg. Also, fiberglass tank, wrap, and cuirass ventilators and pneumobelts all require pressure pumps that weigh 10 to 20 kg.

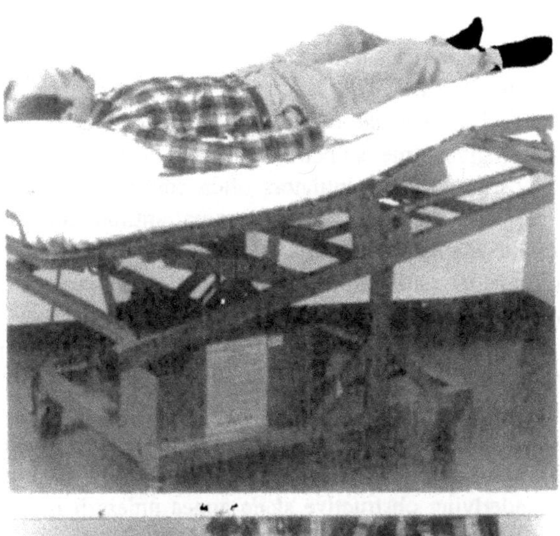

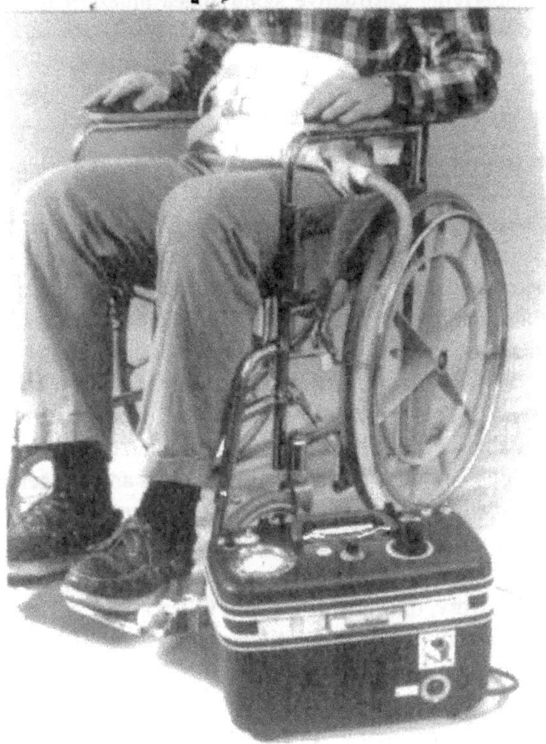

Figure 9 (Top) Rocking bed shown in head-down position. (Bottom) Pneumobelt on subject sitting in wheelchair is shown attached via tubing to positive pressure portable ventilator in foreground.

Second, with the exception of the rocking bed, application of body ventilators is less convenient than NPPV. The patient must be positioned carefully within a device or garment with the need for proper placement of straps or seals, consuming considerable caregiver time, sometimes from multiple caregivers. Third, by restricting body position, these ventilators often contribute to musculoskeletal and back pain, requiring therapy with nonsteroidal antiinflammatory drugs and impeding successful adaptation. Fourth, successful use of "body" ventilators depends on body habitus; patients with severe chest wall deformities or marked obesity are usually not successfully ventilated. Finally, all "body" ventilators and negative pressure ventilators in particular are prone to inducing or at least aggravating obstructive sleep apneas. This phenomenon occurs in normals (49) and may lead to repeated severe oxygen desaturations in the majority of users with neuromuscular diseases such as postpolio syndrome or Duchenne muscular dystrophy (50,51). This precludes use of negative pressure ventilation in patients with significant underlying obstructive sleep apnea unless it is combined with nasal CPAP.

D. Selection of Ventilator Settings

In the absence of controlled studies to guide the selection of settings for noninvasive ventilation, the process is largely an empirical one. The clinician must select initial settings based on the type of ventilator used, the nature of the underlying respiratory impairment, prior experience, patient response to ventilation, and the goals that are prioritized. For example, the clinician must decide on whether to use pressure- or volume-limited ventilation, and whether a backup rate is necessary or not. Most practitioners advise use of a backup rate for patients with neuromuscular disease, but the need for a backup rate has not been established for patients with chest wall deformity or COPD. Further, specific pressure or volume settings depend partly on whether the patient is initiated in a sleep laboratory, where elimination of sleep-disordered breathing events and oxygen desaturations may be prioritized, or in the physician's office or patient's home, where patient comfort is usually prioritized. Typical initial and long-term settings are listed in Table 5.

In a sleep laboratory, once the patient has fallen asleep, inspiratory pressure or tidal volume is gradually increased until hypopneas and REM-associated oxygen desaturations are abolished. If apneas persist, expiratory pressure can then be increased until these are eliminated. Typical inspiratory pressures are 10 to 16 cm H_2O (or tidal volumes 10 to 15 ml/kg) and expiratory pressure are 4 to 8 cm H_2O. In the office or home, ventilation is begun in awake patients and pressures or volumes are titrated mainly to patient comfort. Increases in inspiratory pressure or volume are limited by the patient's tolerance for side effects such as nasal pressure or burning and sinus or ear pain. Typically, when patient

Table 5 Typical Initial and Long-Term Settings for NPPV

	Initial	Long-term
Inspiratory pressure (cm H_2O)	8–10	12–20
Tidal volume (mL/kg)	8–12	10–20
Expiratory pressure	3–4	3–4
If auto-PEEP or obstructive apneas	4–8	5–12
Backup rate/min (if used)	12–20	12–20
Inspiratory duration (sec)[a]	1–2.5	1–2.5
Rise time (sec)[a]	0.3–0.5	0.1–0.5
I/E ratio[a]	0.3–0.5	0.3–0.5

[a]Adjustments not possible on all ventilators.

comfort is prioritized, initial pressures are slightly less than those selected in a sleep laboratory, usually in the 8 to 12 cm H_2O range, and tidal volumes are also slightly lower. Unless the patient is known to have obstructive sleep apnea, the expiratory pressure is usually set at 3 to 4 cm H_2O to assure sufficient expiratory flow to minimize rebreathing (see below).

It is important to recall that the inspiratory inflation pressure (or pressure support) is the difference between the inspiratory and expiratory pressures. Augmentation of tidal volume depends on the magnitude of this difference rather than on the absolute inspiratory pressure. Some clinicians monitor tidal volume when initial settings are being selected, but it should be recognized that this may be misleading. Spontaneously breathing patients sometimes subconsciously alter their breathing pattern during the initial trial, and later, when they relax and have more air leaking during use at home, minute volume may fall. Rather than target a particular minute volume, the initial goal should be to achieve the highest inspiratory pressure that is sensed as tolerable by the patient.

The backup rate, if used, is set slightly below the spontaneous daytime breathing rate to permit patient triggering while awake. If the clinician desires controlled breathing when the patient falls asleep, as is often the case with neuromuscular patients, the rate should be set closer to the spontaneous breathing rate. For patients with COPD or chest wall deformity, on the other hand, the backup rate may be used mainly to prevent apneas or hypoventilation during REM sleep, and a lower rate is often selected. Typical initial rate settings are from 12 to 20/ min.

Some ventilators offer other options for ventilator adjustment, such as adjustable inspiratory triggering and expiratory cycling sensitivities (52). These may be adjusted to enhance patient comfort. Other ventilators offer an adjustable "rise time," the rapidity with which target pressure is reached when pressure-limited ventilation is used. This is related to the inspiratory flow rate and adjustments may aid in achieving patient comfort. For example, dyspneic patients, particularly those with COPD, may prefer a short "rise time" (i.e., 0.1 to 0.2 sec) (53), whereas patients with neuromuscular disease often prefer a longer one (i.e., 0.3 to 0.5 sec). Some ventilators also permit setting of a maximal inspiratory time. This setting should be determined by the backup rate, and should not exceed 50% of the duty cycle. For example, at a rate of 20/min, inspiratory time should not exceed 1.5 sec. Otherwise, the I/E ratio can exceed 1:1 during large leaks, and ventilator efficiency can be reduced by the shortened expiratory time (54).

Oxygenation and Humidification

Oxygen supplementation is usually unnecessary in patients with restrictive thoracic disorders once noninvasive ventilation has successfully lowered $Paco_2$. In patients with underlying parenchymal lung disease, however, the need for continued oxygen supplementation should be determined by periodic daytime measurement of arterial blood gases and monitoring of oximetry during ventilator use. Should oxygen supplementation be deemed necessary, it should be titrated to maintain oxygen saturation above a desired level, such as 90%. Many portable pressure-limited ventilators lack oxygen blenders, so supplementary oxygen is bled directly into the breathing circuit, either by attaching oxygen tubing directly to a nipple on the mask, or to a T-tube attachment inserted into the ventilator circuit. Oxygen liter flow can then be titrated accordingly.

Types of humidifiers include heated or unheated pass-over devices, pass-through devices, and heat and moisture exchangers. With portable pressure-limited ventilators, pass-through humidifiers or heat and moisture exchangers may interfere with air pressure and flow delivery to the interface, so only pass-over humidifiers should be used. Heated pass-over humidifiers are more efficient than unheated ones and are useful when patients complain of nasal dryness or burning. Most patients using long-term NPPV complain of drying of the nasal and oral mucosa at times during ventilator use, particularly during colder months in temperate climates. Control of air leaks may help to alleviate these complaints, but most patients receiving long-term NPPV require some form of humidification. Reimbursement issues should also be considered in that some insurers are reluctant to approve payment for humidifiers unless they are included during initiation.

E. Role of the Clinician

Successful implementation of noninvasive ventilation requires patient motivation and cooperation. The role of an experienced, skilled, and knowledgeable clinician in facilitating this process cannot be underestimated. The skilled clinician engenders the patient's confidence by projecting a relaxed, optimistic attitude, and explaining clearly the overall goals of the therapy as well as the purpose and function of each article of equipment. The clinician gives the patient realistic expectations and warns about potential problems. The patient is also encouraged to express feelings of fear, confusion, or discomfort.

During the initial session, after selecting a mask type and ventilator, the clinician places the mask on the patient's face and assures optimal fit. Having the patient hold the mask in place, if this is possible, may help to bolster the patient's feeling of control. The mask is then connected to the ventilator tubing and the ventilator is turned on. Initially, low inflation pressures (or volumes) are advisable so that the patient can become accustomed to the feeling of airflow from the mask. Coaching with words such as "try to let the ventilator breathe for you" may help the patient coordinate breathing with the ventilator. Pressures (or volumes) are then gradually increased as tolerated by the patient. The ability to augment tidal volume and reduce breathing effort must be balanced against the patient's ability to tolerate the pressure. In the chronic setting, relatively low initial inspiratory pressures, lower than will eventually be needed to ameliorate the respiratory failure (i.e., 8 to 10 cm H_2O), may be advisable to facilitate patient acceptance. Unlike those with acute deteriorations, patients with chronic respiratory failure have time to adapt to noninvasive therapy. Because the aim is to use the therapy long-term, a less aggressive approach that eases the initiation process is likely to yield greater benefits in the long run.

V. Adaptation

Once noninvasive ventilation has been initiated, the patient enters the most important aspect of successful use of noninvasive ventilation: the adaptation phase. Noninvasive ventilation for chronic respiratory failure aims to have the patient sleep with a foreign object strapped over the nose and/or mouth while pressurized air is blown through it. Not surprisingly, most patients encounter difficulty adapting and require frequent attention during the first several weeks. During the initiation visit, patients should be prepared for the adaptation process. They should be told that the process of adaptation may take days, weeks, or even months, and that they should not give up easily. It may be helpful to compare the process to that of learning to play a musical instrument. Patients can appreciate the unfamiliarity of a musical instrument when it is first played, but repeated practice sessions lead to mastery. Likewise, the process of adapting to noninvasive ventilation requires repeated practice sessions before patients become comfortable and are able to sleep through the night.

During the adaptation process, occasional home visits by a skilled respiratory therapist (usually employed by a durable medical equipment vendor) are highly desirable. The vendor should deliver the noninvasive ventilator and other necessary equipment to the home and review, in detail, the operation, application, and maintenance of the equipment. The patient is encouraged to begin using the equipment on the first night and to attempt to fall asleep. If the patient awakens and wishes to remove the mask, he is instructed to do so. Forcing patients to suffer intolerable discomfort while attempting to adapt to noninvasive ventilation is counterproductive. Patients grow to dread use of the device and successful adaptation becomes impossible.

Early on, patients are encouraged to use the ventilator for an hour or two while they are awake during the daytime, to facilitate familiarization. The home respiratory therapist should make several visits during this time to ascertain that the apparatus is being properly used and to make any adjustments or changes necessary to optimize comfort. This includes trying different interfaces or strap systems, and adjusting pressures (or volumes). As noted above, initial pressures are usually relatively low to facilitate adaptation. If the patient complains of ear or sinus pain after the first few sessions, even lower pressures may be necessary temporarily. Usually, after the first week or 10 days, pressures (or volumes) can be gradually increased. As pressures exceed 10 to 12 cm H_2O and hours of use approach 4 to 6/24 hr, patients usually notice improved sleep and energy levels. When this threshold is reached, success becomes a virtual certainty as compliance is reinforced by the symptomatic improvement. Interestingly, although patients are encouraged to use the ventilator during sleep, improvements in gas exchange will occur whether or not ventilator use is nocturnal (27). Thus, patients who are encountering difficulty with nocturnal adaptation should be encouraged to increase hours of daytime use, while reading or watching television.

Communication between the patient, therapist, and physician is crucial during the adaptation process. The physician is appraised of problems as they arise and, in consultation with the therapist, suggests possible solutions based on prior experience. Using this approach in motivated, persistent patients with restrictive thoracic disease who are willing to try a variety of solutions to the problems encountered, adaptation should be successful in the vast majority of appropriate patients. Despite the best efforts, success rates in patients with COPD tend to be lower than in patients with restrictive disease.

VI. Monitoring

Close monitoring is the key to the successful implementation of noninvasive ventilation. The specific parameters monitored follow from the major goals of long-term noninvasive ventilation (Table 6). Monitoring should occur at frequent intervals initially, and then less often as the adaptation progresses. The home respiratory therapist should visit up to several times during the first week or two, and should report problems back to the physician. The physician should see the patient in the office within the first several weeks of initiation, and then as frequently as needed thereafter until adaptation succeeds. Once the major goals have

Table 6 Goals of Long-Term Noninvasive Ventilation

Primary
Alleviate symptoms and signs
Ameliorate gas exchange disturbance, daytime and nocturnal
Secondary
Improve sleep quality
Improve functional status
Improve pulmonary function
Reduce need for hospitalization
Prolong survival

been achieved in stable patients, follow-up need not occur at more frequent intervals than twice or thrice yearly. The following discussions consider aspects of monitoring as they apply to each of the main goals.

A. Alleviation of Symptoms and Signs

Noninvasive ventilation is usually initiated after patients develop symptoms related to hypoventilation and impaired sleep. Hence, monitoring should determine whether symptoms are improved or resolved. As listed in Table 1, these include symptoms attributable to sleep disruption, such as fatigue and daytime hypersomnolence, and to nocturnal CO_2 retention, such as morning headache. Changes in physical findings may also reflect successful use of noninvasive ventilation. Heart rate may drop, and signs of cor pulmonale, including neck vein distention, an increase in the pulmonic component of the second heart sound, liver enlargement, and peripheral edema, may resolve. Simple sleepiness scales, such as the Epworth Sleepiness Scale (55), may be used to monitor responses, as may questionnaires to assess quality of life. The latter are more often used as research tools, however, and do not necessarily add to a simple patient interview by the therapist or physician. When noninvasive ventilation is successful, these symptoms invariably improve, sometimes in dramatic fashion. This improvement also serves as a strong reinforcement for continued use.

In contrast to symptoms attributable to hypoventilation or poor sleep quality, the resolution of dyspnea is not so consistent. As mentioned earlier, patients with severe neuromuscular disease often have no dyspnea, even in the face of severe respiratory failure. Dyspnea is more consistently found in patients with chronic respiratory insufficiency due to chest wall deformity or obstructive lung disease. Unfortunately, institution of noninvasive ventilation may not improve dyspnea in these patients, unless its use is associated with improvements in spontaneous ventilatory capacity.

B. Gas Exchange

Arterial blood gases have long been the gold standard for the assessment of pulmonary gas exchange. Although results will vary from laboratory to laboratory, the standard deviation of $Paco_2$ and Pao_2 measurements has been estimated at ± 3 and $\pm 6\%$, respectively (56). For monitoring purposes in patients using noninvasive ventilation, daytime arterial blood gases are routinely used as the main indicator of improvement in gas exchange. Hypoventilating patients with neuromuscular disease or chest wall deformity invariably register substantial reductions in $Paco_2$ and elevations of Pao_2 when noninvasive ventilation is used successfully. The lack of improvement should trigger additional therapeutic efforts or diagnostic studies to determine the reason for failure (see below).

The ideal target for daytime $Paco_2$ during noninvasive ventilation has not been established, but normalization of daytime $Paco_2$ is neither necessary nor even desirable. In the author's experience, patients experience symptomatic relief and resolution of signs of cor pulmonale even when daytime spontaneous $Paco_2$ cannot be lowered below the mid-50s or even low 60s mm Hg. The patient's ventilatory impairment may make it difficult to lower daytime $Paco_2$ below this level without an increase in inspiratory pressure or a prolongation of the duration of ventilator use that is unacceptable to the patient. In addition, maintenance of a normal $Paco_2$ requires a higher level of alveolar ventilation than an elevated $Paco_2$ and would be potentially more fatiguing to the patient. Thus, the ideal $Paco_2$ level probably differs from one patient to another and in the same patient over time, depending on the severity of the ventilatory impairment and the level of hypercapnia at which symptoms worsen.

Although arterial blood gases provide the most accurate measure of $Paco_2$, they are invasive and require ready access to a blood gas machine, so some clinicians advocate the use of noninvasive measures of gas exchange as a way to monitor responses to noninvasive ventilation (31). Pulse oximetry is adequate to assure a desired level of oxygenation, but even when oxygen saturation is normal, CO_2 retention can be substantial. Unfortunately, noninvasive measures of CO_2 have not proven to be sufficiently accurate to replace blood gases. End-tidal CO_2 measures can be misleading during noninvasive ventilation because of bias flow with some ventilator types and air leaking that may lead to underestimation of the actual CO_2 level. Devices that measure transcutaneous CO_2 tension have been hampered by the need for heated transducers and frequent calibration. In addition, although recent studies suggest that the technology is improving (57), measurements have been imprecise and response times slow (18).

On the other hand, noninvasive measures of gas exchange may be useful for nocturnal monitoring. Continuous nocturnal oximetry has been used to assess responses to nasal CPAP in patients with obstructive sleep apnea, and likewise, it provides an accurate assessment of the adequacy of oxygenation during noninvasive ventilation. Unfortunately, it may not accurately reflect changes in $Paco_2$, particularly during use of supplemental oxygen. Transcutaneous CO_2 monitoring during sleep can be helpful in establishing trends and confirming the adequacy of ventilation over many minutes or hours. Unfortunately, its response time is too slow to detect transient episodes of hypoventilation. Also, patient movements that cause alterations in transducer position may lead to upward or downward drifting in the recorder signal and the need for frequent recalibration. These problems limit the utility of transcutaneous CO_2 recording in busy clinical sleep laboratories, so it has been used largely as a research technique.

C. Sleep Monitoring

Sleep-disordered breathing is an important component of chronic respiratory failure (13), and occasional sleep monitoring for follow-up of noninvasive ventilation has been advocated by most authorities (19,58). However, the specific technique that should be used for sleep monitoring remains a matter of contention. Full facility-based polysomnography remains the gold standard, but as discussed earlier, it is expensive, may be difficult to arrange on short notice, and may be uncomfortable for neuromuscular patients. Simple nocturnal oximetry may suffice as a screening technique to assure adequacy of gas exchange. If abnormalities are detected, then more sophisticated monitoring must be done to identify the cause of the abnormalities. For this purpose, multichannel recorders that monitor nasal airflow, chest wall impedance, the electrocardiogram, and oximetry may be quite useful for home monitoring. These may allow identification of apneic or hypopnic episodes of an obstructive or central nature. However, it must be considered that changes in patient position may alter signal intensity without any change in breathing pattern.

Sleep quality in patients with restrictive thoracic disorders has been shown to deteriorate when noninvasive ventilation is temporarily withdrawn (59). In addition, one of the purported benefits of noninvasive ventilation in patients with severe obstructive lung disease is to lengthen total sleep time (17). The only way to accurately assess effects of noninvasive ventilation on sleep quality and duration is to perform a full polysomnogram, including electroencephalography. However, unless it is demonstrated that such detailed monitoring is necessary to optimize the efficacy of noninvasive ventilation, it is difficult to recommend that full polysomnography be included as part of routine monitoring. From a pragmatic viewpoint, clinicians can probably assume that if symptoms such as fatigue and daytime hypersomnolence resolve with noninvasive ventilation, sleep quality has improved. Furthermore, if nocturnal oximetry or portable multichannel recordings performed in the home show adequate support of gas exchange and amelioration of hypopneas, it is unlikely that findings from full polysomnography will substantially alter the management approach. On the other hand, studies using full polysomnography have demonstrated the occurrence of frequent arousals associated with air leaking through the mouth despite adequate support of gas exchange (60). If techniques are developed that can successfully reduce air leaking and associated arousals, then full polysomnography to assess the frequency of arousals could be useful.

D. Functional Capacity

The main favorable effects of long-term noninvasive ventilation are to improve symptoms and gas exchange; improvements in respiratory or other muscle strength and endurance are not consistently seen. Thus, it is not surprising that improvements in overall functional capacity as determined by treadmill walking time or the 6-min walk distance have been difficult to demonstrate (61–63). These measures are mainly of interest in research studies and need not be done on a routine basis. Furthermore, many of the patients who benefit from long-term noninvasive ventilation have advanced neuromuscular disease and would not be expected to manifest gains on such tests of functional capacity.

E. Pulmonary Function

Pulmonary function should be monitored on a periodic basis. The frequency of monitoring depends on the anticipated rapidity of progression of the underlying respiratory impairment and changes in the patient's clinical state. The spirogram and lung volumes should be measured at baseline, but the latter need not be repeated frequently unless there are concerns about changes in the patient's lung or chest wall compliance. A decline in the vital capacity below 40% of predicted (1 to 1.5 l) has been shown to correlate with CO_2 retention in patients with neuromuscular disease (64), and further declines below this level after initiation of noninvasive ventilation may indicate the need for increasing hours of ventilator use.

Maximal inspiratory and expiratory pressures (MIP and MEP) have also been shown to correlate with the onset of respiratory failure and are commonly measured during follow-up (64). Retention of CO_2 was rare if MIP was above 50% of predicted, but common if MIP was below 33% of predicted. The accuracy of MIP and MEP measurements is less than for vital capacity, however, and combining these measures with vital capacity has not been shown to add any prognostic information. The peak expiratory flow or "peak cough flow" measured using a simple hand-held peak flow meter is also a useful measurement in patients with severe neuromuscular impairment, serving as an objective measure of coughing ability (16). Peak cough flows exceeding 3 L/sec with or without cough-assisting maneuvers have been shown to correlate with successful removal of tracheostomies in patients with chronic respiratory failure (65).

F. Monitoring for Adverse Side Effects and Complications

When patients are properly selected to receive noninvasive ventilation and are managed optimally, adverse side effects and complications should be minor in nature. Nonetheless, certain adverse effects should be anticipated and promptly addressed if success rates are to be maximized. In general, side effects and complications include those associated with the mask and air pressure or flow from the ventilator, failure to improve ventilation, and major complications. These and possible remedial actions have been discussed in more detail elsewhere (66) and in the following section. The discussion focuses on NPPV, but adverse effects of other forms of noninvasive ventilation are considered briefly.

VII. Complications of Noninvasive Ventilation and Possible Remedial Actions

A. Mask-Related Complications

Mask (or interface)-related problems are the most commonly encountered complications during use of NPPV (Table 7). As discussed earlier, different types of interfaces are used to administer NPPV, and the specific problems encountered depend on mask type.

Nasal Masks

Discomfort and redness at areas of skin contact are the most common adverse side effects of nasal masks because of the tension necessary to control air leaks (see Table 7). As would be anticipated, the discomfort depends on the type of mask used, with standard nasal masks applying the most pressure to the bridge of the nose and cheeks, and nasal pillows to the nares. To minimize this problem, proper fitting of the mask and use of the least strap tension that controls air leaks are of paramount importance. For standard nasal masks, the smallest mask size that just encompasses the nose is usually best. The most common errors in administering nasal ventilation are to select a mask that is too large and to apply excess tension on the straps in an effort to eliminate air leaking. Although excessive air leaking may impair the efficacy of NPPV, complete elimination of leaks is usually unnecessary.

Should uncontrollable leaking under the mask occur, the first step should be to ascertain that the mask is optimally fit. Next, the mask should be lifted entirely away from the face and repositioned to assure proper sealing of the silicone flange. If included, forehead spacers should be used and replaced at regular intervals to redistribute pressure away from the nasal bridge. Strap tension should be reduced so that two fingers can be accommodated underneath the straps.

Table 7 Adverse Side Effects and Complications of Interfaces

Type of interface	Adverse effect	Possible remedy
Nasal masks	Discomfort	Optimize fit Try different mask
	Nasal bridge redness or ulceration	Artificial skin; try different mask type Loosen straps; use forehead spacers
	Acneiform rash	Topical antibiotics, steroids
Oronasal mask	Discomfort	Optimize fit
	Nasal bridge redness or ulceration	Loosen straps Artificial skin Try mask with softer seal
	Rebreathing, risk of aspiration	Nonrebreathing valves; rapid release mechanisms
Mouthpiece with lipseal	Discomfort, sores on lips	Readjust straps Remove facial hair
	Interference with swallowing	Strapless mouthpieces
	Hypersalivation	Reassurance
	Dental deformity	Orthodontal consultation

Alternative strap systems can also be tried. Masks with very thin silicone flanges or plastic flaps placed over standard silicone flanges may enhance air sealing at lower strap tensions. Alternatively, nasal "pillows" or "mini-masks" may be used to avoid pressure on the bridge of the nose and cheeks.

Pressure sores on the nasal bridge caused by excessive strap tension occur in up to 10% of patients treated with nasal masks (67), usually during the adaptation period. These can be prevented by minimizing the strap tension needed to achieve an adequate air seal and by having susceptible patients place artificial skin on the nasal bridge. Nasal mini-masks or pillows may be used to avoid contact with the bridge of the nose and cheeks, and the newer "gel" masks are well tolerated by many patients. Sometimes, alternating between different mask types may offer a solution to the problem of persistent pressure sores.

Other complications associated with nasal mask use are listed in Table 7. With the wide variety of nasal masks commercially available, an acceptable mask assembly can usually be found, and custom fitting is rarely necessary. Also, as adaptation progresses and patients become familiarized with the technique, they can be reassured that mask-related problems usually subside.

Oronasal Masks

Oronasal masks also cause discomfort at areas of skin contact and may be even more likely than nasal masks to cause ulcerations on the bridge of the nose. Measures to minimize these are similar to those undertaken with nasal masks. Newer oronasal masks with softer silicone seals may help. Oronasal masks are also more apt to cause claustrophobic reactions than nasal masks, and air leaking at the point of contact with the (highly moveable) lower jaw may be a persistent problem, particularly in edentulous patients.

Vomiting during oronasal ventilation has been raised as a concern, because material retained by the mask could be aspirated. This has led to recommendations that a nasogastric tube be routinely inserted when an oronasal mask is used (68). However, this complication occurs infrequently, even in the acute setting, and insertion of a nasogastric tube is no longer recommended. Overall, complications associated with use of oronasal masks are similar in occurrence to those with nasal masks (see Table 7), but nasal masks are preferred by most patients using long-term noninvasive ventilation because they are less bulky and leave the mouth free for speech and eating.

Lipseals and Mouthpieces

Common problems associated with mouthpiece ventilation include discomfort, interference with swallowing and salivary retention (see Table 7) (31). Pressure sores occur on the cheeks or gums when the lipseal that holds the mouthpiece in place is strapped on too tightly. Air leakage around the lipseal or through the nose may interfere with efficacy, sometimes necessitating use of nose clips or insertion of nasal plugs. Growth of a mustache or beard may also interfere with proper air sealing. Most of these problems can be overcome with fitting adjustments and adaptation, but the author has found that commercially available mouthpieces and lipseals are generally less well tolerated by patients than nasal masks.

Some centers have reported excellent results with custom-made mouthpieces fitted by an oral prosthesis (31). These devices can be fashioned so that straps are unnecessary and they can be expectorated in case of choking or secretion retention, even by quadriplegic patients. In addition to the adverse effects listed in Table 7, these devices elicit occasional allergic reactions to the prosthetic materials. Dental deformity, aerophagia, and 11 deaths have been reported among 257 mouthpiece users with neuromuscular disease (31). Some of the deaths occurred when the mouthpieces accidentally fell out from patients who were dependent on continuous mechanical ventilation, so adequate monitoring and alarms should be used for such patients.

B. Complications Caused by Air Pressure and Flow

Excessive air pressure may cause nasal or sinus pain, burning, or coldness, or ear pain during the initiation of NPPV (Table 8). These can be alleviated by lowering inspiratory pressure during initiation of NPPV. Inspiratory pressures can later be titrated upward as tolerated by the patient to achieve the target level of gas exchange and resolution of symptoms. Nasal congestion and dryness are also common complaints, and may occur at different times in the same patient. Nasal congestion usually responds to nasal steroids or antihistamine/decongestant combinations. Nasal congestion associated with upper respiratory infections probably interferes with the efficacy of NPPV, and temporary use of topical vasoconstrictors may be useful. Nasal dryness, often associated with a sensation of cold or burning, may also respond to use of topical saline or emollient sprays.

Mouth drooling and dryness are also common, the latter usually associated with air leaking through the mouth. High gas flows during nasal ventilation associated with air leaking through the mouth have been shown to increase nasal resistance (69), presumably by cooling the nasal mucosa. This problem may respond to measures aimed at reducing mouth leaking, such as chin straps. However, if dryness persists, heated humidifiers, which have been shown to reverse the increase in nasal resistance (69), should be added to the breathing circuit. When pressure-limited ventilators are used, heated pass-over humidifiers are recommended. Heat and moisture exchangers and pass-through humidifiers can increase resistance in the circuit, reducing delivered pressures and interfering with triggering, so these should be avoided. When nasal dryness becomes severe, epistaxis may occur. This is treated with standard local measures such as emollients and humidification.

Table 8 Adverse Effects of Air Pressure and Flow

Adverse effect	Possible remedy
Sinus, ear pain	Reduce air pressure
Nasal/oral congestion	Topical steroids
	Antihistamine/decongestants
	Short-term topical decongestants during colds
Nasal/oral dryness	Nasal saline, emollients, humidifier
Eye irritation	Check mask fit; try different mask
Gastric insufflation	Simethicone; reduce inflation pressure
Pneumothorax	Reduce inflation pressure

Eye irritation is another adverse effect of air flow and has been reported in up to a third of patients (66). It is caused by leakage of air under the mask on the steep sides of the nose lateral to the nasal bridge, where effective air sealing is difficult. The problem may respond to loosening of head straps because excessive tightening over the bridge of the nose may cause the silicone flanges to splay away from the sides of the nose, exacerbating air leaking. Soothing eye drops may also help. More often, however, an alternative mask must be used to correct the problem. Alternatives include "comfort flaps," "bubble" masks, or nasal "pillows."

Gastric insufflation occurs in up to 50% of patients using NPPV (67), but is usually tolerable. This tolerance may be related to the tonic pressure in the lower esophageal sphincter pressure that is estimated at 10 to 40 mm Hg (70), at or above the peak insufflation pressures commonly used for NPPV. Patients often note increased eructation or flatulence for a few hours in the morning after using NPPV at night, but most patients tolerate the symptom without therapy or respond to agents such as simethicone. The author has encountered only one patient who found these symptoms intolerable. This patient failed to improve after a gastric tube was placed and eventually switched to tracheostomy ventilation (66). Some of her symptoms persisted despite the switch, suggesting that aerophagia unrelated to NPPV was responsible for some of her gastric distension.

Because inflation pressures are usually low (<25 cm H_2O), pulmonary barotrauma is a rare occurrence during NPPV. The author has encountered two patients, brother and sister, who have developed pneumothoraces during long-term use of NPPV (66). These occurred after inspiratory pressure had been increased from 14 to 16 cm H_2O in one and from 18 to 20 cm H_2O in the other. Both had apical blebs that likely predisposed them, but NPPV may have contributed. The sister required closed tube drainage and sclerosis, while the brother required open pleurodesis.

In sum, air pressure and flow can cause numerous adverse effects and complications in users of NPPV. However, these are usually minor and can be ameliorated by making certain that mask fit is optimized. Also, insufflation pressures should be the minimal ones that achieve the desired effect on gas exchange. More consequential complications such as pneumothoraces are, thankfully, unusual. However, in patients who are at increased risk because of bullae or apical blebs, inspiratory pressures should be increased with caution.

C. Failure to Tolerate NPPV

A small minority of appropriately selected patients with chronic respiratory failure due to restrictive thoracic disorders has difficulty tolerating NPPV (perhaps 10%) and may discontinue therapy (67). Intolerance rates tend to be higher among

COPD patients (up to 33%) (62). Mask discomfort and claustrophobia are the most common reasons. With patience and persistence, the experienced practitioner may still be successful in many of these patients, but at the expense of additional time. Proper fit of the mask and optimization of the strap system should first be assured. Different mask sizes and types should be tried if the patient is unable to tolerate the initial choice. Some patients tolerate oronasal masks when nasal masks fail, and vice versa. Other manipulations, such as adjusting body or head position, may occasionally help.

Less often, failure to tolerate NPPV is related to air pressure discomfort or difficulty synchronizing with the ventilator. Although volume- and pressure-limited ventilators appear to be similar in efficacy, some investigators have found that the pressure support mode is better tolerated (37,38). Thus, switching to the pressure support mode may enhance synchronization and acceptance if the patient encounters difficulty using a volume-limited mode. Other ventilator adjustments, such as changes in pressure to optimize comfort, adding positive end-expiratory pressure (PEEP) in patients with presumed intrinsic PEEP, adding humidification in patients with oral or nasal dryness, and silencing alarms in patients whose sleep is disturbed by them, are often useful in facilitating acceptance.

In any event, the patient should be reassured and encouraged not to give up easily. Coaching of breathing pattern and frequent practice sessions may be required, and months may pass before patients become entirely comfortable with the technique. Despite the best efforts, however, some patients (perhaps 10% overall) remain intolerant, objecting to the sensation of a foreign object on the face or of air flow into the nose or mouth. In these few patients, other forms of noninvasive ventilation, such as negative pressure or abdominal ventilation, may be successful when NPPV fails (71).

D. Failure to Adequately Assist Ventilation

Patients who fail to tolerate NPPV derive no improvement in gas exchange. Thus, failure to tolerate may be considered a reason for failure to assist ventilation. However, there are also patients who appear to tolerate NPPV, yet fail to manifest improvements in symptoms or gas exchange. Most commonly, this failure is caused by an insufficient assisted minute volume due to inadequate inflation pressures (or tidal volumes) or backup rate, or too little ventilator use because of patient noncompliance or difficulty (sometimes occult) with adaptation (Table 9). Patient characteristics may also contribute. For instance, a high respiratory impedance caused by increased airway resistance or respiratory system elastance could necessitate the use of higher than usual inflation pressures. Excessive air leaking or rebreathing, two factors that are discussed in detail below, could also play a role.

Table 9 Failure to Adequately Assist Ventilation

Reason	Remedy
Failure to tolerate	Adjust mask, try different mask Adjust pressure Try alternative ventilator
Inadequate inspiratory pressure or tidal volume	Increase inspiratory pressure or V_T as tolerated
Inadequate duration of ventilation	Encourage increased use of ventilator
Difficult patient characteristics	
High impedance	Try higher pressure
Poor compliance, motivation	Encourage greater use
Excessive air leaking	Nocturnal monitoring Chin strap
Rebreathing	Try nonrebreathing valve; increase expiratory pressure

Remedial actions include a gradual upward titration of inspiratory pressure in excess of increases in expiratory pressure (so that the level of pressure support increases). As long as the patient tolerates these changes, tidal volume should be augmented. Patients with neuromuscular disease using volume-limited ventilators may respond to increases in tidal volume and/or backup rate. These patients often breathe at the controlled ventilator rate during sleep (72), so increasing the set ventilator rate (up to a certain point) will augment nocturnal minute volume. This adjustment should lower nocturnal $Paco_2$, helping to lower the respiratory center "set point" for CO_2.

Increasing the duration of ventilator use may also enhance the effectiveness of ventilatory assistance. The minimum duration of ventilation per 24 hr necessary for adequate ventilatory assistance varies among patients, ranging from as little as 3 to 4/24 hr to continuous. Improvements in gas exchange and symptoms are not seen until this threshold is reached, so patients should be encouraged to gradually increase the duration of ventilator sessions while symptoms and gas exchange are monitored.

If no improvement in gas exchange is apparent even after the patient is sleeping through the night using NPPV with an inspiratory pressure support >10 cm H_2O, the patient should be monitored nocturnally using a multichannel recorder, seeking evidence of persisting hypoventilation, apneas, or excessive air leaking. Persisting hypoventilation may respond to further increases in inflation pressure or duration of ventilation. Adding PEEP to splint the upper airway open at the initiation of inspiration may eliminate persisting obstructive apneas and hypopneas. Repeat nocturnal monitoring is indicated to ascertain whether the PEEP level is adequate.

Some patients fail to adequately ventilate after long prior periods of successful ventilatory assistance. Most often, this failure is caused by progression of the underlying disease process. Patients with slowly progressive neuromuscular disease may experience gradual increases in daytime $Paco_2$ as their respiratory muscles weaken, a process that can be slowed or prevented by gradual increases in the duration of ventilator use (such as by having patients take daytime ventilator "naps") and in inflation pressures. If these measures fail, repeat sleep monitoring is indicated to determine whether changes in breathing pattern, apneas, or increased air leaking may be responsible. Some patients fail to realize improvements in ventilation because of inability to clear secretions and mucus plugging. These problems are most apt to occur as neuromuscular diseases progress, weakening the upper airway and expiratory muscles. Ventilatory crises may arise in such patients during acute exacerbations caused by bronchitis or pneumonia, phenomena that are discussed in more detail below.

Even when initial ventilator settings are inadequate to assist ventilation, most patients eventually succeed after inflation pressures are adjusted upward, and mask fit is optimized. However, occasionally, patients will fail despite the best efforts and for these, alternative forms of noninvasive ventilation should be considered and may occasionally be successful. However, particularly in those with secretion retention due to weak cough or swallowing impairment, invasive ventilation will be necessary if prolongation of survival is desired by the patient. Many are willing to try NPPV, but most decline tracheostomy.

E. Air Leaking

Lacking an airtight conduit to the lower airways, the open circuit design of NPPV is inherently leaky. Some air leaking between mask and face is universal, but mask leaks can usually be reduced to acceptable levels. The greater challenge is to achieve adequate alveolar ventilation while relying on upper airway structures to permit air entry into the lungs. Awake, cooperative subjects can usually be coached to allow insufflated air to assist their breathing, but this is nearly impossible in agitated, uncooperative patients. During sleep, the success of NPPV depends on the continued patency of the upper airway. The question might be posed as to how sleeping subjects permit any insufflated air to enter their lungs. The mechanisms by which this is achieved are not fully understood, but recent studies of Jouniaux et al. (73,74), discussed in Chapter 5 on upper airway adaptations during NPPV, offer some insight. These demonstrate that the glottic aperture is important in regulating airflow into the lower airways. For example, hyperventilation induced by volume-controlled NPPV causes glottic narrowing and promotes air leaking. The glottis is probably not the only upper airway structure that plays an important role in conducting air to the lower airways. The soft palate and positioning of oropharyngeal structures are probably important, as well.

In addition to leaks between the mask and skin, air leaks through the mouth are virtually universal during nasal ventilation, and through the nose during mouth ventilation. Some air may enter the esophagus and cause gastric insufflation, although the volume of air entering this pathway is undoubtedly lower than the others because of the impedance posed by the lower esophageal sphincter. In a recent study, air leaking through the mouth was noted during the majority of sleep in seven patients with kyphoscoliosis receiving volume-limited nasal ventilation (75). An association was detected between leak and sleep fragmentation, characterized by lightening of sleep stage and brief arousals. These arousals were most apt to occur during brief oxygen desaturations associated with the leaking, so hypoxemia was presumed to be the mechanism for the arousals. Another investigation on six patients using pressure-limited ventilation, most with neuromuscular disease, also found leaking during the majority of sleep (76). The prevalence of leaking was associated with sleep stage, occurring less often (62%) during stage 1 sleep and most often (100%) during slow wave sleep (SWS, stages 3 and 4). This latter study also found an association between air leaking and arousals.

These studies demonstrate that despite the universality of air leaking, it does not always impair efficacy. In the Meyer et al. (76) study, ventilation and oxygenation were adequately supported despite prolonged periods of air leaking. Sleep fragmentation due to leak-associated arousals appears to be the major adverse consequence of leaking in most patients. However, when air leaking compromises the effectiveness of NPPV, a number of strategies may help to compensate for the leak. First, switching to a ventilator that has good leak compensating capabilities (such as a portable pressure support ventilator) may help. In addition, adding chin straps may reduce leaking through the mouth during nasal ventilation. Alternatively, switching to an oronasal mask or mouthpiece may ameliorate the problem, although leaking can occur with any mask type. Increasing insufflation pressure or tidal volume to compensate for leaks may not always be the best strategy, because this could lead to glottic narrowing and exacerbate the leak. Firm recommendations on the best way to deal with air leaking await more studies on the responses of the upper airways to NPPV, and on the effectiveness of ways to cope with leak.

F. Rebreathing

Some rebreathing occurs normally as CO_2 reenters the lungs from the dead space in the upper airways with each breath. Nasal and oronasal masks contribute to this dead space, although this contribution has not been measured precisely. In addition, portable pressure support ("bilevel") ventilators have been reported to contribute to rebreathing. This phenomenon was first described during use of the bilevel positive airway pressure (BiPAP) ventilator (33), which, like most bilevel devices, uses a single tube for both inspiratory and expiratory flow. To minimize rebreathing, these ventilators use expiratory bias flow to flush exhaled CO_2 out through a fixed exhalation valve that connects the tubing to the mask. Certain connectors, such as the Whisper Swivel that is often used with the BiPAP device, contribute to more rebreathing than connectors specifically designed to eliminate rebreathing, particularly when expiratory pressures are low (<4 cm H_2O) (33). The Whisper Swivel connector has carefully engineered parallel slits that provide a fixed leak throughout the respiratory cycle, but flow of gas through them may be insufficient to exhaust all exhaled CO_2 when expiratory pressure and hence bias flow is low. In one study, the rebreathing was enough to prevent reduction in CO_2 among patients during a brief daytime trial (33).

The problem of rebreathing may be ameliorated by maintaining adequate bias flows with expiratory pressures >4 cm H_2O or by using nonrebreathing exhalation valves. Nonrebreathing valves eliminate the problem, but may increase the expiratory work of breathing (77). In addition, the clinical significance of rebreathing has not been established in long-term studies. One recent preliminary field study suggests that rebreathing may not be as much of a problem as feared in long-term NPPV users, even when low expiratory pressures are used. Much of the exhaled gas exits via mask or mouth leaks, mitigating the effects of rebreathing (34).

G. Major Complications

Complications that lead to significant medical morbidity are unusual with NPPV if the modality is properly applied in appropriately selected patients. Particularly in long-term applications, the usual major complications of mechanical ventilation such as adverse hemodynamic effects or barotrauma are distinctly unusual (see above), presumably because most patients are adequately hydrated and inflation pressures are usually lower than during invasive positive pressure ventilation. Perhaps the greatest concern during long-term noninvasive ventilation is mucus plugging associated with acute respiratory infections, because NPPV provides no direct airway access to aid in secretion removal. This is of particular concern in neuromuscular patients with severely impaired cough mechanisms who may plug suddenly, leading to respiratory crises. Such crises were thought to be responsible for the greater mortality observed among patients with Duchenne muscular dystrophy randomized to use prophylactic NPPV, compared with conventionally treated controls (78). It was speculated that patients using NPPV were given a false sense of security, causing them to delay seeking medical attention when they developed respiratory infections, and permitting the retention of excessive secretions. An approach to dealing with this problem is discussed below.

H. Adverse Side Effects and Complications During Use of "Body" Ventilators

Negative pressure and abdominal displacement ventilators are much less often used currently than at times in the past. Nonetheless, for the patient who fails a trial of NPPV in whom a trial of "body" ventilation may be warranted, knowledge of the potential complications is useful. As with NPPV, the most common problems with negative pressure ventilation are related to improper fitting and discomfort during use (Table 10) (79). With tank negative pressure ventilators, the only fitting consideration is to select an appropriate length if a fiberglas chamber is to be used. However, patients often have to overcome feelings of claustrophobia when using this device, and the restriction of movement caused by the need to lie supine on the mattress contributes to musculoskeletal pain. Restricted movement also contributes to musculoskeletal pain during wrap ventilation, particularly of the back and shoulders. Nonsteroidal antiinflammatory drugs (NSAIDs) are often necessary to help patients cope with this problem until they adapt. The cuirass restricts movement less; patients may use the device while lying on their side or sitting up. However, pain or even skin abrasions may occur at points of skin contact, necessitating fitting adjustments or strategic placement of gauze or foam rubber.

Other problems with negative pressure ventilation include air leaks at points of contact with the skin that reduce the efficiency of ventilation. These are often effectively eliminated by minor fitting or strap adjustments. However, patients with severe chest wall or spinal deformities may be very difficult to fit properly. These patients are usually poor candidates for "body" ventilators, even with custom-built devices. Their poor chest wall compliance renders the efficiency of

Table 10 Adverse Effects and Complications of "Body" Ventilators

Problem	Possible remedy
Negative pressure ventilators	
Discomfort	Assure proper fit, positioning
Musculoskeletal pain	NSAIDs, repositioning
Skin abrasions	Strategically placed padding
Air leaking	Assure proper fit
Obstructive apneas	CPAP if NPPV has failed
Pneumobelt	
Skin abrasions	Proper fit, strap tension
Abdominal discomfort	Adjust strap tension
Rocking bed	
Motion sickness (unusual)	Scopolamine until adapted
Inability to ventilate	May increase rate, arc of rocking

"body" ventilators low, and they commonly have underlying obstructive sleep-disordered breathing. As discussed previously, negative pressure ventilators are apt to exacerbate obstructive apneas (50,51). Thus, use of negative pressure ventilation in patients with moderate to severe obstructive sleep apnea is contraindicated unless combined with CPAP that is demonstrated to adequately eliminate apneas.

The pneumobelt and rocking bed are tolerated by most patients, but their ability to assist ventilation requires a nearly normal body habitus. Also, they are most effective in patients with significant diaphragm dysfunction, so few patients stand to benefit substantially from their use. Although these ventilators have limited efficacy, ventilatory assistance can be increased with the pneumobelt by raising bladder inflation pressures to as high as 60 or 70 cm H_2O. With the rocking bed, assisted ventilation can be enhanced by raising rocking rate (although tidal volumes may drop at rates over 16/min) (80) or increasing the arc of rocking. Their limited efficacy may be problematic during lower respiratory tract infections, when alternative means of ventilatory assistance are often required to avert respiratory crises.

The pneumobelt must be properly fit, and some patients cannot be adequately accommodated by the variety of sizes commercially available. Even when fit is good, abrasions are common after prolonged use at points of skin contact, and added padding is often necessary. This problem generally subsides with continued use, but strap wear and failure may require frequent replacement in long-term users. The rocking bed is perceived as comfortable by most patients who use it, and adaptation is usually quite simple. Occasionally patients may develop motion sickness, but the major complaints are usually related to the lack of portability and noisy operation.

I. Avoidance of Complications

Although knowledge of potential complications is essential for the successful management of patients using NPPV, the best course of management is to anticipate and avoid complications altogether, if possible. In this regard, a thorough familiarity with masks and strap systems is helpful. As emphasized above, one of the most common errors is to use an ill-fitting mask and then to tighten the straps excessively in an attempt to reduce air leakage. Careful attention to optimizing mask fit and minimizing strap tension will usually eliminate this problem. Also of critical importance is gaining experience and skill in the implementation of NPPV and being able to apply these when working with new patients. Relative to invasive ventilation, NPPV affords patients a high degree of control, but using it successfully requires learning. Patients must learn to relax their breathing muscles and position their upper airway structures to permit airflow into the lungs. Having an experienced practitioner available who can spend the time to optimize comfort and help patients to relax and synchronize their breathing with the ventilator often makes the difference between success and failure.

Another extremely important aspect of avoiding complications during use of NPPV is to exclude inappropriate patients. As discussed earlier, the likelihood of failure is so high in certain situations as to render a trial of NPPV futile, and certain patients with respiratory failure could be harmed if invasive ventilation is inappropriately delayed. Patients who are agitated or incapable of cooperating cannot be successfully ventilated noninvasively. Likewise, the inability to fit a mask due to anatomic abnormalities precludes the use of NPPV. Also, severe compromise of the ability to protect the airway presages failure. Nonetheless, a trial of noninvasive ventilation may still be worthwhile even when patients have bulbar involvement. One study on patients with motor neuron disease showed improved survival among those who tolerated NPPV compared to those who didn't despite the presence of bulbar dysfunction (81).

VIII. Management of Acute Exacerbations During Long-Term Noninvasive Ventilation

Patients with chronic respiratory failure may be stabilized for long periods of time by using noninvasive ventilation, sometimes for many years. However, acute episodes of bronchitis or pneumonia may threaten the stability, particularly if the cough mechanism is impaired. Secretions may accumulate in the airways, increasing the breathing load and interfering with gas exchange. Unless corrective measures are promptly undertaken, respiratory collapse may ensue, followed by endotracheal intubation or even death in patients who have declined intubation.

Bach et al. (35) have proposed a way of managing these situations without requiring hospitalization or invasive ventilation. Patients increase the duration of NPPV use to 24 hr/day to avoid respiratory muscle fatigue. Manually assisted coughing is used to assist with secretion removal, often in combination with the cough in–exsufflator. These may be used as needed, sometimes as frequently as every 10 minutes. Patients are not given oxygen supplementation and are advised to monitor themselves continuously with a pulse oximeter. If O_2 saturation falls below 95%, they are instructed to increase their minute ventilation by using bag ventilation and to proceed with secretion removal techniques until saturation returns to the upper 90s. If O_2 saturation cannot be returned to this level, then hospitalization is advised.

Although this approach has not been evaluated in a prospective fashion, the authors report that very few patients have failed (35). Whether or not a pulse oximeter is necessary in all cases has not been established, but some modification of this approach seems prudent in patients with chronic respiratory failure and cough impairment, particularly the extended duration of noninvasive ventilation and the increased application of cough assistance techniques. The approach presumes that the other usual therapeutic measures for respiratory infection will be applied, including adequate hydration and antibiotics. It is also important to bear in mind that this approach applies to patients with restrictive thoracic processes and has not been evaluated in those with chronic obstructive diseases.

IX. Summary and Conclusions

Over the past decade, the increasing use of noninvasive ventilation, NPPV in particular, has revolutionized the care of patients with chronic respiratory failure. NPPV has replaced negative pressure and tracheostomy ventilation as the ventilator modality of first choice for these patients, greatly enhancing convenience and portability, adding to the quantity as well as the quality of their lives, and all at a lower cost. However, to realize these advantages, NPPV must be administered to appropriately selected patients by clinicians knowledgeable and experienced in its application.

The clinician must be familiar with the wide range of interface and ventilator choices available as well as their advantages and limitations. Patients to receive NPPV must be selected carefully, and must be properly instructed on what to expect. The initiation and adaptation processes are critical to success, and the patient must receive an optimally fit interface with appropriate initial ventilator settings. The clinician must impart a sense of optimism and confidence to the patient, and must be readily available to the patient should problems arise. Monitoring should encompass the main goals of mechanical ventilation, including the symptomatic and gas exchange responses, as well as anticipated complications that are handled in a proactive rather than reactive fashion.

If managed according to the approach outlined above, NPPV should succeed in the vast majority of cases. However, in the event of failure, the clinician should be prepared to try alternative noninvasive ventilators. Tracheostomy should be considered only if noninvasive options have been tried and failed, ventilatory support is required most or all of the time and the patient would rather use invasive than noninvasive ventilation, or airway protective mechanisms are compromised and the patient desires maximum prolongation of survival.

References

1. Wilson JL. Acute anterior poliomyelitis. N Engl J Med 1932; 206:887–893.
2. Alba A, Khan A, Lee M. Mouth IPPV for sleep. Rehabilitation Gazette 1984; 24: 47–49.
3. Curran FJ. Night ventilation by body respirators for patients in chronic respiratory

failure due to late stage Duchenne muscular dystrophy. Arch Phys Med Rehabil 1981; 62:270–274.

4. Garay SM, Turino GM, Goldring RM. Sustained reversal of chronic hypercapnia in patients with alveolar hypoventilation syndromes. Long-term maintenance with noninvasive nocturnal mechanical ventilation. Am J Med 1981; 62:270–274.
5. Splaingard ML, Frates RC Jr, Harrison GM, et al. Home-positive-pressure ventilation: Twenty years' experience. Chest 1983; 84:376–384.
6. Colbert AP, Schock NC. Respirator use in progressive neuromuscular diseases. Arch Phys Med Rehabil 1985; 66:760–762.
7. Sullivan CE, Issa FG, Berthon-Jones M, et al. Reversal of obstructive sleep apnea by continuous positive airway pressure applied through the nares. Lancet 1981; 1: 862–865.
8. Bach JR, Alba A, Mosher, et al. Intermittent positive pressure ventilation via nasal access in the management of respiratory insufficiency. Chest 1987; 94:168–170.
9. Kerby GR, Mayer LS, Pingleton SK. Nocturnal positive pressure ventilation via nasal mask. Am Rev Respir Dis 1987; 135:738–740.
10. Ellis ER, Bye PT, Bruderer JW, et al. Treatment of respiratory failure during sleep in patients with neuromuscular disease. Positive-pressure ventilation through a nose mask. Am Rev Respir Dis 1987; 135:148–152.
11. American Respiratory Care Foundation. Consensus conference: Non-invasive positive pressure ventilation. Respir Care 1997; 42:364–369.
12. American College of Chest Physicians. Mechanical ventilation beyond the intensive care unit. Chest 1998; 113:S289–S344.
13. McNicholas WT. Impact of sleep in respiratory failure. Eur Respir J 1997; 10:920–933.
14. Hill NS. The cardiac exam in lung disease. Clin Chest Med 1987; 8:273–285.
15. Braun NMT, Arora NS, Rochester DF. Respiratory muscle and pulmonary function in polymyositis and other proximal myopathies. Thorax 1983; 38:616–623.
16. Bach JR. Update and perspective on noninvasive respiratory muscle aids. Part 2. The expiratory aids. Chest 1994; 105:1538–1544.
17. Meecham Jones DJ, Paul EA, Jones PW. Nasal pressure support ventilation plus oxygen compared with oxygen therapy along in hypercapnic COPD. Am J Respir Crit Care Med 1995; 152:538–544.
18. Sanders MH, Kern NB, Costantino JP, et al. Accuracy of end-tidal and transcutaneous Pco_2 monitoring during sleep. Chest 1994; 106:472–483.
19. Piper AJ, Sullivan CE. Effects of long-term nocturnal nasal ventilation on spontaneous breathing during sleep in neuromuscular and chest wall disorders. Eur Respir J 1996; 9:1515–1522.
20. Kramer N, Meyer TJ, Meharg J, et al. Randomized, prospective trial of noninvasive positive pressure ventilation in acute respiratory failure. Am J Respir Crit Care Med 1995; 151:1799–1806.
21. Mehta S, Hill NS. Noninvasive ventilation in acute respiratory failure. Respir Care Clin N Am 1996; 2:267–291.
22. Raphael JC, Chevret S, Chastang C, et al. French multicenter trial of prophylactic nasal ventilation in Duchenne muscular dystrophy. Lancet 1994; 343:1600–1604.
23. Meduri GU, Abou-Shala N, Fox RC, et al. Noninvasive face mask mechanical venti-

lation in patients with acute hypercapnic respiratory failure. Chest 1991; 100:445–454.

24. Soo Hoo GW, Santiago S, Williams J. Nasal mechanical ventilation for hypercapnic respiratory failure in chronic obstructive pulmonary disease: Determinants of success and failure. Crit Care Med 1994; 27:417–434.
25. Bach JR. A comparison of long-term ventilatory support alternatives from the perspective of the patient and care giver. Chest 1993; 104:1702–1706.
26. Bach JR, Intintola P, Alba AS, Holland I. The ventilator-assisted individual cost analysis of institutionalization versus rehabilitation and in-home management. Chest 1992; 101:26–30.
27. Schonhofer B, Geibel M, Sonneborn M, Haidl P, Kohler D. Daytime mechanical ventilation in chronic respiratory insufficiency. Eur Respir J 1997; 10:2840–2846.
28. Parreira VF, Delguste P, Jounieaux V, Aubert G, Dury M, Rodenstein DO. Effectiveness of controlled and spontaneous modes in nasal two-level positive pressure ventilation in awake and asleep normal subjects. Chest 1997; 112:1267–1277.
29. Drinkwine J, Kacmarek RM. Noninvasive positive pressure ventilation: Equipment and techniques. Respir Care Clin NA 1996; 2:183–194.
30. Criner GJ, Travaline JM, Brennan KJ, et al. Efficacy of a new full face mask for noninvasive positive pressure. Chest 1994; 106:1109–1115.
31. Bach JR, Alba AS, Saporito LR: Intermittent positive pressure ventilation via the mouth as an alternative to tracheostomy for 257 ventilator users. Chest 1993; 103: 174–182.
32. Strumpf DA, Carlisle CC, Millman RP, et al. An evaluation of the Respironics BiPAP bi-level CPAP device for delivery of assisted ventilation. Respiratory Care 1990; 35:415–422.
33. Ferguson GT, Gilmartin M. CO_2 rebreathing during BiPAP ventilatory assistance. Am J Respir Crit Care Med 1995; 151:1126–1135.
34. Hill NS, Carlisle CC, Kramer NR. Does the exhalation valve really matter during bilevel nasal ventilation? Am J Respir Crit Care Med 1997; 155:A408.
35. Bach JR, Ishikawa Y, and Kim H. Prevention of pulmonary morbidity for patients with Duchenne muscular dystrophy. Chest 1997; 112:1024–1028.
36. Kacmarek RM, Stanek KS, McMahon K, et al. Increased work of breathing during synchronized intermittent mandatory ventilation (SIMV) in home care ventilators. Am Rev Respir Dis 1988; 137:64.
37. Vitacca M, Rubini F, Foglio K, Scalvini S, Nava S, Ambrosino N. Noninvasive modalities of positive pressure ventilation improved the outcome of acute exacerbations in COLD patients. Intensive Care Med 1993; 19:450–455.
38. Girault C, Richard J-C, Chevron V, Tamion F, Pasquis P, Leroy J, Bonmarchand G. Comparative physiologic effects of noninvasive assist-control and pressure support ventilation in acute hypercapnic respiratory failure. Chest 1997; 111:1639–1648.
39. Restrick LJ, Fox NC, Braid G, Ward EM, Paul EA, Wedjicha JA. Comparison of nasal pressure support ventilation with nasal intermittent positive pressure ventilation in patients with nocturnal hypoventilation. Eur Respir J 1993; 6:365–370.
40. Meecham-Jones DJ, Wedzicha JA. Comparison of pressure volume and volume preset nasal ventilator systems in stable chronic respiratory failure. Eur Respir J 1993; 6:1060–1064.

41. Schonhofer B, Sonneborn M, Haide P, Bohrer H, Kohler D. Comparison of two different modes for noninvasive mechanical ventilation in chronic respiratory failure: Volume versus pressure controlled device. Eur Respir J 1997; 10:184–191.
42. Dalziel J. On sleep and apparatus for promoting artificial respiration. Br Assoc Adv Sci 1938; 1:127.
43. Corrado A, Gorini M, Villella G, DePaola E. Negative pressure ventilation in the treatment of acute respiratory failure: An old noninvasive technique reconsidered. Eur Resir J 1996; 9:1531–1544.
44. Montserrat JM, Martos JA, Alarcon A, et al. Effect of negative pressure ventilation on arterial blood gas pressures and inspiratory muscle strength during an exacerbation of chronic obstructive lung disease. Thorax 1991; 46:6–8.
45. Miller HJ, Thomas E, Wilmot CB: Pneumobelt use among high quadriplegic population. Arch Phys Med Rehabil 1988; 69:369–372.
46. Hill NS. Use of negative pressure ventilation, rocking beds, and pneumobelts. Respir Care 1994; 39:532.
47. Abd AG, Braun NMT, Baskin MI, et al. Diaphragmatic dysfunction after open heart surgery: Treatment with a rocking bed. Ann Intern Med 1991; 111:881–886.
48. Bach JR, Alba AS. Noninvasive options for ventilatory support of the traumatic high level quadriplegic. Chest 1990; 98:613–619.
49. Levy RD, Bradley TD, Newman SL, et al. Negative pressure ventilation: Effects on ventilation during sleep in normal subjects. Chest 1989; 95:95–99.
50. Bach JR, Penek J. Obstructive sleep apnea complicating negative pressure ventilatory support in patients with chronic paralytic restrictive ventilatory dysfunction. Chest 1991; 99:1386.
51. Hill NS, Redline S, Carskadon MA, Curran FJ, Millman RP. Sleep-disordered breathing in patients with Duchenne muscular dystrophy using negative pressure ventilators. Chest 1992; 102:1656–1662.
52. Hill NS, Mehta S, Carlisle CC, McCool FD. Evaluation of the Puritan-Bennett 335 portable pressure support ventilator: Comparison with the Respironics BiPAP S/T. Respir Care 1996; 41:885–894.
53. Bonmarchand G, Chevron V, Chopin C, Jusserand D, Girault C, Moritz F, Leroy J, Pasquis P. Increased initial flow rate reduces inspiratory work of breathing during pressure support ventilation in patients with exacerbation of chronic obstructive pulmonary disease. Intensive Care Med 1996; 22:1147–1154.
54. Mehta S, McCool FD, Hill NS. Leak compensation in portable positive pressure ventilators. Resp Crit Care Med 1997, 155:A407.
55. Johns MW. A new method for measuring daytime sleepiness: The Epworth Sleepiness Scale. Sleep 1991, 14:540–545.
56. American Thoracic Society Statement. Standards for diagnosis and care of patients with chronic obstructive pulmonary disease. Respir Crit Care Med 1995; 152(5): S77–S120.
57. Janssens JP, Howarth-Frey C, Chevrolet JC, Abajo B, Rochat T. Transcutaneous Pco_2 to monitor noninvasive mechanical ventilation in adults: Assessment of a new transcutaneous Pco_2 device. Chest 1998; 113:786–773.
58. Strumpf DA, Millman RP, Hill NS. The management of chronic hypoventilation. Chest 1990, 948:474–480.

59. Jimenez JFM, de Cos Escuin JS, Vicente CD, et al. Nasal intermittent positive pressure ventilation. Analysis of its withdrawal. Chest 1995;107:382–388.
60. Meyer TJ, Pressman MR, Benditt J, et al. Mouth leaking during nocturnal nasal ventilation: Effect on sleep quality. Am J Respir Crit Care Med 1995; 151:A423.
61. Zibrak JD, Hill NS, Federman ED, et al. Evaluation of intermittent long-term negative pressure ventilation in patients with severe chronic obstructive pulmonary disease. Am Rev Respir Dis 1988; 138:1515–1518.
62. Strumpf DA, Millman RP, Carlisle CC, et al. Nocturnal positive-pressure ventilation via nasal mask in patients with severe chronic obstructive pulmonary disease. Am Rev Respir Dis 1991; 144:1234–1239.
63. Shapiro SH, Ernst P, Gray-Donald K, et al. Effect of negative pressure ventilation in severe chronic obstructive pulmonary disease. Lancet 1992; 340:1425–1429.
64. Braun NMT, Arora NS, Rochester DF. Respiratory muscle and pulmonary function in polymyositis and other proximal myopathies. Thorax 1983; 38:616–623.
65. Bach JR, Saporito LR. Criteria for extubation and tracheostomy tube removal for patients with ventilatory failure: A different approach to weaning. Chest 1996; 110: 1566–1571.
66. Hill NS. Complications of noninvasive positive pressure ventilation. Respir Care 1997; 42:432–442.
67. Leger P, Bedicam JM, Cornette A, et al. Nasal intermittent positive pressure. Long-term follow-up in patients with severe chronic respiratory insufficiency. Chest 1994; 105:100–105.
68. Meduri GU, Abou-Shala N, Fox RC, et al. Noninvasive face mask mechanical ventilation in patients with acute hypercapnic respiratory failure. Chest 1991; 100:445–454.
69. Richards GN, Cistulli PA, Ungar G, Berthon-Jones M, Sullivan CE. Mouth leak with nasal continuous positive airway pressure increases nasal airway resistance. Am J Respir Crit Care Med 1996; 154:182–186.
70. Christensen J. Motor functions of the pharynx. In: Johnson LR, ed. Physiology of the Gastrointestinal Tract. 2nd ed. New York: Rawson Press, 1987.
71. Hill NS. Use of the rocking bed, pneumobelt and other noninvasive aids to ventilation. In: Tobin MJ, ed. Principles and Practice of Mechanical Ventilation. New York: McGraw Hill, 1994; 413–425.
72. Hill NS, Eveloff SE, Carlisle CC, et al. Efficacy of nocturnal nasal ventilation in patients with restrictive thoracic disease. Am Rev Respir Dis 1992; 101:516–521.
73. Jouniaux V, Aubert G, Dury M, et al. Effects of nasal positive-pressure hyperventilation on the glottis in normal awake subjects. J Appl Physiol 1995; 79:176–185.
74. Jouniaux V, Aubert G, Dury M, Delguste P, Rodenstein DO. Effects of nasal positive-pressure hyperventilation on the glottis in normal sleeping subjects. J Appl Physiol 1995; 79:186–183.
75. Bach JR, Dominique R, Leger P, et al. Sleep fragmentation in kyphoscoliotic individuals with alveolar hypoventilation treated by NPPV. Chest 1995; 107:1552–1558.
76. Meyer TJ, Pressman MR, Benditt J, McCool FD, Millman RP, Natarajan R, Hill NS. Air leaking through the mouth during nocturnal nasal ventilation: Effect on sleep quality. Sleep 1997; 20:561–569.
77. Lofaso F, Brochard L, Thierry H, Hubert L, Haref A, Isabey D. Home versus inten-

sive care pressure support devices. Experimental and clinical comparison. Am J Respir Crit Care Med 1996; 153:1591–1599.

78. Raphael JC, Chevret S, Chastang C, et al. French multicenter trial of prophylactic nasal ventilation in Duchenne muscular dystrophy. Lancet 1994; 343:1600–1604.
79. Hill NS. Clinical applications of body ventilators. Chest 1986; 90:897–905.
80. Bryce-Smith R, Davis HS. Tidal exchange in respirators. Curr Res Anaesth Analg 1954, 33:73–85.
81. Aboussouan LS, Khan SU, Meeker DP, Stelmach K, Mitsumoto H. Effect of noninvasive positive pressure ventilation on survival in amyotrophic lateral sclerosis. Ann Intern Med 1997; 127:450–453.

11

Conversion from Invasive to Noninvasive Ventilation

JOSEPH VIROSLAV and RANDALL L. ROSENBLATT

St. Paul Medical Center
University of Texas Southwestern Medical School
Dallas, Texas

I. Introduction

The use of mechanical aids to assist patients with chronic respiratory insufficiency, especially those with neuromuscular diseases, has increased over the past few years. Initially, patients were ventilated with negative pressure tanks, which were quite popular during the polio epidemics (1). With the development and increasing sophistication of positive pressure ventilators and the concerns about their effects on upper airway function (2–4), negative pressure ventilators were either discarded or delegated to storage. Positive pressure ventilation via tracheostomy became the method of choice for chronic conditions; but during the last 20 years, the use of the "old style" techniques of negative pressure ventilation and the acceptance of positive pressure ventilation without the need for a tracheostomy or an endotracheal tube have been reexamined.

This chapter is designed to discuss the concepts and techniques used in treating patients with chronic respiratory failure without an endotracheal tube or a tracheostomy, with an emphasis on the methodology of transitioning patients from invasive to noninvasive ventilation.

II. Historical Notes

During the polio epidemics, the iron lung was the ventilator most commonly used to support patients during the acute phase of the illness. Fortunately, most patients recovered sufficient muscle function to support adequate spontaneous ventilation; but in those patients with insufficient function, a variety of mechanical devices were improvised to enable patients to return home. The pneumobelt, rocking bed, cuirass, and pneumosuit were all utilized to support these patients (5–7). In patients with marginal respiratory muscle function, intermittent ventilation (ventilation for portions of each day) was recognized as a method for maintaining respiratory muscle function and strength (5,6,8). Thus, the concept of resting the respiratory muscles in chronic diseases was appreciated even 50 years ago.

During the 1950s, vaccination eliminated the polio epidemics, but the techniques and ingenuity developed for home ventilation have since been adapted for patients with chronic respiratory failure resulting from inherent lung diseases, muscle diseases, and neurologic conditions (1,7,9,10–14). Ventilation can be enhanced by either negative or positive pressure techniques, although the latter are more commonly used today in the treatment of acute respiratory failure (15,16). The negative pressure devices, however, are still readily accepted by patients with neurologic disorders such as postpolio syndrome or muscular dystrophies (3).

III. Advantages and Disadvantages of Ventilators Used for Long-Term Ventilatory Support

Negative pressure ventilation has fallen into disfavor because of the bulkiness of the machines, the difficulty with nursing care, and the tendency to induce or exacerbate upper airway obstruction (2–4). Some of the nursing issues and the concerns about the size of the tank ventilators were addressed by the development of the cuirass ventilator and body wrap techniques. Positive pressure ventilators, on the other hand, are smaller and more convenient to use. However, they require an interface between the patient and the machine. With invasive ventilation, initially an endotracheal tube is utilized and then converted to a tracheostomy tube for chronic use. These interfaces, however, may be associated with significant complications. Barotrauma, vocal cord injury, an increase in bronchial secretions, bleeding (especially innominate artery erosion), the need for humidification, the propensity for infection, and interference with the ability to speak are all significant concerns (17–19). Furthermore, many patients with chronic disabilities view the tracheostomy as a death-prolonging measure rather than a technique utilized to improve the quality of their lives.

Because of these problems, our institution developed a program to ventilate patients without using a tracheostomy. The presence of the tracheostomy tube was associated with a loss of self-esteem, an increase in secretions, the occurrence of hemoptysis from tracheal injury, and the need for increased frequency of suctioning and respiratory therapy. Frequent suctioning traumatizes the tracheal and bronchial mucosa, contributing to an increased incidence of bacterial colonization and respiratory infections. Thus, we postulated that removal of the tracheostomy tube would not only allow the patients improved communication abilities by restoring their ability to speak but also would decrease the number of respiratory infections and airway complications (17,20,21).

The initial attempts to use these noninvasive techniques were in patients with traumatic tetraplegia who were being chronically ventilated with positive pressure ventilation via a tracheostomy tube. These efforts were well received by the patients and successful in decreasing the number of hospital admissions and respiratory complications (17).

IV. General Considerations

Respiratory failure should be viewed as an inability of the respiratory system to meet the ventilatory and/or oxygen needs of the body. The causes of respiratory failure that respond to noninvasive ventilation include an unresponsive respiratory center, abnormalities of lung parenchyma or airway function, skeletal abnormalities, muscle weakness, and neurologic diseases (Table 1). The type of support selected to prevent or treat respiratory failure is determined by the primary injury

Table 1 Types of Respiratory Failure and Amenability to Switching to Noninvasive Ventilation

	Amenable	Nonamenable
Neuromuscular	Poliomyelitis	Guillain Barré syndrome
	Muscular dystrophies	Myasthenia gravis
	Spinal cord injuries	
	Amyotrophic lateral sclerosis	
	Multiple sclerosis	
Musculoskeletal	Chest wall deformities	
Sleep apnea	Central or obstructive apnea	
Parenchymal lung disease	COPD	Interstitial lung disease
Neurological	Central apnea	

or abnormality. For example, patients with a sudden loss of functioning respiratory muscles, as seen in spinal cord injuries or Guillain-Barré syndrome, essentially have normal lungs, normal airway function, normal chest wall mechanics, and normal respiratory centers. The basic defect is a loss of the bellows function of the respiratory muscles. Consequently, these patients can easily be ventilated noninvasively as long as their bulbar function remains intact and is not impaired.

Patients with chronic myopathies and/or skeletal abnormalities have abnormal chest wall mechanics and reduced respiratory system compliances, which markedly alter their ventilatory requirements and ventilation perfusion relationships (21,22). These patients have hypoxemia and hypercarbia from inadequate expansion of the lungs and atelectasis. The normal compliance of the respiratory system in acute injuries or diseases allows for easy expansion of the lung and reversal of the atelectasis, whereas the patients with chronic diseases have immobile or stiff chest walls that impair adequate lung expansion (22).

Patients with high cervical spinal cord injuries experience acute respiratory failure via the loss of respiratory muscle function. The major muscle of inspiration, the diaphram, derives its innervation from C3, C4, and C5 nerve roots. The major muscles of forced expiration are the abdominal muscles. The intercostal muscles function by stabilizing the chest wall. Thus, assuming that there has been no associated chest wall trauma or significant cardiac injury, the lung itself should be normal. Assisted ventilation is usually easily accomplished with either negative or positive pressure techniques. The level of spinal cord injury correlates with the need for ventilation. A patient with injuries below C5 should not require chronic assistance, assuming previously normal lungs and an intact respiratory center (17). However, these patients do have a high incidence of gastric acid aspiration, which may cause significant parenchymal injury. Also, patients with muscle abnormalities or weakness are prone to atelectasis because of their inability to "sigh," their inability to cough and adequately clear secretions without intact respiratory muscles, and because of shallow tidal volumes (23). All of these factors increase the likelihood of developing respiratory infections. Consequently, early and aggressive respiratory management can address these conditions and prevent the associated complications of atelectasis and infection.

The presence of abnormal chest wall or lung mechanics impairs the normal treatment regimen. Muscle fatigue develops in these patients because of the low respiratory system compliance that increases the work required to maintain adequate ventilation. Usually, tidal volumes are reduced, and the respiratory rate is increased in order to maintain an adequate V_E. Furthermore, atelectasis and retained secretions result in an increased dead space and a higher V_E requirement in order to maintain a normal P_{CO_2} (24). Consequently, these patients are more difficult to manage even with assisted ventilation. When these patients are admitted to an acute care facility, the physicians, in the past, have recommended a tracheostomy.

These patients, however, are still good candidates for conversion to noninvasive ventilation. The presence of some respiratory muscle activity will allow for spontaneous ventilation for short periods of time. This is a distinct advantage when transferring patients from tracheostomy ventilation to noninvasive ventilation. Restoring the chest wall compliance and lung function toward normal helps to decrease the workload imposed on the respiratory muscles. This requires aggressive chest wall stretching (25) and respiratory muscle rest (26–29).

Patients with neurologic abnormalities such as Guillain-Barré syndrome, amyotrophic lateral sclerosis, or multiple sclerosis should have normal chest wall and lung mechanics. However, their muscular function or strength cannot be improved and may be worsened by our techniques of resistance training of muscles (30). Additionally, pain in these patients may limit the effectiveness of assisted cough and other methods necessary to clear secretions. In general, these patients tolerate these techniques less well than spinal cord injury patients who lack sensation below the neck. The assisted cough technique, for example, utilizes forceful thrusts into the upper abdomen at the beginning of expiration that can be quite uncomfortable if sensation is intact.

V. Contraindications to Noninvasive Ventilation

Unfortunately, not all patients are candidates for noninvasive ventilation and are better served with a tracheostomy. Prior to considering noninvasive ventilation, careful evaluation of the following is essential: the level of cognitive ability, dysphagia, upper airway function, age, the sophistication of the caregiver, and the patient's ability to breathe spontaneously.

A. Cognitive Function

The patients must comprehend the prescribed treatment. They must be able to assist in the maneuvers to expand lung volume, to cooperate with the assisted cough techniques, to recognize respiratory distress, and to learn techniques to sustain spontaneous ventilation for short periods of time, such as glossopharyngeal breathing, in the event of a mechanical ventilator failure (31–33).

B. Swallowing Dysfunction

Dysphagia is common in patients with neuromuscular disorders, although it is rarely a problem with spinal cord injuries. The ability to handle oropharyngeal secretions and an intact swallowing mechanism are essential to prevent aspiration. The lung defense mechanisms are impaired by the inability to spontaneously cough and clear secretions. Some patients will require placement of a jejunostomy tube to deliver adequate nutrition, but this should not interfere with plans for noninvasive ventilation. Patients with early amyotrophic lateral sclerosis can use these noninvasive techniques but should be assessed periodically for their ability to handle their oral secretions and risk for aspiration, since their disease is usually progressive.

C. Upper Airway Function

Upper airway function should be carefully evaluated. Patients with tracheostomies or long-term intubations may have tracheal stenosis, tracheomalacia, granulation tissue, or vocal cord dysfunction that could interfere with the effectiveness of noninvasive ventilation. If there is any question concerning the adequacy of the airway, then fiberoptic laryngoscopy and/or bronchoscopy should be performed. Negative pressure ventilation requires stabilization of the larynx and contraction of the genioglossus muscle in order to maintain an adequate airway during inspiration (2,34). Thus, those patients who develop functional upper airway obstruction during negative pressure ventilation should be treated with positive pressure modalities. The addition of continuous positive airway pressure (CPAP) to the negative pressure modality is an alternative consideration but requires a nasal or oral interface and additional equipment.

D. Age

Advanced age is not a contraindication to noninvasive ventilation for patients with chronic respiratory failure. However, older patients, in most circumstances, do not have adequate support at home or in their postdischarge environment to successfully manage assisted ventilation. Also, depression is common in older persons and may be a significant inpediment to educating these patients (35,36). Other complicating factors, such as hypertension, cardiovascular disease, and diabetes, commonly seen in older patients result in lower long-term survival rates.

E. Caregiver Availability

The caregiver is one of the most important components for the successful delivery of noninvasive ventilation. Patients often require assistance that is not easily provided by a nursing home environment. Consequently, those patients who are obligated to go to nursing homes are not good candidates for noninvasive ventilation. The caregiver must be able to provide nursing care, deliver an assisted cough, be capable of utilizing the various protocols to expand lung volumes, and be available full time. With an inadequate caregiver, the technique of noninvasive ventilation is doomed to fail.

F. Spontaneous Ventilation

Patients being considered for a switch to noninvasive ventilation must be able to sustain some ventilation on their own for 30 minutes (17). This allows for the patients to be transferred from the bed to a chair, take baths, etc. and allows for a safeguard in the event of a power failure or failure of the caregiver to adequately respond. Many patients with adequate oral motor function learn the technique of glossopharnygeal breathing (GPB), which was initially used during the polio epidemics. This technique consists of short "gulps" of air that are stacked. The normal "gulp" is 50 to 180 cc of air and is repeated 10 to 12 times to achieve a normal tidal volume. Passive relaxation of the chest allows for exhalation. Each sequence occurs 10 to 14 times per minute resulting in a VE of 5 to 8l (33,37). Many patients learn this technique on their own, but it requires intact oropharyngeal muscle function. Patients who experience paralysis of the respiratory muscles and who require continuous ventilatory support may spontaneously develop glossopharyngeal breathing. Most of the time this becomes a learned technique. At our facility, we teach glossopharyngeal breathing to all ventilator-dependent patients who are being considered for noninvasive ventilation.

Glossopharyngeal breathing is taught by imitating the movements, motions, and sounds of the instructor. The development of strength and endurance, after the basic techniques has been learned, takes time. Much like any training, patients undergo GPB practice sessions several times per day to build strength and endurance. When the patient is discharged, daily use of GPB is required to maintain proficiency.

VI. Patient Selection

When selecting patients for conversion to noninvasive ventilation, several factors should be considered. First and foremost, the goals of ventilation need to be identified: the prevention of respiratory muscle fatigue, the maintenance of adequate lung function, the prevention of nocturnal hypoventilation, or the fulfillment of baseline respiratory demands (13,30,38,39). Chronic respiratory failure patients are often excellent candidates for noninvasive support, but they should have acceptable lung or chest wall mechanics to allow a reasonable minute volume to adequately meet respiratory demands; adequate financial, family and caretaker support; and motivation to use this technique instead of a tracheostomy.

The type of ventilation used depends on several factors discussed above: (1) the amount of support needed; (2) upper airway function; (3) type of mask; (4) nursing care needs; and (5) preference of the patient. The algorithms in Figures 1 and 2 outline the steps used in our facility for transition from invasive to noninvasive ventilation. Figure 1 depicts the use of noninvasive ventilation to completely wean

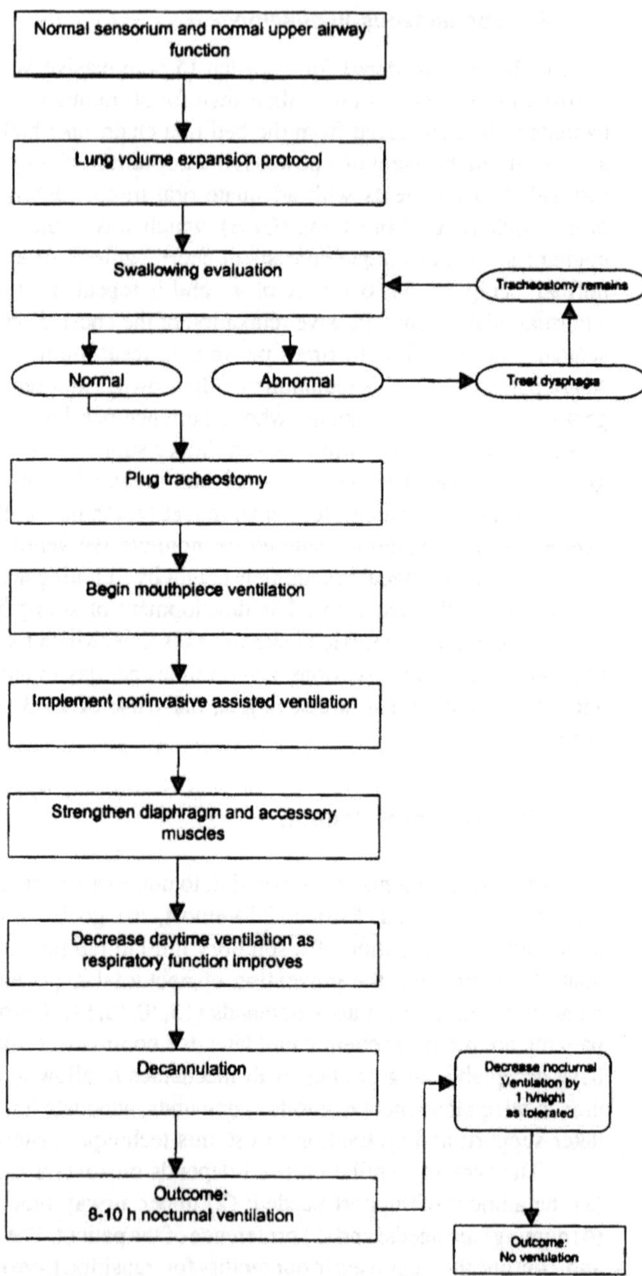

Figure 1 Weaning from a tracheostomy using noninvasive ventilation: eventual complete ventilation weaning.

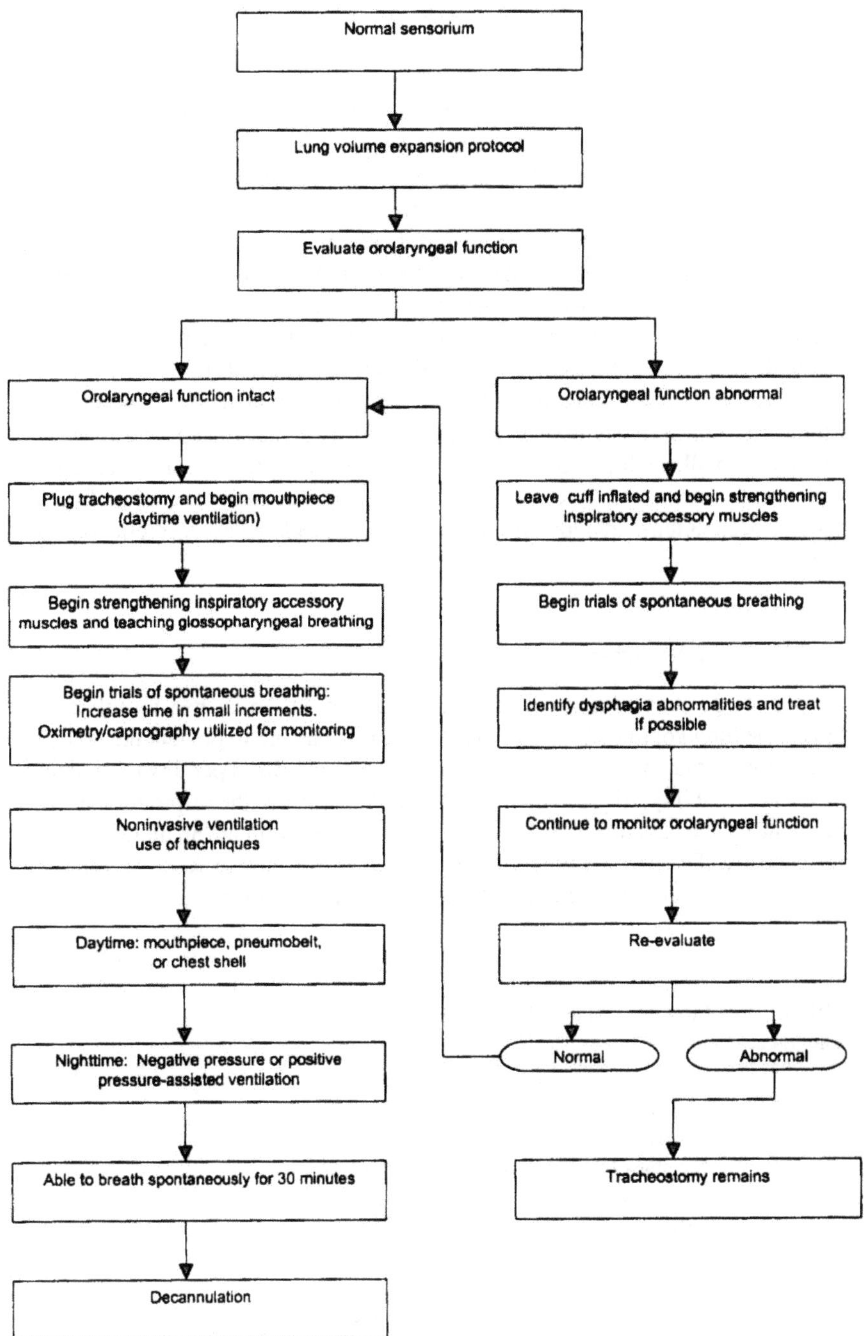

Figure 2 Switching from tracheostomy ventilation to noninvasive ventilation.

from ventilatory assistance. Figure 2 depicts switching from tracheostomy ventilation to noninvasive ventilation. Negative pressure ventilators, although effective, are less popular than in the past for reasons enumerated earlier.

Positive pressure ventilators are effective but require patient cooperation. The interfaces now used include commercial or custom-made nasal masks, oral masks that fit in the mouth using a custom made mouthpiece, or oronasal masks (Table 2). Air may leak around these masks resulting in an inadequate $\dot{V}_E$. Pressure necrosis of the skin on the bridge of the nose occurs with improper or excessively tight fittings. Aerophagia and gastric distention may occur, usually associated with excessive pressure settings on the ventilator (40,41).

Positive pressure ventilation is now the preferred method for intermittent ventilation, as it is less cumbersome, avoids the potential for upper airway obstruction, and allows for easier delivery of nursing care. The algorithms used rely on a team approach with integration of the nursing, respiratory therapy, physical therapy, occupational therapy, speech therapy, and behavioral medicine departments.

A. Lung Volumes

Intermittent positive pressure breathing (IPPB) or an Ambu bag is utilized to expand the lung volume. A 40-cm pressure limit is utilized to prevent the complication of barotrauma. This therapy is performed 4 to 6 times per day to maintain chest wall flexibility, to prevent atelectasis, and to improve the respiratory system compliance. The patient's exhaled volume is compared with the predicted inspiratory capacity. The optimal lung volume desired is assumed to be 80 to 100% of the predicted inspiratory capacity. This allows for maximum elastic recoil to help

Table 2 Interfaces for Commonly Used Noninvasive Ventilation

Appliances	Types
Nasal	Pillows
	Standard Goldseal™ (Respironics, Inc., Pittsburgh, PA)
	Custom
Oral	Bennett seal
Oronasal	SONI[a]
Full face	Standard Goldseal™ (Respironics, Inc.)
Mouthpiece	Curved tip mouthpiece

[a]Strapless oronasal interface.

with clearing of secretions, and the improvement in respiratory compliance allows for easier ventilation (42,43).

B. Oxygenation

Assuming that the patient had normal pre-morbid lung function and does not have significant problems with aspiration, the oxygen (O_2) saturation should be normal. Hypoxemia, thus, is secondary to ventilation-perfusion ratio (V/Q) abnormalities from atelectasis, inadequate lung expansion, and retained secretions. Oxygen supplementation is not unusual early on but should not be necessary after aggressive therapy.

C. Swallowing Evaluation

Prior to removal of the tracheostomy, adequate oropharyngeal function must be demonstrated to ensure that patients can manage their own secretions and not aspirate their feedings. The first step in determining oropharyngeal function involves a "blue dye test." This is performed by placing blue dye on the posterior portion of the tongue, deflating the tracheostomy cuff, and observing the tracheal secretions. If blue dye does not appear in the tracheostomy secretions, then the patients are assumed to have the ability to handle their own secretions.

Following an adequate blue dye test, a more formal examination of oromotor function is performed to determine the ability of the patients to eat. This examination, performed by the speech therapy department, consists of administering foods of various consistencies and textures mixed with contrast material to the patients who are being monitored by fluoroscopic techniques while swallowing. The patients with neurologic deficits from muscular dystrophy or postpolio syndrome are best studied late in the day to detect the effects of fatigue on muscular function. More recently, direct fiberoptic laryngoscopy also has been helpful in determining the function of the posterior pharynx and larynx.

Patients who aspirate their oral secretions are not candidates for decannulatization. Patients who handle their own secretions but demonstrate aspiration of food consistencies may be decannulated as long as they are not fed orally and have an adequate cough. These patients may, at first, have a tracheostomy button placed to allow urgent placement of the tracheostomy tube should the patients demonstrate aspiration that was not initially detected on the screening examination.

Should the patients continue to show drooling and lack of adequate oropharyngeal function, then the use of the foam-filled self-inflating tracheostomy tubes is effective in reducing aspiration and reducing the damage to the tracheal mucosa.

D. Behavioral Intervention

As discussed above, the cognitive level of the patient is critical to the success of noninvasive ventilation. Many of these patients have concurrent depression, especially in view of their long-term prognosis. Giving them the ability to talk and the potential for removal of the tracheostomy are invaluable for improvement in their self-esteem and sense of accomplishment (17).

E. Caregivers and Home Environment

The weaning process requires a concentrated effort by the patient and future caregiver. The present health care delivery system has insisted on shorter inpatient rehabilitation stays and more home therapy. Nursing homes cannot commit the necessary personnel to make this aggressive approach worthwhile. Consequently, if the postrehabilitation planning includes discharge to a nursing home, removal of a tracheostomy in a ventilator-dependent patient is not realistic.

F. Assisted Cough Techniques

Patients with neuromuscular weakness have difficulty clearing secretions. To assist in clearing secretions, two techniques are utilized. The assisted cough, as discussed earlier, is quite effective at enhancing the expectoration of secretions. With this method, the patients' lungs are expanded with IPPB or an Ambu bag to total lung capacity (TLC). The patient keeps the glottis closed between breaths to allow the breaths to be "stacked." Then, once TLC is reached, the therapist holds the chest wall with one forearm for stabilization and forcefully thrusts the other hand in the epigastric area, resulting in an increase in intra-abdominal pressure, which forces the diaphragm cephaled. This increases the alveolar pressure and results in a sudden increase in airflow (17,44,45).

A number of mechanical devices can also be used to enhance cough and secretion removal. One such device is the In-Exsufflator (J. H. Emerson Co., Cambridge, MA). This device insufflates the lungs with a positive pressure of 40 cm or more and then drops the pressure rapidly below atmospheric pressure (46–48) (see Chapter 12 for details).

Measurements of inspiratory and expiratory forces and lung volumes are helpful in guiding the need for ventilation. These measurements are also useful in judging the adequacy of therapy and in monitoring the status of these patients. For example, a drop in measured exhaled lung volume or inspiratory forces would suggest progressive muscle weakness and/or atelectasis.

The type of prescribed ventilation is dependent on the disease process. Partial ventilation is utilized to prevent carbon dioxide (CO_2) retention in patients with neuromuscular disorders. These patients typically are ventilated at night with a nasal, an oral, or an oronasal mask using positive pressure ventilation. Their clinical course is followed with arterial blood gases, spirometry, chest xrays, and measurement of inspiratory and expiratory forces. Full-time ventilation can be accomplished in several ways. Positive pressure ventilation may be achieved with a mouthpiece during the day and with a mask at night. Other patients may choose a cuirass ventilator or pneumobelt during the day and an iron lung, pneumowrap, or a shell ventilator at night when sleeping.

An important aspect of the transfer to noninvasive ventilation is respiratory muscle training, assuming that the primary disease is not a degenerative neuropathy or myopathy. Most often, respiratory muscle exercises utilize progressive resistance valves to train the muscles to be more efficient and powerful. These exercises are especially helpful in building the sternocleidomastoid, the scalenus, and the other accessory muscles of inspiration. These exercises are not indicated in patient with muscular dystrophy, amyotrophic lateral sclerosis, or postpolio syndrome because they cause more fatigue; however, they are extremely helpful in spinal cord injury patients (30). Inspiratory training techniques are also useful in patients with chronic obstructive lung disease.

We define inspiratory muscle weakness as the inability to generate at least 80% predicted maximal inspiratory force at residual volume. The diaphragm is the major contributor to this effort. Expiratory muscles are mostly abdominal muscles, intercostals, and sometimes the latissimus dorsi and pectoralis. Similarly, expiratory muscle weakness is defined as the inability to generate at least 80% of predicted maximum expiratory force. If patient's chest wall and lung mechanics are normal, gas exchange will not be significantly altered until the inspiratory force is reduced to 25% of its predicted value. The inspiratory capacity is not reduced unless the inspiratory force is less than 40 cm H_2O. Atelectasis tends to develop when the patient is unable to sigh fully. Similarly, if the expiratory force is decreased, the inability to cough and clear secretions may interfere with airflow and increase the likelihood of atelectasis and pulmonary infections.

We also utilize the inspiratory training techniques in patients with COPD. The exercise program consists of a volume spirometer for visual feedback and resistance valve devices calibrated from 5 to 80 cm H_2O/L/sec. Inspiratory exercises performed with graded resistance increase the inspiratory capacity (IC) by improving inspiratory muscle strength. Expiratory exercises utilizing graded resistance will help improve expiratory muscle strength and thus the efficacy of the cough.

The following calculations determine the resistance values utilized in respiratory muscle training. Pulmonary function tests and inspiratory and expiratory forces are obtained every 2 wk to adjust the values. To determine the inspiratory resistance values, the maximum inspiratory force obtained at residual volume (MIP) is multiplied by 10, 20, and 40% to obtain the low, medium, and high resistance values, respectively.

Example: MIP = 20 cm
[MIP] [%] = inspiratory resistance value

Values utilized:

Low resistance value	20 cm × 0.1 = 2 cm/L/sec
Medium resistance value	20 cm × 0.2 = 4 cm/L/sec
High resistance value	20 cm × 0.4 = 8 cm/L/sec

The expiratory resistance training values are determined by subtracting the patient's inspiratory capacity mulitpled by 10 from the maximum expiratory force at total lung capacity (MEP) and then multiplying that value by either 25, 75, or 100%.

Example: MEP = 20 cm
IC = 1.0 liter
Values utilized:

[MEP − (IC) (10)] [%] = expiratory resistance value
[20 cm − (1.0 l) (10)] [0.25] = 2.5 cm/L/sec low resistance valve
[20 cm − (1.0 l) (10)] [0.75] = 7.5 cm/L/sec medium resistance valve
[20 cm − (1.0 l) (10)] [1.00] = 10 cm/L/sec high resistance valve

This accessory muscle training program is performed twice daily. Too much resistance could result in fatigue of the accessory muscles.

Upon discharge, patients who cannot obtain their predicted normal volumes and have not reached a plateau in their strength or exhaled volumes are sent home on a program utilizing a disposable incentive spirometer (4000 ml capacity) and precalibrated (10 cm H_2O) resistive valves. The home program is monitored closely to prevent muscle fatigue. The patient is instructed to perform the exercise program daily. Spirometry and forces are tested during routine outpatient appointments.

VII. Tracheostomy Weaning

Ventilator-dependent patients with normal swallowing evaluations and who achieve 80 to 100% of their predicted lung volumes on the lung volume expansion protocol may be trained in mouthpiece ventilation with a curved mouthpiece that is connected to a positive pressure ventilator. The tidal volume is usually set at 5 to 6 ml/kg, the respiratory rate is set at 10 to 14 breaths per minute, and the tracheostomy is plugged. The patients utilize this mouthpiece ventilation technique for 10 to 15 min and then increase the time, as their tolerance allows.

Glossopharyngeal breathing is also taught during this time period as discussed above. Once this can be maintained for 30 min, aggressive efforts to remove the tracheostomy begin. During the day, different types of ventilation are introduced to assess their effectiveness.

At night, a nasal mask is usually tried first. If there is significant discomfort

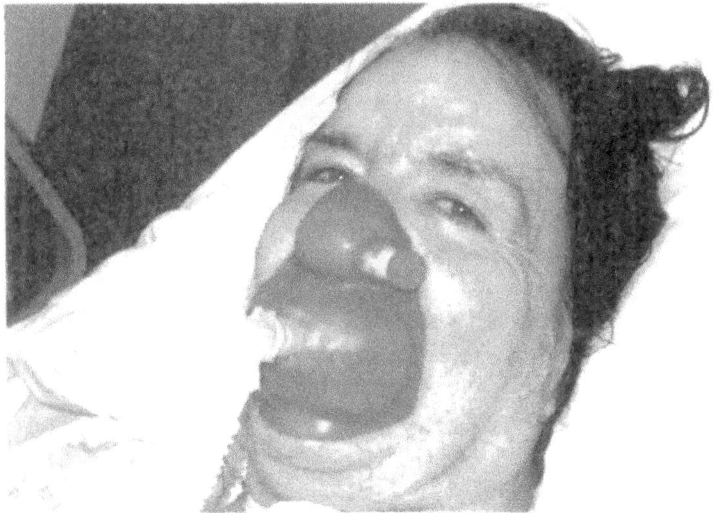

Figure 3 Strapless oral nasal interface (front view).

or leaks occur around the mask, then a custom nasal mask is fashioned. If there are oral leaks, a chin strap is applied. An oronasal mask is used when the oral leaks cannot be corrected. The oronasal mask consists of a bite wing, which is similar to a bite block that football players wear, that is connected to a molded acrylic cover. The strapless mask is held in place by placing the bite wing around the patient's teeth and is removed by opening the mouth and pushing the bite wing out with the tongue (Figs. 3 and 4). The original oral masks covered both the nose and the mouth and were strapped in place. However, they were somewhat dangerous if the patients had a mucus plug or vomited.

Once it is determined that the patient can be ventilated successfully with this technique, the tracheostomy tube is capped. Until the patient gains confidence, noninvasive ventilation is used during waking hours with the patient's cooperation. The time period is gradually increased until the patient is able to be fully ventilated using noninvasive means. The daytime techniques vary with the type of neurologic or muscle injury. For instance, a mouthpiece ventilator cannot be used effectively in patients who use a sip-and-puff wheelchair.

A pneumobelt is quite effective in daytime ventilation. It fits around the abdomen and contains an inflatable rubber bladder. When the bladder is inflated by the positive pressure ventilator, it compresses the abdominal viscera, forcing the diaphragm upward, causing exhalation. Gravity then returns the diaphragm to its resting level, which results in inspiration as it causes a negative pressure

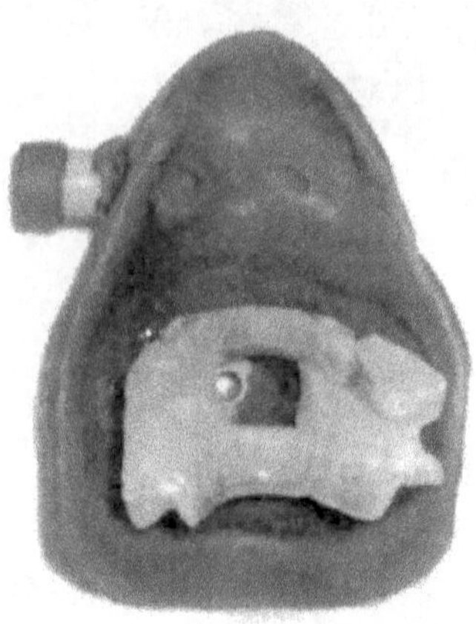

Figure 4 Strapless oral nasal interface (inside view).

in the alveolus. To be effective, the patient must be in a sitting position, or at least in a 30° reclining position (49).

A cuirass ventilator can be used in a sitting or supine position. The shell fits around the chest and is connected to a negative pressure generator (3). The amount of negative pressure required is dependent on the compliance of the respiratory system. (Table 3)

Once the patient has demonstrated the ability to be ventilated round the clock with the tracheostomy cannula capped, the cannula is removed. A tracheos-

Table 3 Commonly Used Ventilators for Conversion to Noninvasive Ventilation

Type of ventilator	Examples
Negative pressure	Iron lung
	Poncho
	Shell
Positive pressure	Bilevel PAP
	Volume-cycled/time-cycled
Abdominal displacement	Pneumobelt
	Rocking bed

tomy "button" is placed to keep the stoma open for emergency placement of an airway and to reassure the patient that a tracheostomy cannula could be emergently replaced. After several days, with the patient's permission, the "button" is subsequently removed. Only those patients who can sustain adequate ventilation on their own for at least 30 min are decannulated (see Figs. 1 and 2).

As the nutritional status, chest wall compliance, and accessory muscle strength improve, spontaneous breathing trials are introduced. These are gradually increased as tolerated, assuming that patients do not have a progressive neurologic disease. Patients who require only intermittent ventilation are treated in much the same manner but can be converted to noninvasive ventilation much more rapidly because they have some capability of spontanous ventilation function.

Patients with acute spinal cord injuries can be treated with noninvasive techniques to obviate a tracheostomy altogether. Since our institution is a rehabilitation center, the patients are usually transferred several days to weeks after their acute injury, but a tracheostomy can be deferred even in the acute setting if patients are able to handle their oral secretions, have adequate cognitive function, and do not have significant O_2 needs. Patients can be placed in an iron lung with the endotracheal tube still in place, rather than undergo a tracheostomy. If they can easily be ventilated in the iron lung, then the endotracheal tube can be removed. Patients using the iron lung must be carefully observed for signs of upper airway obstruction once the endotracheal tube is removed. Mouthpiece ventilation is introduced so patients can be switched to positive pressure ventilation and improve accessibility to nursing care.

The types of ventilators and ventilation interfaces for noninvasive intermittent positive pressure ventilation for any particular patient are chosen with input from the therapists, care providers, and the patients. Daytime ventilation is usually achieved using a mouthpiece or a pneumobelt. This is accomplished with the use of a portable ventilator. We like to use battery-powered systems that can be transported on the back of a wheelchair. In our facility, we have experience with portable volume-limited and pressure-limited ventilators. For patients requiring nocturnal ventilation only, a bilevel PAP unit may be adequate to support their ventilation needs, assuming normal lung compliance.

After assessing the patient's tolerance for cuff deflation, the patient is introduced to mouthpiece ventilation and insufflation IPPB techniques. Most patients prefer using the pneumobelt as a method of alternative ventilation during the daytime hours. The pneumobelt may be concealed under clothing and also allows patients to talk and use their mouths for activities such as operating a sip-and-puff wheelchair or a computer mouth stick.

For nocturnal ventilation, most patients prefer positive pressure ventilation through a nasal or oronasal interface. A selection of nasal pillows, nasal masks, and full-face masks are available in the market today. For patients with significant oral air leaks, a soft collar, padded wire collar (Freeman collar), or a chin strap may be used. If the leak persists and ventilation is not effective, we will try to use an oronasal mask, and in some occasions we will use a strapless oronasal mask.

Patients are initially placed on a nasal mask during the daytime hours when attempting nasal ventilation. This trial may last from 5 min to as long as 1 to 2 hr. Once the patient has demonstrated the ability to use a nasal interface for 1 hr, a nocturnal ventilation trial will then be instituted. A commercial nasal mask is initially used to evaluate the patient's tolerance to this ventilation modality. Considerations for interface selection include skin integrity, amount of leakage, ventilation pressure, compliance, and patient ability to remove the interface.

We utilize two styles of custom masks at our facility. The most common mask is the "Lyon" nasal mask created of a puttylike silicone material (Otoform-K) and directly molded by placing the material over the patient's nose to form an impression. The Lyon mask is held in place by two elastic straps creating a less restrictive headgear and is more comfortable. The custom fit of the Lyon mask reduces the risk of skin breakdown and encourages patient compliance. This mask remains functional for 1 to 3 yr before it needs to be replaced.

The customized Strapless Oral Nasal Interface (SONI) is utilized for patients who desire more independence in their ventilation management. Patients with significant oral leakage that cannot be managed by the traditional chin strap and/or collar for support may also be candidates for this custom mask. There are three parts to the production of this mask. First a dental impression is obtained to create the "bite splints" that hold the mask in place. Then an impression of the patient's face is molded using Alginate and Dentsone. Once dried, Triad Composite (hybrid) is added and cured with an ultraviolet light. In the final step, the bite splint is attached to the custom mask. It is important that the patient be able to remove the mask by using the tongue to dislodge the teeth from the bite splint. The life expectancy of the SONI is approximately 1 to 2 yr.

VIII. Conclusion

Overall, noninvasive ventilation is a successful modality in patients with chronic respiratory failure. It allows patients the ability to maintain the integrity of the upper airway, to humidify the air and filter particles, and to preserve the ability to speak, while decreasing the risk of respiratory infections and tracheal complications. Noninvasive ventilation in selected ventilator-dependent patients improves their quality of life without increasing the risk of respiratory complications.

References

1. Hill NS. Clinical applications of body ventilators. Chest 1986; 90:897.
2. Bach JR, Penek J. Obstructive sleep apnea complicating negative pressure ventilatory support in patients with chronic paralytic restrictive ventilatory dysfunction. Chest 1991; 99:1386.
3. Shneerson JM. Negative pressure ventilation. Home Mechanical Ventilation. Proceedings of the 4th International Conference on Home Mechanical Ventilation, March, 1993, Lyon, France.
4. Hill NS, Redline S, Carskadon MA, et al. Sleep-disordered breathing in patients with Duchenne muscular dystrophy using negative pressure ventilators. Chest 1992; 102:1656.
5. Brown L, Kinnear W, Sergeant KA, Shneerson JM. Artificial ventilation by external negative pressure: A method for manufacturing cuirass shell. Physiotherapy 1985; 71:181–183.
6. Spalding JMK, Opie L. Artificial respiration with the Tunnicliffe breathing-jacket. Lancet 1985; 1:613–615.
7. Curran JF, Colbert AP. Ventilator management in Duchenne muscular dystrophy and postpoliomyelitis syndrome: Twelve years' experience. Arch Phys Med Rehabil 1989; 70:180–185.
8. Shneerson JM. Disorders of Ventilation. Oxford: Blackwell Scientific, 1988.
9. Alba AS, Khan A, Lee M. Mouth IPPV for Sleep. Rehabil Gazette 1981; 24:47–49.
10. Bach JR, Alba AS, Bohatiuk G, Saporito L, Lee M. Mouth intermittent positive pressure ventilation in the management of postpolio respiratory insufficiency. Chest 1987; 91:859–864.
11. Baydur A, Gilgoff I, Prentice W, Carlson M, Fisher DA. Decline in respiratory function and experience with long-term assisted ventilation in advanced Duchenne muscular dystrophy. Chest 1990; 97:884–889.
12. Segall D. Noninvasive nasal mask-assisted ventilation in respiratory failure of Duchenne muscular dystrophy. Chest 1988; 93:1298–1300.
13. Anthonisen NR. The Intermittent Positive Pressure Breathing Trial Group. Intermittent positive pressure breathing therapy of chronic obstructive pulmonary disease. Ann Intern Med 1983; 99:612–620.
14. Fabbri M, Galavotti V, Sturani C, Bassein L, Fasano L, Bunella G. Long-term home treatment with noninvasive mouth positive pressure ventilation in COPD patients with chronic alveolar hypoventilation. Consensus Conference on Recommendation for Home Mechanical Ventilation, Arona, Italy, February 7–8, 1991.
15. Rigaud-Bully C. Comparison of methods of organization of home mechanical ventilation in different countries. Home Mechanical Ventilation. Proceedings of the 4th International Conference on Home Mechanical Ventilation, March, 1993, Lyon, France.
16. Hill NS. Noninvasive nasal positive pressure ventilation: Management and monitoring. Home Mechanical Ventilation. Proceedings of the 4th International Conference on Home Mechanical Ventilation, March 1993, Lyon, France. Arnette Blackwell SA.

17. Viroslav J, Rosenblatt RL, Tomazevik S. Respiratory management, survival, and quality of life for high-level traumatic tetraplegics. Respir Care Clin North Am 1996.
18. Stauffer JL, Olson DE, Petty TL. Complications and consequences of endotracheal intubation and tracheostomy: A prospective study of 150 critically ill adult patients. Am J Med 1981; 70:65–76.
19. Niederman MS, Ferranti RD, Ziegler A, et al. Respiratory infection complicating long-term tracheostomy: The implication of persistent gram-negative tracheobronchial colonization. Chest 1984; 85:39–44.
20. Buckwalter JA, Sasaki CT. Effect of tracheotomy on laryngeal function. Otolaryngol Clin North Am 1984; 17:41–48.
21. El-Kilany SM. Complications of tracheostomy. Ear Nose Throat J 1980; 59:123–129.
22. Sinha R, Bergofsky EH. Prolonged alteration of lung mechanics in kyphoscoliosis by positive pressure hyperinflation. Am Rev Respir Dis 1972; 106:47–56.
23. Jackson AB, Groomes TE. Incidence of respiratory complications following spinal cord injury (abstr). J Am Paraplegia Soc 1991; 14:87.
24. Lisboa C, Moreno R, Fava M, Ferretti R, Ganz E. Inspiratory muscle function in patients with severe kyphoscoliosis. Am Rev Respir Dis 1985; 132:48–52.
25. Estenne M, Heilporn A, Delhez L, Yernault JC, de Troyer A. Chest wall stiffness in patients with chronic respiratory muscle weakness. Am Rev Respir Dis 1983; 128:1992–1997.
26. Ellis ER, Grunstein RR, Chan S, Bye PT, Sullivan CE. Noninvasive ventilatory support during sleep improves respiratory failure in kyphoscoliosis. Chest 1988; 94: 811–815.
27. Leger P, Jennequin J, Gerard M, Robert D. Home positive pressure ventilation via nasal mask for patients with neuromuscular weakness or restrictive lung or chest wall deformities. Respir Care 1989; 34:73–77.
28. Goldstein RS, Derosie JA, Avendano MA, Domage TE. Influence of noninvasive positive pressure ventilation on inspiratory muscles. Chest 1991; 99:408–415.
29. Hill NS, Eveloff SE, Carlisle CC, Goff SG. Efficacy of nocturnal nasal ventilation in patients with restrictive thoracic disease. Am Rev Respir Dis 1992; 145:365–371.
30. Aubier M. Physiological basis of noninvasive ventilation. Negative pressure ventilation. Home Mechanical Ventilation. Proceedings of the 4th International Conference on Home Mechanical Ventilation, March, 1993, Lyon, France.
31. Lerman RM, Weiss MS. Progressive resistive exercises in weaning high tetraplegics from the ventilator. Paraplegia 1987; 25:130–135.
32. Gilgoff IS, Barras DM, Jones MS, et al. Neck breathing: A form of voluntary respiration for the spine-injured ventilator-dependent quadriplegic child. Pediatrics 1988; 82:741–745.
33. Bach JR, Alba AS, Bodofsky E, et al. Glossopharyngeal breathing and non-invasive aids in the management of post-polio respiratory insufficiency. Birth Defects 1987; 23:99–113.
34. Strohl KP, Redline S. Nasal CPAP therapy, upper airway muscle activation, and obstructive sleep apnea. Am Rev Respir Dis 1986; 135:555–558.

35. Lundqvist C, et al. Spinal cord injuries. Spine 1991; 16:78–83.
36. DeJong G, Wenker T. Attendant care of a prototype independent living service. Caring 2:26–30.
37. Dail CW, Affeldt JR, Collier CR. Clinical aspects of glossopharyngeal breathing. JAMA 1953; 158:445.
38. Vitacca M, Rubini F, Foglio K, et al. Noninvasive modalities of positive pressure ventilation improved the outcome of acute exacerbations in COLD patients. Intens Care Med 1993; 19:450.
39. Marrleo W. Intermittent volume cycled mechanical ventilation via nasal mask in patients with respiratory failure due to COPD. Chest 1991; 99:681–684.
40. Bach JR, Alba AS, Saporito LR. Interfaces for non-invasive intermittent positive pressure ventilatory support in North America. Eur Respir Rev 1993; 3:254.
41. Bach JR, McDermott I. Strapless oral-nasal interfaces for positive pressure ventilation. Arch Phys Med Rehabil 1990; 71:908–911.
42. Barois A, Estournet-Mathiaud B. Ventilatory support in children with spinal muscular atrophies. Eur Respir Rev 1992; 2(10):319–322.
43. Duvre-Beaupere G, Barois A, Quinet I, Estournbet B. Les problemes thoraciques rachidiens et respiratories de l'enfant atteint d'amyotrophie spinale infatile á évolution prolongéem. Arch Fr Pdiatr 1985; 42:625–634.
44. Jaeger RJ, Turba RM, Yarkony GM, et al. Cough in spinal cord injured patients: Comparison of three methods to produce cough. Arch Phys Med Rehabil 1993; 75: 1358.
45. Massery MP. An innovative approach to assistive cough techniques. Top Acute Care Trauma Rehabil 1987; 1:73.
46. Bach JR. Mechanical insufflation-exsufflation: Comparison of peak expiratory flows with manually assisted and unassisted coughing techniques. Chest 1993; 104:1553.
47. Barach AL, Beck GJ. Exsufflation with negative pressure: Physiologic and clinical studies in poliomyelitis, bronchial asthma, pulmonary emphysema and bronchiectasis. Arch Intern Med 1954; 93:825.
48. Bach JR, Smith WH, Michaels J, et al. Airway secretion clearance by mechanical exsufflation for post-poliomyelitis ventilator-assisted individuals. Arch Phys Med Rehabil 1993; 74:170.
49. Adamson JP, Lewis L, Stein JD. Application of abdominal pressure for artificial respiration. JAMA 1959; 169:1613.

35. Lundqvist C, et al. Spinal cord injuries. Spine 1991; 16:78–83.
36. [illegible] long-term care of a [illegible] patient using [illegible] [illegible]
37. Dail CW, Affeldt JE, Collier CR. Clinical aspects of glossopharyngeal breathing. JAMA 1955; 158:445.
38. Vitacca M, Rubini F, Foglio K, et al. Non-invasive modalities of positive pressure ventilation improve the outcome of acute exacerbations in COLD patients. Intens Care Med 1993; 19:450.
39. Marino W. Intermittent volume cycled mechanical ventilation via nasal mask in patients with respiratory failure due to COPD. Chest 1991; 99:681–684.
40. Bach JR, Alba AS, Saporito LR. Interfaces for non-invasive intermittent positive pressure ventilatory support in North America. Eur Respir Rev 1993; 3:254.
41. [illegible]
42. [illegible]
43. [illegible]
44. [illegible]
45. Massery M. [illegible]
46. [illegible]
47. [illegible]
48. Bach JR, Smith WH, Michaels J, et al. Airway secretion clearance by mechanical exsufflation for post-poliomyelitis ventilator assisted individuals. Arch Phys Med Rehabil 1993; 74:170.
49. [illegible] Application of [illegible] pressure for artificial respiration. JAMA 1939; [illegible]

12

Use of Respiratory Muscle Aids in Prevention of Respiratory Failure

JOHN R. BACH and ALICE C. TZENG

University of Medicine and Dentistry–New Jersey Medical School
Newark, New Jersey

I. Definition of the Problem

Although normal tidal volumes are under 1000 mL, an average cough involves the expulsion of 2.3 to 2.5 L of air. To achieve these volumes the vital capacity (VC) should, therefore, be at least 2.5 L (1). Normal peak cough flows (PCFs) are 6 to 16 L/sec and minimum PCFs of 160 L/m are required to cough out airway secretions (2). To achieve normal cough flows, the abdominal, internal intercostal, and accessory expiratory muscles normally generate over 200 cm H_2O of thoracoabdominal pressure to create the forces required to expel air at these flows upon glottic opening. Although patients with chronic obstructive pulmonary disease (COPD) can usually attain adequate inspiratory volumes for coughing, the inspissation of airway secretions and the collapse of airways with the generation of high thoracoabdominal pressures often prevent them from adequately expelling airway mucus. Very often, airway collapse in these patients prevents PCFs from attaining 160 L/m, the minimum flow necessary to eliminate airway secretions (2). For the majority of patients with the conditions listed in Table 1, however, the lungs and airways are normal, but inspiratory and expiratory muscle weakness results in failure to autonomously attain adequate PCFs to effectively eliminate airway secretions.

Table 1 Conditions Causing Primarily Ventilatory Impairment with Functional Bulbar Musculature

Myopathies
Muscular dystrophies
Dystrophinopathies—Duchenne and Becker dystrophies
Other muscular dystrophies—limb-girdle, Emergy-Dreifuss, facioscapulohumeral, congenital, childhood autosomal recessive, and myotonic dystrophy
Non-Duchenne myopathies
Congenital, metabolic, inflammatory
Diseases of the myoneural junction like myasthenia gravis
Neurologic disorders
Anterior horn cell diseases, such as spinal muscular atrophy, motor neuron disease, and poliomyelitis
Neuropathies such as Guillain-Barré Syndrome
Central nervous system disorders such as multiple sclerosis and Friedrich's ataxia
Myelopathies, including spinal cord injury
Restrictive lung disorders
Obesity hypoventilation syndrome
Following lung resection
Primary skeletal deformity, as from kyphoscoliosis or osteogenesis imperfecta
Central and congenital hypoventilation syndromes

There is much debate in the medical literature about the indications for introduction of nocturnal nasal intermittent positive pressure ventilation (IPPV) for patients with inspiratory muscle dysfunction. There is also considerable debate concerning how to use noninvasive IPPV to avoid intubation, when tracheostomy tubes should be placed for ventilatory support, and to what degree financial and ethical issues should be taken into regard when making these decisions (3). All of these questions fail to consider that the acute respiratory failure that develops during intercurrent upper respiratory tract infections in patients with severe respiratory muscle dysfunction because of inability to effectively cough out airway secretions can most often be managed noninvasively in the home (4).

For patients with COPD and restrictive pulmonary diseases such as pulmonary fibrosis, the use of inspiratory and expiratory muscle aids has not been shown to improve long-term clinical outcomes. However, for patients with primarily ventilatory impairment, unless inspiratory and expiratory muscle aids are used, secretions are retained in the lungs, atelectasis occurs, oxyhemoglobin saturations (Sao_2) levels decrease, pneumonia develops, and the patient seeks attention for acute respiratory failure. Thus, expiratory muscle dysfunction, which is usually more severe than inspiratory muscle dysfunction (5), most often plays the key role in the development of acute respiratory failure. Patients with most of the diagnoses listed in Table 1 are at risk for episodic respiratory failure in this manner. For the great majority of these patients, proper use of respiratory muscle aids can eliminate episodes of respiratory failure and the need for hospitalization or intubation with eventual tracheostomy.

II. Conventional Management

For patients with severe respiratory muscle dysfunction at risk of developing life-threatening "chest colds" with profuse airway secretion, current management strategies include:

1. Not treating hypercapnic ventilatory insufficiency and expiratory muscle dysfunction at all but, rather, obtaining a "living will" or other decree interdicting the use of invasive interventions
2. Not treating hypercapnic ventilatory insufficiency and expiratory muscle dysfunction until an episode of acute respiratory failure leads to hospitalization and intubation, and tracheostomy becomes the most palatable ethical option, after management with some combination of oxygen, bronchodilators, theophylline, chest physical therapy, intubation, and attempts at ventilator meaning fail
3. The use of "prophylactic" tracheostomy
4. Using nocturnal nasal IPPV to possibly delay tracheostomy

The first two strategies, the most commonly used in the past (6), essentially ignore the problem. In a recent survey that we performed of Jerry Lewis Muscular Dystrophy Association clinic directors, we found that with few exceptions nothing is being done to prevent episodes of respiratory failure. More clinic directors reported being biased against the use of ventilators than being favorably disposed or impartial to their use. Many directors are now using nocturnal low span bilevel positive airway pressure but are not using full noninvasive ventilatory support or noninvasive expiratory as well as inspiratory aids during respiratory tract infections. Most directors still usually associate ventilator use with intubation and tracheostomy. Thus, the great majority of patients are not fully informed about noninvasive treatment options when consenting to or refusing endotracheal intubation or tracheostomy. Those who refuse "prophylactic" tracheostomy must inevitably develop respiratory failure.

It is inappropriate to treat patients with primarily ventilatory impairment as though they have primarily lung disease or oxygenation impairment. Methylxanthine administration does not alleviate "diaphragm fatigue" or make any clinical difference for patients with primarily ventilatory impairment (7). Indeed, in the presence of hypercapnia and hypoxia, theophylline appears to delay recovery from diaphragm fatigue (8) and side effects are common. Bronchodilators are frequently used despite a lack of subjective or objective benefits for most of these patients. Bronchodilators often cause anxiety by worsening the tachycardia that is most often present in these patients, many of whom have cor pulmonale or cardiomyopathy on the basis of generalized myopathic disease.

Although it significantly improves the survival of hypoxic patients with COPD, oxygen administration to patients whose hypoxia is secondary to inspiratory muscle weakness results in exacerbation of hypercapnia and symptoms of hypercapnia, and an increased incidence of respiratory failure, hospitalizations, and hospitalization days by comparison with patients who are treated with respiratory muscle aids or who are not treated at all (4). Instead of the primary focus being on chest physical therapy, the focus should be on helping the patient generate sufficient PCF to eliminate airway secretions. Likewise, since ventilator users with indwelling tracheostomy tubes have a higher incidence of respiratory complications and hospitalizations than patients who use either part-time or full-time noninvasive IPPV (4), and since only a small minority of patients with neuromuscular disease should ever require an indwelling tracheostomy tube, prophylactic tracheostomy is inappropriate.

Although there are numerous publications concerning the nocturnal use of nasal IPPV by patients with hypercapnia secondary to inspiratory muscle weakness, nocturnal nasal IPPV is often used at inadequate bilevel positive airway pressure spans to adequately assist inspiration as generalized muscle weakness progresses. Likewise, as weakness progresses, daytime inspiratory muscle assistance becomes necessary and expiratory muscles need to be assisted to clear airway secretions during intercurrent chest colds. It is not surprising that studies limited to nocturnal-only nasal IPPV that ignore the need to assist clearance of airway secretions fail to demonstrate avoidance of tracheostomy or death for patients with primarily ventilatory impairment (9,10).

III. Patient Evaluation

The evaluation of patients with respiratory muscle weakness includes the use of spirometry to measure VC (in sitting and recumbent positions), maximum insufflation capacity (MIC), glossopharyngeal breathing (GPB) tidal volumes and maximum GPB single breath capacity, assisted PCF, Sao_2, and end-tidal Pco_2. The VC in the supine position is important because, in the presence of predominantly diaphragm weakness, it is much less than when one is sitting. Since patients' hypoventilation is often worse during sleep than when awake, this VC measurement tends to better signal the need to introduce nocturnal noninvasive IPPV.

The MIC is the maximum volume of air that can be stacked into the lungs or the maximum single breath insufflation that the patient can receive and hold with a closed glottis. It can also be attained by using GPB or some combination of GPB and air stacking. Air stacking is the receiving and holding of consecutive volumes of air delivered via a manual resuscitator or volume-triggered ventilator.

Peak cough flow is measured by having the patient cough through a peak flow meter (Fig. 1). If the lips are too weak to grab a mouthpiece to cough through, the patient can cough through an anesthesia mask. Once unassisted PCF is noted, assisted PCF is measured. Since patients with severe respiratory muscle impairment almost always require assistance to cough out airway secretions, the assisted rather than the unassisted PCF is the most important. Anyone with a VC below 1.5 L first air stacks or receives a maximal insufflation, holds it with a closed glottis, then expels it as the expiratory muscles are manually assisted (see later section on expiratory muscle aids).

Besides measuring the Sa_{O_2} and end-tidal P_{CO_2} with the patient awake, nocturnal Sa_{O_2} monitoring is also warranted to justify the institution of nocturnal noninvasive IPPV for symptomatic patients with ventilatory impairment. Oximeters that monitor and print out trends should be used. An appropriate oximeter

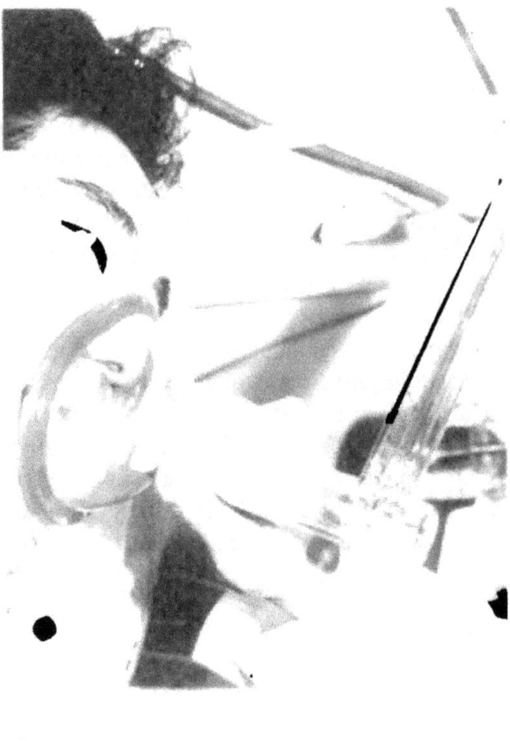

Figure 1 Both autonomous and assisted PCF are measured by having the patient cough through a peak flow meter. For the latter, an abdominal thrust is timed to glottic opening after a maximal insufflation has been provided.

(e.g., Datex-Ohmeda 3760, Louisville, CO) will give the percentages of time that Sao_2 is less than 90, 85, 80, and 70%, as well as the low Sao_2s and the hourly and nocturnal saturation means.

Full polysomnography is warranted for patients with progressive neuromuscular disease only when they are complaining of symptoms characteristic of sleep-disordered breathing in the presence of a normal daytime Sao_2 and end-tidal Pco_2 and a VC that is too high to explain the symptoms. This is rare for patients with neuromuscular conditions but it can occur for patients with spinal cord injury (SCI). Since respiratory failure almost invariably occurs during intercurrent respiratory tract infections and patients usually have minimal symptoms until these occur, and since many will eventually require continuous noninvasive IPPV for the rest of their lives, it is important not to encumber them with nocturnal continuous positive airway pressure (CPAP) or ventilator use too early because of asymptomatic sleep-disordered breathing.

IV. Respiratory Muscle Aids

Inspiratory and expiratory muscle aids are devices and techniques that involve the manual or mechanical application of forces to the body or intermittent pressure changes to the airway to assist inspiratory or expiratory muscle function. The devices that act on the body include the negative pressure body ventilators that create atmospheric pressure changes around the thorax and abdomen, body ventilators and exsufflation devices that apply force directly to the body to mechanically displace respiratory muscles, and devices that apply intermittent pressure changes directly to the airway.

Certain positive pressure ventilators or blowers have the capacity to deliver CPAP. Likewise, certain negative pressure generators or ventilators that can be used to operate a chest shell or tank-style ventilator can create continuous negative extrathoracic pressure (CNEP). Continuous positive airway pressure and CNEP act as pneumatic splints to help maintain airway and alveolar patency and to increase functional residual capacity. They do not directly assist respiratory muscle activity. These techniques are ineffective for patients with primarily ventilatory impairment and will no longer be considered in this chapter.

A. Glossopharyngeal Breathing

Both inspiratory and, indirectly, expiratory muscle function can be assisted by glossopharyngeal breathing (GPB) (11). This technique, first recognized and described in the early 1950s as an aid for coughing (12,13), involves the use of the glottis to add to the inspiratory effort by projecting (gulping) boluses of air into the lungs. The glottis closes with each "gulp." One GPB breath usually consists of 6 to 9 gulps of 60 to 100 mL each. During the training period, the efficiency of GPB can be monitored by spirometrically measuring the milliliters of air per gulp, gulps per breath, and breaths per minute (Fig. 2).

Glossopharyngeal breathing can provide up to many hours of freedom from the ventilator for individuals with no ventilator-free breathing ability and safety in the event of sudden ventilator failure day or night (11,14). Although severe oropharyngeal muscle weakness can limit the usefulness of GPB, we and others (15) have reported its effective use in some Duchenne muscular dystrophy ventilator users and many others with very weak bulbar musculature. Approximately 60% of ventilator users with no ventilator-free breathing ability and good bulbar muscle function (14,16) can have ventilator-free periods by using GPB.

Although potentially extremely useful, GPB is rarely taught since there are few health care professionals familiar with the technique. Glossopharyngeal breathing is also rarely useful in the presence of an indwelling tracheostomy tube. It cannot be used when the tube is uncapped, as it is during tracheostomy IPPV. Even when the tube is capped, the gulped air tends to leak around the outer walls of the tube and out through the stoma as airway volumes and pressures increase

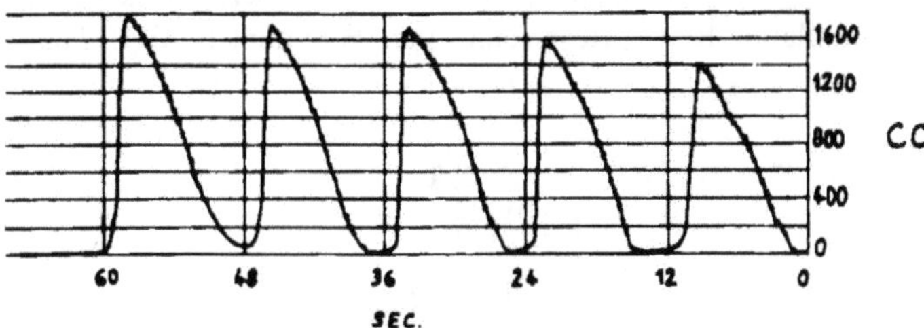

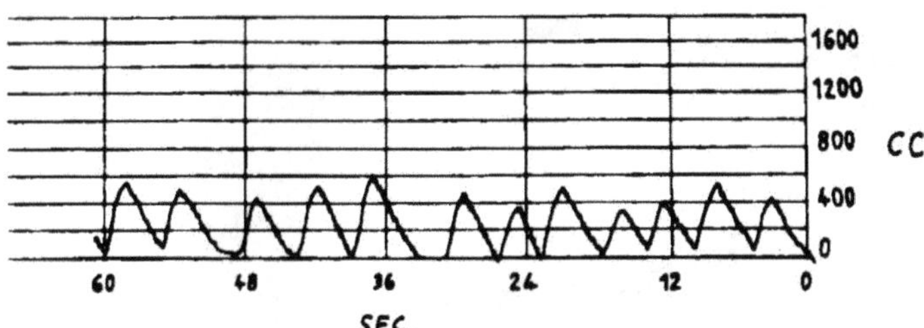

Figure 2 (Top) Maximal GPB minute ventilation 8.39 L/min, GPB inspirations average 1.67 L, 20 gulps, 84 mL/gulp for each breath in a patient with a vital capacity of 0 mL. (Bottom) Same patient, regular GPB minute ventilation 4.76 L/min, 12.5 breaths, average 8 gulps per breath, 47.5 mL/gulp performed over a 1-min period. (From Ref. 11.)

during the air stacking process of GPB. The safety and versatility afforded by effective GPB are key reasons to eliminate tracheostomy in favor of noninvasive aids.

B. Inspiratory Muscle Aids

Body Ventilators

Inspiratory muscle aids are used as an alternative to endotracheal delivery of IPPV for both ventilatory support and to provide the deep breaths needed to facilitate coughing, to raise voice volume, and to expand the lungs. Although the rocking bed and negative pressure body ventilators (Fig. 3) are noninvasive aids and were the first widely used ventilatory support methods, their use is rarely warranted at this time except during tracheal extubation and conversion to noninvasive IPPV methods (17), and possibly as a break from noninvasive IPPV for infants requiring continuous noninvasive IPPV.

The intermittent abdominal pressure ventilator (IAPV) or "pneumobelt" is a respiratory muscle aid that can provide normal alveolar ventilation for some individuals with little or no measurable VC. It involves the intermittent inflation of an elastic air sac that is contained in a corset worn beneath the patient's outer clothing (Exsufflation Belt™, Respironics Inc., Westminster, CO). The sac is in-

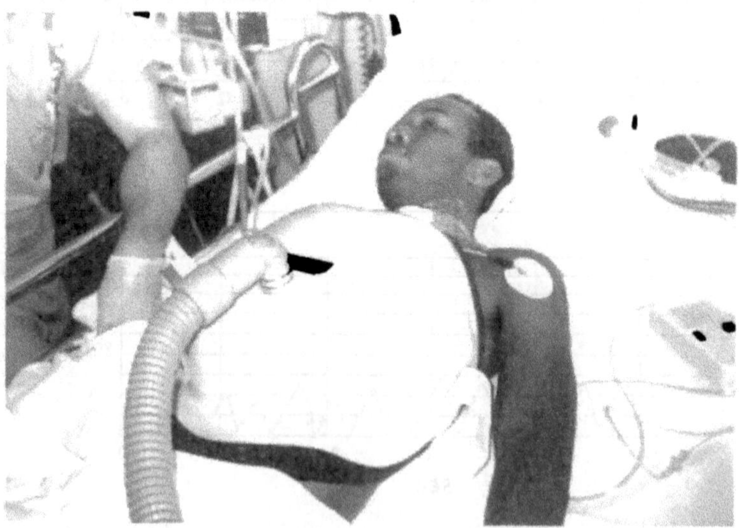

Figure 3 A chest shell ventilator is an example of a negative pressure body ventilator. The subatmospheric pressure generated around the chest and abdomen causes air to enter the patient's lungs.

flated by a positive pressure ventilator. Bladder action moves the diaphragm upwards causing a forced exsufflation. During bladder deflation the abdominal contents and diaphragm return to the resting position and inspiration occurs passively. A trunk angle of 30° or more from the horizontal is necessary for it to be effective. If patients have any inspiratory capacity or are capable of GPB, they can add autonomously generated tidal volumes to the mechanically assisted inspiration. The IAPV generally augments tidal volumes by about 300 ml, but volumes as high as 1200 mL have been reported (18). When sitting, patients with less than 1 hr of ventilator-free breathing ability usually prefer to use the IAPV rather than noninvasive methods of IPPV (18). The IAPV optimizes patient appearance, function, and mobility. It is often inadequate in the presence of scoliosis or obesity. It has the advantage of freeing the mouth from mouthpiece IPPV for the performance of mouth stick activities.

Mouthpiece IPPV

Noninvasive IPPV methods are better tolerated, more effective, and more convenient than negative pressure body ventilators. As opposed to negative pressure body ventilator use, which tends to cause obstructive apneas during sleep (19), noninvasive IPPV methods tend to stabilize the airway by creating a positive pressure upper airway splint.

Intermittent positive pressure ventilation delivered via a mouthpiece has been used by many individuals with progressive neuromuscular conditions for up to 24-hr ventilatory support for decades (20). Because of its versatility, effectiveness, practicality, and convenience for up to 24 hr of use, mouthpiece IPPV may be the most important method of noninvasive ventilation for patients requiring continuous ventilatory support. Along with use of the intermittent abdominal pressure ventilator, it is the method of choice for daytime ventilatory support.

The mouthpiece should be fixed onto the motorized wheelchair chin, tongue, or sip-and-puff controls. For wheelchairs not having these controls, it should be positioned adjacent to the mouth and held in place by a gooseneck clamp attachment to the wheelchair frame (Fig. 4). With progression of weakness, and perhaps guided by oximetry feedback (21), patients require additional hours per day of mouthpiece IPPV use each year to maintain adequate ventilation during daytime hours.

Ventilator users may also choose to use mouthpiece IPPV overnight with lipseal retention (Fig. 5) (20). The lipseal retains the mouthpiece firmly in the mouth during sleep and it can seal off the mouth to prevent oral leakage of ventilator-delivered air (insufflation leakage). In our experience, this technique has the advantage of normalizing alveolar ventilation during sleep. Fewer oxyhemoglobin desaturations occur than with nocturnal use of nasal IPPV, although the two have not been compared in a controlled study (20). Likewise, sleep quality may

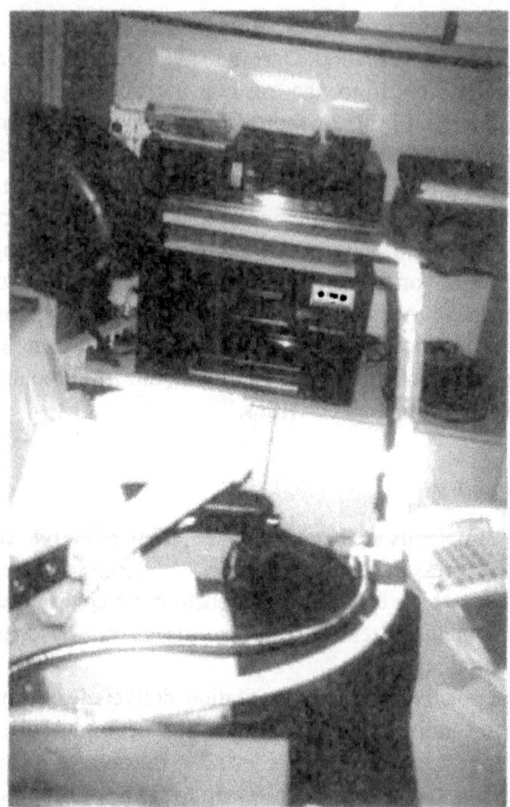

Figure 4 The delivery of mouthpiece IPPV via a mouthpiece fixed in place on a wheelchair to be within grasp of the patient's mouth.

be better when using lipseal IPPV than with the open system of nasal IPPV. For a few patients, seal of the nostrils with cotton pledgets has been used to create a closed system of ventilatory support, similar to that of tracheostomy IPPV with an inflated cuff.

Nasal IPPV

Patients usually prefer to use nasal rather than lipseal IPPV for nocturnal ventilatory support (22). In 1982, as an alternative to mouthpiece IPPV for "resting" the inspiratory muscles of muscular dystrophy patients in France, DeLaubier, Rideau, and Bach delivered IPPV via the nostrils (23). In 1984, nasal IPPV was first used for 24-hr ventilatory support for a patient with a VC of 100 ml and no

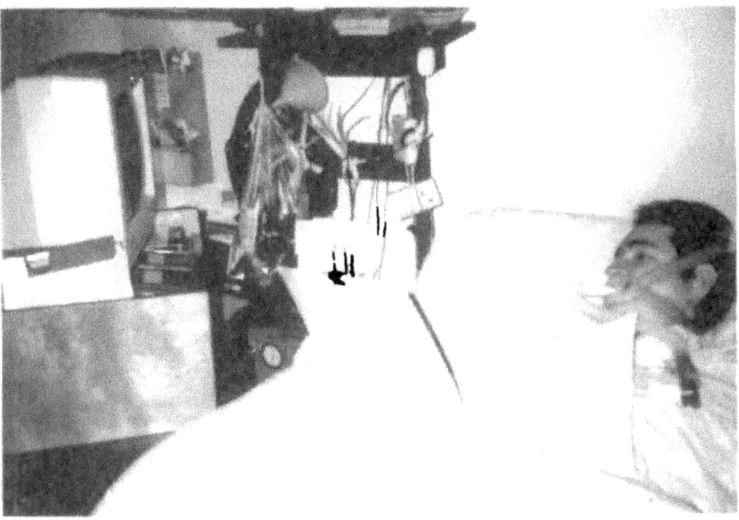

Figure 5 Mouthpiece IPPV with lipseal retention.

ventilator-free breathing ability (24). Nasal CPAP masks (nasal interfaces) also became commercially available in 1984. Commercially available nasal interfaces now include numerous varieties and sizes. Each design applies pressure differently to the nasal area. It is impossible to predict which one will be preferred by any particular nasal IPPV user. The user should, therefore, have the opportunity to try at least three or four varieties of nasal masks to determine the ones that are most comfortable and leak-free while acknowledging that the complete elimination of leak around the mask is unnecessary. Many people alternate nasal interfaces nightly to vary skin contact pressure. Skin contact pressure and insufflation leakage into the eyes, common complaints with several of these generic models, may warrant the fabrication of custom-molded nasal interfaces and oral–nasal shells (Fig. 6) (25). Custom-molded nasal interfaces can now be obtained both commercially (SEFAM Co., distributed by Respironics, Inc., Pittsburgh, PA) and individually (see Fig. 6) (25). Although usually only preferred for nocturnal use or when the patient is in bed, nasal IPPV has been used for up to 24 hr a day by ventilator users whose lips or neck are too weak to accommodate daytime mouthpiece IPPV.

Strapless Oral–Nasal Interfaces

In addition to the possibility of offering mouthpiece and nasal IPPV alternatives to intubation and tracheostomy, strap-retained oral–nasal interfaces and custom-

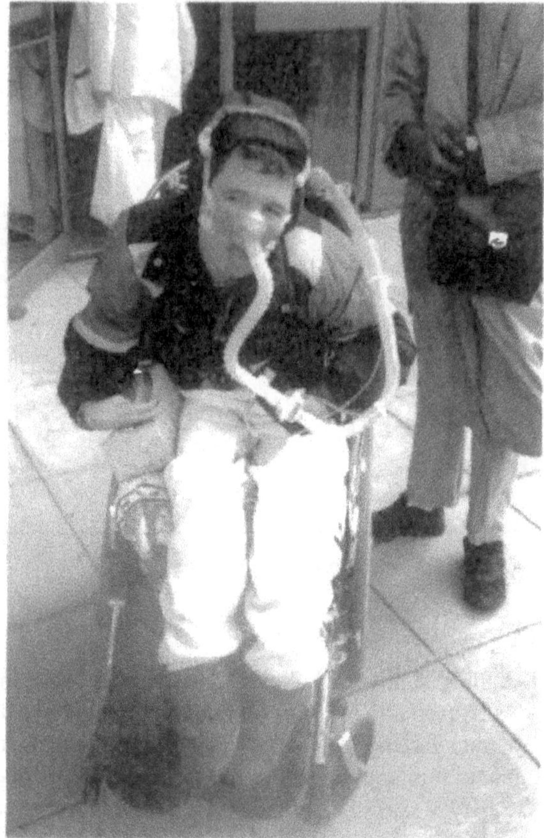

Figure 6 Custom acrylic low-profile nasal interface (25).

molded strapless acrylic oral-nasal interfaces have been used for nocturnal support (25). The latter are retained by a bite-plate that is fastened to an outer shell, essentially an acrylic lip and nose seal, by metal clasps. It may be thrust out of the mouth by simple tongue movement. This interface is indicated for ventilator users who live alone and who have some upper extremity function but insufficient function to don the straps of strap-retained interfaces. The disadvantages are expense and need for stable dentition.

Ventilators for Noninvasive IPPV

The great majority of earlier publications on noninvasive IPPV used portable volume-triggered ventilators. Most recent publications, however, have used portable pressure-limited devices such as the BiPAP® (Respironics, Inc.) devices to deliver nocturnal nasal ventilation (26). These devices were developed to improve compliance in patients with obstructive sleep apneas requiring high CPAP levels. By using higher inspiratory pressures and minimizing expiratory pressures, it became apparent that these machines could function as ventilators. For some patients, such as those with obesity hypoventilation with severely restricted VC, with inspiratory muscles inadequate to maintain normal lung ventilation, and inability to tolerate high expiratory pressures, pressure-limited ventilators have limitations. Even using the maximum inspiratory pressures available from these devices may be inadequate to normalize alveolar ventilation for these patients, many of whom eventually develop respiratory failure and undergo tracheostomy.

The use of portable volume-triggered ventilators, on the other hand, can deliver set volumes of air under high pressures. Not only can this be important for patients with stiff lungs or chest walls who require air delivery at higher pressures to normalize lung ventilation, but it is also important to provide the deep insufflations that are intermittently needed to expand the lungs to raise voice volume, maintain lung compliance, prevent atelectasis, and augment PCF. The advantages and disadvantages of portable pressure-limited versus volume-limited ventilators are noted in Table 2.

C. Expiratory Muscle Aids

The expiratory (cough) muscles can be manually or mechanically assisted. One manually assists expiratory muscle function by giving a sharp thrust to the abdomen (Fig. 7) after the patient has taken a breath to over 2.5 L or receives a maximal insufflation. Usually, the palms of each hand are placed under the rib cage on each side and the thrust is posterior and cephalad. If the patient is sitting or has a small abdomen, a thrust from the palm of one hand placed on the epigastrum might be sufficient. Counterpressure across the chest can also increase assisted PCF for some patients. Practice coordinating the care provider's abdominal thrusts to the patient's glottic opening following a maximal insufflation is important to maximize cough flows. Assisted PCFs are often many times greater than unassisted PCFs for patients with respiratory muscle weakness (27).

Patients for whom PCFs cannot exceed 270 L/m are at high risk of developing pneumonia and acute respiratory failure during intercurrent chest colds (21). Although most patients with advanced neuromuscular weakness or SCI cannot independently generate PCFs of over 270 L/m, most can do so with assistance. Patients who cannot generate PCFs of over 160 L/m, even with manually assisted coughing, will require intubation to clear airway secretions when present and will often be better off undergoing tracheostomy (2). The inability to generate over 160 L/m of assisted PCF despite having an MIC greater than 1 L usually indicates upper airway obstruction or severe bulbar muscle weakness and hypo-

Table 2 Portable Pressure- Versus Volume-Targeted Ventilators

Advantages of volume ventilators
1. Can deliver higher pressures to achieve higher volumes as needed for patients with poor lung compliance
2. Have adjustable flow rates for comfort
3. Use 3 to 8 times less electricity for comparable air delivery, permitting greater patient mobility for the same battery capacity
4. Quieter than some pressure-limited devices
5. Permit air stacking to obtain maximum insufflations for raising voice volume and increasing cough flows
6. Some can be used to operate intermittent abdominal pressure ventilators as well as for noninvasive IPPV
7. Have alarm system that can enhance safety during use of continuous noninvasive IPPV

Disadvantages of volume ventilators
1. Heavier
2. Annoying alarms (low-pressure alarm can be eliminated by setting alarm to minimum and using flexed mouthpiece or a regenerative humidifier)
3. More complicated to use

Advantages of BiPAP® (Respironics Inc., Pittsburgh, PA)
1. No annoying alarms
2. Lightweight, more portable
3. Less cost
4. Can compensate for insufflation leaks

Disadvantages of BiPAP
1. Inability to air stack
2. High flow rates during leaks can cause mouth drying and arousals from sleep
3. High power utilization limits duration under battery power
4. Inadequate pressure generation capabilities for some patients
5. Lack of alarms may be less safe in patients requiring continuous IPPV
6. Some devices are noisier
7. Significant CO_2 rebreathing may occur; this can be corrected by using a nonrebreathing valve at the cost of greater expiratory resistance

Source: Adapted from Ref. 55.

pharyngeal collapse. Vocal cord adhesions or paralysis may have resulted from a previous transtracheal intubation or tracheostomy. Since some lesions, especially the presence of obstructing granulation tissue, are amenable to surgical correction, laryngoscopic examination is warranted. When PCFs can exceeed 160 L/m, safe tracheostomy tube removal and conversion to noninvasive ventilatory support is possible irrespective of the extent of respiratory muscle dysfunction (14,16).

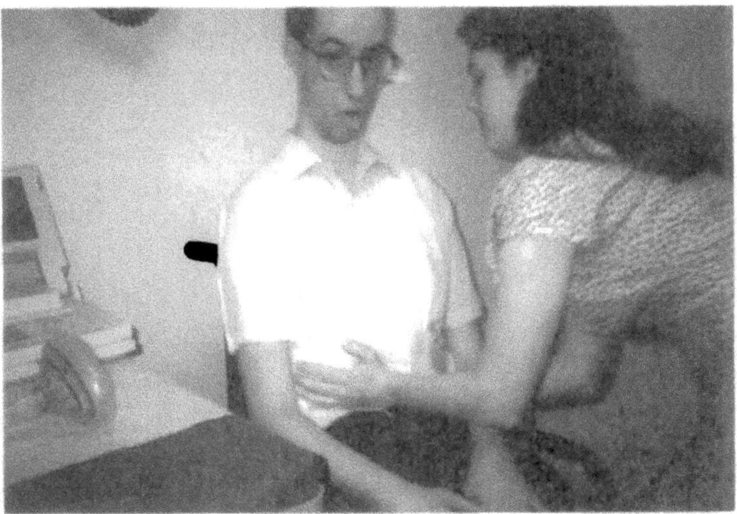

Figure 7 A manually assisted cough.

For patients with respiratory muscle weakness, both assisted and unassisted PCFs are diminished following general anesthesia and during intercurrent chest colds because of fatigue, and temporary weakening of both inspiratory and expiratory muscles (28), and bronchial mucus plugging. These factors can decrease VC and Sao_2. Concomitant weakness of oropharyngeal muscles exacerbates the problem. The higher the assisted PCFs and the better the function of the bulbar musculature, the greater the ability to clear airway secretions. This enhances the long-term prospects for using noninvasive IPPV alternatives to tracheostomy. The attainment of adequate PCFs is the most important goal for preventing serious pulmonary complications in these patients (2).

Patients with severe scoliosis may also have poor PCFs because of a combination of restricted lung capacity and the inability to effect sufficient diaphragm movement by abdominal thrust because of severe rib cage deformity. Unlike patients with fixed upper airway obstruction, these patients can often benefit considerably from the use of mechanical insufflation–exsufflation.

Mechanically Assisted Coughing

Mechanical insufflation–exsufflation (In-Exsufflator, J. H. Emerson Co., Cambridge, MA) involves the use of a device to deliver a deep insufflation (Fig. 8) followed by a rapid exsufflation. Typically, pressures range from +40 cm H_2O during insufflation to −40 cm H_2O during exsufflation or a drop of about 80 cm

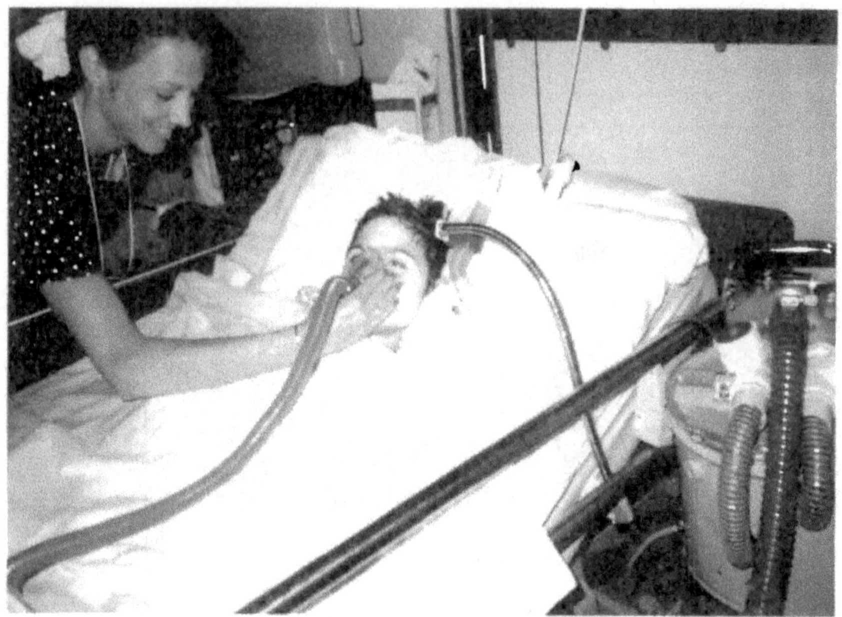

Figure 8 The application of mechanical insufflation–exsufflation via the upper airway.

H_2O. The resulting 6 to 10 L/sec of expiratory flow expulses airway debris and secretions (27). In doing so, the VC and Sao_2 increase to pre–mucus plug levels. For most patients, unless a meal has been taken during the previous hour or two, an abdominal thrust should also be timed with the exsufflation phase (27).

The mechanical insufflation–exsufflation can be delivered via an oral–nasal interface, mouthpiece, or endotracheal or tracheostomy tube. When provided via an indwelling tube it can be more effective than suctioning because suction catheters usually fail to enter the left mainstem bronchus so it is difficult to clear the left airways (29). When used via a tube, the tube's cuff should be inflated.

Mechanical insufflation–exsufflation should be used with caution for acutely injured high-level spinal-cord–injured individuals, who are susceptible to suction-induced bradycardias, and the insufflation pressures should be increased gradually for patients who have not been receiving maximal insufflations. Failure to perform the latter can result in painful intercostal muscle pulls. Despite hundreds of patient-years of experience in its use and many thousands of applications, however, no serious untoward effects have been reported.

Mechanical Oscillation Techniques

Chest wall oscillation was first used for patients with chronic bronchial asthma and emphysema in 1966 (30). Oscillation applied to the chest, adbdomen, or directly to the airway has been noted to enhance mucociliary transport (31). High-frequency chest wall compression to anesthetized dogs at 11 to 15 Hz was found to increase the tracheal mucus clearance rate (32). For the Hayek oscillator, a device that can apply high-frequency chest wall oscillation, the inspiratory–expiratory ratio (I/E) can be adjusted to permit asymmetric inspiratory and expiratory times and pressures, e.g. +3 to −6 cm H_2O, that bias exsufflation to enhance secretion mobilization. Baseline pressures can be set at negative, atmospheric, or positive values to provide oscillation above, at, or below the functional residual capacity. Mucociliary clearance in anesthetized sheep receiving exsufflation-biased oscillation to the airway at 15 Hz with peak expiratory flows of 3.8 L/sec and peak inspiratory flows of 1.3 L/sec was greatly affected by posture. It was 3.5 mL/10 min in the horizontal position and 11 mL/10 min with a head-down tilt. No clearance occurred with inspiratory-biased high-frequency oscillation during head-down tilt (33). Using a hand-held internal airway percussor (Bird Corp., Exeter, UK) that delivers 30-mL sine wave oscillations through a mouthpiece at 20 Hz improved tracheobronchial clearance significantly as measured by inhaled radioaerosol (34).

Intrapulmonary percussive ventilation (IPV) has been reported to be more effective than chest percussion in the treatment of postoperative atelectasis and secretion mobilization in COPD patients (35). The Percussionator, Impulsator, and Spanker respirators (Percussionaire Corp., Sandpoint, Idaho) can deliver aerosolized medications while providing high flow mini-bursts of air to the lungs at a rate of 2 to 7 Hz. In one study on 20 patients, sputum volume and forced vital capacity increased during regular use of IPV and the majority of the patients felt that the treatments were helpful (36). Intrapulmonary percussive ventilation is being used in certain centers by patients with neuromuscular weakness; however, no studies have compared IPV with mechanical insufflation–exsufflation, a modality that can be used manually at the same pressures and frequencies. Further study is needed to establish how the theoretical benefits of high-frequency oscillations and related techniques will translate to clinical benefits for humans.

V. Clinical Goals

A. Prevention of Chest Tightness

Although incentive spirometers are often given to patients with restrictive pulmonary syndromes, their use has never been shown to be beneficial for these patients.

On the other hand, a basic physical medicine intervention is to provide range of motion exercises to hypomobile tissues; that is, to put each joint through what would be its normal range of motion. This principle is particularly important to apply to the lungs and chest walls of patients with diminishing VC.

A program of providing increasing insufflations with the goal of attaining the patient's predicted inspiratory capacity is often warranted. Short periods of mild mechanical hyperinflation can briefly increase dynamic pulmonary compliance (37). However, late in the course of the disease, the static compliance of the lung tissues themselves has not been shown to improve by applying range of motion to musculoskeletal articulations of the chest wall (38). Thus, although confirmatory data are lacking, maximum insufflations are recommended on a daily basis earlier in the course of the disease before the VC decreases below 50% of predicted.

Deep insufflation methods include air stacking by GPB, air stacking using a manual resuscitator or volume-targeted ventilator delivered tidal volumes (11), and the delivery of maximal single insufflations from a portable volume-targeted ventilator. The air can be delivered via a mouthpiece, nasal interface, or mouthpiece with a lipseal if the buccal muscles and glottis are too weak to grasp a mouthpiece or retain a deep insufflation with open delivery systems. Insufflation volumes should be increased gradually as tolerated to approach the predicted normal inspiratory capacity (39,40). There is some evidence that regular lung hyperinflation can have a beneficial effect on VC (41,42).

B. Protocol to Maintain Normal Lung Ventilation and Clear Airways

"Permissive hypercapnia" may be a useful strategy in mechanically ventilating patients with severe lung pathology. However, for patients with primarily ventilatory impairment, hypercapnia sufficient to decrease baseline Sa_{O_2} below 95% usually results in symptoms and greatly increases the risk of pulmonary morbidity and hospitalizations for acute respiratory failure (4). Whether or not used in conjunction with nocturnal noninvasive IPPV, sedatives, narcotics, and oxygen should be used only with extreme caution in such patients, and should rarely be administered in the home. Oxygen should not be used as an alternative to noninvasive IPPV. These modalities should usually only be considered when intubation is indicated. One should always first attempt to correct hypoxia by normalizing blood CO_2 levels with noninvasive IPPV before considering oxygen supplementation or intubation for IPPV.

As lung restriction and hypoventilation progress, respiratory chemoreceptors reset, ventilatory drive falls, right ventricular strain occurs, and resort to noninvasive IPPV used only at night becomes less successful. Noninvasive IPPV, the most practical and effective noninvasive method of ventilatory support, works in concert with central-nervous-system–mediated muscle activity that is depressed in the presence of hypercapnia (43). Thus, the primary goal of physical medicine intervention is to maintain adequate alveolar ventilation around the clock by noninvasive means. The oximeter can be used to estimate alveolar ventilation and screen for severe hypercapnia provided that supplemental oxygen is not administered.

A management protocol has been developed and shown to be effective (21) for avoiding episodes of acute respiratory failure and the need for hospitalization and tracheostomy for patients with the diagnoses listed in Table 1 who can attain at least 160 L/m of assisted PCF. These patients are taught that decreases in Sao_2 below 95% indicate either hypoventilation or bronchial mucus plugging and that these must be corrected to prevent atelectasis, pneumonia, and respiratory failure. To accomplish this, the following is instituted:

1. As the VC decreases to 50% of predicted, the patient is instructed to air stack or use multiple maximal insufflations from a manual resuscitator three times a day to maintain pulmonary compliance and maximum insufflation capacity. It is important for the clinician to know that patients who can air stack via a mouthpiece or nasal interface are capable of using noninvasive IPPV for up to 24 hr a day, as necessary, as an alternative to intubation for IPPV.
2. When assisted PCF decreases to 270 L/m or below, patients are trained in manually assisted coughing and in mechanical insufflation-exsufflation. They are also prescribed an oximeter and instructed to check the Sao_2 whenever short of breath, unusually fatigued, and most importantly, during intercurrent respiratory infections. It not already using noninvasive IPPV, they are promptly provided with a portable volume ventilator, various mouthpieces, nasal interfaces, a lipseal, and a mechanical insufflator-exsufflator (21). They are instructed to immediately reverse all decreases in baseline Sao_2 below 95% by using ventilatory assistance and assisted coughing. In this manner, most potential hospitalizations are avoided. There are now many long-term 24-hr ventilator users who have never been hospitalized or undergone tracheostomy.

Following continuous use of noninvasive IPPV during respiratory infections, patients often wean to nocturnal noninvasive IPPV, or occasionally they discontinue ventilator use until their next episode of profuse airway secretion and ventilatory failure. It is at this time that oximetry feedback can be especially useful to signal how much daytime aid is required to maintain normal Sao_2, and by presumption, adequate alveolar ventilation.

Patients who hypoventilate can have prolonged periods of Sao_2 less than 95%. Patients are shown that by increasing breathing rate, depth, or both, the Sao_2 can be normalized, and alveolar ventilation, therefore, improved. Patients learn that they cannot keep up the effort required to accomplish this all day without using noninvasive IPPV. As weakness progresses over time and relief of chronic fatigue by noninvasive IPPV is appreciated, many individuals gradually use these techniques for increasing periods of time as they age. They see that with occasional deep insufflations they can maintain Sa_{O_2} over 95%. During the training period, an alarm can be set to sound when the Sa_{O_2} decreases below an unacceptable level, for example 95%, to remind the patient to take a few mouthpiece IPPV–assisted breaths.

Overnight ventilatory assistance is usually needed when the supine VC diminishes to about 30% of predicted (44). In reality, however, most individuals remain free of ventilator use, albeit at the expense of hypercapnia and fatigue, until a chest cold causes respiratory distress and signals the need for noninvasive IPPV. Patients are motivated to use nocturnal noninvasive IPPV on an ongoing basis only when they have obvious symptomatic relief or when nocturnal mean Sa_{O_2} is demonstrated to have increased. Although, with time, the need for noninvasive IPPV often extends to 24 hr a day, this is neither felt to cause significant inconvenience for the ventilator user (45), nor does it necessitate institutionalization (4). Thus, most of our patients use noninvasive IPPV for the first time during intercurrent respiratory tract infections and gradually increase use on their own.

VI. Sudden Onset of Physical and Ventilatory Disability

The most common conditions that cause sudden onset and permanent respiratory muscle dysfunction are traumatic SCI, Guillain-Barré syndrome, and acute poliomyelitis, rarely seen today. Respiratory complications are the most common causes of death in the acute post-SCI period and account for 14% of long-term mortality for SCI individuals (46). For all SCI patients, regardless of spinal level, the incidence of ventilatory failure is 22.6% and it develops an average of 4.5 days following admission (47). Ventilatory failure lasts an average of 5 wk. About 4% of ventilator-supported patients remain ventilator-dependent. Long-term SCI tracheostomy IPPV users have been reported to have 67% mortality by 5 yr post-discharge (46).

Of the over 500,000 people afflicted with paralytic poliomyelitis in the United States from 1928 through 1962 (48), about 15% developed ventilatory failure, severe swallowing impairment, or both (49). About 12.5% of these remained ventilator-assisted (49). Today, however, there are many more late-onset postpolio ventilator users than people who have remained ventilator users since the onset of polio (50).

A. Preventive Interventions

Most SCI patients who experience ventilatory failure do so 12 or more hr after hospital admission. Thus, noninvasive IPPV can be used to avoid intubation provided that the patient is cooperative and medically stable, does not have severe lung trauma or disease, and the upper airway is clear to facilitate the use of manually and mechanically assisted coughing as needed. Spirometry should be performed every 8 hr and oximetry monitored continuously. Patients with decreasing VC, especially below 1500 mL, should be placed on regular maximum tolerated insufflations via a mouthpiece for regular lung expansion. If dyspnea and hypercapnia occur, the patient should also be assisted by mouthpiece or nasal IPPV as needed. Oxygen therapy should be avoided unless the Sao_2 baseline decreases despite the effective use of noninvasive IPPV and assisted coughing, or hypoxia associated bradycardia occurs. Continuous SaO_2 monitoring serves as an indicator of lung ventilation and the extent of airway mucus plugging provided that oxygen administration is avoided. When oxygen supplementation is also usually indicated. However, for many SCI patients and others with sudden onset ventilatory failure, intubation can be avoided by this protocol of noninvasive IPPV and manually and mechanically assisted coughing. Even if intubation and ultimately tracheostomy are deemed necessary, the patient should be considered for decannulation and transition to noninvasive IPPV once clinical stability has been restored.

VII. Ventilator Weaning by Decannulation

In the mid-1950s a long debate ensued as to whether tracheostomy or body ventilators were preferable for long-term ventilatory support. In 1955, an International Consensus Symposium defined the indications for tracheostomy as the combination of respiratory insufficiency with swallowing insufficiency and disturbance in consciousness or vascular disturbances (51). "If a patient is going to be left a respirator cripple with a very low VC, a tracheotomy may be a great disadvantage. It is very difficult to get rid of a tracheotomy tube when the VC is only 500 or 600 cc and there is no power of coughing, whereas, as we all know, a patient who has been treated in a respirator (iron lung) from the first can survive and get out of all mechanical devices with a VC of that figure" (51). It was recognized that once an individual with a low VC underwent tracheostomy, the person was very likely to quickly become dependent on ventilatory support around the clock, whereas an individual with the same VC who used a body ventilator overnight could often go without ventilatory assistance throughout daytime hours. Unfortunately, this phenomenon is not widely appreciated.

There are many reasons that patients receiving IPPV via indwelling tracheostomy tubes require more prolonged ventilator use than patients receiving noninvasive IPPV. Patients receiving tracheostomy IPPV often tend to develop high minute ventilation requirements. This results in chronic hypocapnia that the patient finds impossible to maintain when not using the ventilator (52). Patients with tracheostomy tubes also have chronic production of airway secretions that hamper autonomous breathing efforts. There may also be a tendency for patients receiving tracheostomy IPPV to have deconditioning of inspiratory muscles because they initially receive IPPV for longer periods than necessary, whereas mouthpiece IPPV users take assisted breaths only when THEY feel the need. For all of these reasons, once a patient has an episode of acute respiratory failure and undergoes tracheostomy, the patient very often becomes dependent on continuous ventilatory support. Patients who have no ventilator-free breathing ability while invasively ventilated most often wean to nocturnal-only use after then are extubated or decannulated and switched to noninvasive IPPV. Following decannulation, many of these patients with as little as 10 to 20% of predicted normal VC wean entirely from daytime use of mechanical ventilation. Although they tend to be mildly hypercapnic during daytime hours, their Sao_2s remain within normal limits provided that they continue to use noninvasive IPPV every night. Any patients who have had complications related to their indwelling tracheostomy tubes should be considered candidates for decannulation and transition to using noninvasive IPPV. However, this approach is particularly attractive for patients who have the potential to master GPB. It should also be strongly considered for all patients with SCI, non-Duchenne myopathies, non-infantile spinal muscular atrophies, and nonbulbar amyotrophic lateral sclerosis.

VIII. Conclusion

In summary, tracheostomy and intubation are rarely necessary unless PCF is below 160 l/m. Noninvasive IPPV methods are the preferred methods of ventilatory support by patients and caregivers (53) and can greatly reduce the cost of home mechanical ventilation (54). Adaptive equipment and other assistive devices can facilitate activities of daily living for even the most severely affected individuals (55). Ventilator users with primarily ventilatory impairment express greater life satisfaction and have less risk of pulmonary morbidity and need for hospitalization when maintained by noninvasive rather than tracheostomy IPPV (45).

References

1. Leith DE. Cough. In: Brain JD, Proctor D, Reid L, eds. Lung Biology in Health and Disease: Respiratory Defense Mechanisms. Part 2. New York: Marcel Dekker, 1977; 545–592.
2. Bach JR, Saporito LR. Criteria for extubation and tracheostomy tube removal for patients with ventilatory failure: A different approach to weaning. Chest 1996; 110: 1566–1571.

3. Bach JR, Barnett V. Ethical considerations in the management of individuals with severe neuromuscular disorders. Am J Phys Med Rehabil 1994; 73:134–140.
4. Bach JR, Pansit R, Ballanger F, Kulessa R, Ishikawa Y. Neuromuscular ventilatory insufficiency: The effect of home mechanical ventilator use vs. oxygen therapy on pneumonia and hospitalization rates. Am J Phys Med Rehabil (in press).
5. Johnson E, ed. Profiles of neuromuscular diseases. Am J Phys Med Rehabil 1995; 74:S70–159.
6. Bach JR. Ventilator use by muscular dystrophy association patients: An update. Arch Phys Med Rehabil 1992; 73:179–183.
7. Moxham J: Aminophylline and the respiratory muscles: An alternative view. Clin Chest Med 1988; 9:325–336.
8. Esau SA: The effect of theophylline on hypoxic, hypercapnic hamster diaphragm muscle in vitro. Am Rev Respir Dis 1991; 143:954–959.
9. Raphael J-C, Chevret S, Chastang C, Bouvet F. Randomised trial of preventive nasal ventilation in Duchenne muscular dystrophy. Lancet 1994; 343:1600–1604.
10. Bach JR: Misconceptions concerning nasal ventilation (letter). Lancet 1994; 344: 752.
11. Bach JR, Alba AS, Bodofsky E, Curran FJ, Schultheiss M. Glossopharyngeal breathing and non-invasive aids in the management of post-polio respiratory insufficiency. Birth Defects 1987; 23:99–113.
12. Dail CW, Affeldt JE: Glossopharyngeal breathing (video). Los Angeles: Department of Visual Education, College of Medical Evangelists, 1954.
13. Feigelson CI, Dickinson DG, Talner NS, Wilson JL: Glossopharyngeal breathing as an aid to the coughing mechanism in the patient with chronic poliomyelitis in a respirator. N Engl J Med 1956; 254:611–613.
14. Bach JR: New approaches in the rehabilitation of the traumatic high level quadriplegic. Am J Phys Med Rehabil 1991; 70:13–20.
15. Baydur A, Gilgoff I, Prentice W, Carlson M, Fischer A: Decline in respiratory function and experience with long-term assisted ventilation in advanced Duchenne's muscular dystrophy. Chest 1990; 97:884–889.
16. Bach JR: New approaches in the rehabilitation of the traumatic high level quadriplegic. Am J Phys Med Rehabil 1991; 70:13–20.
17. Bach JR. Update and perspectives on noninvasive respiratory muscle aids. Part 1. The inspiratory muscle aids. Chest 1994; 105:1230–1240.
18. Bach JR, Alba AS. Total ventilatory support by the intermittent abdominal pressure ventilator. Chest 1991; 99:630–636.
19. Bach JR, Penek J. Obstructive sleep apnea complicating negative pressure ventilatory support in patients with chronic paralytic/restrictive ventilatory dysfunction. Chest 1991; 99:1386–1393.
20. Bach JR, Alba AS, Saporito LR. Intermittent positive pressure ventilation via the mouth as an alternative to tracheostomy for 257 ventilator users. Chest 1993; 103: 174–182.
21. Bach JR, Ishikawa Y, Kim H. Prevention of pulmonary morbidity for patients with Duchenne muscular dystrophy. Chest 1997; 112:1024–1028.
22. Bach JR, Sortor S, Saporito LR. Interfaces for non-invasive intermittent positive pressure ventilatory support in North America. Eur Respir Rev 1993; 3:254–259.

23. Delaubier A. Traitement de l'insuffisance respiratoire chronique dans les dystrophies musculaires. In: Memoires de certificat d'etudes superieures de reeducation et re-adaptation fonctionnelles. Paris: Universite R Descarte, 1984; 124.
24. Bach JR, Alba AS, Mosher R, Delaubier A. Intermittent positive pressure ventilation via nasal access in the management of respiratory insufficiency. Chest 1987; 92: 168–170.
25. McDermott I, Bach JR, Parker C, Sortor S. Custom-fabricated interfaces for intermittent positive pressure ventilation. Int J Prosthodont 1989; 2:224–233.
26. Bach JR. Conventional approaches to managing neuromuscular ventilatory failure. In: Bach JR, ed. Pulmonary Rehabilitation: The Obstructive and Paralytic Conditions. Philadelphia: Hanley & Belfus, 1996; 285–301.
27. Bach JR. Mechanical insufflation-exsufflation: Comparison of peak expiratory flows with manually assisted and unassisted coughing techniques. Chest 1993; 104:1553–1562.
28. Mier-Jedrzejowicz A, Brophy C, Green M. Respiratory muscle weakness during upper respiratory tract infections. Am Rev Respir Dis 1988; 138:5–7.
29. Fishburn MJ, Marino RJ, Ditunno JF. Atelectasis and pneumonia in acute spinal cord injury. Arch Phys Med Rehabil 1990; 71:197–200.
30. Beck GJ. Chronic bronchial asthma and emphysema rehabilitation and use of thoracic vibrocompression. Geriatrics 1966; 21:139–158.
31. Chang HK, Harf A. High-frequency ventilation: A review. Respir Physiol 1984; 57: 135–152.
32. King M, Phillips DM, Gross D, Vartian V, Chang HK, Zidulka A. Enhanced tracheal mucus clearance with high frequency chest wall compression. Am Rev Respir Dis 1983; 128:511–515.
33. Freitag L, Long WM, Kim CS, Wanner A. Removal of excessive bronchial secretions by asymmetric high-frequency oscillations. J Appl Physiol 1989; 67:614–619.
34. George RJD, Geddes DM. High frequency oscillations and mucociliary transport. Biomed Pharmacother 1989; 43:25–30.
35. Toussaint M, De Win H, Steens M, Soudon P. A new technique in secretion clearance by the percussionaire for patients with neuromuscular disease (abstr). In: Programme des Journées Internationales de Ventilation à Domicile. Lyon, France: Hopital de la Croix Rousse, 1993; 27.
36. McInturff SL, Shaw LI, Hodgkin JE, Rumble L, Bird FM. Intrapulmonary percussive ventilation in the treatment of COPD. Respir Care 1985; 30:885.
37. Sinha R, Bergofsky EH. Prolonged alteration of lung mechanics in kyphoscoliosis by positive pressure hyperinflation. Am Rev Respir Dis 1972; 106:47–57.
38. De Troyer A, Deisser P. The effects of intermittent positive pressure breathing on patients with respiratory muscle weakness. Am Rev Respir Dis 1981; 124:132–137.
39. O'Donohue W. Maximum volume IPPB for the management of pulmonary atelectasis. Chest 1976; 76:683–687.
40. Huldtgren AC, Fugl-Meyer AR, Jonasson E, Bake B. Ventilatory dysfunction and respiratory rehabilitation in post-traumatic quadriplegia. Eur J Respir Dis 1980; 61: 347–56.
41. Houser CR, Johnson DM. Breathing exercises for children with pseudohypertrophic muscular dystrophy. Phys Ther 1971; 51:751–759.

42. Adams MA, Chandler LS. Effects of physical therapy program on vital capacity of patients with muscular dystrophy. Phys Ther 1974; 54:494–496.
43. Bach JR, Robert D, Leger P, Langevin B. Sleep fragmentation in kyphoscoliotic individuals with alveolar hypoventilation treated by nasal IPPV. Chest 1995; 107: 1552–1558.
44. Bach JR, Alba AS. Management of chronic alveolar hypoventilation by nasal ventilation. Chest 1990; 97:52–57.
45. Bach JR, Barnett V. Psychosocial, vocational, quality of life and ethical issues In: Bach JR, ed. Pulmonary Rehabilitation: The Obstructive and Paralytic Conditions. Philadelphia: Hanley & Belfus, 1996; 395–411.
46. Wicks AB, Menter RR. Long-term outlook in quadriplegic patients with initial ventilator dependency. Chest 1986; 90:406–410.
47. Jackson AB, Groomes TE. Incidence of respiratory complications following spinal cord injury. Arch Phys Med Rehabil 1994; 75:270–275.
48. Historical Statistics of the United States: Colonial Times to 1970. Bicentennial Edition. Part 1. Washington, DC: U.S. Department of Commerce, Bureau of the Census, 1975; 8, 77.
49. Lassen HCA. The epidemic of poliomyelitis in Copenhagen, 1952. Proc R Soc Med 1953; 47:67–71.
50. Bach JR, Tilton M. Pulmonary dysfunction and its management in post-polio patients. NeuroRehabilitation 1997; 8:139–153.
51. Hodes HL. Treatment of respiratory difficulty in poliomyelitis. In: Poliomyelitis: Papers and Discussions Presented at the Third International Poliomyelitis Conference. Philadelphia: Lippincott, 1955; 91.
52. Haber II, Bach JR. Normalization of blood carbon dioxide levels by transition from conventional ventilatory support to noninvasive inspiratory aids. Arch Phys Med Rehabil 1994; 75:1145–1150.
53. Bach JR. A comparison of long-term ventilatory support alternatives from the perspective of the patient and care giver. Chest 1993; 104:1702–1706.
54. Bach JR, Intintola P, Alba AS, Holland I. The ventilator-assisted individual: Cost analysis of institutionalization versus rehabilitation and in-home management. Chest 1992; 101:26–30.
55. Valenza J, Guzzardo SL, Bach JR. Functional interventions for individuals with neuromuscular disease. In: Bach JR, ed. Pulmonary Rehabilitation: The Obstructive and Paralytic Conditions. Philadelphia: Hanley & Belfus, 1996; 371–394.

13

Costs and Reimbursement Issues in Long-Term Mechanical Ventilation of Patients at Home

JOHN J. DOWNES and MARTHA M. PARRA

The Children's Hospital of Pennsylvania
Philadelphia, Pennsylvania

I. Introduction

Scientific and technological advances in the care of critically ill and injured individuals of all ages have resulted in an unprecedented improvement in their survival and subsequent quality of life. Concomitant with these improvements have come rapid increases in the costs of health care (1), and the emergence of a relatively small but increasing number of persons living with severe disability. Most striking among these disabled persons are those with chronic respiratory failure requiring long-term mechanical ventilation. We, as well as others (2), consider chronic respiratory failure (CRF) to be a condition persisting for greater than 1 mo in which the impairment of ventilation requires that the patient receive mechanical ventilatory assistance, during part or all of the day, to provide adequate gas exchange for the support of vital functions.

Persons with CRF reside in acute or intermediate intensive care units, rehabilitation hospitals, sub-acute or long-term care facilities and in homes. Assignment of the individual with CRF to one of these venues should depend primarily on health status and family human resources, with cost a secondary consideration. Unfortunately, our experience and that of others (3) indicates that cost, as perceived by some health insurance entities, can become the determining factor governing the venue and extent of care. Articulate physicians, nurses, social workers, lawyers, political representatives, and other advocates who are committed to achieving the best overall plan for the individual patient often can negotiate successfully with upper management of insurance companies to meet the patient's needs.

Published national data on the incidence, prevalence, mortality, and health care costs of individuals with CRF appear to be lacking (2). Several reports provide some data and discuss these issues at the national level (4) and at state levels for New York, Illinois, Pennsylvania, and Minnesota (5–8). Others describe the experiences of children with CRF in institutions (9) as well as in the home (7,10–14). Several authors have reviewed the voluminous literature on the medical aspects of long-term mechanical ventilation in adults outside the acute intensive care unit (2,15–16).

Published data on costs of care in institutions, in the home, and comparison of the two reveal extraordinary variation in levels of care provided and the costs assigned to these levels. Some authors report actual expenditures while others describe charges or payments by insurance entities. These are particularly difficult data to obtain with accuracy and to compare among institutions or programs. The recent comprehensive report of the 1998 Consensus Conference of the American College of Chest Physicians entitled "Mechanical Ventilation Beyond the Intensive Care Unit" cited this issue as follows: "A lack of detailed information on costs, length of stay, and outcome of patients receiving prolonged mechanical ventilation is a major obstacle in setting a national policy for reimbursement . . ." (2).

Despite the lack of epidemiologic and economic information, in the past 15 years comprehensive guidelines have been developed for managing the transition from hospital to home, and for the ongoing home care of ventilator assisted adults (17–18) and children (12,19,20). These guidelines include recommendations for 1) selecting appropriate patients for home care, 2) preparing and training family members to become caregivers, 3) arranging for home nursing care, medical equipment and adjunctive therapies at home, 4) ensuring appropriate physician referral, direction and coverage, 5) identifying community resources, and 6) advocating for the patient and family to ensure adequate funding.

In this chapter we have been selective rather than exhaustive in citing the literature. We present the limited information available in the current literature and from our own experience that describes 1) the costs of care for patients requiring long-term mechanical ventilation at home and in other locations, 2) the available funding mechanisms, 3) the value of nonprofessional caregivers in the home, and 4) the ethical issues regarding care versus costs that confront the physician and other health professionals in providing services to the ventilator-assisted person. We conclude with our recommendations that should help resolve many of the economic and related inequities encountered by severely disabled persons, especially those requiring mechanical ventilation, and their families.

II. Funding Sources

Funding for home care services of children and adults who require mechanical ventilation comes from three major sources: public, private, or a combination of public and private. Publicly funded programs include state and federal programs such as Medicare and Medicaid. Private payment sources encompass all third party payors who provide insurance coverage to groups and individuals, as well as the private not-for-profit organizations such as the Muscular Dystrophy Association (MDA). These organizations provide funding for specific patient care services as defined by the organization.

Title XIX of the Social Security Act of 1965 established the Medicaid and Medicare as entitlement programs. Since its enactment, Medicaid has been a major source of health insurance in the United States. In 1997, Medicaid covered 41 million people and spent $160 billion for services of low-income persons who were elderly, blind, disabled, receiving public assistance or among the working poor (21). Medicaid, jointly financed by the federal and state governments, provides services to individuals who meet specific eligibility criteria. The Early and Periodic Screening, Diagnosis and Treatment (EPSDT) program, legislated in 1967, is a special health care program under Medicaid for children from birth through 21 years of age. This program, in theory, has the potential to provide comprehensive screening for children and the necessary services to treat the diagnosed condition, whether or not the services are included in the state's Medicaid plan. Thus, EPSDT provides an extremely important source of funding for children with complex medical needs because it offers a source of payment for home nursing services.

Medicaid waivers are another source of public funding for home care services of children requiring prolonged mechanical ventilation. In 1982 President Reagan approved the "Katie Beckett waiver" as a mechanism for funding home and community-based services for severely disabled children requiring technological support. This new type of waiver was developed in response to the Beckett family's desire to care for their daughter in the home. The Reagan administration deemed home care to be less restrictive as well as less expensive than the cost of hospitalization. The Health Care Financing Administration (HCFA) issued the "Katie Beckett waiver" until states could begin applying for the "2176 waiver" which involved a lengthy and complex application process (22). The two unique features of the "2176 waiver" are that a state determines the specific population to be served by the waiver, including age and specific disability, and that parental income will not be considered for eligibility purposes (22). In effect, only the child's personal financial resources (usually none) are considered, thus expanding Medicaid eligibility for children from middle and upper income families who have exhausted their private insurance benefits, or whose policy benefits do not include reimbursement for home care services (13).

Since 1980, states increasingly have relied on managed care corporations to serve Medicaid recipients. Currently, every state except Alaska has some form of managed care in place for the Medicaid population. The number of enrollees nationwide has increased from 2.7 million in 1991 to 15.3 million in 1997 (21). Medicaid covers a broad range of services with nominal cost sharing by beneficiaries. This package of benefits, especially for the disabled, exceeds that of Medicare and many employer-sponsored programs (21).

Medicare is administered by the Health Care Finance Administration (HCFA) to provide funding for the health care of citizens 65 years of age and older. This program pays a major portion of bills for hospitalization, physician services, and nursing home care, but offers relatively little for the patient being cared for in their own home. Unlike the Medicaid program, Medicare does not provide benefits for continuous home care services, limiting reimbursement to intermittent home health care visits.

Although most Americans rely on health insurance benefits provided through employer-sponsored programs, we are witnessing an increasing number of individuals who no longer have access to this type of funding. Factors contributing to this problem include rising premiums, both for persons who have insurance through their employers and for those who individually purchase it. Temporary and part-time employment, a current trend, seldom includes health insurance benefits (23). Lower income Americans bear a disproportionate share of health care costs because they are more likely to work for employers who do not provide health care coverage or who require employees to make larger contributions for health insurance (23). Also, the rising premiums that beneficiaries must pay for prescription medications (23) add further economic burdens to many families of ventilator-assisted persons.

Families with children who require long-term mechanical ventilation usually exhaust their private insurance benefits and personal resources within 1 or 2 yr. Nursing and other home care services are then paid for through Medicaid until the child reaches age 21. At that point, funding for most home health care services, including daily nursing care, ceases. The family then either pays for such services from their own funds, assumes all of the daily care burdens, or places the newly adult patient in a Medicaid-funded nursing home. None of these options assures the combination of appropriate care of the disabled persons and least restrictive environment without an unreasonable burden on nearly every family. This policy of Medicaid, in fact, appears to be in direct conflict with the mandates of the Americans with Disabilities Act of 1990 (ADA) and a 1999 United States Supreme Court decision. This decision upheld the provisions of the ADA requiring that disabled persons of any age be cared for in the community insofar as their condition permits (see later section on ethical and legal considerations related to home care).

Other funding sources that provide reimbursement for home care services include the Social Security Act Title V programs for Children with Special Health Care Needs administered by the Federal Bureau of Maternal and Child Health, Social Security income (SSI) for the disabled of all ages, and public school systems. These programs, although valuable for their specific financial contributions, do not provide adequate funding for the comprehensive home care of severely disabled individuals. An important legal decision was reached by the United States Supreme Court in March, 1999, in the case of Garret F. v. Cedar Rapids Community School District. This decision changed the responsibility of school systems by mandating the provision of funding for the nursing services of school age children who require prolonged mechanical ventilation (24). In this case, the Supreme Court 'ed that states receiving assistance under the Individuals with Disabilities Education Act are required to provide a student who is ventilator-dependent with personal nursing services during school hours (24).

However, funding for the home care of ventilator-assisted individuals (VAIs) across the United States varies widely depending on the patient's age, financial status, diagnostic category, and state of residence. The gaps in this patchwork system seem most striking for persons requiring prolonged mechanical ventilation who are over 21 years of age and who lack comprehensive private health insurance; they are denied funding for nursing care or even trained assistants at home.

III. Costs of Home Care

Each year a growing number of individuals across the nation who require long-term mechanical ventilation are being discharged from the hospital to the home. In 1993, for example, the Respiratory Rehabilitation Unit of The Children's Seashore House in Philadelphia, a pediatric rehabilitation hospital, had an average length of stay of 8 mo for ventilator-assisted children; following discharge nearly all patients received mechanical ventilation at home for extended periods. By 1997, the average length of stay had been reduced to 4 mo (25). By reducing or denying payments, private and public health insurers have pressured hospitals to reduce overall costs, especially for these patients deemed ready for home care.

Other contributing factors to shortened lengths of hospital stay include 1) willingness of insurance companies to fund home care, at least for a time following discharge, 2) increased awareness of home health nursing agencies and durable medical equipment companies regarding the care of VAIs, 3) improved skills of hospital case managers with the discharge process for these patients, and 4) parental awareness of this option and the advantages to the child of living at home. In some geographic areas, parents have been forced to accept home care by physicians, hospital administrators and insurance companies, not only to achieve reduction in costs, but also because alternative sites for chronic care were not available.

Home care of VAIs is not a new notion, having been employed in the 1930s through 1950s for victims of severe poliomyelitis. Some of these patients still live with ventilatory support at home. The overall financial cost of this care, however, remains poorly defined. This can be attributed, in part, to a lack of consensus about the specific elements that constitute home care costs. Some have considered the relevant costs of home care to be only direct costs, while others (4,13) have incorporated both direct and indirect costs. In this regard, the works of Sevick et al. (4) and Dranove (13) are benchmark studies despite the significant limitations that are acknowledged by the authors. Their comprehensive analyses of the many factors involved in cost estimates of care for these patients provide a basis for understanding the total costs of home care (Table 1).

Sevick et al. (4) included both direct medical and nonmedical costs of home care in their analysis as well as the indirect costs that are associated with lost wages as a result of caregiving. Potential participants for Sevick's study (4) were selected from patients served by three respiratory care companies. A total of

Table 1 Components of Home Care Costs

Direct Costs
Physician fees
Formal services purchased by family
Hospital and skilled nursing facility inpatient days
Medications
Equipment rental
Oxygen
Ambulance
Medical supplies
Extra utility charges
Major one-time purchases or remodeling
Indirect Costs
Alterations in employment
Lost wages resulting from caregiving

Source: Adapted from Ref. 13.

1404 primary family caregivers of VAIs were sent detailed survey questionnaires designed for this study. Of this group, 277 caregivers (20%) responded with complete or nearly complete surveys, and 239 provided suitable data for analysis.

The patients lived in 37 states and ranged in age from less than 21 yr (25%) to over 65 yr (28%) with 46% between 21 and 65 yr (4). All diagnostic categories were included, but the majority (59%) suffered degenerative neuromuscular disorders or spinal cord injury. Seventeen percent had chronic lung disease, 8% congenital malformations, and only 1.7% had sleep apnea. Long-term tracheostomy was a factor increasing the complexity and costs of care in 74% of these individuals. Patients living independently with hired attendants providing all the care were excluded from the study; these are considered in the next section of this chapter.

Utilizing the 1993 Medicare schedule for home health agency costs, Sevick et al. (4) estimated the direct health care costs at home, including skilled nursing, and physical and occupational therapies. These estimates averaged $5265/mo (median $2344, range $0 to 28,794) at licensed practical nurse (LPN) rates, and $6892/mo (median $2432, range $0 to 38,500) at rates for a registered nurse (RN). Medications, equipment rental, supplies, ambulance service, and out-of-pocket expenses were estimated to average an additional $2059/mo (median $1545, range $0 to 17,534). While nursing is the most costly aspect of home care, Sevick's study (4) does not indicate the hours per day of home nursing support utilized by families. However, only a small number (4 to 14%) of respondents indicated that they provide all the care for the patient with no professional nurse or attendant services. Sevick (4) also does not compare the costs of care for children as opposed to adults in the home. From our observations, adult patients receive fewer home nursing services when compared with infants and children, and thus their home care costs should be less.

Evaluating home care cost data proves difficult because of the various definitions of "cost" (this may include actual expenditures, scheduled reimbursement, charges, direct and indirect expenses) and the host of variables affecting actual costs. In a 1986 study, Dranove (13) interviewed 34 selected families enrolled in a federally funded program for children requiring ventilator assistance at home in Illinois, Maryland, and Louisiana. This program included 141 children, of whom 42% had bronchopulmonary dysplasia, 20% central nervous system disorders, 18% congenital anomalies, and 20% other causes of respiratory failure.

Dranove reviewed virtually all the factors, except for individual diagnoses, that might contribute to the costs of caring for each of 34 selected children in the hospital and subsequently at home. These included nursing care, developmental therapies, physician services, equipment rental, supplies, medications, hospital readmissions, and indirect costs to the family. Each case served as its own control for analyses of cost over time. Hospital "costs" were derived from "charges" and the hospital's cost-to-charge ratio, and they were adjusted for factors that included severity of illness.

Dranove (13) also added a new dimension to these calculations, that of "maturation" or changes in costs associated with changes in medical status (either improving or deteriorating) during the period of the study. Further, he considered the initial discharge from the hospital to home as an "irreversible" step for purposes of cost analyses; subsequent hospitalizations, whether due to the primary illness, for respiratory management, or for other reasons were treated as part of home care costs. If the physicians caring for the child in an acute ICU thought that the child could be cared for in a "step-down" unit, the cost was adjusted to 75% of the ICU cost. Data were obtained from hospital records, parental interviews, home medical equipment providers, and physicians. Proportionately, nursing and physician costs were the highest, accounting for 65% of all

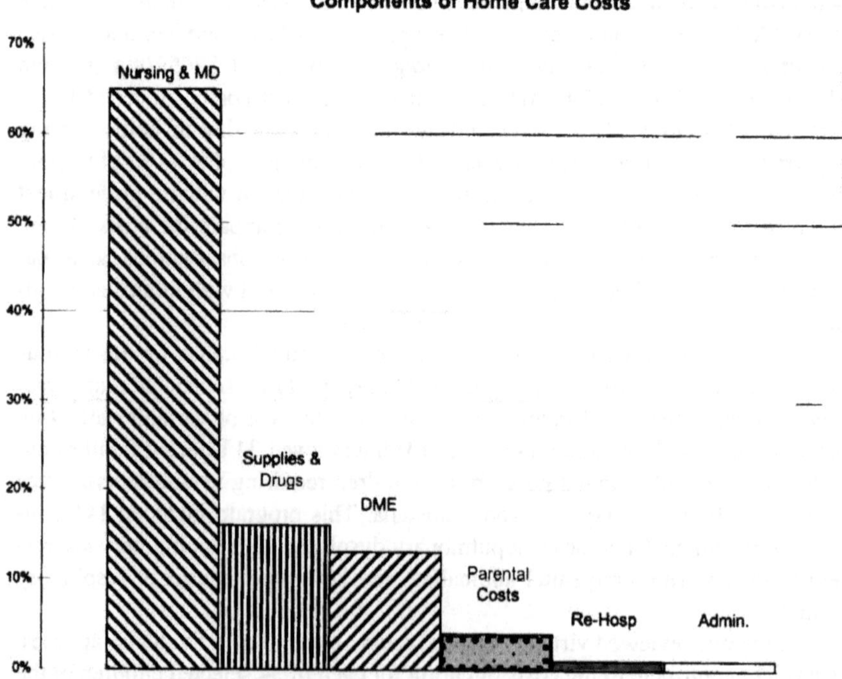

Figure 1 The components of home care costs of ventilator-assisted children derived from analysis of data from 34 selected families in three states. See text for details. DME, durable medical equipment costs; Re-Hosp, cost of rehospitalization after initial discharge to home; Admin, cost of administrative services. (Adapted from Ref. 13.)

costs. Figure 1 shows the components of home care costs as a percentages of the total per diem cost.

The Ventilator Assisted Children's Home Program (VACHP), funded by the Commonwealth of Pennsylvania through the Department of Health, provides advocacy, case management, and respite care services for infants and children under age 21 and their families. All children who require prolonged mechanical ventilation and are residents of Pennsylvania are eligible for program services, regardless of parental income or the primary funding source. Of the 200 children currently enrolled in the program, 50% receive funding for home care services through Medicaid and 50% have private funding sources. Referrals to the program are obtained from hospitals throughout Pennsylvania, as well as from hospitals in neighboring states that are caring for a child whose home is in Pennsylvania.

Between 1997 and 1999, the costs of 10 representative VACHP home care cases from across the state were reviewed. At the median of 16 hr/day and $40/hr, the average cost of nursing was $19,276/mo (range $16,800 to 21,120) or $231,312/yr. The average monthly cost of the respiratory equipment rental and supplies was $4377 (range $3000 to 6333) or $52,527/yr. Thus, the average total cost for nursing and the equipment and supplies was $23,653/mo or $283,836/yr.

As mentioned previously, there exists a wide range in the reported costs of home care of ventilator-dependent children and adults. A number of reasons can be cited for this, including a lack of agreement on criteria for discharge from the hospital and the absence of national standards for care of these patients at home. Since nursing is the most costly component of this care at home, variations in the hours of professional nursing care or the use of nonlicensed attendants will significantly affect costs. In most states, only a licensed nurse (RN or LPN) can provide this care according to the state's nurse practice act as well as standards set by some third party payors (2). O'Donohue (17) cited these limitations by third party payors as greatly increasing the cost of care. In 1988, Plummer (18) and a nationwide group of experts with extensive experience in caring for VAIs at home met to identify problems related to equipment, levels of care, individual needs assessment, and reimbursement. They recommended flexibility in reimbursement policy to allow for a variety of caregivers, including both licensed and unlicensed but formally trained personnel. The use of unlicensed but trained personnel would require carefully prepared and effectively conducted programs to ensure an acceptable quality of patient care skills. Such programs (26) can be successful but appear to be few in number at this time. Additionally, a high degree of complexity in the patient's medical condition or extreme dependency (as with infants and small children), will usually demand high-caliber professional nursing care to achieve appropriate levels of safety and comprehensive care.

IV. Comparison of Costs: Institutions Versus Home

As discussed above, assessing the costs of caring for ventilator-assisted individuals is complex because of variable definitions of "cost" and the myriad factors affecting expenditures. Comparisons of costs, therefore, between the different locations and levels of care will be subject to considerable variation and possible misinterpretation. Nonetheless, several studies have provided valuable information and insight which can serve as the basis for more extensive research that should enable the health professions, insurers, and communities to plan effectively for the humane support of these disabled individuals and their families in the future.

As described in the previous section, Sevick (4) considers the many elements that definitely constitute health care costs and the other factors that can add economic burden to the family and perhaps to the community. In her study (4) hospital in-patient cost estimates were based on Medicare prospective payments (1994) and yielded a per diem of $1353 ($40,590/mo). Skilled nursing facility costs were considered but not assigned a specific estimate.

Combining estimated costs of home care, and assuming 50% RN and 50% LPN skilled nursing rates, as cited in their report, Sevick's data (4) yield a median of $3933 with a range from $0 to 33,650 for monthly direct costs. This constitutes a *median reduction of 90% in costs by providing care at home* rather than in the ICU of a general hospital.

As Sevick et al. (4) acknowledge, their analysis underestimates the true costs of both inpatient and home care when compared with other studies because it relies on Medicare payments alone, and these do not ordinarily fully reimburse total costs. They cite other reports providing cost data converted to 1994 dollars for comparison, indicating home care expenditures for VAIs that range from $7814 to 40,678/mo. Costs varied widely from patient to patient, depending on the complexity of illness, the extent of disability, and the hours per day of mechanical ventilation required.

In the previously mentioned 1986 study by Dranove (13), the hospital-adjusted per diem costs for the entire group of 34 children averaged $784 ($23,520/mo) with variation in individuals from $411 to $1377. By comparison, home care costs per day for all children averaged $490 ($14,700/mo) with a range of $121 to 923/day. The average per diem costs for the individual states, with 37 states represented, ranged from $329 to 611 ($9870 to 18,330/mo). Thus, *home care costs averaged 38% less than hospital care*, even if that care was in a step-down unit. On examination of the various cost factors, it becomes clear that the principal factor responsible for lower costs ($329/day) was the total substitution of family members for professional nurses or other paid caretakers.

Bach et al. (26) reported on 20 adults with severe neuromuscular or spinal cord impairment who received noninvasive mechanical ventilation 24 h/day while residing independently in their homes in New York City. They had been trained for independent living in one of two rehabilitation hospital-based programs, and were being followed by a dedicated community agency with daily assistance from noncertified home care attendants trained by the agency or by the patient. The average cost of care of these patients in a respiratory unit at one of the two rehabilitation hospitals was $719/day ($21,570/mo) compared with a total estimated cost of home care and other living expenses of $235/day ($7050/mo). Funding for home care in each case was provided by Medicaid (health-related costs) and SSI payments (general support).

This *67% reduction in costs at home compared with hospital* was achieved because of several factors: 1) preparation of the patients by providing an excellent training program in independent living and supervision of their own respiratory care, 2) no need for a tracheostomy due to the nonpulmonary nature of their disorders, 3) substitution of home care attendants for professional nurses and the support of a dedicated home care agency funded by Medicaid, and 4) the cooperation of the New York state Medicaid program. Success in enhancing the quality of life for the patients and reducing the costs depended on the convergence of all these factors. According to these authors (26), innovative programs involving Medicaid for similar patients have been initiated in Massachusetts and Colorado. In our opinion, exceptional vision, effort, and sustained commitment will be required to replicate the success of the New York City program in other locations. Nonetheless, this should be vigorously pursued for this group of patients who represent a large number of VAIs.

In statewide surveys of long-term care units and home medical equipment providers in Minnesota in 1986 and again in 1992, Adams et al. (8) found that the number of VAIs outside of acute intensive care units had increased from 103 to 216 (110%) over the 6 yr. The ages of the patients were not specified, but presumably most were adults, and the majority had underlying neuromuscular or neurologic disorders resulting in respiratory failure. Patients receiving mask ventilation were excluded for unstated reasons, but those maintained with negative pressure ventilators were not. Curiously, in 1986, 81% of these patients were at home, whereas in 1992 only 65% resided at home with the remainder in long-term care facilities. The causes for the shift to long-term care facilities are unclear.

In 1986 but not in 1992, these investigators (8) conducted a detailed study of the costs of care for eight selected patients whose complete data were available as they progressed from the ICU to a long-term care facility and eventually to home. Monthly hospital charges in the acute ICU averaged $64,513, in the long-term care facility $19,351, and at home $6557 (all in 1986 dollars). The home care charges included the patients' living expenses and taxes. This indicates that *home care resulted in reduction in expenditures of approximately 90% compared with care in a general hospital ICU, and 66% compared with costs of residence in a long-term care facility.* The authors, however, point out that this striking reduction in costs occurred because only two patients had licensed nurses caring for them; three had unlicensed personal care attendants, and three had their family members providing all the care.

Fields et al. (14) evaluated costs of care in the mid-1980s, for six children requiring long-term mechanical ventilation. They analyzed the projected Maryland Medicaid reimbursement for institutional care, and compared it with the actual Medicaid reimbursement over 2 yr (1985 to 1987) for home care of these children. The projected institutional reimbursements were 96% of charges for this type of care in two regional pediatric long-term care facilities. Four of the six children at home received professional nursing care 16 to 24 hr/day, 7 days/wk, while two received less nursing care. Nurses were paid $18/hr for home care. The mean cost (±SD) for institutional care (1985 to 1987 dollars) was $190,000 (20,000), and for home care $110,000 (21,000), *a savings of 42% on average with home care* in this limited sample. Nursing care accounted for 69% of the total reimbursement, which also included short-term hospital care after discharge to home and other costs, such as durable medical equipment, supplies, developmental or rehabilitation therapies, case management, outpatient physician visits, drugs, and transportation. In fact, nursing costs were significantly less than projected because some agencies could not fill the approved hours all the time. The authors (14) acknowledge that they did not include indirect costs of home care paid by the families, such as structural adaptation of the home, increased utility expenses, and lost income. Nonetheless, the savings achieved by home care remain appreciable on the basis of this study.

Moss et al. (27) compared the average costs of 50 patients receiving mechanical ventilation for respiratory failure caused by amyotrophic lateral sclerosis (ALS) in an institution and at home. Fourteen patients resided in long-term care facilities and 36 were cared for at home. Patients at home rated their quality of life significantly higher than those in an institution, and their average annual expenses were significantly less at $136,560 compared with $366,852. Thus, *home care created an average savings of 63% in this special group with ALS.*

Parra et al. (28) at the previously mentioned Pennsylvania Department of Health's Ventilator Assisted Children's Home Program (VACHP) assessed the costs of home nursing care (averaging 16 hr/day and $40/hr), as well as respiratory equipment and supplies in 10 representative children between 1997 and 1999. The nursing care costs averaged $19,276/mo. Since nursing care constituted approximately 65% of home care costs in a similar pediatric population (13), we can estimate that the average total cost of home care, including equipment, supplies, drugs, developmental therapies, nutrition, and indirect costs in these 10 children would be $30,119/mo or $361,425/yr.

Chalom and colleagues (29) analyzed the individual and total costs of care for 1376 children (6605 patient days) in various diagnostic categories admitted to the multidisciplinary Pediatric Intensive Care Unit of the Children's Hospital of Philadelphia (PICU) from July, 1993 through June, 1994. Physician fees were not included. The average cost per day was $2264, or $69,052/mo. Nursing compensation and administration, associated with an average of 16.5 hr of nursing care per child per day, constituted 54% of this cost. A few of the children developed chronic respiratory failure with ongoing instability and required lengths of stay exceeding 1 mo. In contrast, the average cost in a respiratory unit devoted to children with chronic respiratory failure located in a pediatric rehabilitation hospital was determined to be $1200/day, or $36,600/mo with an average length of stay of 8 mo (30).

After adjusting the cost data from these two institutions for an average of 5% annual inflation of health care costs between 1994 and 1998 (1), monthly costs in the PICU would be $82,862, and in the respiratory unit $43,920. *Thus, home care, even at $30,119/mo, results in estimated monthly savings of $52,743 (64%) compared with the PICU and $13,801 (31%) compared with the pediatric rehabilitation hospital respiratory unit (Fig. 2).*

In conclusion, for both adult and pediatric patients who require prolonged mechanical ventilation, home care is substantially less costly than hospital care, with figures ranging from 31% to 90% in the studies we reviewed. The magnitude of savings varies considerably from state to state and patient to patient. Within a specific health insurance plan, the savings will be driven primarily by the hours of skilled nursing care provided in the home. This, in turn, will depend on the degree of dependency of the patient, the complexity of medical care, and the availability and competency of family members other or nonprofessional attendants to assist in the care. Unfortunately, comparisons of home care costs with those of subacute or long-term care facilities are limited by the lack of recent peer-reviewed publications or books dealing with the costs of prolonged mechanical ventilation in subacute or long-term care facilities. These data would be very useful in determining further if the value of home care is more economical than these alternative sites.

V. Caregiver Value

The economic value of nonprofessional caregivers, usually family members, in reducing the total cost of home care of the VAI seldom receives recognition by the insurance companies or analysis by investigators. Wegener (31) and Sevick and Bradham (32) are exceptions. Using the same 1986 database as Dranove (13), Wegener computed the contribution of parents caring for infants and children requiring mechanical ventilation in 36 households. She found that the family contribution was equivalent to $19 per day ($580 monthly in 1986 dollars). This figure included increased utility expenses, lost income from outside work, transportation, babysitting, and the amortized cost of home remodeling to accommo-

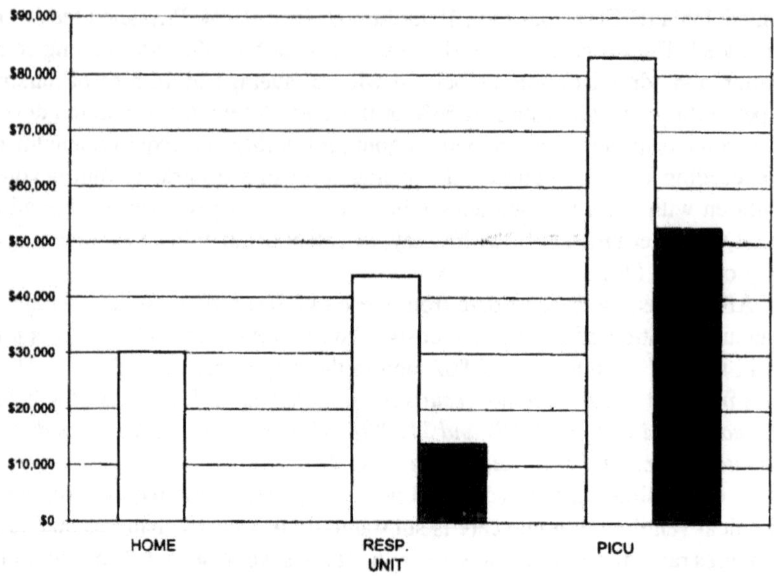

Figure 2 Comparison of the average costs per month for care of a child with chronic respiratory failure requiring long-term mechanical ventilation who is: 1) at home with 16 hr/day of professional nursing care (HOME); 2) in a pediatric rehabilitation hospital's respiratory unit (RESP. UNIT); and 3) in a children's hospital acute pediatric intensive care unit (PICU). Savings (black columns) are computed against the costs in the PICU. See text for details. (Adapted from Refs. 28–30.)

date the patient. However, the dollar value of the parent's time spent caring for the child's medical needs was not reported or estimated.

Sevick's survey of 277 VAIs in 37 states (4), provided the database for determinating the relative economic contribution of the family to the patient's overall costs of care in the home (32). Recall that this patient group did not include individuals with chronic respiratory failure living independently with the aid of paid attendants. The typical caregiver in Sevick's sample was white (90%), female (74%), spouse, partner, or parent (86%), had some college education (55%), and a median age of 52 (range 23 to 96), and lived with the patient (97%). The majority (65%) of the caregivers had been gainfully employed outside the home prior to becoming a caregiver. Fifty percent of them quit their jobs and 34% decreased their hours at the job to care for the patient. This resulted in a median loss of monthly income of $1125 (range $75 to $30,000).

Most patients in the Sevick et al. (4,32) studies had a degenerative neuromuscular (46%) or spinal cord (18%) disorder, or chronic lung disease (15%). The patients ranged from age 1 to 92 (median 45), 83% had tracheostomies, and they required a median of 20 hr/day of mechanical ventilation, with 44% needing continuous assisted ventilation. Mechanical ventilation had been utilized for a median of 4 years (range 2 months to 60 years). Without question, these patients were highly dependent on caregiver support.

Computation of the value of the caregiver's time, as Sevick and Bradham (32) point out, depends on the skills required to care for the specific patient and the prevailing market compensation for persons possessing those skills. Thus, any one figure as the value per hour for the caregiver's time spent caring directly for the patient can only be a rough estimate. Nonetheless, if we value that time at the rate of a professional nurse, which Sevick and Bradham (32) estimate at \$38 per hour (1995 dollars), and pay this for at least 16 hr/day (the amount of care a highly dependent patient might need), \$18,544 per month will be added to the home care cost. If, on the other hand, we set the value of this service at the rate of an unlicensed attendant, approximately \$10.54 per hour (1995 dollars), the caregiver's direct patient care portion of the cost adds only \$2572 per month, an 84% reduction in the value of care. These estimates serve as the lower and upper estimates of what might be anticipated for any given patient. If we include the estimated median lost income of caregivers (\$1125), we add further to the actual monthly costs of home care. In such calculations, it should be noted that the primary caregiver does not have any days off, thus providing care for even more hours per week, unless a respite program is in place, which rarely occurs.

Thomas et al. (33) compiled responses to questionnaires and to trained personal interviews of 44 caregivers who provided care in their homes for 29 ventilator-assisted persons (mean age 43, range 1 to 83). Among the caregivers' gravest concerns, beyond the immediate safety of the patient, were maintaining closeness among family members, assuring that someone would assume the role as caretaker if they became incapacitated, worrying that the family's needs were not being met, getting adequate sleep, and having time for leisure activities and to talk with family and friends. These findings indicate that these are substantial nonfinancial costs to caregivers for VAIs.

In another survey of 27 families caring for VAIs at home, Sevick et al. (34) found that despite the difficulties of assuming the burdens of complex, highly technical care for over 8 hr/day, caregivers viewed the experience in a positive light. The authors point out that this response contradicts the common perception of health care professionals that the emotional and other burdens assumed by families of VAIs cause extreme stress.

Quint et al. (35) performed structured interviews and assessed parental responses to a questionnaire, the Impact on Family Scale, in 18 Northern California families caring for a child receiving mechanical ventilation at home. Although families showed considerable resilience over time, coping skills of the primary caretaker (usually the mother) who had endured over 2 yr of home care were significantly less than those with a shorter experience.

Downes and Hock-Long (36) studied the responses of 85 families across the state of Pennsylvania who were caring for children requiring long-term mechanical ventilation at home. The children received a median of 16 hr/day of professional nursing care. The scores on standardized tests completed by the primary caregiver, usually the mother, to evaluate family functioning and the caregiver's mood states did not differ significantly from published norms. Interpartner relationships, subsequent to the child's arrival at home needing mechanical ventilation, were strengthened in 22% of families, unchanged in 34%, strained in 25%, and ended in 17%. The findings were not significantly altered by the length of home care, thus differing from the observations of Quint et al. (35) despite similarities in the patients and families observed. Although this type of care places extraordinary burdens on all families, and the noneconomic costs occasionally can be devastating, the majority of families appear to cope quite effectively and deeply cherish their disabled child or partner.

In conclusion, as Sevick and Bradham (32) point out, health care professionals "should be sensitive to the impact of caregiving on employment and the long term effects on the financial independence of caregivers." Furthermore, the economic and psychological vulnerability of families caring for persons needing mechanical ventilation at home demands that health care professionals carry out their responsibilities with utmost compassion and understanding, especially when dealing with those caregivers who have more problems coping and prove to be more difficult and unappreciative.

VI. Ethical and Legal Considerations Related to Home Care

The management of an adult or child at home who requires complex care involving professional personnel and life-support equipment poses at least two ethical problems for families, physicians, and society. The first problem concerns the imposition of extraordinary burdens on the primary caregiver as well as other family members (37). Currently, our health care system requires that most families provide some, and occasionally all, of the nursing care as well as general support of the VAIs without financial compensation. For the patient, under most circumstances, home will be the least restrictive environment; for the family, the care and economic burdens can be quite restrictive.

As discussed above, most families welcome their incapacitated loved one home and willingly deal effectively with the responsibilities of care and support. On the other hand, for numerous reasons, some families are not able to cope with these burdens. Placement of the patient in a subacute care or long-term care facility that is equipped and staffed to care for individuals requiring complex respiratory care may prove best for all concerned. The availability of such facilities, however, remains quite limited throughout the country. In the case of children, the additional option of carefully selected voluntary medical foster care can provide a beneficial solution.

The other ethical problem concerns not only home care but also the entire concept of devoting exceptional resources and technology to the long-term support of adults and children who suffer from severe disabilities. Our Western economic and legal philosophy, in part, derives from the doctrine of *utilitarianism*. This doctrine states that, in a virtuous society, one should seek the "*greatest happiness for the greatest number*" (38). Various philosophers in the eighteenth and nineteenth centuries promulgated this doctrine, but its most influential promoter was Jeremy Bentham (1748–1832). Bentham, a well known English philosopher and jurist in his time, promoted this doctrine as "*the greatest good for the greatest number*" through publications and establishment of a reform political party (39). This doctrine has influenced British and American law regarding social policy and economics ever since, and laid a foundation for socialist philosophy and social reforms of the late nineteenth century.

At about the same time, the idea of *individual rights* was proposed by John Locke and other philosophers of the English and French enlightenment (40). This idea inspired and sustained Thomas Jefferson and other revolutionaries in America and France. The concept was anathema to Bentham, however, who in 1805 bluntly characterized individual rights as "nonsense" (38). He held to this despite the recent victory of the concept, if not the fact, of individual rights and freedom culminating in the American and French Revolutions. Bentham set forth the dilemma in stark terms, and the struggle between "individual rights" and the "greatest good for the greatest number" continues in Western democracies to this day.

One of the frontiers of this struggle is health care, especially as it concerns the expenditure of large sums of money and resources for the care of a small number of individuals. The doctrine of utilitarianism applied to disabled infants, children, and adults appears to underlie the recent arguments of Peter Singer, a widely recognized and controversial Australian bioethicist at Princeton University (41). Dr. Singer reasons that the suffering incurred by a person with a severe disability, as well as the burden on the family and society, far outweighs the benefits of providing that person with long-term complex care and support. Needless to say, many disabled individuals and their families vigorously oppose this view. The debate over whose life merits extraordinary care and commitment from society has continued throughout this century, but in the last 20 years has become more focused on specific cases and conditions. Differences of opinion will undoubtedly become more strident as medical progress further complicates our lives while conferring its benefits.

At the heart of this health care dilemma lies another important concept closely related to individual rights, that is, the health care professional's *imperative to rescue.* When professionals undertake responsibility for the health and ultimately the life of a person, they have a contract with that person to do all in their power to maintain or restore health, provide comfort, and act according to that person's stated directives. This obligation for the physician, nurse, or other professional does not end if this care becomes quite expensive or extends over months or years. Indeed, the only release from this obligation comes with the death of the person or their wish to transfer that responsibility to another professional. From our observations, few outside the health care professions fully grasp the profundity of this relationship and responsibility. Presently, this obligation conflicts with efforts by health care management organizations, health insurance corporations, and the government that advocate, overtly or covertly, for strict limitations on funds for those dependent on expensive, long-term care for their survival. Until this conflict is resolved, health care practitioners will continue to be caught in a bind where they perceive that their efforts to provide optimal care for VAIs are stymied by these imposed limitations on financial and other resources.

Ultimately, the underlying philosophical principles held by a society will determine how that society acts. Fortunately, in the United States, the Bill of Rights in our Constitution and our legal code strongly support individual rights, especially regarding preservation of life and liberty. This is well exemplified in the Americans with Disabilities Act of 1990 (ADA), although the law faces constant challenges from many quarters. In June, 1999, the United States Supreme Court, in Olmstead v. L.C. and E.W., held that Title II of the ADA requires that long-term services to the disabled must follow the ADA's integration mandate. The court ruled that unjustified retention of disabled persons in institutions with limitation of their exposure to the community constitutes a form of discrimination (42).

Our nation's current acquiescence to the extraordinary expenditures required to treat and maintain VAIs, and continued enforcement of the ADA, represents an expression of national commitment to a person's right to life with a decent quality of existence. The number of persons in the United States needing mechanical ventilation while living at home is estimated at some 6000 to 8000 thousand. Their overall cost to society is almost trivial in a nation of 270 million citizens spending over $1 trillion annually on health care. Since 1950, the gross domestic product of the United States has steadily expanded and now exceeds $8 trillion, by far the largest in the world. Severely disabled persons, including those requiring ventilatory assistance, will not bankrupt our economy or the health care system. Their expenses can, however, bankrupt a family or the health benefits plan of a small, self-insured business. Thus, a plan to finance this exceptionally costly care equitably needs to be developed.

VII. Conclusion

Reported estimates of the costs of home care vary widely from one study to another because of a number of factors. These factors include 1) the complexity and severity of the patient's medical condition, especially the level of respiratory and other vital system support, and the degree of dependency on others for basic activities of life, 2) the number of nursing care hours assumed by the family without compensation, 3) the availability of funds to pay for professional or attendant care, and 4) the availability of professional nurses even when funds are provided. Additionally, each of the reports on home care costs uses differing methodology to compute the expenditures. This variability also occurs with the computation of inpatient costs of ventilator-assisted persons in intensive care units, in subacute care, and in long-term care facilities.

Our review of the recent literature and our own experience and data clearly indicate that, even with inclusion of indirect expenses and lost wages in total home care expenditures, the management and support of ventilator-assisted persons costs significantly less in the home than in any other setting. Furthermore, for nearly every child or adult requiring long-term mechanical ventilation, the home provides the least restrictive and most fulfilling environment. The exceptions would be individuals whose family cannot cope with the demands of their care, or whose family is fragmented or nonexistent.

Available data indicate that the number of children and adults with chronic respiratory failure necessitating long-term mechanical ventilation and other support has been steadily increasing over the past 25 years, with a more rapid increase in the past decade, especially in children. Children, however, lose most of their nursing and other home care benefits at age 21, imposing further burdens and restrictions on the patients and their families. As mentioned above, this regulation of Medicaid and most private insurance plans appears to be in violation of the spirit, if not the exact stipulations, of the Americans with Disabilities Act.

Our lack of comprehensive nationwide information about ventilator assisted persons with chronic disabilities impedes our ability to establish policies in each state that would ensure funding for nursing care and other needed services at home. Extensive research at a national level should be conducted to investigate the epidemiology of chronic respiratory failure, clinical management and outcomes, and the economic and psychosocial effects of these conditions on the patients, their families, and the community. Utilizing data from such studies as well as our own extensive experience, those of us who care for ventilator-assisted children and adults should join with other groups to advocate for a national policy that would assure provision of adequate and equitably distributed funding for their proper care in the least restrictive setting.

References

1. Igelhart JK. The American health system—Expenditures. N Engl J Med 1999; 340: 70–76.
2. Make BJ, Hill NS, Goldberg AI, Bach JR, Criner GJ, Dunne PE, Gilmartin ME, Heffner JE, Kacmarek R, Keens TG, McInturff S, O'Donohue WJ, Oppenheimer E, Robert D. Mechanical ventilation beyond the intensive care unit: Report of a consensus conference of the American College of Chest Physicians. Chest 1998; 113:289S–344S.
3. DeWitt PK, Jansen MT, Davidson Ward SL, Keens TG. Obstacles to discharge of ventilator-assisted children from the hospital to home. Chest 1993; 103:1560–1565.
4. Sevick MA, Kamlet MS, Hoffman LA, Rawson I. Economic cost of home-based care for ventilator-assisted individuals: A preliminary report. Chest 1996; 109:1597–1606.
5. Kurek CJ, Dewar D, Lambrinos J, Booth FVMcL, Cohen IL. Clinical and economic outcome of mechanically ventilated patients in New York state during 1993. Chest 1998; 114:214–222.
6. Goldberg AI, Frownfelter D. The ventilator-assisted individuals study. Chest 1990; 98:428–433.
7. Downes JJ, Parra MM, Costarino AT. Home care of children with chronic respiratory failure: Etiologic categories and overall outcomes. Crit Care Med 1999; 27(suppl): A164.
8. Adams AB, Whitman J, Marcy T. Surveys of long-term ventilatory support in Minnesota: 1986 and 1992. Chest 1993; 103:1463–1470.
9. Shreiner MS, Downes JJ, Kettrick RG, Ise C, Voit R. Chronic respiratory failure in infants with prolonged ventilator dependency. JAMA 1987; 258:3398–3404.
10. Burr BH, Guyer B, Todres ID, Abrahams B, Chiodo T. Home care for children on respirators. N Engl J Med 1983; 309:1319–1323.
11. Frates RC, Splaingard ML, Smith EO, Harrison GM. Outcome of home mechanical ventilation in children. J Pediatr 1985; 106:850–856.
12. Shreiner MS, Donar ME, Kettrick RG. Pediatric home mechanical ventilation. Pediatr Clin North Am 1987; 34:47–60.
13. Dranove D. What impact did the programs have on the costs of care for ventilator assisted children? In: Aday LA, Aitken MJ, Wegener DH. Pediatric Home Care: Results of a National Evaluation of Programs for Ventilator Assisted Children. Chicago: Pluribus Press, University of Chicago, 1988; 295–321.
14. Fields AI, Rosenblatt A, Pollack NM, Kaufman J. Home care cost-effectiveness for respiratory technology-dependent children. Am J Dis Child 1991; 145:729–733.
15. Make BJ, Gilmartin ME. Mechanical ventilation in the home. Crit Care Clin 1990; 6:785–796.
16. Dasgupta A, Rice R, Mascha E, Litaker D, Stoller JK. Four-year experience with

a unit for long-term ventilation (respiratory special care unit) at the Cleveland Clinic Foundation. Chest 1999; 116:447–455.

17. O'Donohue WJ, Giovannoni RM, Goldberg AI, Keens TG, Macke BJ, Plummer AL, Prentice WS. Long-term mechanical ventilation: Guidelines for management in the home and at alternate community sites. Chest 1986; 90:1S–37S.
18. Plummer AL, O'Donohue WJ, Petty TL. Consensus conference on problems in home mechanical ventilation. Am Rev Respir Dis 1989; 140:555–560.
19. Eigen H, Zander J. Home mechanical ventilation of pediatric patients: Official statement of the American Thoracic Society. Am Rev Respir Dis 1990; 141:258–259.
20. Panitch HB, Downes JJ, Kennedy JS, Kolb SM, Parra MM, Peacock J, Thompson MC. Guidelines for home care of children with chronic respiratory insufficiency. Pediatr Pulmonol 1996; 21:52–56.
21. Iglehart JK. The American health care system—Medicaid. N Engl J Med 1999; 340: 403–408.
22. Murray JE. Payment mechanisms for pediatric home care. Caring Magazine, October 1989; 33–35.
23. Kuttner R. The American health care system—Health insurance coverage. N Engl J Med 1999; 340:163–168.
24. United States Supreme Court. Cedar Rapids Community School District v. Garret F. No. 96-1793, decided March 3, 1999.
25. Dougherty JM, personal communication, 1999.
26. Bach JR, Intintola P, Alba AS, Holland IE. The ventilator-assisted individual: Cost analysis of institutionalization vs rehabilitation and in-home management. Chest 1992; 101:26–30.
27. Moss AH, Oppenheimer EA, Casey P, Cazzolli PA, Roos RP, Stocking CB, Siegler M. Patients with amyotrophic lateral sclerosis receiving long-term mechanical ventilation. Advance care planning and outcomes. Chest 1996; 110:249–255.
28. Parra MM, personal communication, 1999.
29. Chalom R, Raphaely RC, Costarino AT. The hospital costs of pediatric intensive care. Crit Care Med 1999; 27:2079–2085.
30. Downes JJ, Dougherty JM, personal communication, 1999.
31. Wegener DH. What impact did the programs have on the adaptation of families of ventilator assisted children? In: Aday LA, Aitken MJ, Wegener DH. Pediatric Home Care: Results of a National Evaluation of Programs for Ventilator Assisted Children. Chicago: Pluribus Press, University of Chicago, 1988; 263–294.
32. Sevick MA, Bradham DD. Economic value of caregiver effort in maintaining long-term ventilator-assisted individuals at home. Heart Lung 1997; 26:148–157.
33. Thomas VM, Ellison K, Howell EV, Winters K. Caring for the person receiving ventilatory support at home: Care givers' needs and involvement. Heart Lung 1992; 21:180–186.
34. Sevick MA, Sereika S, Matthews JT, Zucconi S, Wielobob C, Puczynski S, Ahmad SM, Barsh LF. Home-based ventilator-dependent patients: Measurement of the emotional aspects of home caregiving. Heart Lung 1994; 23:269–278.
35. Quint RD, Chesterman E, Crain LS, Winkleby M, Boyce WT. Home care for ventilator-dependent children. Psychosocial impact on the family. Am J Dis Child 1990; 144:1238–1241.

36. Downes JJ, Hock-Long LE. Home care of children with chronic respiratory failure: Impact on families. Crit Care Med 1999; 27(suppl):A147.
37. Lantos JD, Kohrman AF. Ethical aspects of pediatric home care. Pediatrics 1992; 89:920–924.
38. Russell B. The Utilitarians. In: Russell B. A History of Western Philosophy. New York: Simon and Schuster, 1945; 773–782.
39. Brehier E. The Scottish School and English Utilitarianism from 1800 to 1850. In: Brehier E. The Nineteenth Century: Period of Systems, 1800–1850. Chicago: University of Chicago Press, 1968; 95–109.
40. Durant W, Durant A. English philosophy. In. Durant W, Durant A. The Age of Louis XIV. The Story of Civilization: Part VIII. New York: Simon and Schuster, 1963; 548–597.
41. Will GF. Life and death at Princeton. Newsweek, September 13, 1999; 80–82.
42. Gold S. Supreme Court to rule on rights of people with disabilities. Caring Magazine, July 1999; 26–27.

14

New Ventilator Options for Long-Term Mechanical Ventilation in the Home

ROBERT M. KACMAREK

Harvard Medical School
Massachusetts General Hospital
Boston, Massachusetts

I. Introduction

The number of patients requiring long-term mechanical ventilation (LTMV) in the home has markedly increased over the last 10 years. Along with this increase has been a demand for better, more versatile ventilators for use in the home. The advent of bilevel pressure devices has greatly expanded the ventilator choice available for long-term mechanical ventilation. In addition, within the last few years a number of new volume-/pressure-targeted home care ventilators have entered the market. These ventilators are much more responsive than previous volume-targeted home care ventilators and most are also capable of providing invasive pressure-targeted ventilation. All of these additions have increased the options available for both practitioner and patient and have made LTMV in the home more feasible.

II. Clinical Application of Mechanical Ventilation

The choice of mechanical ventilator and the method of application in the home depend upon numerous factors: presence of an artificial airway, the need for continuous ventilation, inability to sustain even short periods of time ventilator independent, and the pathology requiring ventilatory support. Generally, LTMV patients can be divided into four groups: 1) elective noninvasive mechanical ventilation, 2) mandatory noninvasive mechanical ventilation, 3) elective invasive (via tracheostomy) mechanical ventilation, and 4) mandatory invasive (via tracheostomy) mechanical ventilation (1).

A. Elective Noninvasive Intermittent Positive Pressure Ventilation

The question of what type of patient benefits most from elective noninvasive LTMV is still controversial. It is my opinion that elective support benefits primarily patients with neuromuscular and neurologic disease and patients with disturbed sleep who have loss of energy and an inability to perform functions of daily living due to ventilatory dysfunction and carbon dioxide (CO_2) elevation. This is particularly true if the process is nonreversible and progressive. Whether elective noninvasive LTMV benefits patients with chronic obstructive lung disease is still very controversial (see Chapters 5 and 8).

The goals of elective noninvasive LTMV include rest and partial unloading of the ventilatory muscles for about 6 to 12 hr/day (2), avoiding excessive hypoventilation and improving oxygenation during sleep, improving baseline CO_2 levels, and increasing daytime energy levels (2–4). To achieve these goals, care

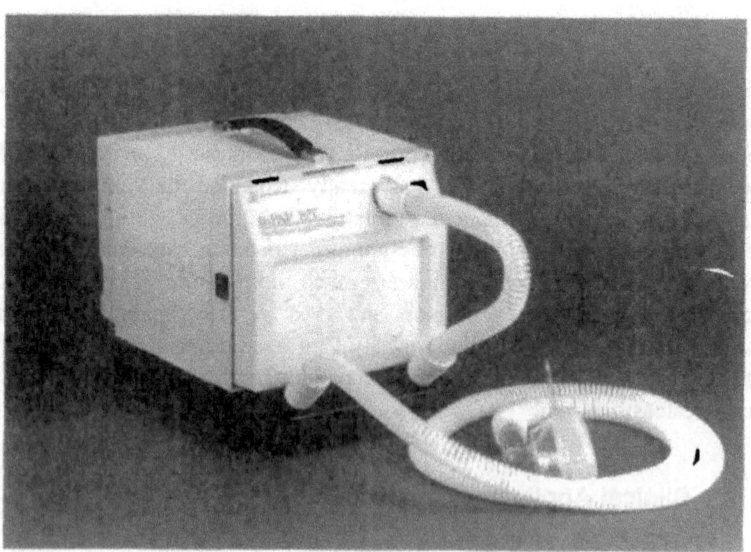

Figure 1 Original BiPAP ventilator (Respironics, Inc., Pittsburgh, PA).

must be taken to ensure that application of positive pressure is comfortable and capable of meeting the patient's ventilatory demands (see later sections).

Although negative pressure ventilation, pneumobelts, and rocking beds are feasible in this setting, noninvasive positive pressure ventilation (NPPV) via nasal mask using a bilevel pressure ventilator is preferable (Fig. 1). In some patients, acceptance of nasal NPPV delivered by volume-cycled ventilators is less than with pressure-limited ventilators because of the higher peak airway pressure generated and the inability of delivered flow to vary with patient demand (5). Noninvasive positive pressure ventilation can be delivered with volume-limited ventilation but setting the ventilator is more difficult (Fig. 2). With all approaches, air leaks of varying sizes occur on a breath-to-breath basis. The ability of bilevel pressure ventilators to compensate for leaks makes them ideal for this type of NPPV (6). With volume-limited ventilators, leak compensation is poor and quantification of actual tidal volume difficult because of air leaks. With volume-limited ventilators, a tidal volume of about 10 to 12 mL/kg is large enough to compensate for leaks, resulting in an actual patient tidal volume of about 6 to 8 mL/kg (5).

With volume-limited ventilation, the clinician directly sets the inspiratory time or sets the peak inspiratory flow indirectly setting the inspiratory time (7).

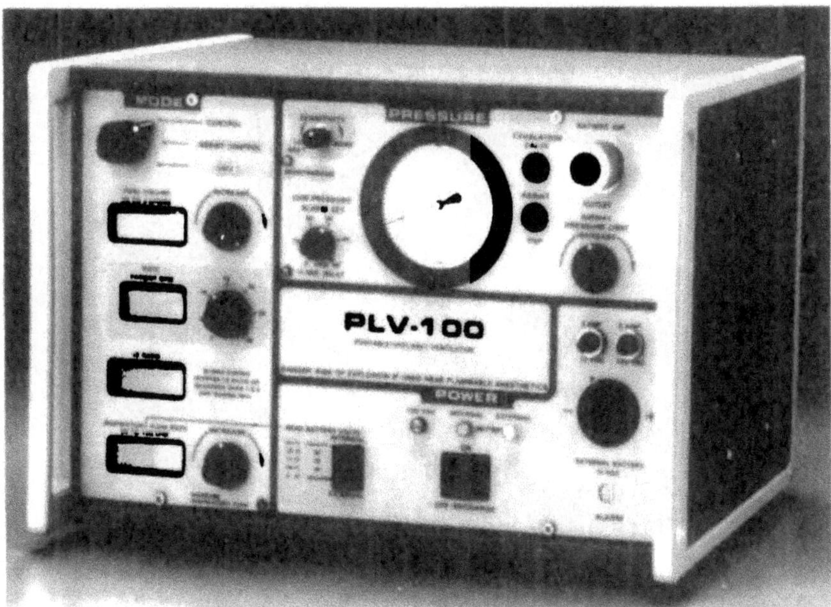

Figure 2 Lifecare PLV-100 (Respironics, Inc., Pittsburgh, PA) volume-targeted home care ventilator.

Appropriate setting of inspiratory time is critical to ensuring patient ventilator synchrony. If the patient desires an inspiratory time of 1.0 sec and the ventilator delivers the gas volume in 1.5 sec, dyssynchrony is inevitable (8). Therefore, the patient's unassisted inspiratory time should be determined and the ventilator set accordingly. Generally, most patients require an inspiratory time of <1.0 sec. In patients with a variable ventilatory drive, the mode used should always be assist/control (A/C) with the backup rate set to ensure a minimum acceptable respiratory rate (≥10/min). With pressure assist/control, inspiratory time is determined by the setting of inspiratory time, but with pressure support, inspiratory time is determined by the reduction of peak inspiratory flow. Inspiration with pressure support is terminated when peak flow decreases to a set level (i.e., 25% of peak flow). With many of the newer ventilators, the flow cycling criteria in pressure support can be adjusted.

B. Noninvasive Mandatory Ventilatory Support

The provision of mandatory NIPPV to patients in the home requires careful monitoring of the patient and equipment. Most clinicians prefer to provide ventilator support invasively in these settings. However, Bach and Alba (9,10) and others (11,12) have nicely demonstrated the effective use of both noninvasive positive

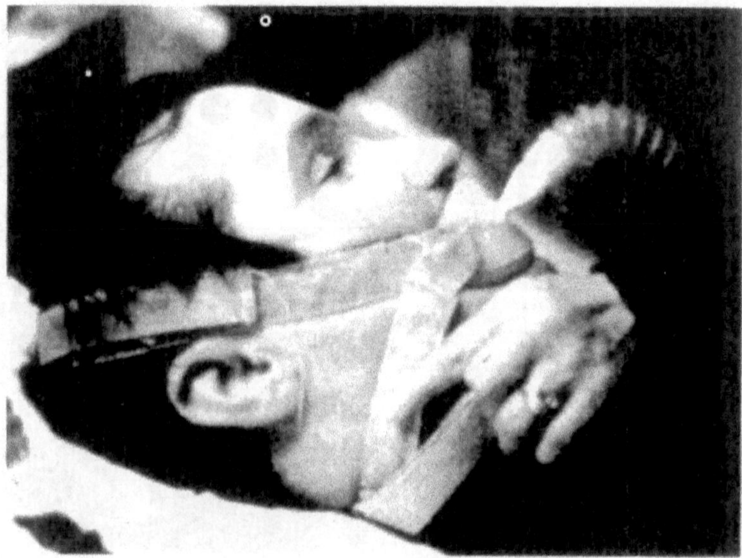

Figure 3 Patient with a vital capacity less than 10 mL set up for overnight MIPPV with the mouthpiece supported firmly in the mouth by the Bennett lipseal. (From Ref. 3.)

pressure (9) and non–positive pressure techniques (10) in large numbers of patients requiring ventilatory support. In this setting, a mouthpiece and lipseal (Fig. 3), a nasal mask, or a full-face mask have been used to interface the patient with the ventilator.

C. Elective Ventilation Via Tracheostomy

Although the use of elective ventilation via a tracheostomy is rare, some individuals require a tracheostomy for bulbar or upper airway disorders and also benefit from elective intermittent ventilatory support while others continue with elective

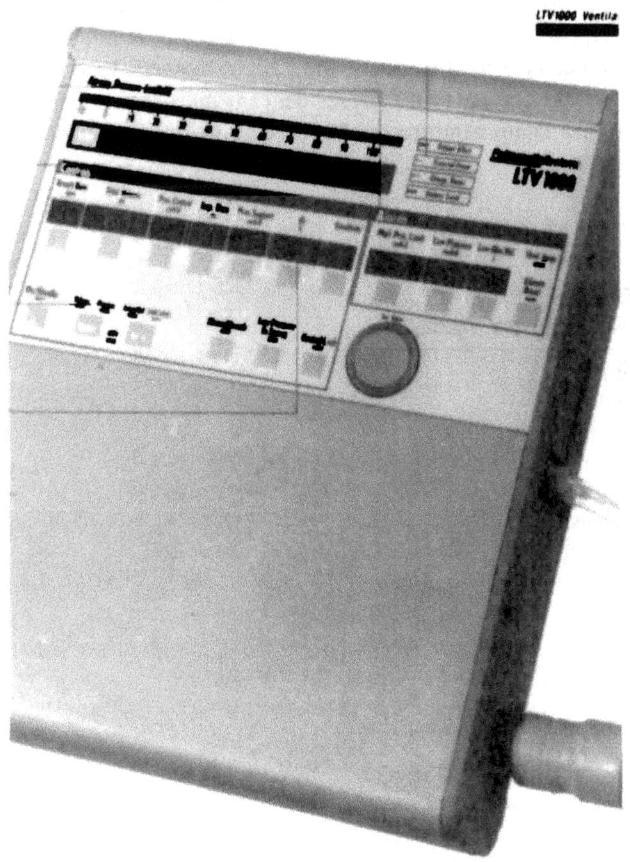

Figure 4 Pulmonetics LTV 1000 ventilator (Pulmonetics, San Diego, CA).

support after recovering from an episode of acute respiratory failure. In this setting, a ventilator should be selected based on its monitoring and alarm capabilities because, unlike NPPV, the closed invasive ventilatory system requires accurate monitoring of tidal volume and pressure (Fig. 4). In general, this means that volume-limited ventilators are preferred because bilevel pressure ventilators designed for the home lack sufficient monitoring or alarm capabilities for invasive ventilation.

D. Invasive Mandatory Ventilatory Support

Because of the potentially life-threatening consequences of ventilator disconnection or malfunction, only ventilators with appropriate monitoring and alarms should be used for this indication. Many patients requiring home mechanical ventilatory support must have a secondary or backup ventilator. Generally, a backup ventilator is recommended if the patient requires 16 or more hours of ventilatory support per day or if their residence is more than 4 hr from a hospital (13). Additional equipment frequently needed by these patients is listed in Table 1.

Table 1 Equipment Required During Invasive Positive Pressure Ventilation

Primary ventilator
Back-up ventilator[a]
System humidifier
Ventilator circuits
Oxygen source
Suction apparatus
Suction equipment
Spare tracheotomy tube
Remote alarm
Battery
Battery charger
Manual ventilator
Compressor for aerosol medications[b]
Small volume nebulizer[b]
Electrical generator[a]

[a]Only necessary if greater than 16 hours per day ventilator support required, or located more than four hours from a hospital.
[b]Only necessary if aerosol medication ordered.

III. Positive Pressure Ventilators for Home Use

Today, numerous positive pressure ventilators whether classified as bilevel pressure ventilators (Fig. 5), volume ventilators, or combined volume/pressure-targeted ventilators (Fig. 6) are available for home use. Because of the microprocessor design of these units, features and capabilities of these devices change very rapidly. In this section, available ventilators are reviewed along with issues and problems specific to the ventilator or class of ventilators. However, because of rapid upgrades, the capabilities of these ventilators change rapidly and may differ from those discussed.

A. Bilevel Pressure Ventilators

The design of most of the ventilators in this group is very similar (Fig. 7). The ventilator uses a compressor/blower system to generate flow and incorporates a fast-response flow control valve that modulates delivered flow (Fig. 8). The Respironics units (Respironics Inc., Pittsburgh, PA) are the prototype of this

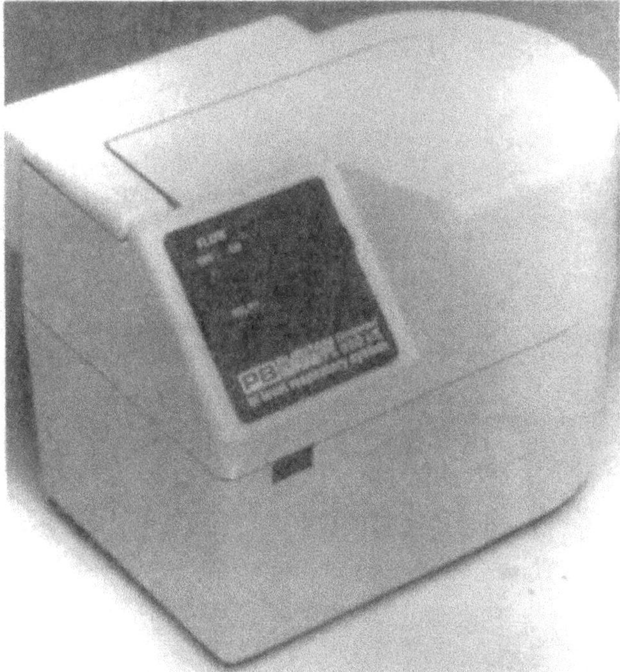

Figure 5 Puritan-Bennett 320 I/E ventilator (Mallinkrodt, St. Louis, MO).

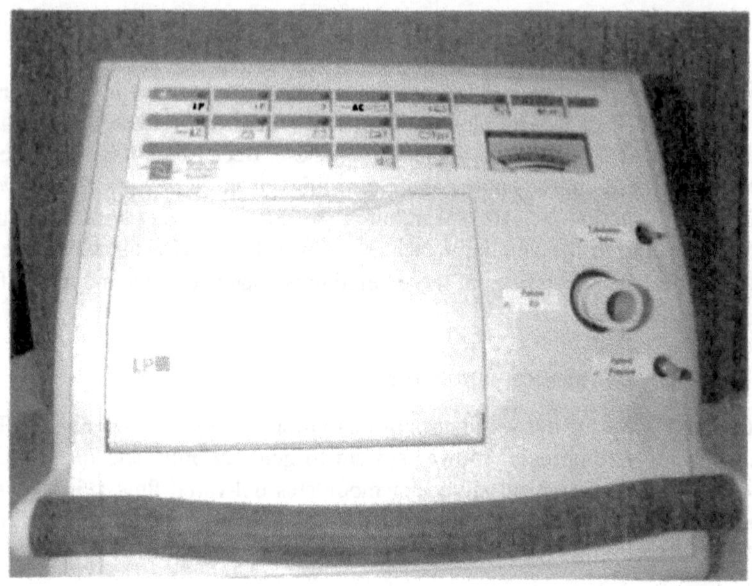

Figure 6 Nellcor Puritan-Bennett Achieva™ ventilator (Mallinkrodt, St. Louis, MO).

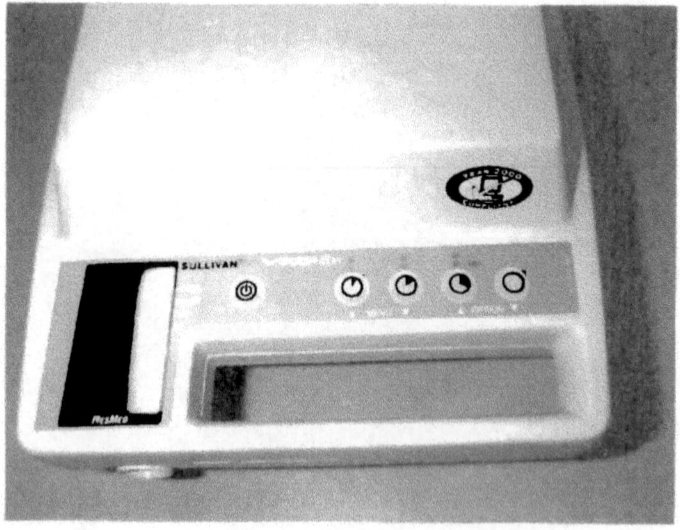

Figure 7 Sullivan VPAP II ventilator (ResMed, San Diego, CA).

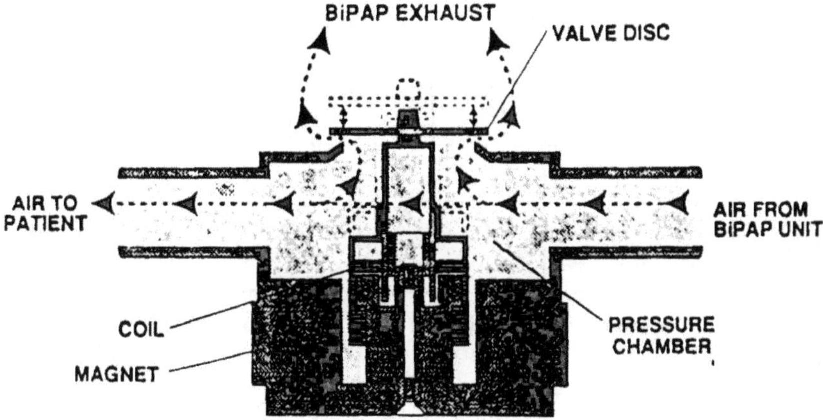

Figure 8 Respironics BiPAP ventilator flow control valve. (Courtesy of Respironics, Inc., Pittsburgh, PA.)

group; their valve opens when 40 ml/sec flow change for 30 msec is identified (5). The gas delivery circuit is a single, large-bore tube with a small-bore hole at the patient end to establish a fixed leak and to allow exhalation. The units are all small (≤12″ × 18″ × 7″), lightweight (≤20 lb), and designed for home use. In addition, all these ventilators are capable of compensating for leaks. This is accomplished by the flow control valve (in a few breaths) learning the level of leak present by measuring flow at end exhalation during the previous few breaths and readjusting trigger sensitivity to the new baseline flow. This occurs on an ongoing basis to insure minimal effort to trigger inspiration and to enhance patient–ventilator synchrony.

The pressure and flow patterns normally established with these units are illustrated in Figure 9. As noted, these units attempt to provide a constant inspiratory pressure with a variable gas flow, similar to that provided by all pressure-targeted modes. The actual volume, airway pressure, and flow patterns delivered depend upon the set inspiratory pressure and the impedance (compliance and resistance) to ventilation (6). The greater the set pressure and the lower the impedance to ventilation, the greater the tidal volume. Depending upon the specific unit, the mode of ventilation may be either continuous positive airway pressure (CPAP), assist, assist/control, or control. Alternative terminology is used by some manufacturers (spontaneous, spontaneous/timed, timed), however, the actual operation of these modes is the same as with the classic terminology (14). Table 2 lists available modes on select bilevel pressure ventilators. Similar to pressure support ventilation, in assist and assist/control inspiration ends when the patient's

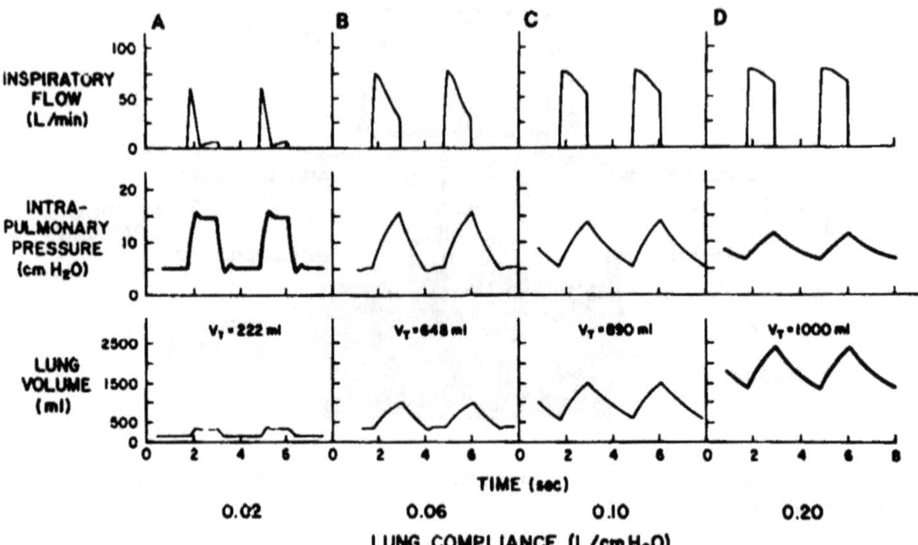

Figure 9 Pressure, flow, and volume vs. time waveforms developed by bilevel pressure ventilators under different lung model compliance settings: (A) compliance 0.02 mL/cm H_2O, (B) 0.06 mL/cm H_2O, (C) 0.10 mL/cm H_2O, and (D) 0.20 mL/cm H_2O. As with all pressure-targeted breaths, a greater volume and greater likelihood for airtrapping occurs in the very compliant system. (From Ref. 6.)

inspiratory flow decreases to a predetermined level, equal to the end inspiratory flow criteria (15). As noted in Table 2, several companies have numerous models of the same basic machine type. The primary differences in models are available modes, pressure limits (some can provide peak pressure up to 35 cm H_2O, as opposed to 20 to 25 cm H_2O in most) and the presence of gas delivery modifiers (rise time, variable inspiratory termination criteria, ramp/delay) (Table 3).

Figures 10 and 11 illustrate a comparison of inspiratory time delays and inspiratory trigger pressures in a series of bilevel pressure ventilators compared with the Puritan-Bennett® 7200ae with flow triggering (Mallinkrodt, St. Louis, MO). As is obvious from these illustrations, this group of ventilators responds as well to patient effort as a typical intensive care unit (ICU) ventilator. Most of these units have highly sensitive inspiratory triggers that are preset.

Inspiratory flow waveforms from a group of bilevel pressure ventilators are illustrated in Figure 12. These waveforms can vary considerably from ventilator to ventilator. However, all are capable of pressurizing the ventilated system as rapidly as the PB7200ae. Figure 13 also shows that these ventilators vary

Table 2 Modes of Ventilation Available on Select Bilevel Pressure Ventilators

Ventilator	Company	CPAP	Assist	A/C	Control
ST-30	Respironics[a]	X	X	X	X
ST-ST	Respironics	X	X	X	X
Tranquility™	Respironics	X	X	—	—
Quantum™	Respironics	X	X	X	X
320 I/E	Puritan-Bennett[b]	X	X	—	—
320 B	Puritan-Bennett	X	X	X	—
335	Puritan-Bennett	X	X	X	—
Comfort	ResMed[c]	X	X	—	—
VPAP II	ResMed	X	X	—	—
VPAP II S/T	ResMed	X	X	X	X
VPAP II-A	ResMed	X	X	X	X
VPAP MAX	ResMed	—	X	X	X

[a]Respironics, Inc., Pittsburgh, PA.
[b]Mallinkrodt, Inc., St. Louis, MO.
[c]ResMed, San Diego, CA.

Table 3 Ventilators with Variable Inspiratory Sensitivity, Rise Time, and Termination Criteria

Ventilator	Company	Inspiratory sensitivity	Rise time	Adjustable termination criteria
320 I/E	Puritan-Bennett[a]	X	—	X
320 B	Puritan-Bennett	X	—	X
335	Puritan-Bennett	X	X	X
VPAP II	ResMed[b]	—	X	—
VPAP II S/T	ResMed	—	X	—
VPAP II S/T-A	ResMed	—	X	—
VPAP MAX	ResMed	—	X	—
Tranquility™	Respironics[c]	—	X	—
Quantum™	Respironics	—	X	—

[a]Mallinkrodt, Inc., St. Louis, MO.
[b]ResMed, San Diego, CA.
[c]Respironics, Inc., Pittsburgh, PA.

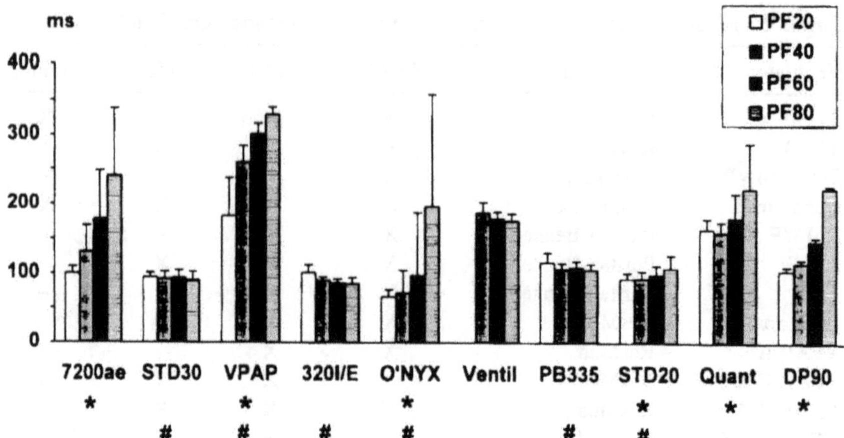

Figure 10 Effects of inspiratory flow demand (PF) at various settings (20 = 20 L/min, 30 = 30 L/min, etc.) on inspiratory time delay (D-I). Mean ± SD across all experimental settings. Asterisk indicates $p < 0.05$ among PF; number sign, $p < 0.05$ vs. 7200ae. (From Ref. 15.)

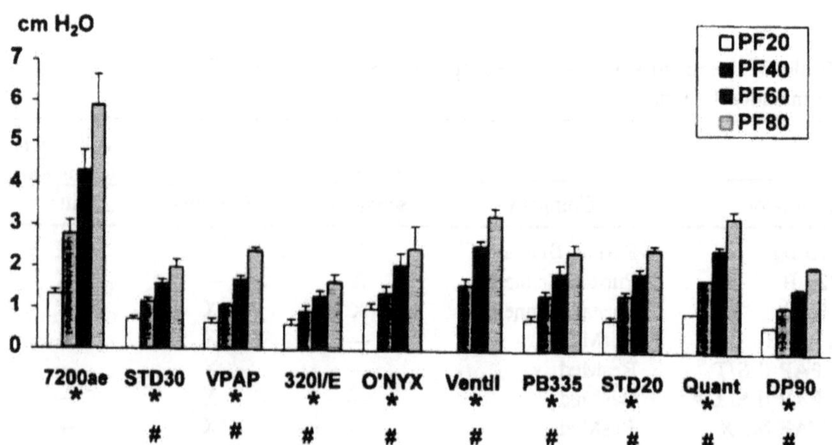

Figure 11 Effect of inspiratory flow demand (PF) at various settings (20 = 20 L/min, 30 = 30 L/min etc.) on inspiratory trigger pressure (P-I). Mean ± SD across all experimental settings. Asterisk indicates $p < 0.05$ among PF; number sign, $p < 0.05$ vs. 7200ae. (From Ref. 15.)

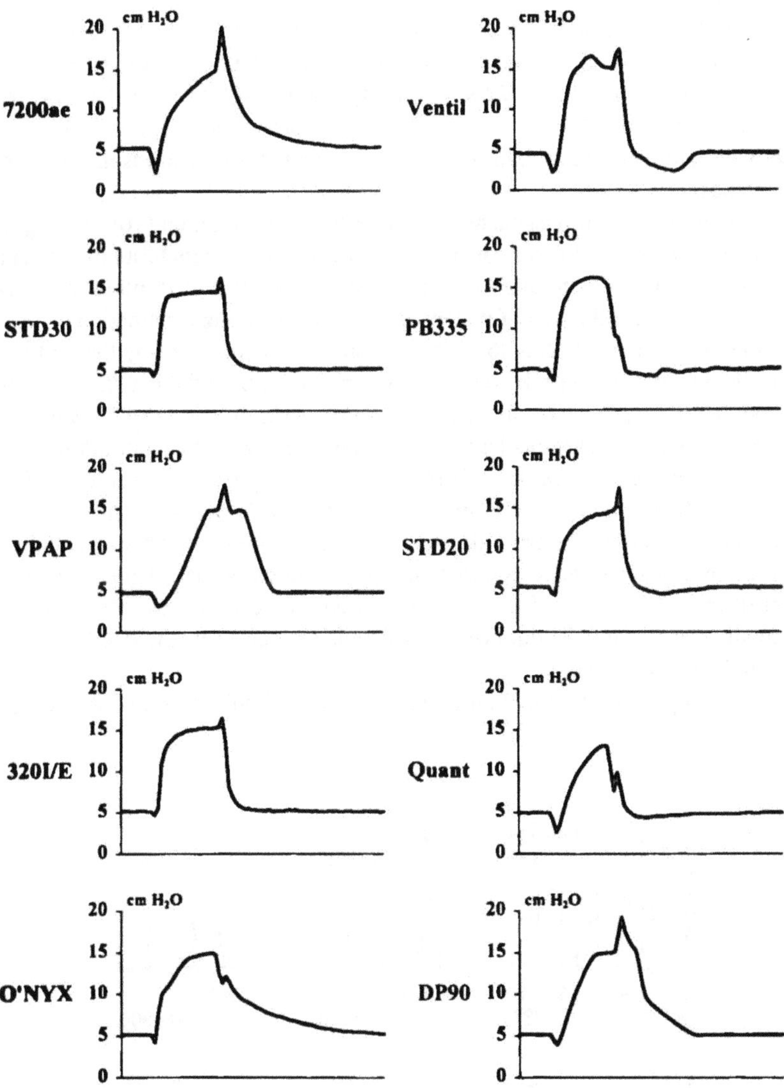

Figure 12 Airway pressure vs. time for various bilevel pressure ventilators. Lung model peak flow at 60 L/min, model compliance 50 mL/cm H_2O, PEEP 5 cm H_2O, inspiratory pressure 10 cm H_2O. Ventil (Sefam, Nancy, France); DP90 (Taema, Antony Cedex, France); VPAP (ResMed, San Diego, CA); O'NYX, 3201E, 7200ae, PB335 (Mallinkrodt, Inc., St. Louis, MO); Quant, STD20, STD30 (Respironics, Inc.). (From Ref. 15.)

considerably in how they cycle to exhalation. Whenever pressure increases above the set level at end exhalation, the ventilator cycles to exhalation (15). Normally, a smooth decrease in airway pressure should occur (as with the PB335). However, Figure 13 shows that the O'NYX and the Quantum cycled to exhalation before the lung model (notch in initial expiratory pressure waveform) and all of the other ventilators cycled to exhalation after the lung model (end inspiratory pressure spike).

Patient ventilator dyssynchrony during NPPV is common (16). After gross air leak, the two major factors causing dyssynchrony are the inability of the ventilator to meet patient inspiratory flow demands at the onset of inspiration (17,18) and the lack of coordination of patient and ventilator during termination of inspiration (19). Problems with both of these issues can be resolved by the ability to adjust the rate of rise to peak pressure (rise time) (15,20) and the ability to adjust the end inspiratory flow threshold that terminates each breath (15,17). A number of bilevel pressure ventilators have incorporated these variables, permitting clinicians the opportunity to set them based on patient response (see Table 3). However, it is difficult to accurately set these variables without visual observation of the airway pressure waveform. Ideally, the rise time should be set so that a linear increase in airway pressure occurs without overshooting the set pressure at the onset of inspiration (21). If the airway pressure curve is concave, the rise time is too slow, whereas if initial pressure exceeds the set level, the rise time is set too rapid (Fig. 13) (20).

The inspiratory termination criteria (cycling) should be set so that the pa-

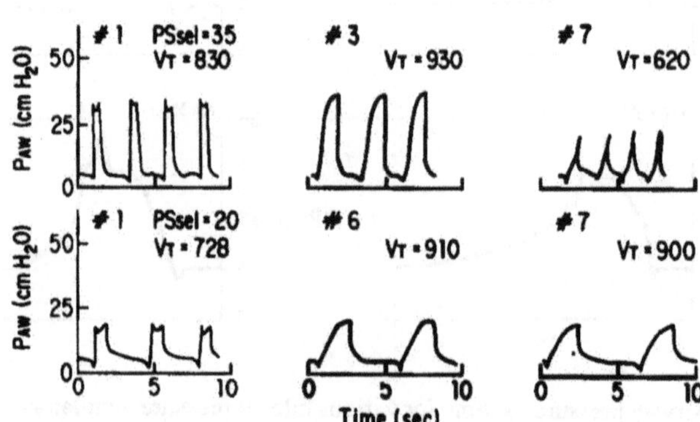

Figure 13 Airway pressure waveforms from two patients at various rise time settings. The setting on the left is too high a flow, the setting on the right is too low a rise time, the middle setting is the ideal rise time. (From Ref. 20.)

tient and ventilator inspiratory times are equal and transition to exhalation is synchronous. If the patient terminates inspiration before the ventilator, patient–ventilator dyssynchrony is induced because accessory muscle of expiration must be recruited at the end of mechanical inspiration to force a transition to exhalation (22). In general, patients with chronic obstructive pulmonary disease (COPD) require a higher inspiratory termination threshold setting (greater percentage of peak flow) than patients with neuromuscular disease, since COPD patients have a higher end inspiratory flow than patients without intrinsic lung disease (22). The use of a set inspiratory time instead of the normal end inspiratory flow terminating criteria can vastly improve patient–ventilator synchrony during NIPPV (Fig. 14) (17). However, as with rise time, it is difficult to set this variable without visual observation of the airway pressure waveforms.

Some bilevel pressure ventilators incorporate a delay time option for reaching target peak inspiratory pressure (PIP) and a ramp increase in pressure to the targeted level. This feature allows a gradual buildup of pressure in the system, avoiding high initial pressure on the first breath. The delay time/ramp can range

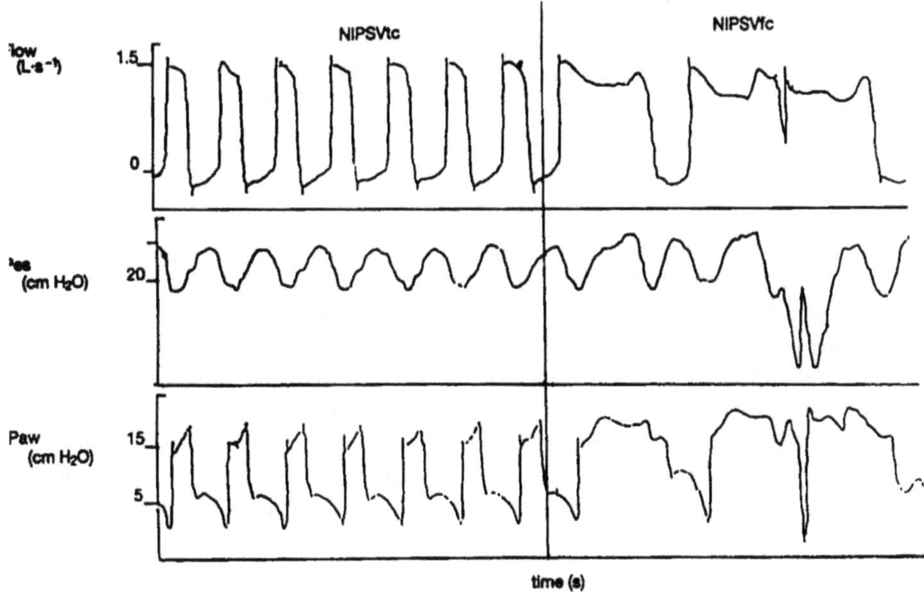

Figure 14 Synchronous (left) and asynchronous (right) triggering to exhalation during NIPPV. (From Ref. 19.)

on some models from 0 up to 20 to 30 min (VPAP II S/T, 335, Tranquility™), but most neuromuscular disease patients do not use this feature, preferring high initial pressures.

Delivery of Oxygen

None of the ventilators designed for home use allows precise delivery of increased inspired oxygen (F_{IO_2}) (5,14). Oxygen is added to the inspiratory circuit via an attachment at the ventilator or to the mask itself. It has been our experience that these ventilators function appropriately with added oxygen flows up to 8 L/min. However, because of the variable flow delivered by all bilevel pressure ventilators, the actual delivered F_{IO_2} is variable throughout the breath and impossible to estimate accurately. Setting of the delivered flow of oxygen depends upon the response of the patient.

Aerosol Therapy

None of the bilevel pressure ventilators is deigned to accommodate the delivery of inhaled aerosolized pharmacologic agents (5,14). However, the delivery of aerosol therapy during ventilation does not appear to adversely affect ventilator operation. Either metered dose inhaler (MDI) adapters or small-volume nebulizers can be placed between the ventilator large-bore tubing and the exhalation orifice or face mask. Adapters can be removed from the circuit between treatment periods.

Carbon Dioxide Rebreathing

A potentially significant problem with all bilevel pressure ventilators that have a single gas delivery circuit is the retrograde movement of exhaled gas into the ventilator circuit and rebreathing of CO_2. These ventilators have very low internal resistance flow control values that allow retrograde movement of gas all the way into the ventilator (5,14). As shown in Figure 15, unless positive end-expiratory pressure (PEEP) is set $\geq$5 cm H_2O or an isolation/exhalation valve is added to the system, exhaled gas can be rebreathed. The use of PEEP increases the ventilator-to-patient pressure gradient preventing gas from entering the inspiratory limb. In any system, CO_2 rebreathing is of greater concern with full-face masks than with nasal masks, since with full-face masks, all exhaled gas must exit from the small exhalation orifice.

Humidification

Although most of the bilevel pressure ventilators are designed to operate without the use of a humidifier, all operate adequately with a passover humidifier added to the inspiratory limb. Both bubble-through, and heat and moisture exchanger

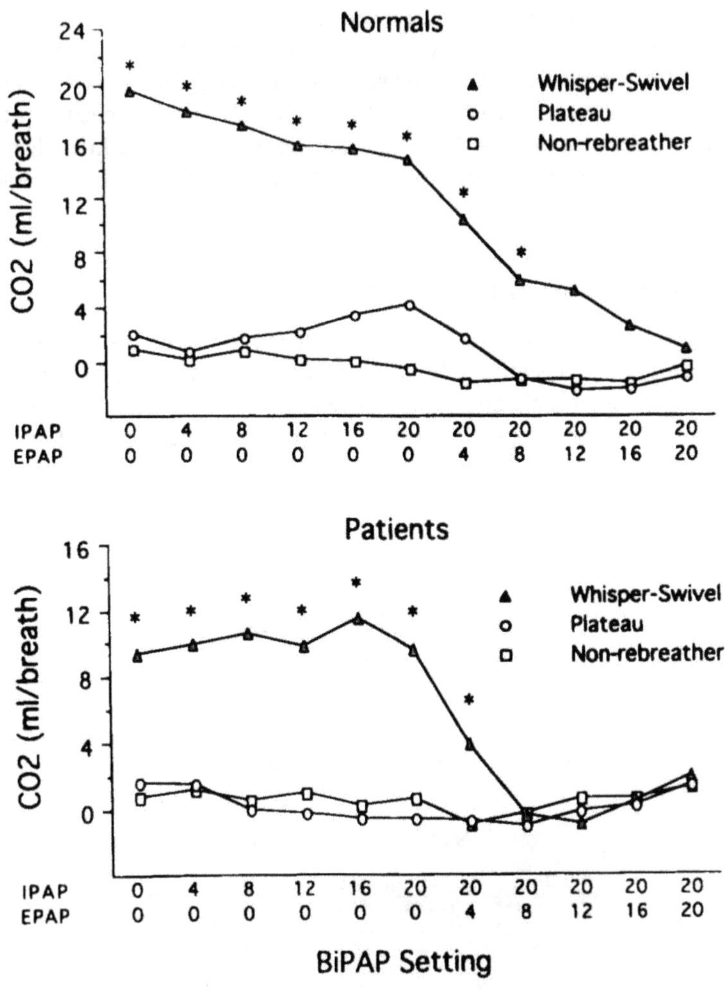

Figure 15 The effect of inspiratory pressure, PEEP level, and type of exhalation system on rebreathing of CO_2 during bilevel pressure ventilation with the Respironics ST-D ventilator (Respironics, Inc., Pittsburgh, PA). Carbon dioxide rebreathing was prevented by PEEP ≥ 5 cm H_2O and the use of an isolation/exhalation valve. (From Ref 23.)

(HME) humidifiers should be avoided. Bubble-through humidifiers, because they increase resistance to flow, may interfere with the operation of the ventilator. Heat and moisture exchanger humidifiers do not grossly interfere with the operation of bilevel pressure ventilators but have limited effectiveness in the presence of leaks, because all exhaled gas must be exhaled through the HME for it to effectively remove water vapor to be added to the next breath. Usually, the passover humidifier does not need to be heated, but a heating element may be added if patients complain of persisting dryness. Since the upper airway is intact, a limited amount of added water vapor is all that most patients require, unless there are large air leaks.

B. Volume-Targeted Home Care Ventilators

Historically, the most common ventilator designed for home use was a piston-driven volume-limited ventilator (Fig. 16). Based on this design, these ventilators have several inherent limitations. Gas delivery must follow a square or sine wave delivery pattern, rendering them unable to respond to patient demand. None of

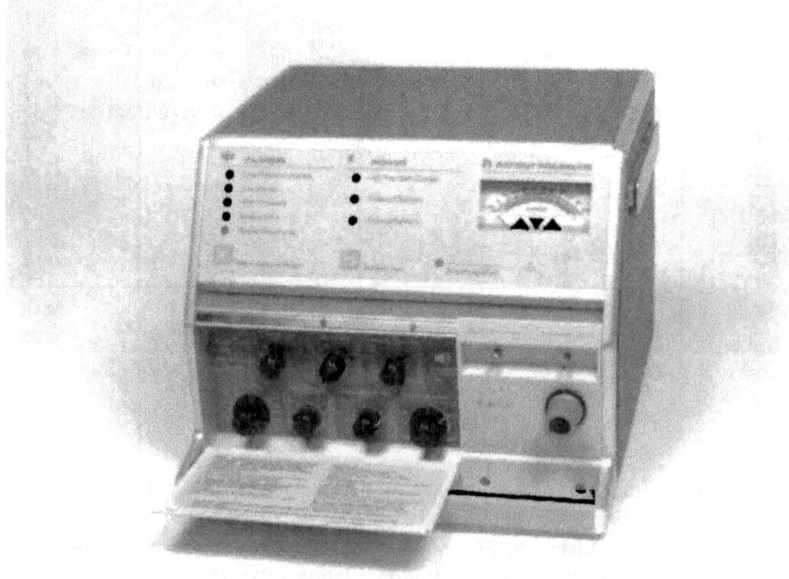

Figure 16 The LP-6 volume ventilator from Aequiton™ (Nellcor Puritan-Bennett, Mallinkrodt, Inc., St. Louis, MO).

these ventilators incorporates PEEP or a demand delivery system, but all include synchronized intermittent mandatory ventilation (SIMV) (5,14). In addition, these ventilators are well alarmed and adequately monitor patients. All can be attached to external batteries and each includes an internal battery allowing about 1 hr of operation (Table 4).

Delivery of Supplemental Oxygen

The typical home volume-limited ventilator is not designed to provide a precise FIO_2 above 0.21. The reason for this is that few patients receiving home ventilation require a precise or high FIO_2. Typically, an FIO_2 of 0.25 to 0.35 is needed and a 0.05 variation in FIO_2 is generally clinically acceptable. Only the Lifecare PLV-102 (Respironics, Inc., Pittsburgh, PA), by the use of a proportioning solenoid valve, is capable of setting and maintaining a precise FIO_2. The other ventilators increase FIO_2 by the attachment of an O_2 accumulator to the gas entry port or the titration of O_2 into the inspiratory limb between the ventilator and the humidifier. An O_2 accumulator is a large rectangular box attached to the gas entry port within which oxygen and room air mix to establish a desired FIO_2. Oxygen is bled into the accumulator while room air is drawn into the accumulator during the backstroke of the piston. All manufacturers provide elaborate formulas or tables to calculate FIO_2 delivered in this way, but these are only correct if the patient is ventilated in the control mode. Variation in the ventilator rate, tidal volume, oxygen flow, and level of spontaneous breathing all affect the breath-by-breath FIO_2 delivered. Oxygen accumulators are available on most of these ventilators.

The FIO_2 may be increased in all units (including pressure-limited units) by the use of an O_2 delivery elbow (Fig. 17) between the ventilator and the humidifier. As with the O_2 accumulator, the FIO_2 delivered is affected by all ventilatory variables. In general, a more stable FIO_2 is possible with the accumulator than with the O_2 delivery elbow. In addition, a bias flow added at the outflow port of the ventilator increases the effort required to trigger inspiration during assist/control ventilation.

SIMV/IMV and Work of Breathing

None of the volume-controlled home care ventilators incorporates a demand system (Fig. 18). Thus, during the spontaneous breathing phase of SIMV, the patient must draw gas from either the piston chamber, a piston chamber bypass valve, or through the exhalation valve (24). As a result, even with the use of an optimal humidifying system (passover humidifier), a large amount of work is imposed by the ventilator. This work increases as patient peak spontaneous inspiratory flow rate increases or if a bubble-through humidifier is in use. A bubble through

Table 4 Gas Delivery Features of Select Volume-Targeted Home Care Ventilators

	Aequitron™ LP-6[a]	Aequitron™ LP-10[a]	Aequitron™ LP-6 Plus[a]	Lifecare PLV-100[b]	Lifecare PLV-102[b]	Nellcor[f] Puritan-Bennett 2801[a]	Nellcor Puritan-Bennett 2500[a]	Intermed Bear 33
Tidal volume, mL	100–2200	100–2200	100–2200	50–3000	50–1800	50–2800	50–2500	100–2200
Inspiratory time, sec	0.5–5.5	0.5–5.5	0.5–5.5	—	—	—	0.8–1.5	0.25–4.99
Peak flow, L/min	—	—	—	10–120	10–120	20–120	—	20–120
Rate, per min	1–38	1–38	1–38	2–40	2–40	1–69	<4–>20	2–40
Battery life, min	Up to 60	Up to 60	Up to 60	Up to 60	Up to 60	20–60	20–60	Up to 60
Modes	C, A/C, press limited after plateau, SIMV	C, A/C, press limited before and after plateau, SIMV	C, A/C, press limited after plateau, SIMV	C, A/C, SIMV	C, A/C, SIMV	C, A/C, SIMV, press limited with plateau	C, A/C	C, A/C, SIMV
Sensitivity, cm H_2O	−10 to +10	−10 to +10	−10 to +10	−6 to +3	−6 to +18	−10 to +10	−1 preset	−9 to +9

[a]Mallinkrodt, Inc., St. Louis, MO.
[b]Respironics, Inc., Pittsburgh, PA.

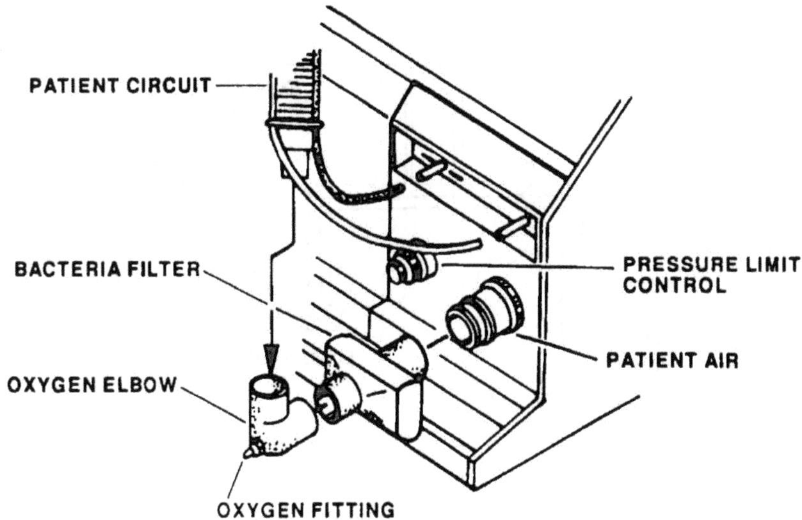

Figure 17 Oxygen delivery elbow used on the LP series ventilators; however, this type of adapter may be used on any of the home care ventilators. Oxygen is titrated directly into the inspiratory limb, bypassing the piston chamber. (From Aequitron LP-6 compact Volume Ventilator: User's Guide and Instruction Manual. Minneapolis, MN: Aequitron Medical Inc., 1985.)

humidifier can more than double the work imposed by the ventilator during the spontaneous breathing phase of SIMV (24).

Whenever the SIMV mode is used, a passover humidifier should be connected to the ventilator via a one-way H-valve. This reduces the inspiratory work imposed during the spontaneous breathing phase of SIMV (24). If an increased FIO_2 is required, a reservoir bag system should be added to the H-valve setup (Fig. 19). The addition of a one-way H-valve, particularly if an increased FIO_2 is desired, complicates the ventilator setup, limits portability, and wastes oxygen. Because of the difficulty in oxygen delivery and the increased workload, the use of the SIMV mode on home care ventilators should be avoided. Until these units incorporate demand systems that reduce the imposed work of breathing, it seems best to maintain patients at home in the assist/control mode.

Humidification

Three basic humidification systems may be used with volume-limited home care ventilators: bubble, passover, and artificial noses. Bubble humidifiers should

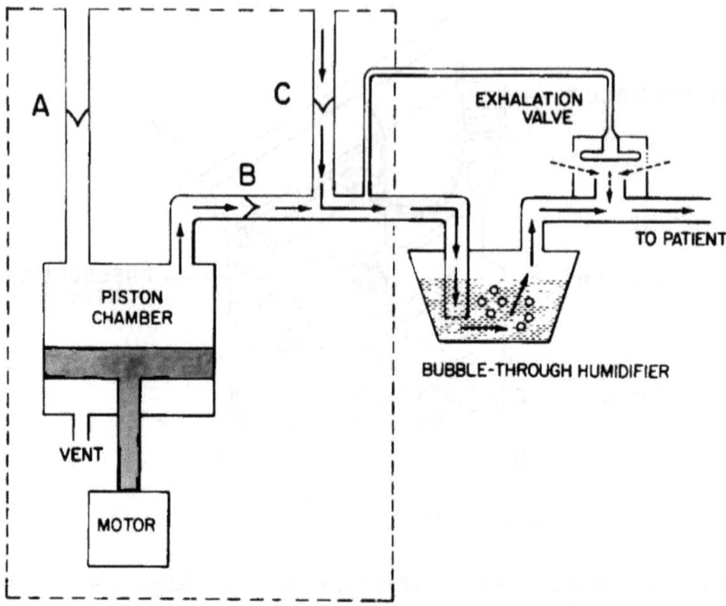

Figure 18 Diagram of gas flow during mechanical ventilation and spontaneous inspiration through a typical home care ventilator: (A) One-way check valve allows gas entry into the piston chamber during piston backstroke. (B) One-way check valve prevents subatmospheric pressure from developing the ventilator circuit during backstroke of piston. (C) One-way check valve allows patient to inspire spontaneously during closure of B when piston backstroke is in progress. Some gas may enter system at the exhalation valve. Arrows depict gas flow during spontaneous inspiration. (From Ref. 24.)

never be used during SIMV. During control and assist/control ventilation, bubble humidifiers function well. Artificial noses, although not recommended on a continuous basis, are very useful during transport and periods away from home. The use of these devices greatly simplifies the ventilator setup on a wheelchair or in a car. When the patient returns home, changing to a bubble or passover humidifier is recommended. The ventilatory load of artificial noses increases with time and varies from one unit to another (25). There are no published data to support the use of artificial noses as the sole source of humidity for mechanically ventilated patients in the home.

Application of PEEP

A PEEP device can be added to the ventilator circuit of any volume-limited home care ventilator. However, the work of breathing is increased unless the control

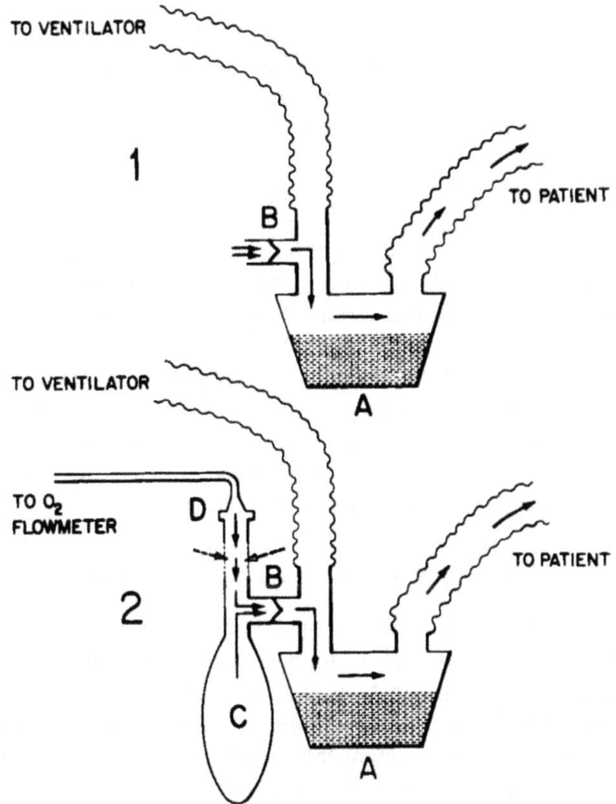

Figure 19 Diagram of one-way H-valve systems: (1) Valve open to atmosphere; (2) valve with 3-L reservoir bag attached to 28% oxygen air-entrainment device, powered by 4/min oxygen. A, Passover humidifier; B, one-way valve; C, reservoir; D, 28% oxygen air-entrainment valve. Arrows depict gas flow during spontaneous inspiration. (From Ref. 24.)

mode is used because none of these units automatically compensates for PEEP (5,14). In the assist/control mode, the sensitivity must be adjusted to decrease the pressure gradient necessary to trigger the ventilator. That is, if 5 cm H_2O PEEP is applied, the sensitivity must be set to approximately 4 cm H_2O (1 cm H_2O below the baseline required to trigger inspiration). However, many patients at home do not maintain a seal at the tracheostomy cuff, which increases the likelihood of auto-triggering when PEEP is used.

Positive end-expiratory pressure should not be used in the SIMV mode.

Appropriate setting of the sensitivity may allow for triggering during positive-pressure breaths. However, the work of breathing during spontaneous breaths is markedly increased. The pressure gradient required to inspire is increased by the amount of PEEP applied. If PEEP is indicated, the assist/control mode with an appropriate sensitivity setting is recommended.

Pediatric Ventilation

The ventilation of pediatric patients has been a challenge with volume-limited home care ventilators (26,27). Systems almost always require modifications to ensure proper gas delivery. Pressure-limited ventilation is the most commonly desired mode, which is unavailable on most of these ventilators. Pop-off or pressure-limiting valves inserted into the circuit between the ventilator and humidifier are used to achieve pressure-limited ventilation. With many small infants, the addition of a continuous flow system is essential (24). None of these ventilators is designed for pediatric patients and extreme care and diligent monitoring are required for successful ventilation of this population.

C. Pressure/Volume-Targeted Home Care Ventilators

The above discussion highlights the fact that both pressure- and volume-limited ventilators have limitations when used for home care. Although these older ventilators are capable of ventilating patients with neuromuscular/neurologic disease, they clearly have problems ventilating patients with primary pulmonary disease or pediatric patients. Recently, a number of new home care ventilators have been introduced. These ventilators are very similar to ICU ventilators and yet they are compact, lightweight, and portable (Table 5). These ventilators also make it possible to appropriately ventilate pediatric patients in the home by the use of pressure-targeted modes.

Table 5 Pressure/Volume-Targeted Ventilators

Company	Ventilator	Availability
Bird Products[a]	Legacy	Available
Pulmonetics[b]	LTV	Available
Nellcor Puritan-Bennett [c]	Achieva	To be introduced late 1999 or 2000
VersaMed[d]	I-Vent 201	To be introduced 1999

[a]Bird Corporation, Palm Springs, CA.
[b]Pulmonetics, San Diego, CA.
[c]Mallinkrodt, Inc., St. Louis, MO.
[d]VersaMed, Hackensack, NJ.

Legacy T-Bird

The Legacy (Bird Corporation, Palm Springs, CA) (Fig. 20) was the first of these new ventilators to become available. Its external dimensions are 12.6" W, 14.0" D, 13.0" H and its weight is 42 lb without the high-pressure oxygen connection and 43 lb with the oxygen connection (28). The only distinction between models (Legacy and Legacy O_2) is the ability of the Legacy O_2 to deliver 21 to 100% O_2. Gas drawn from ambient air via filters or from the O_2 blender (Legacy O_2 only) is pressurized for delivery to the patient by a rotary turbine. Pressure sensors are located at the inlet and outlet of the turbine to allow precise control of delivered gas flow during both pressure- and volume-targeted ventilation and during spontaneous demand flow breathing. In both CPAP and SIMV the turbine provides demand flow in the same manner as ICU ventilators. The modes of ventilation available are volume control, volume assist/control, volume SIMV and CPAP. In addition, pressure support is available as an independent mode or with volume SIMV. A backup ventilation mode is also available (Table 6) and PEEP

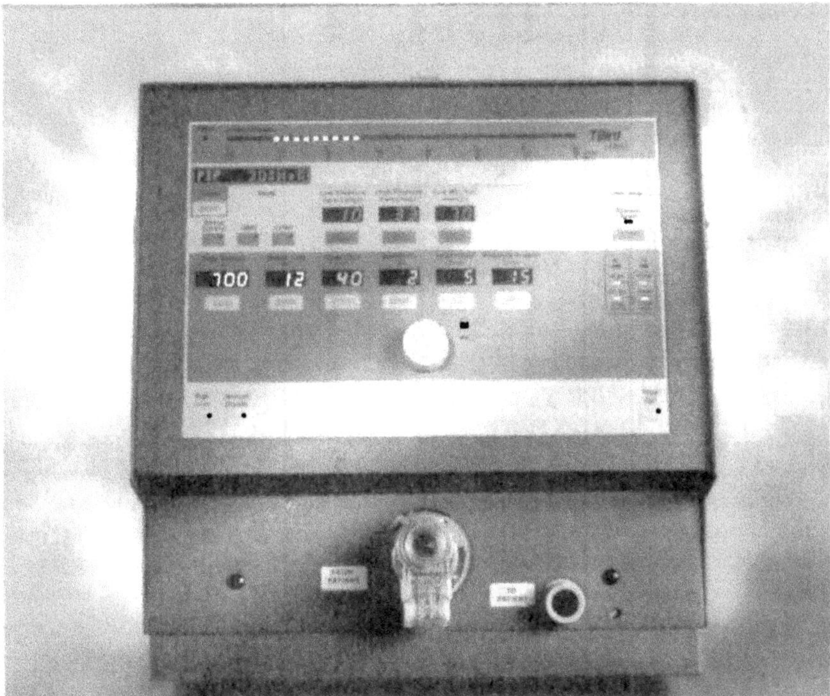

Figure 20 The Legacy T-Bird. (Courtesy of the Bird Corporation, Palm Springs, CA.)

Table 6 Pressure/Volume-Targeted Ventilators: Modes of Ventilation

Legacy[a]	LTV[b]	Achieva[c]	I-Vent 201[d]
Control (V only)[e]	Control (V&P)[e]	—	—
Assist/control (V only)	Assist/control (V&P)	Assist/control (V&P)[e]	Assist/control (V&P)[e]
SIMV (V only)	SIMV (V&P)	SIMV (V only)	SIMV (V&P)
CPAP	CPAP	CPAP	CPAP
Pressure support	Pressure support	Pressure support	pressure support
(Alone or with SIMV)	(Alone or with SIMV)	(Alone or with SIMV)	(Alone or with SIMV)
Sigh breaths	—	—	—
—	NPPV	—	—
Apnea ventilation	Apnea ventilation	Apnea ventilation	Apnea ventilation
—	—	—	Preset ventilation by patient weight

[a]Bird Corporation, Palm Springs, CA.
[b]Pulmonetics, San Diego, CA.
[c]Mallinkrodt, Inc., St. Louis, MO.
[d]VersaMed, Hackensack, NJ.
[e]V, volume-targeted ventilation; P, pressure-targeted ventilation.

is adjustable from 0 to 30 cm H_2O (Table 7). An electromagnetic exhalation valve controls the PEEP level. This valve has both a flow transducer and differential pressure transducer to monitor both pressure and gas flow. Numerous patient ventilator monitors and alarms are available. Inspiratory sensitivity is automatically adjusted to the set PEEP level.

With the Legacy O_2, a high and low FIO_2 alarm is added. In addition, the Legacy O_2 has an internal blender with two high-pressure O_2 attachment ports. The blender operates with only one of the ports active, however, the use of both is recommended to maintain FIO_2 in the setting of high patient inspiratory demand. This model also has a 100% O_2 control (3 min) for use during suctioning. During assisted or spontaneous breathing, breath activation is by flow sensitivity. The sensitivity can be set at off or 1 to 8 L/min. Flow sensitivity operates at the exhalation valve by detecting a change in the bias flow (10 to 20 L/min) equal to the sensitivity setting.

Pressure support is provided in a manner similar to ICU ventilators. The breath is terminated when peak flow decreases to 25% of the set level. Neither the rise time nor the inspiratory termination criteria can be adjusted. Sigh breaths can be delivered at a rate of one every 100 breaths or every 7 min, whichever comes first. When sigh breaths are delivered, the ventilator increases the tidal

Table 7 Gas Delivery Features of Pressure/Volume-Targeted Ventilators: Operating Limits

	Legacy[a]	LTV[b]	Achieva[c]	I-Vent 201[d]
Tidal volume, mL	50–2000	50–2000	50–2200	100–2000
Rate, per min	2–80	1–80	1–80	1–50
Peak flow, L/min	10–140	—	—	—
PEEP/CPAP, cm H_2O	0–30	0–20[e]	0–20	5–20
Pressure support, cm H_2O	1–60	1–60	1–50	1–60
Pressure control, cm H_2O	—	1–60	1–50	1–60
Bias flow, L/min	10–20	10	Not available	Not available
Inspiratory time, sec	—	0.3–9.9	0.2–5.0	—
Inspiration termination criteria	—	10–40%	—	—
Variable rise time	—	1–9	—	—
Variable time duration, sec	—	1.0–3.0	—	—
I/E ratio	—	—	—	1:4 to 2:1

[a]Bird Corporation, Palm Springs, CA.
[b]Pulmonetics, San Diego, CA.
[c]Mallinkrodt, Inc., St. Louis, MO.
[d]VersaMed, Hackensack, NJ.
[e]Control by mechanical spring at exhalation valve.

volume, breath period, inspiratory time, and high-pressure alarm limit by 50%. Inspiratory time is limited to 5.5 sec and high airway pressure to 120 cm H_2O. The Legacy can be operated by an internal battery that lasts up to 25 min, an external battery, or a standard AC current.

Pulmonetic Systems LTV™

Two models of this ventilator are available, the LTV 900 and LTV 1000 (see Fig. 4). The 1000 provides pressure control ventilation and allows high-pressure O_2 as a source gas, insuring precise FIO_2 up to 100%. Otherwise, the models are equivalent. This is the most compact of all the home care ventilators, weighing only 12.6 lb and measuring 10″ × 12″ × 3″, the size of large laptop computer. The LTV ventilator utilizes an electromechanical pneumatic system under the control of a microprocessor (29). Room air enters the ventilator via a foam inlet filter and enters an accumulator/silencer where it mixes with oxygen delivered from an oxygen blender. Gas from the blender enters the turbine (rotary compressor) where energy is added to the gas to increase pressure and flows as necessary for gas delivery. Gas leaving the turbine enters the flow valve where delivered pressure and flow are modulated. A differential pressure transducer is used to regulate gas flow delivery and an airway pressure transducer (at the circuit wye) measures airway pressure and provides feedback signals during the delivery of positive pressure breaths.

Control, assist/control or SIMV modes can be delivered as volume- or pressure-targeted breaths. In addition, CPAP and pressure support modes are available, the latter either as a stand alone mode or with SIMV. During pressure support, a maximum inspiratory time limit can be adjusted (1.0 to 3.0 sec) as well as the inspiratory flow termination criteria (10 to 40%). Cycling to exhalation occurs when either of these limits is reached. The inspiratory flow rise time may also be varied. An apnea backup mode and NPPV mode are included. In the NPPV mode, which can be activated during use of the control, assist/control, or pressure support modes, a number of alarms are inactivated. Only the high pressure, apnea ventilation, line disconnect, ventilator inoperative, and power failure alarms remain functional. Positive end-expiratory pressure (0 to 20 cm H_2O) is set by adjustment of the exhalation valve. When PEEP is used, inspiratory trigger sensitivity must be carefully adjusted.

Supplemental oxygen may be administered via the low-pressure O_2 source, where gas from a flow meter is titrated into the room air entering the ventilator, or via the use of a high-pressure blender (model 1000 only). As with the older home care volume ventilators, FIO_2 depends upon O_2 liter flow and patient ventilatory pattern. The FIO_2 may vary considerably when the low-pressure O_2 source is selected. When this option is selected, the high- and low-O_2-inlet-pressure alarms are inactive and the % O_2 control is inactive. When oxygen is delivered via the high-pressure O_2 source, oxygen is blended with room air as it enters the turbine and the % O_2 control and high- and low-inlet-pressure alarms are active.

The ventilator is normally flow triggered at 1 to 9 L/min or by a default pressure trigger at -3 cm H_2O. A manual breath option is available, which can only be activated during exhalation and delivers a breath of the type set on the ventilator. The LTV ventilators are capable of operating on standard AC power, an external battery, or an internal battery that lasts up to 60 min.

Nellcor® Puritan-Bennett® Achieva™

The Achieva (see Fig. 6) is an upgrade of the Aequitron LP series ventilators that were acquired by Mallinkrodt, Inc. (St. Louis, MO). This is the only one of the four new ventilators in this group that still uses a piston. The Achieva weighs 32 lb and its external dimensions are 10″ × 13″ × 15″ (30). It differs from earlier piston units by incorporating a patient flow sensor and pressure transducer in the gas delivery path and the use of a microprocessor to coordinate gas delivery ensuring that desired gas delivery patterns are achieved. The PEEP level is microprocessor controlled by varying inflation of a mushroom-type exhalation valve, and trigger sensitivity is PEEP compensated. The three models of the Achieva are the Achieva, Achieva X, and Achieva PS. The Achieva X and PS include an internal O_2 blender and the Achieva PS also offers pressure support with or without SIMV.

Increased F_{IO_2} can be delivered by a high-pressure gas source directly attached to the back of the ventilator (X and PS only) or by adding a 90° elbow oxygen fitting to the gas outlet of the ventilator (see Fig. 19). In addition, an oxygen entrainment kit (reservoir) can be added to the room air inlet of the ventilator that allows delivery of variable F_{IO_2} up to about 40%.

Room air enters the ventilator through a 0.3-micron inlet filter during the back stroke of the piston. After passing an inlet check valve, gas enters the piston and mixes with gas from the oxygen blender (X and PS models only). Gas from the piston is then delivered to the patient after first passing through two additional filters. In the event of a power loss or complete ventilator failure, gas bypasses the piston chamber and can be inspired spontaneously by the patient. Assist/control (pressure- or volume-targeted), SIMV (volume-targeted only), pressure support, and CPAP modes are available. All models offer both flow or pressure triggering; flow sensitivity is adjustable from 3 to 25 L/min and pressure triggering between 1 to 15 cm H_2O. The ventilator can be operated by standard AC power, external battery, or an internal battery that lasts 1 to 4 hr.

VersaMed I-Vent 201

This is a compact, microprocessor-controlled ventilator that weighs 13.2 lb without its internal battery and 18.7 lb with the battery. Its external dimensions are

8.6″ × 11.4″ × 9.8″ (31). The I-Vent 201 is the only ventilator designed for home use that incorporates a screen with a display of airway pressure and flow waveforms. In addition, set and monitored variables are displayed on the screen as well as alarms when activated. Ambient air is drawn into the ventilator through a 5-micron filter and supplemental O_2 is supplied via a high-pressure blender. The ventilator microprocessor controls gas entry from both areas and titrates the gases to maintain a stable F_{IO_2} despite variations in inspired gas flow. Mixed gas enters a turbine that consists of a variable speed DC motor and a rotary compressor. A differential pressure sensor is attached to the turbine and is used to measure flow. Gas leaves the turbine via an electromechanical valve that controls gas flow and operates as a demand valve during CPAP. A fixed orifice differential pressure transducer is attached to the patient breathing circuit at the airway to monitor delivered gas volumes and flows. Oxygen can be delivered not only via the internal high-pressure blender but also via an elbow attached to the outflow port of the ventilator (see Fig. 19). Volume- or pressure-targeted assist control, SIMV, CPAP, and pressure support with or without CPAP or SIMV are available modes. This ventilator also has a backup apnea mode and a preset ventilation mode based on patient weight that are provided in the volume assist/control format.

The parameters that can be set with this ventilator differ somewhat from those in other ventilators. Tidal volume and inspiratory–expiratory ratio (I/E) are set during volume-limited ventilation, and I/E and pressure limit are set in pressure-limited ventilation. The PEEP is controlled between 5 and 20 cm H_2O (sensitivity adjusted automatically). Inspiratory triggering is achieved by flow, pressure, or a combination of the two triggers (whichever occurs first). The ventilator can be operated by a standard AC current, an external battery, or an internal battery that lasts for 1.5 to 3 hr.

IV. Non–Positive Pressure Techniques

Positive pressure ventilation has become the standard for LTMV in the home. However, there are non–positive pressure techniques that may be options for a limited number of patients. These techniques include negative pressure ventilation, pneumobelts, and rocking beds. Indications for use of these approaches is limited to patients with neuromuscular/neurologic diseases. These ventilators may be used as the sole means of ventilator support in select patients or alternated with invasive or noninvasive positive pressure ventilation to free the upper airway for communication during the day. Details on these techniques have been presented in Chapter 10.

V. Selection of a Home Care Ventilator

When selecting a ventilator for use in the home, the clinician has a number of options are available: bilevel pressure, volume-limited, or combined pressure/

Table 8 Comparison of Positive Pressure Home Care Ventilators

	Volume ventilators	Pressure ventilators	Combined pressure/volume-ventilators
Versatility of modes	+[a]	+	+++
Monitoring	++	+	+++
Alarms	+	+	+++
Delivery of oxygen	+	+	+++
Compensation for leaks	+	+++	++
Internal battery	++	+	+++
Rise time	++	+	++
Inspiration termination criteria	++	+	++
Cost	++	+	+++

[a]+, Lowest rating; +++, highest rating.

volume-limited ventilators, as well as non–positive pressure devices. Based on the design and capabilities of these machines as summarized in Table 8, the following are recommendations for use of each. The bilevel pressure ventilators are primarily indicated for noninvasive application on an elective basis. The primary reasons for this limited application are the lack of monitors, alarms, or an internal battery. In the few patients with neuromuscular/neurologic disease who are managed with noninvasive mandatory ventilatory support, the volume-limited ventilators work well and are recommended because of their greater alarm and monitoring capabilities, although some of these patients may benefit from the versatility of modes available with the combined pressure/volume-limited ventilators. The volume-limited ventilators have been and remain the primary ventilator of choice for invasive mandatory ventilation for the vast majority of LTMV patients in the home. The patients who stand to benefit the most from the expanded capabilities of the combined pressure/volume-limited ventilators are infants and pediatric patients as well as adult patients with intrinsic lung disease who have problems with patient–ventilator synchrony. The non–positive pressure devices have the most limited application and are best used as part-time alternates to positive pressure ventilation in patients with neuromuscular/neurologic disease.

VI. Ventilator Settings

As with all ventilated patients, the setting of the mechanical ventilator is dependent on gas exchange requirements, lung mechanics, and patient–ventilator synchrony. During noninvasive ventilation using bilevel pressure ventilators or invasive ventilation with the combined pressure/volume-limited ventilators, PEEP is set to counterbalance the effect of auto-PEEP on ventilator triggering. In COPD patients, this may require a PEEP of 5 to 8 cm H_2O, whereas in patients with neuromuscular diseases, PEEP is normally not required. The pressure support or pressure assist/control ventilating pressure is adjusted to tidal volume delivery. A tidal volume of 5 to 6 mL/kg is usually adequate in both neuromuscular and COPD patients ventilated noninvasively. In these patients, pressure support levels of 8 to 15 cm H_2O are usually adequate. When pressure- or volume-limited A/C is used, inspiratory time should be set equal to the patient's spontaneous inspiratory time, or about 0.7 to 1.0 sec.

If rise time adjustment is available, it should be set based on patient comfort. Most unstressed patients feel comfortable with a moderate rise time (0.3 to 0.5 sec), however, some COPD patients prefer a rapid rise time (0.1 to 0.3 sec). In all patients, rise time should be fast enough to ensure a linear rise in airway pressure without peak pressure exceeding the set level. End-inspiratory flow threshold adjustment in pressure support is most critical in patients with COPD. Because of high end-inspiratory flow, a high flow threshold (25 to 40% of peak flow) is most likely to ensure expiratory synchrony.

During volume ventilation, regardless of ventilator type, tidal volume is set to ensure adequate gas exchange and patient comfort. In most patients, this is a delivered tidal volume of 6 to 12 mL/kg, although some patients with neuromuscular disease prefer larger tidal volumes. As with acute applications, peak alveolar pressure should be limited to <30 cm H_2O, regardless of mode.

In all patients, a backup respiratory rate sufficient to ensure adequate CO_2 elimination should be set if the patient's ventilatory drive is inadequate and whenever invasive ventilatory support is provided. Finally, FIO_2 should be adjusted to ensure a target PaO_2 or SaO_2.

VII. Preparing the Patient to Go Home

Successful transition of a LTMV patient to home requires a coordinated effort by hospital staff and the home care providers. Ideally, the patient should be switched to the ventilator to be used at home as early as possible before hospital discharge. Preparation requires education of all caregivers in the home, assessment of the home for safety, and assurance that financial difficulties have been addressed.

Patient/family/caregiver education should be provided by both hospital- and home-based practitioners to ensure a smooth transition of the patient into the home. Operational and safety issues should be reviewed repeatedly and in depth to assure that all caregivers are fully versed in these areas. In addition, tracheostomy care and suctioning training must be provided to caregivers of all patients with artificial airways. Families/caregivers should be prepared to provide manual ventilation wherever necessary and should be taught to recognize the signs and symptoms of respiratory distress or acute illness and to deal effectively with commonly encountered technical problems.

The home should be carefully assessed for suitability to accommodate patient needs such as wheelchair access and electrical support for the ventilator and related equipment. Ideally, the ventilator should be on a separate circuit with backup power available for patients who are unable to breathe for even short periods without ventilatory support. Local emergency medical service (EMS) systems should be notified of the patient's ventilatory support needs and the potential for problems. Social services/case management should carefully evaluate the financial status of the family and formulate plans to provide adequate support for long-term ventilation. It should be acknowledged that home placement is often not feasible, either for financial reasons or because of inadequate caregiver support. Finally, all involved should be fully aware of the problems and difficulties of maintaining a LTMV patient in the home. The more complete the planning and education prior to transition, the greater the likelihood of success.

VIII. Summary

Ventilator options for patients receiving LTMV in the home have rapidly expanded in recent years. Appropriately designed ventilators that can provide either volume- or pressure-targeted ventilation are now available. The abundant assortment of bilevel pressure ventilators and the new pressure/volume-targeted ventilators have raised the capabilities of home ventilators to a new and most welcomed level. Patients with a wide variety of ventilatory needs can now be accommodated with ventilators that have expanded mode and monitoring capabilities, and increase the likelihood of improved patient–ventilator synchrony, comfort, and success.

References

1. Kacmarek RM. The practical application of home mechanical ventilatory equipment. J Neurol Rehabil 1992; 6:103–112.
2. Braun NMT, Marino WD. Effect of daily intermittent rest of respiratory muscles in patients with severe chronic airflow limitation (abstr). Chest 1984; 85:59S.
3. Bach JR, Alba AS, Bohatiuk, et al. Mouth intermittent positive pressure ventilation in the management of postpolio respiratory insufficiency. Chest 1987; 91:859–864.
4. Bach JR, Alba AS. Tracheostomy ventilation: A study of efficacy with deflated cuffs and cuffless tubes. Chest 1990; 97:697–703.

5. Hess DR, Kacmarek RM. Noninvasive ventilation. In: Branson R, Hess DR, Chatburn R. Respiratory Care Equipment. Philadelphia: Lippincott, 1995; 593–612.
6. Strumpf DA, Carlisle CC, Millman RP, et al. An evaluation of the Respironics Bi-PAP Bilevel CPAP device for delivery of assisted ventilation. Respir Care 1990; 25:415–422.
7. Kacmarek RM. Home mechanical ventilation equipment. In: Branson R, Hess DR, Chatburn R. Respiratory Care Equipment. Philadelphia: Lippincott, 1995; 567–592.
8. Yamada Y, Du H-L. Effects of different pressure support termination criteria on patient-ventilator synchrony. Respir Care 1998; 43:1048–1057.
9. Bach JR, O'Brien J, Krotenberg R, Alba A. Management of end stage respiratory failure in Duchenne muscular dystrophy. Muscle Nerve 1987; 10:177–182.
10. Bach JR, Alba AS. Intermittent abdominal pressure ventilator in a regimen of noninvasive ventilatory support. Chest 1991; 99:630–636.
11. Goldstein RS, Molotiu N, Skrastins R, et al. Reversal of sleep-induced hypoventilation in chronic respiratory failure by nocturnal negative pressure ventilation in patients with restrictive ventilatory impairment. Am Rev Respir Dis 1987; 135:1049–1055.
12. Curran FJ, Colbert AP. Ventilator management in Duchenne muscular dystrophy and postpoliomyelitis syndrome: Twelve years' experience. Arch Phys Med Rehabil 1989; 70:180–185.
13. Gilmartun ME. Long-term mechanical ventilation outside the hospital. In: Pierson DJ, Kacmarek RM. Foundations of Respiratory Care. New York: Churchill Livingstone, 1992; 1185–1204.
14. Kacmarek RM, Hess DR. Equipment required for home mechanical ventilation. In: Tobin MJ. Principles and Practice of Mechanical Ventilation. New York: McGraw-Hill 1994; 111–155.
15. Bunburophong T, Imanaka H, Nishimura M, et al. Performance characteristics of bilevel pressure ventilators: A lung model study. Chest 1997; 111:1050–1060.
16. Kacmarek RM. NIPPV: Patient-ventilator synchrony, the difference between success and failure? Intens Care Med 1999; 25:645–647.
17. Bonmarchard G, Chevron V, Minard J-F, et al. Effects of pressure ramp slope values on the work of breathing during pressure support ventilation in restrictive patients. Crit Care Med 1999; 27:715–722.
18. Branson RN, Campbell KS, Davis K, et al. Altering flow rate during maximum pressure support ventilation (PSV_{MAX}): Effects on cardiorespiratory function. Respir Care 1990; 35:1056–1064.
19. Calderini E, Confalonieri M, Puccio PG. Patient-ventilator synchrony during noninvasive ventilation: The role of the expiratory trigger. Intens Care Med 1999; 25: 662–667.
20. MacIntyre NR, Ho L-I. Effects of initial flow rate and breath termination criteria on pressure support ventilation. Chest 1991; 99:134–138.
21. McIntyre N, Nischimura M, Usada Y, et al. The Nagoya conference on system design and patient-ventilator interactions during pressure support ventilation. Chest 1990; 97:1463–1467.
22. Jubran A. van de Graaff WB, Tobin MJ. Variability of patient-ventilator interaction

with pressure support ventilation in patients with chronic obstructive pulmonary disease. Am J Respir Crit Care Med 1995; 152:129–136.

23. Ferguson GT, Gilmartin M. CO_2 rebreathing during BiPAP ventilatory assistance. Am J Respir Crit Care Med 1995; 151:1126–1135.
24. Kacmarek RM, Stanek KS, McMahon KM, et al. Imposed work of breathing during synchronized intermittent mandatory ventilation provided by five home care ventilators. Respir Care 1990; 35:405–414.
25. Ploysongsang Y, Branson RD, Rashkin MC, et al. Effect of flow rate and duration of use on the pressure drop across six artificial noses. Respir Care 1980; 34:902–907.
26. Kacmarek RM, Thompson JE. Respiratory care of the ventilator-assisted infant in the home. Respir Care 1986; 31:605–614.
27. Kacmarek RM. Home mechanical ventilatory assistance for infants. Respir Care 1994; 39:550–565.
28. [Product Literature] T-Bird Legacy and Legacy O_2 ventilator systems: Operator's Manual L1405 Rev A, 1998.
29. [Product Literature] Pulmonetic Systems LTV™ Series Ventilator. Operator's Manual P/N 10664 Rev B, 1999.
30. [Product Literature] Achieva™ ventilators. Nellcor® Puritan-Bennett L-007481-000 Rev A, 1998.
31. [Product Literature] SmartVent 201. Operators Manual, VersaMed, Inc. Rev 9906a (draft) 1999.

with pressure support ventilation in patients with chronic obstructive pulmonary disease. Am J Respir Crit Care Med 1995; 152:129–136.

23. Ferguson GT, Gilmartin M. CO_2 rebreathing during BiPAP ventilatory assistance. Am J Respir Crit Care Med 1995; 151:1126–1135.

24. [illegible] RM, [illegible] KS, [illegible], et al. Inspiratory work of patients during synchronized intermittent mandatory ventilation [illegible]. [illegible] Respir Care 1990; [illegible].

25. [illegible] Y, [illegible], et al. [illegible] and triggering of [illegible] pressure [illegible]. [illegible] 1990; [illegible]–937.

26. [illegible] RM, [illegible] of the [illegible] assisted [illegible] Respir Care 1990; [illegible].

27. [illegible] RM. [illegible] Respir Care 1994; [illegible].

28. [illegible] Laggner O, ventilator [illegible] 1990; [illegible].

29. [illegible].

30. [illegible] 1998.

31. [illegible].

15

Health Care Networks for Long-Term Mechanical Ventilation

ALLEN I. GOLDBERG

Loyola University Chicago
Pediatric Home Health
Loyola University Health Systems
Maywood, Illinois

I. Introduction

The establishment of long-term mechanical ventilation (LTMV) provides important insights about the organization and development of systems of health care and social service delivery in the community (1,2). The evaluation of LTMV programs and systems in different nations, and the analysis of political, cultural, social, and economic influences on their evolution provide an understanding of how communities can identify and meet growing health care needs of patients with complex chronic health conditions that generate catastrophic health care and social costs (3,4).

The purposes of this chapter are to provide the reader with 1) an understanding about the current state of *community health networks*: private-public-partnerships established in communities to assess, plan, and evaluate community health and social needs and to integrate health and human services into collaborative caring systems, 2) an appreciation of why community health networks are solutions to meet growing population-based health and social needs within the constraints of predefined and/or limited resources, 3) a review of how LTMV developed as "informal" community health networks and how they will continue to evolve in the future, 4) an understanding of the cultural basis and ethical foundation of home care essential for development of community health networks, and 5) a conceptual framework for "futures thinking" and "visioning" and the practical considerations necessary to understand the processes required to develop community health networks for LTMV.

II. Community Health Networks

Health care networks represent recent local and regional initiatives to meet global health and social needs of individuals, families, and communities. These associations of organizations vary in location (rural, urban, mixed), purpose, membership composition, design, and target patient population(s) to be served. They are community-based and usually focus on 1) major public health or health planning issues of concern to multiple public/private constituencies in their communities or 2) comprehensive integrated health care system development. These community partnerships generally develop from grass-roots efforts of multiple sectors: private, voluntary, public, government, academic, and consumer. They consequently pose enormous design and operational challenges to the individual participating organizations and the alliances and coalitions that subsequently form (5,6).

In the United States, the recent growth in number and variety of community health networks began in the early 1980s as a response to changing demographics and health needs of communities and the increasing constraints on resources of health care and social service organizations to meet them. The desire to satisfy community needs and increased health and social costs of more adult and elderly persons with chronic illnesses and disabilities encouraged cooperation among organizations and willingness to leverage their limited resources.

The Community Medical Alliance in Boston exemplifies one approach to the successful integration of health care delivery services (7). This community health network adapted to prepaid managed care by redesigning health care services for people with severe physical disability and late-stage AIDS within the constraints of a fixed payment plan. By establishing effective primary and specialty care coordination and individual case management and by contracting with a complete spectrum of community-based services, the alliance delivered comprehensive health care and services in the community and the home settings. This approach fostered self-care and independence of patients and families and reduced the utilization of expensive institution-based acute care resources. This resulted in significant economic savings, enhanced quality of life, and greater user satisfaction (8).

The Chicago Asthma Consortium is another specific example of a functional community health network directly related to long-term breathing. The impetus for its formation in 1996 was based on recognition of community need to better understand and reduce the alarming increased morbidity and mortality of asthma in Chicago. This was to be accomplished by improved communication, coordination, and integration of education, care, and management of asthma among physician groups, health care institutions, managed care organizations, and community-based organizations, including public and voluntary agencies and the public school system. The network evolved from a common vision shared by leaders from multiple sectors of the local community: public health (Chicago Board of Health), voluntary association (American Lung Association of Metropolitan Chicago), professional association (American College of Chest Physicians), and philanthropic organization (Otho S. A. Sprague Memorial Institute) (9). Leaders identified and invited open community participation essential for success: patients and families, local community activists, health care and educational professionals, public health officials, health service researchers, local school representatives, and public and private health care funding agencies including managed care organizations. The specific parts of this grass-roots network interact ''bottom-up'' by involving all participants in standing committees where the real work gets done by community members with first-hand insights of reality-based needs and with the passion to find meaningful solutions. These committees are designed to have impact *in their local communities*, where differences can be made that will directly affect outcome. In only two years, major improvements in public school health policies, emergency room and health care practices, and professional and patient education were instituted and their impact evaluated. Members also interact and network at quarterly meetings always, held in different locations in Chicago, where recent committee accomplishments are summarized and educational programs offered to enhance members' skills and understanding. Overall function and integration of network efforts are governed by an executive group of committee and community leaders. Initial problems that arose in network development included ''cultural misunderstandings'' of the perspectives of participants from different community sectors, fragmentation of accomplishments due to inadequate formulation a common shared vision, and insufficient management of financial planning for sustained operations. Current program evolution has reached the stage when independent operational (501-c-3) status is being entertained (10).

A major stimulus for more recent growth of community health networks has been change driven by the failure of health care reform by the Clinton Administration. The lack of reform by public policy has created a vacuum that has been met, in part, by further growth of community health networks. The prevalence and diversity of members and purposes of community health networks can be appreciated by a review of the Community Care Network (CCN) Demonstration Program (11,12). The CCN Demonstration Program has provided a means for both the development and evaluation of a variety of ''formal'' community partnerships that link health care, business, government, and community organizations in a wide range of settings and fulfill the CCN's four principal goals:

1. *A focus on the health issues of communities*, not just patients who receive care or enrollees of a health plan;
2. *A seemless continuum of care*, with mechanisms that facilitate service delivery at the right time in the most appropriate setting based on patient need;
3. *Management within fixed resources* as achieved through capitated payments or global budgets based on the costs of efficient care delivery;
4. *Community accountability*.

Outcomes were evaluated at a national conference, "Building Healthier Communities, Ten Years and Learning" (13). The coalition of sponsors of this evaluation also represent multiple sectors of society: government, private, public, and voluntary. Unfortunately CCN data are only kept on demonstrations funded by the program. In the United States, we do not really know the total number, types, and rate of proliferation of networks, alliances, and coalitions that have been established as "locally based health care reform." The CCN Program follows only the 25 demonstration sites originally funded among 283 "serious applicants." Successful projects have had clear vision, goal-focused accomplishments, and sustained funding support strategies.

Community health networks are not limited just to the United States. The availability of advanced information and communication technologies and the global need to contain health care costs that are becoming a rising percentage of social budgets have stimulated their development in other nations as well. For example, a recent provincewide interactive telecommunications network has linked every hospital in Nova Scotia, Canada (14). The 43-site Nova Scotia Tele-Health Network represents one of the world's largest tele-medicine projects and demonstrates how networks can be formed from government, public, and private sector collaboration. In France, the need for stricter fiscal policies and limitation of social expenditures because of the adoption of a common European currency required the French Ministry of Social Service to adopt a "zero sum budget" for 1999 (15). This effort has encouraged the development of formal "reseaux de soins" (care networks) (16). In France, however, informal "care networks" for long-term mechanical ventilation had already been in existence for nearly 40 years. Long-term mechanical ventilation networks had developed regionally in the 1960s and nationally in the 1980s (1,2). The national network is now being further extended by a multisector tele-management initiative (17,18).

III. Long-Term Mechanical Ventilation in the Community

Communities have always had informal care networks of private, public, and government organizations serving the needs of patients requiring long-term mechanical ventilation (19–21). Studies of individual LTMV networks reveal certain patterns of development. Each network responds to national priorities and regional needs and reflects their own unique history, tradition, culture, politics, and specific local realities (1,2,4,22–24). A major international analysis at the Max Planck Institute for Social Science Research (Köln) revealed that community solutions evolve mainly due to national culture and local availability of resources rather than the kind of finance system in place (25). Community networks also demonstrate universal principles that transcend nations, cultures, and finance systems. During the current transformation of society from the industrial era to the information age and beyond, knowledge management and communication are keys to network development. This development will be facilitated by a new concept of health care (as an "information business") and of community (as both local and global).

A. The Past

Long-term mechanical ventilation was occasionally delivered in the homes of patients who had families with economic means after iron lungs became commercially available during the early 1930s (26,27). However, community-based LTMV became more prevalent only in the last half of the twentieth century with the improvement of the iron lung (28), invention of the modern positive pressure mechanical ventilator (29), and the application of tracheostomies (30). These technologies were developed in response to the global epidemic crisis of poliomyelitis, which peaked in the 1950s (19). Later innovations in upper airway management and mechanical ventilation, as well as advances in neonatal, pediatric, and adult critical care and rehabilitation medicine, have permitted home management of survivors of other life-threatening medical and surgical conditions (31).

In different nations, use of LTMV at home arose from the collaborative local initiatives of health care professionals, community leaders (including public agencies), and ventilator users (consumers). All the original programs around the world were designed for and with polio patients' involvement. Mechanical ventilation at home became the solution for regional health centers to meet the health and social needs of these ventilator users and families. In addition, it permitted the more appropriate allocation of expensive regional critical care beds for new patients with acute life-threatening illnesses. Initial home mechanical ventilation experiences reduced long-term care expenditures of public and private reimbursement agencies for patients with sequelae of poliomyelitis. Later, home mechanical ventilation was offered to patients with conditions resulting in chronic respiratory insufficiency due to disorders of the central nervous system (e.g., central hypoventilaton syndrome), neuromuscular conditions (e.g., muscular dystrophies, hypotonias, amyotrophic lateral sclerosis), skeletal disorders (kyphoscoliosis, sequelae of tuberculosis), and cardiopulmonary causes (congestive heart failure, chronic obstructive pulmonary disease).

Although designated associations developed these local and regional solutions in their respective communities, no one organization had sufficient resources to serve the needs of all their constituents (32). Rather, informal community health networks spontaneously arose and evolved in localities as determined by participants who defined the need. Successful networks always involved essential individuals and organizations required for their planning and operation: government, public/social agencies, health care facilities, and ventilator users and groups in each locality (1,2). Networks were practical solutions that pooled locally available resources. They were started and developed in each country in ways determined by national traditions and culture as well as local community need (1,2,4). In the United States, individuals in the communities worked with support from a nonprofit association (National Foundation for Infantile Paralysis—March of Dimes) with the spirit of challenge by new frontiers. In France, existence of nonprofit associations and participant involvement reflected the French core values of fraternity, equality, and liberty for all citizens. Similar associations did not develop in other nations, despite need and similar finance systems, without such cultural and traditional influences.

B. The Present

Today's user of home mechanical ventilation requires medical, psychosocial, environmental, technological, organizational, and financial support. Home mechanical ventilation exists in many nations but varies in each locality in regard to patient access and specific applications. Where and when available, services and financing for home mechanical ventilation remain fragmented and uncoordinated in most communities since organizations compete for limited resources that are targeted only for designated purposes. The best local and regional solutions still result from people who informally join together in networks. Networks work where more traditional approaches of public, private, and voluntary sectors cannot or do not respond alone.

Home mechanical ventilation illustrates all issues of what has been defined by industry and public policy as "high-technology" home care: the prolonged use of complex life-sustaining medical technology in the home that requires intermittent or continuous support of community resources. High technology home care exists all over the world, only limited by available financial, technological, and human resources. In the United States, high technology home care now represents the fastest growing health expenditure, stimulated by the development of a home care industry (33), education of health care professionals, and the preference of consumers (34). Such growth has raised ethical debates regarding the appropriateness of high technology home care and the "medicalization of the home" (33,35).

The following are some questions raised in the debate. Is it right to submit families to complex medical technological interventions in the sanctity of their own homes? Is it just to spend finite resources intended for the good of society for the limited benefit of a few private individuals who may (or even may not) want to go home? Is mechanical ventilation at home based on medical necessity as determined by physicians or on proposed benefit as suggested by representatives of a growing industry who profit by increased utilization?

C. The Future

Persons who require LTMV in the community will face exciting opportunties and dangerous threats. The wide availability of needed health care information will enhance possibilities. Ventilator users, health care professionals, and others will use global information networks and interactive telecommunications as personal and system management tools to support health, social, and technical needs. Risk will result from shifting national priorities from solving domestic social concerns to meeting new challenges created by the global market and recognition of inabilities to serve community needs with existing public models. This will stimulate further development of health community networks.

IV. Cultural Concerns: The Basis of Ethical Issues

In order to understand how community health networks evolve for LTMV, it is important to clarify how home care differs from the more traditional ways of delivering health care.

A. The "Medical Model" vs. the Home Care Culture

Home care should not be considered an extension of the "medical model" into the home. In the "medical model," the physician commands the situation, with the patient and family dependent upon professional authority for decisions and actions. When receiving care in a hospital or ambulatory care setting, the patient and family remain at a power disadvantage and cannot be in control. Patients are more likely to accept medical decisions based on scientific and technical information, which may not always take into account their own wishes and desires. In these settings, physicians and other health professionals control decisions and management, with success dependent on patient compliance. The goals are the reversal of illness and possible cure.

Home care represents a culture with attitudes, beliefs, values, and norms of behavior that differ from the more traditional "medical model." Service providers and others involved with delivery of home care must accept this different "mind set" from the institutional way of thinking and relating to patients. Home care demonstrates a social concept typified by the independent living movement of persons with disabilities. In this model, physicians serve as collaborators of care and invited care partners. The patient and family are conceived of as persons who want to be active in decision-making, plan implementation, and outcome evaluation. In person-directed, family-centered care, the person and family members are central and in charge. They consider multiple options because they have been empowered by the information necessary to make good decisions. Their knowledge comes from self-help and mutual aid groups and from global information networks and health portals to the worldwide web established to aid health care consumers seeking to obtain reliable information to take charge of their own health. For examples, ventilator users have benefitted for over 30 years from reading the *Rehabilitation Gazette*, an international journal by and for persons with long-term ventilator needs, which has now evolved into the International Ventilator Users Network (36).

More recently, former U.S. Surgeon General C. Everett Koop, a strong believer of self-help, established an Internet-based portal to reliable health information including "virtual community" interaction on line (37). Persons and families focus more on wellness and desire to improve their health status and life situation rather than expect a total cure. They are active participants who take responsibility for their own health. They have important management insights and can make decisions that enhance safety, reduce risk, improve quality, and reduce costs. This makes them essential participants in self-care and case management. Table 1 presents a comparison of the medical model and the home care culture (38).

Table 1 Medical Model vs. Home Care Culture

	Medical	Home care
Process	Command/control	Collaboration
Focus	Professional focus	Person-centered
	Patient focus	Family-centered
Emphasis	Illness (episodic)	Health-wellness (continuous)
		Health promotion/prevention
Goal	Curing	Caring
Fosters	Dependency	Independency
Decisions	Receptive	Participative
Communication	One-way	Two-way
Response	Reactive	Proactive
Respect	Professional wisdom	Person/family insights
Environment	Clinical, invasive	Dignified, private
Ethical foundation	Beneficence	Autonomy

Source: Ref. 38.

B. Differing Ethical Perspectives

Ethical conflicts result from efforts to design community health networks when multiple ethical principles must be considered. What judgment principles are relevant to LTMV? The following are commonly accepted notions of the ethical considerations about health care in general. They reflect the different perspectives of those participants involved and affected by the decisions (39,40).

Beneficence-Based Judgment. If a treatment has merit and meets the individual's health need, it ought to be instituted and continued. Only harmful interventions ought to be stopped; there is no obligation to continue nonbeneficial intervention. Minimal benefit interventions may be continued or stopped, but intervention ought to be instituted or continued if clinical judgment determines more than minimal benefit. *This is the ethical principle used by professionals when deciding on treatment options they offer to individual patients with less concern for societal needs or the individual patient's desires.*

Autonomy-Based Judgment. Only interventions based on informed opinion, desired by the person/family, and in the best interest of the person/family perspective are justified. The person's and family members' wants are valued, person- and family-centered care is a core belief, and independent decisions made by the person/family are the chief determinants of care. *This is the ethical principle used by persons/families who require and want to be supported by life-sustaining technology at home.*

Justice-Based Judgment. Only interventions that result in social utility are justified since finite resources must be distributed equitably for the most good for society. *Given that freedom-based, merit-based, and needs-based interests all generate justice-based obligations, there is no uncontended theory of justice that prevails.*

These ethical principles result in conflict regarding what the professional wants to do, what the patient (person) and family want to have done, and what society can afford to do. Since one option demands tradeoff with another, LTMV stimulates an ethical debate. These ethical concerns raise the more difficult and larger practical issue of allocation of finite resources for the entire population. This debate becomes more critical in a managed care environment that may further limit resources for long-term mechanical ventilation. These ethical principles also highlight some of the organizational challenges to establishing more formal and universal community health networks (5,6).

V. The Futurist Approach: The Concept of Vision

Success of community health networks depends upon formulation of a commonly desired future that is shared among all participants. "Futures thinking" can help those who learn how to use it in this endeavor. With "futures thinking" users can anticipate likely future directions of health care delivery by their analysis of current trends and subsequent design of possible scenarios. This helps them to define and achieve shared visions for more healthy communities (41). "Futures thinking" can be useful to anticipate the evolution of LTMV community health networks.

A vast multidisciplinary experience exists with analysis of social and technological trends for the purpose of making such informed forecasts. In addition, rigorous methodology exists to help users of information about future possibilities make intelligent decisions for their own direction and that of their organizations. Futurist thinkers first define a vision to guide their strategic planning. One global organization unifying such people from all nations and walks of life is the World Future Society. Hundreds of such thinkers join at the Society's annual meeting to consider the future of many aspects of modern life. The Society also provides access to wide body of literature and scholarly research about the future and publishes *The Futurist*, a monthly magazine that provides forecasts, trends, and ideas about the future.

A. Futurist Assumptions

Two basic assumptions can be made about the future that are not necessarily mutually exclusive:

1. The future is uncertain. There is no single, certain forecast. There are multiple possible futures and we can take steps to anticipate them and possibly affect positively the chance of their actually happening.
2. We chose and create major aspects of our future by what we do or fail to do. There *are* large aspects of the future that we *can* influence. We can make intelligent choices for strategic planning based upon careful analysis of available information. "Visions and strategies linked to a clear sense of trends and scenarios make us better able to shape the future we prefer" (42).

B. Futurist Techniques

Four primary tools have been proposed to deal with future uncertainty (42):

1. *Trends*: The observer must focus on that which is specific and important to them and then determine patterns of significant changes in *what is happening* over time. Trends alert us to threats and opportunities. Conflicting trends can be identified and modified. Favorable changes can be accelerated if we look ahead to what should be changed.
2. *Scenarios*: These are descriptions of *what might happen*: the path into the future taken by a set of interacting forces. Scenarios represent compilations of trends that present differing, more comprehensive images

of a possible future (what might be likely). Scenarios consider how interacting sets of trends might lead to a range of conditions in the future. They describe images of a plausible future and a broad range of other possibilities under different situations (if an unexpected turn of events were to occur).

3. *Vision*: For the purpose of planing, this is a compelling, inspiring statement of *what we want to have happen*. The vision represents the preferred future shared by those who want to create it. These are the best outcomes that might be accomplished by working interdependently and in synergy.
4. *Strategies*: These are action plans that focus efforts on achieving the vision. Strategies highlight the major things we must do to achieve our vision . . . *to make it happen*.

"Futurist thinkers" have recently attempted to make informed predictions about health care in general to formulate a future vision for the United States. One of the most outstanding attempts to define a future vision for individual, family, and community health was made by 18 of the leading thinkers of our time who met in 1994 and defined *The Belmont Vision for Health Care in America: Healthy People in a Healthy World* (41). In the foreword, former U.S. Surgeon General C. Everett Koop recognizes that "vision is a powerful tool" for a healthier society. He encourages us to "use vision to explore your own sense of the best that health care can be and to focus on what you want to create." He states that "the discussion of health care reform in the United States must begin to focus on our visions in addition to our plans for reform" (41).

VI. Developing Health Care Networks for LTMV

A. Describing Trends Relevant to LTMV

"Futurist thinking" can be useful to better understand the future of more specific areas of health care, including community health networks for LTMV. In order to describe trends that are relevant to development of health care networks for LTMV, some terms and concepts must be defined.

Network: A chain of interconnected people and/or operations (43).

Integrated Delivery System: a network of healthcare organizations that provides or arranges to provide a coordinated continuum of services to a defined population. The system commits to be held clinically and fiscally accountable for the outcomes and health status of the population served (44).

Community Health Network: People and community organizations that comprise a social network at the local level, working together to enhance health and well-being of individuals, families, and the community.

Managed Care: A health plan that usually focuses on provision of insurance for the greatest value (defined as quality/cost) to a target population. This is accomplished by assessment of financial risk, collection of funds, design of health care delivery systems, allocation of designated resources, management of costs, and consideration of continuous quality improvement and satisfaction of customers, users, and all other participants.

Care Management: Clinical management by health care professionals (physicians, nurses, therapists, social workers) working with family members and others to coordinate comprehensive patient care plans, expedite achievement of target outcomes, monitor and guide patient progress, and maximize the patient's and family's self-care potential.

Case Management: Healthcare administration, often provided by nurses, who are assigned to evaluate benefits vs. needs and determine mechanisms to provide ''medically necessary'' services as determined by ''gatekeepers'' using ''standards'' and managed by guidelines for resource utilization.

Capitated Payment: Fixed amount of health care financing (per patient per unit of time) designated for comprehensive health care services to be delivered by a system that includes physicians, ambulatory care, home health services, hospitals, and long-term care.

Global Budget: A finite, but all-encompassing, public budget for a designated social purpose such as health, education, housing, or employment.

B. Determining the Actors

Networks for LTMV will only be successful if they consider and integrate the perspectives of all the essential participants. All beneficiaries with a stake in the success of the network must be included: patients and family members, consumers and users, buyers and payers, suppliers, distributors, providers of services and products, professionals, and policy leaders. They must all be involved with the initial planning, implementation, evaluation, modification and improvement of the network. ***In sum, establishment of integrated community networks requires that patients, providers, and payers work together in partnership.***

Representatives from multiple sectors must contribute their invited perspectives. Each sector differs in purpose, organization, and function. Each sector's role must be understood for how it functions and recognized for the value of their contribution to network development.

Role of Government

Governmental agencies allocate financial resources collected for the public good, set standards for resource distribution and how the network may function, and oversee network operations. The government makes social and economic policies that may encourage or discourage network development. Government agencies may serve the social good directly (as providers) or indirectly (as facilitators for network development or financial resource development). Government functions are authorized by laws and regulations determined for the common good by elected officials and public service workers.

Role of the Private Sector

For-profit organizations access financial markets and leverage fiscal resources that are invested in activities with expected returns on their investments. Purpose-driven activities of private sector organizations are set by organizational mission, goals, and objectives. Private sector organizations do not highly prioritize social purposes, but that might change in the future. These organizations will face greater societal demands and recognize their potential for increasing their share of the market by demonstrating more social responsibility to the public. The private sector functions by legal authority and with accountability to owners and shareholders who may demand more social consciousness in the future.

Role of the Public Sector

The nonprofit (voluntary) sector utilizes privileged, tax-exempt resources that are donated and designated for the societal improvement (such as education, social services, and health). Activities of nonprofit organizations are purpose-driven as defined by mission, goals, and objectives. The public sector serves social purposes to enhance human potential and well-being and to improve the community. It functions by legal authority and with accountability to donors and volunteers who provide financial and human resources, to the government that grants tax-exempt status, and to the users of their services (patients and families).

Integrated community network systems development requires transsector collaboration among government, private, and public sectors.

C. Directing the Focus

Community Health Networks must focus on larger issues in order to get needed attention and resources. Although the number of people who require LTMV is not large, their needs generate catastrophic costs for their communities. They are considered ''expensive outliers'' by traditional health care finance approaches. However, if funds are made available that target such ''high-risk'' populations, systems of care and services can be designed that improve quality of care and life, enhance satisfaction of all users, and contain costs (7,8). Due to the complexity of their situation, their needs have universal solutions that when put in place may also benefit others. Thus, focusing local community health networks on people with such conditions is justifiable (45).

Since persons who require LTMV are worldwide and many of their needs are informational, the meaning of "community" takes on a more global perspective. Many individuals who require LTMV and their families have access to internet information which they must use with circumspection to determine that the source of information is reliable. Excellent networking tools include web pages designed by well-known and dedicated supporters of long-term mechanical ventilation. One such tool is the health portal "drkoop.com" created by C. Everett Koop, former Surgeon General of the United States (37). While he was Surgeon General, Dr. Koop focused attention on public policy and the community needs of LTMV users, an action that has benefitted all children with special needs (46). Dr. Koop strongly supported development of self-help networks and understood the need for access to reliable information so that patients and families could take charge of their own health management (47). Another important informational resource for long-term ventilator users, families, providers, and others concerned with LTMV is the International Ventilator Users Network (IVUN) of the Gazette International Networking Institute, which was established to honor the late Gini Laurie, publisher of the *Rehabilitation Gazette* and pioneer of informational resources for ventilator users all over the world (36). The IVUN represents a network of ventilator users enthusiastic to share their extensive experience and insights with others.

D. Determining the Process

Networks must provide structure and establish mechanisms to identify and encourage participation of all potential beneficiaries (48–50). Involved participants develop motivation, commitment, and a sense of "ownership," which are key factors in the success of network development. Working together synergistically, participants can accomplish more together in a community partnership than with the sum of individual or single organizational efforts. At the local level, all sectors face resource constraints and seek creative means to obtain and leverage local diversified resources.

Local community leaders must develop innovative processes that reward interactive team efforts applied to partnership goal accomplishment. The challenges of doing this at the local level have been well reviewed in recent evaluations of the Community Care Network Demonstration Programs (5,6). At the national level, participants (including the government) may establish evaluation standards for defined expected outcomes. This is practicable when the standards are based on universal principles and require revenues collected for the national public good. However, proper program planning, implementation, and modification based on feedback and experience can only be accomplished at the *local* level.

VII. Creating Community Health Visions

A. Role of Communities in Designing Health Care Systems and Networks

Today, communities provide health care without a systems approach. This will no longer be possible due to the constraints of limited financial resources. Communities need shared visions to accomplish more than just incremental reform of a broken "non-system." Communities must go beyond mere design of a system to the achievement of even larger goals: health and quality of life. This is *critical* for conditions that pose catastrophic cost issues, such as those that require LTMV, since health care expenditures will undergo greater scrutiny as they will continue to represent a growing percentage of social budget.

Much can be learned from reviewing past and current ways that local communities and regions have served persons who require LTMV. This is best done by reviewing current general health care trends and developing a common vision of the future that can be shared and supported by the community.

What is the most desirable scenario that will guide a "future vision" for long-term mechanical ventilation under anticipated changes?

1. *LTMV networks must become a component of a more global community, family-centered, integrated service delivery system that will operate within finite predetermined financial constraints.* The financial risk to manage available resources and respond to the multiple needs of all beneficiaries will be the burden of the system. Community-based solutions serving targeted populations (such as users of LTMV) cannot survive if they cost more than institutional-based alternatives.

2. *The community health system must be operated by an integrated management approach that involves and links all stakeholders in system development.* Stakeholders include health care, social service, rehabilitation, and educational professionals, patients and families, payers, community-based providers, social agencies, and funding sources. Ethical, organizational, and management conflicts can be resolved by a process of planning, implementing, evaluating, and modifying the system in response to multiple viewpoints and perspectives. In this way, the evolution of the system will be flexible, adaptable, and cognizant of the individual needs of each participant. This can be accomplished more effectively within a network that aims to maximize the utilization of resources. The system will not survive if it is fragmented, inflexible, and lacks the capacity for innovation.

3. *The system must be designed "smartly" utilizing available information and advanced telecommunications that can extend the reach of each participant.* Each person using LTMV and family member has valuable insight and skills in self-management that warrant a central role in system design and program management.

4. *The system must integrate a variety of services targeted to meet multiple needs.* The system must present a total service package with options depending upon the needs of each individual patient. Such an integrated system must be designed and operated locally. Success will be based on dedicated collaborative efforts of multiple participants who will collectively benefit if given the opportunity to work together within the constraints of managed care, global budgets, or capitation.

5. *The system must responsibly accomplish multiple goals: universal access, necessity as determined by system criteria, continuous quality improvement, and cost containment.* The system must prove itself by presetting desirable outcomes and acceptable indicators of variance. Only by achieving desired results as determined by rigorous evaluation and comparison to objective standards, practices, and reasonable benchmark experiences will the system justify the resources required for further growth and development.

VIII. Summary and Conclusions

With only 50 years of history, LTMV represents a modern phenomenon. Its past, present, and preferred future can be understood in context of the framework of community health networks. Global health networks are informal arrangements that evolve spontaneously in response to health and social needs and perceived solutions by multiple actors in different sectors of the community. Networks develop in stages that must overcome participants' "cultural misunderstandings" of each other and their organizations. They can overcome barriers facing more limited approaches to community health. Better outcomes result from the diversity of grass-roots participants and their needs-based perspectives and real-world understanding of workable solutions.

Long-term mechanical ventilation will continue to be provided by these networks due to the lack global health reform and public policy to address these patients', their families' and their communities' needs. These networks are visionary "experiments in action" that must remain sensitive to ethical perspectives and cultural elements of all participants. They will succeed if they involve all essential participants in all stages of development. Networks will accomplish multiple benefits including leverage of limited resources and synergy of diverse viewpoints. They must constantly adapt to change by planning for their future via trend analysis, scenario determination, and visionary action.

References

1. Goldberg AI. Home care services for severely physically disabled people in England and France. Case example: The ventilator dependent person. International exchange

of experts and information in rehabilitation. Fellowship Report. New York: World Rehabilitation Fund, 1983.
2. Goldberg AI. Home care and alternatives to hospitalization in France for medical technology dependent children and adults with severe chronic respiratory insufficiency: the associative system. Fellowship Report. Geneva, Switzerland: World Health Organization, 1986.
3. Goldberg AI. Mechanical ventilation and respiratory care in the home in the 1990s: Some personal observations. Respir Care 1990; 35(3):247–259.
4. Goldberg AI. Home care for life-supported persons: The French system of quality control, technology assessment, and cost containment. Public Health Rep 1989; 104(4):329–335.
5. Weiner BJ, Alexander JA. The challenges of governing public-private community health partnerships. Health Care Manage Rev 1998; 23(2):39–55.
6. Alexander JA, Comfort ME, Weiner BJ. Governance in public-private community health partnerships: Evidence from the Community Care Network Demonstration. Non-Prof Manage Leadership 1998; 8(4):311–332.
7. Master RJ, Dreyfus T, Connors S, Tobias C, Zhou Z, Kronick R. The Community Medical Alliance: An integrated system of care in Greater Boston for people with severe disability and AIDS. Managed Care Q 1996; 4(2):26–37.
8. Berwick D. Changing the boundaries of health care. (Institute for Health Care Improvement: Highlights of Keynote Address. International Society for Quality in Health Care, 5/96) Qual Connect 1996: 5(3):1–2.
9. Wolf RL. Chicago Asthma Consortium. Curr Opin Pulm Med 1998; 4:49–53.
10. Addington WW, Weiss K, guest eds. Asthma in Chicago. Chest 1999; 116(4 suppl): 129S–236S.
11. Bazzoli GJ. Public-private collaboration in health and human service delivery. Milbank Q 1997; 75(4):533–561.
12. Bogue RJ, Antia M, Harmata R, Hall CH. Community experiments in action: Developing community-defined models for reconfiguring health care delivery. J Health Polit Policy Law 1997; 22(4):1051–1076.
13. Building healthier communities: Ten years and learning. 104th National Conference on Governance. Fourth National Community Care Network Conference, Washington, DC: November 13–15, 1998. Contact: Frances S. Margolin, American Hospital Association Health Research Education Trust, Tel: (312)422-2612, FAX: (312)422-4568.
14. Nova Scotia, Canada: Canada's first provence-wide telemedicine network announced. Telemed Today 1996; June:10.
15. Sécu: Martine Aubry. Sur le déficit zéro pour 2000. Liberation 1998; 23 Sep:2.
16. Médecins, médicaments: l'encadrement des dépenses de santé des renforcé. Les Echoes 1998; 23 Sep:3.
17. Dautzenberg B, Henry M, Ludot A, Lyon-Caen Y, Salès A. Télésurveillance appliquée à l'insuffisance respiratoire chronique grave traitée à domicile: Rapport 1: Choix des matériels et logiciels. 30 sep 95. Téléport: Paris Ile-de-France, August, 1997.
18. Dautzenberg B, Henry M, Ludot A, Lyon-Caen Y, Salès A. Télésurveillance appliquée à l'insuffisance respiratoire chronique grave traitée à domicile. Rapport 2: Équipement des patients, recueil des données. Préfiguration du surveur régional. 28 mar 97. Téléport: Paris Ile-de-France, August, 1997.

19. Faure EAM, Goldberg AI, eds. Proceedings of an international symposium: Whatever happened to the polio patient? Chicago: Northwestern University Press, 1982.
20. Goldberg AI. Home care for a better life for ventilator-dependent people. Chest 1983; 84:365–366.
21. Goldberg AI. The regional approach to home care for life-supported persons. Chest 1984; 86:345–346.
22. Goldberg AI, Faure EAM. Home care for life-supported persons in England: The Responaut program. Chest 1984; 86:910–914.
23. Goldberg AI, Faure EAM. Home care for life-supported persons in France: The regional association. Rehabil Lit 1986; 47(3–4):60–64, 103.
24. Goldberg AI. Home care for life-supported persons: Is a national approach the answer? Chest 1986; 90:744–748.
25. Goldberg AI. Home health care for the chronically ill in the United States: The market-oriented system. In: Hollingsworth JR, Hollingsworth EJ, eds. Care of the Chronically and Severely Ill: Comparative Social Policies. New York: Aldine de Gruyter, 1994.
26. Hawkins LC, Lompask M. The Man in the Iron Lung: The inspiring story of Frederick B. Snite. England: Kingswood, 1957.
27. Drinker F, Shaw LA. An apparatus for the prolonged administration of artificial ventilation. J Clin Invest 1929; 7:229–247.
28. Maxwell JH. The iron lung: Halfway technology or a necessary step. Milbank Quart 1986; 84(1):3–29.
29. Engström CG. Treatment of a severe case of respiratory paralysis by the Engström Universal Respirator. Br Med J 1954; 2:666.
30. Kristensen HS, Neukirch F. Very long-term articial ventilation (28 years). In: Rattenborg CC, Via-Requé, eds. Clinical Use of Mechanical Ventilation. Chicago: Year Book, 1981; 220.
31. Goldberg AI. Pediatric high-technology home care. In: Rothkopf MM, Askanazi J, eds. Intensive Homecare. Baltimore: Williams & Wilkins, 1992.
32. Laurie G. Introductory remarks. In: Faure EAM, Goldberg AI, eds. Proceedings of an international symposium: Whatever happened to the polio patient? Northwestern University Press, Chicago, 1982.
33. Arras JD. Bringing the hospital home: Ethical and social implications of high-tech home care. Baltimore, MD: Johns Hopkins University Press, 1995.
34. Managed Care News. January, 1997:1.
35. Special Supplement. The technological tether: An introduction to ethical and social issues in high-tech home care. Hastings Ctr Rep 1994; 24(5):S1–S28.
36. gini_intl@msm.org http://www.post-polio.org/ivun.html.
37. http://www.drkoop.com.
38. Goldberg AI, Faure EAM, O'Callaghan JJ. High-technology home care: Critical issues and ethical choices. In: Monagle JF, Thomasma DC, eds. Health Care Ethics: Critical Issues for the 21st Century. Gaithersburg, MD: Aspen, 1998.
39. McCullough LB. A primer on bioethics. In: Preparation Course for the American Board of Medical Management Examination. National Institute on Healthcare Leadership and Management. Tampa: American College of Physician Executives, 1992.

40. McCullough LB. An ethical model for improving physician-patient relationships. Inquiry (Blue Cross/Blue Shield Association) 1992; 25:454–468.
41. Carlson RJ, Ellwood PM, Etzioni A, Goldbeck WB, Gradison B, Johnson KE, Kitzhaber J, Koop CE, Lee DR, Lewin LS, McNerney WJ, Ray RD, Riley T, Schmoke KL, Thier SO, Tilson HH, Tuckson RV, Warden GL. The Belmont Vision for Health Care in America: Healthy People in a Healthy World. Alexandria, VA: Institute for Alternative Futures, 1994.
42. Bezold C. Your health in 2010: Four scenarios. Futurist 1996; 30(5):35–39.
43. Oxford American Dictionary. New York: Oxford University Press, 1980.
44. Shortell SM, Gillies RR. Creating organizational delivery systems: The barriers and facilitation. Hosp Health Serv Admin 1993; 38(4):447–466.
45. Genry C. Big HMO's new affiliate makes hard cases easier. Wall Street Journal, Nov. 19, 1997; NE1, NE3.
46. Report of the Surgeon General's Workshop on Children with Handicaps and Their Familes. Case-Example: The Ventilator-Dependent Child. Department of Health and Human Services publication DHSS-PHS-83-50194. Washington, DC: U.S. Government Printing Office, 1983.
47. The Surgeon General's Workshop on Self Help and Public Health. Department of Health and Human Services publication DHHS-PHS-224-250-88. Washington, DC: U.S. Government Printing Office, 1988.
48. Egan G. The skilled helper: a problem management approach to helping. ed 5. Pacific Grove, CA: Brooks/Cole, 1994.
49. Egan G. Adding Value: A Systematic Guide to Business-Driven Management and Leadership. San Francisco, CA: Jossey-Bass, 1993.
50. Emery M, Purser RE. The Search Conference: A Powerful Method for Planning Organizational Change and Community Action. San Francisco, CA: Jossey-Bass, 1996.

16

Weaning from Long-Term Mechanical Ventilation

DOUGLAS R. GRACEY and ROLF D. HUBMAYR

Mayo Clinic and Mayo Foundation
Rochester, Minnesota

I. Introduction

The physician concerned with weaning a patient from mechanical ventilation must address two important questions: 1) When is it appropriate to initiate the weaning process? and 2) Which of the many weaning strategies is most efficacious? During the past five years, several prospective controlled randomized clinical trials have address questions of weaning strategy and outcomes. However, the relevance of these trials for weaning from long-term mechanical ventilation is not clear because most of the study participants had acute and imminently reversible forms of respiratory failure.

There is no universally accepted definition of "long-term" mechanical ventilation nor is there a central database to track such patients. Therefore, the scope of the problem in the United States and its economic impact cannot be fully assessed. The Health Care Financing Administration (HCFA) defined chronic ventilator dependency for the Demonstration Project for Chronic Ventilator Dependent Units in 1990 as mechanical ventilation for 21 days or longer. There are thought to be 14,000 such patients in the United States, who consume $8.8 million per day in health care costs. Data from chronic ventilator-dependent units suggest that it costs $65,000 per hospital stay to care for each patient who remains ventilator dependent, whereas the cost drops to $14,490 for each patient who can be liberated from mechanical ventilation. Data from 1987 and 1989 show that hospital financial losses from chronic ventilator-dependent patients under Part A Medicare were substantial before as well as after the revision of the Prospective Payment System (1,2). The availability of alternate sites to provide long-term mechanical ventilation has in recent years given some hospitals relief from the financial burden of caring for such patients.

II. Causes of Long-Term Ventilator Dependence

Causes of long-term ventilator dependence fall into three general categories: (1) preexisting cardiopulmonary diseases, such as chronic obstructive pulmonary disease (COPD), that are exacerbated by an intercurrent illness or a surgical complication, (2) a catastrophic medical or surgical insult that leads to multiorgan failure, and (3) neuromuscular diseases with varying degrees of rehabilitation potential. Given the complexity of insults encountered in long-term ventilator-dependent patients, the pathophysiology of respiratory failure in them is rarely simple and as a rule involves the lungs as well as the ventilatory pump (3). One need only recall that long-term ventilator-dependent patients are at increased risk for nosocomial pneumonia and that many ventilator-dependent patients suffer neuromuscular complications of acute and prolonged critical illness (4–6).

Prolonged mechanical ventilation itself can decrease diaphragm strength and endurance. Anzueto et al. (7) have shown in a baboon model that mechanical ventilation for 11 days causes a 25% decrease in maximum transdiaphragmatic pressure and a 36% decrease in diaphragmatic endurance. Maher et al. (6) analyzed the records of 40 patients admitted to a critical care/trauma center in whom a respiratory assessment suggested one or more neuromuscular causes of prolonged ventilator dependence. Twenty-five had critical illness polyneuropathy, two had Guillain-Barré syndrome, four had diabetic and critical illness polyneuropathy, two uremic and critical illness neuropathy, ten had an abnormality of central respiratory drive, five a unilateral phrenic nerve palsy, three a neuromuscular transmission defect, and five had a primary myopathy. Patients with more severe neuromuscular dysfunction took longer to wean (a mean of 136 days vs. 52 days). We have found polyneuropathy of critical illness to be present in a significant number of ventilator-dependent patients admitted to our chronic ventilator-dependent unit (8). Clinical evaluation usually suggests this problem and electromyographic examination usually confirms it. In addition, we see a number of patients who present with unilateral, and rarely bilateral, phrenic nerve paralysis complicating open heart surgery or thoracic trauma. Many of these patients have additional co-morbidities, such as chronic obstructive or restrictive lung disease. Insufficient inspiratory drive may also contribute to ventilator dependence. It is a common occurrence in acute care units, where use of sedative drugs, sleep deprivation, and nutritional deficiencies interact to compound this problem (9–11).

III. When Is It Appropriate to Initiate the Weaning Process?

Stroetz and Hubmayr (12) asked intensivists to predict whether their patients would be able to complete a 1-hr T-piece trial and then proceeded to test the accuracy of these predictions using a weaning protocol of graduated pressure support withdrawal (12). Failure criteria had been established prospectively and were based primarily on the intensity of respiratory sensations (dyspnea scores ≥18 using a modified Borg scale), tachypnea (respiratory rate ≥35/min), and cardiovascular response parameters indicative of a hyperdynamic state. The results of this small survey are shown in Table 1 and illustrate that physicians tend to underestimate the short-term weaning potential of their patients. Based on this information, it might be more appropriate to rephrase the question and ask when it might *not* be prudent to initiate the weaning process. This is important because delays in weaning not only have an adverse financial impact but also unnecessarily extend the patients' risk for mechanical ventilation–associated complications, such as nosocomial pneumonia and barotrauma. Consistent with this hypothesis, Nava et al. (13) reported that patients with respiratory failure from COPD who were extubated early to noninvasive mechanical ventilation had a lower in-hospital mortality than those who remained intubated until they were able to sustain breathing without ventilatory assistance.

Table 1 Prediction of Weaning Outcome

	Clinical prediction		
Test results	Failure	Success	Total
Failure	11	3	14
Success	11	6	17
Total	22	9	31

False positive, 0.65.
False negative, 0.21.
Sensitivity, 0.79.
Specificity, 0.35.
Positive predictive value, 0.5.
Negative predictive value, 0.67.

Source: Adapted from Ref. 12. © American Lung Association.

There is little reason to think that subjecting patients to unsuccessful weaning trials has adverse long-term consequences, provided one avoids certain pitfalls. For example, it is unwise to impose a weaning stress on patients with active ischemic heart disease knowing that systemic oxygen demand and cardiac output can increase substantially during the transition from controlled mechanical ventilation to spontaneous breathing. Patients must be prepared psychologically that other than premature extubation, failing a single weaning trial has no bearing on their ultimate prognosis. Finally, it seems prudent to guarantee sufficient respiratory muscle rest after an episode of weaning-induced ventilatory pump failure. Although there is considerable controversy about the role of respiratory muscle fatigue in the pathogenesis of ventilatory failure syndromes, patients should probably not undergo more than one (failed) weaning trial in any 24-hr time span.

Yang and Tobin (14) have provided the most comprehensive account of the sensitivity and specificity of commonly used weaning parameters. Table 2 has been adapted from their study and shows both threshold values and the accuracy of indices used to predict weaning outcome. Results are based on a prospec-

Table 2 Threshold Values and Accuracy of the Indices Used to Predict Weaning Outcome

Index	Value[a]	Positive predictive value[b]	Negative predictive value[b]
Expired ventilation (L/min)	≤15	0.55	0.38
Respiratory frequency (breaths/min)	≤38	0.65	0.77
Tidal volume (mL)	≥325	0.73	0.94
Tidal volume (mL)/patient's weight (kg)	≥4	0.67	0.85
Maximal inspiratory pressure (cm H_2O)[c]	≤−15	0.59	1.00
Dynamic compliance (mL/cm H_2O)	≥22	0.65	0.58
Static compliance (mL/cm H_2O)	≥33	0.60	0.53
P_{AO_2}–Pa_{O_2} ratio	≥0.35	0.59	0.53
Frequency–tidal volume ratio (breaths/min/L)	≤105	0.78	0.95
CROP index (mL/breath/min)[d]	≥13	0.71	0.70

[a] Threshold values were those that discriminated best in the training data set between the patients who were successfully weaned and those in whom a weaning trial failed: ≥ and ≤ indicate whether the values above the threshold value or those below it are those that predicted a successful weaning outcome.

[b] Values shown were derived from the complete prospective-validation data set, comprising 36 successfully weaned patients and 28 patients in whom weaning failed.

[c] To convert value to kilopascals, multiply by 0.09807.

[d] A weaning outcome index that integrates thoracic compliance, respiratory rate, arterial oxygenation, and PImax

Source: Adapted from Ref. 14.

tive validation data set of 64 patients, 28 of whom failed weaning. Although the authors emphasized the value of the frequency–tidal volume ratio (f/V_T), it should be noted that a V_T ≥325 ml was almost as good a predictor of weaning success as a f/V_T ≤105. Observing patients during extended trials of unassisted breathing (e.g., during a 30 to 120 min T-piece trial) increases the predictive value of f/V_T, further reducing the reintubation rate (false positive rate) below 20% (15–19). One should recall that Yang and Tobin made their measurements with a hand-held spirometer after disconnecting patients from the ventilator and allowing them to breathe room air. The simplicity of this approach is of obvious appeal to the clinician, although one may question to what extent hypoxemia affected the measurements. This is important because many care providers use ventilator-based instrumentation to measure V_T during unassisted breathing on morning rounds before they establish a weaning plan. This is often done without disconnecting the patient or changing the inspired oxygen concentration and may or may not include the use of continuous positive end-expired pressure (CPAP) and low levels of pressure support ventilation (PSV). The predictive value of the f/V_T under those circumstances is certainly less. Furthermore, V_T measurements that are derived from ventilator-based instrumentation are not as accurate as those reported in a research paper. For example, in one small survey, 25% of ventilator-derived V_T estimates (means of 6 breaths) had a greater than 10% error (R. W. Stroetz, personal communication, 1994).

As already pointed out, there are important differences between the type of patient studied by Yang and Tobin and patients admitted to long-term ventilator-dependent units. Scheinhorn et al. (20) evaluated predictors of weaning after 6 wk of mechanical ventilation in 565 patients and found that the alveolar-arterial oxygen tension gradient, blood urea nitrogen, and gender were the most reliable predictors of continued ventilator dependence. On the basis of these observations, they proposed a simple scoring system, the A+B+G score, which had 68% accuracy in a post hoc analysis. The formula used for scoring patients is shown in Figure 1. In a prospective study of 163 consecutive mechanically ventilated patients, Leitch et al. (21) found that expired ventilation ($\dot{V}_E$) and f/V_T had moderate sensitivity and specificity as predictors of need for reintubation 60 min after extubation. These authors concluded that clinical judgment produces satisfactory weaning outcomes and that measurements of respiratory pressures and volumes have limited utility. In a retrospective analysis of 174 ventilator-dependent subjects (120 of whom were weaned from mechanical ventilation), Clochesy et al. (22) found no differences in maximum inspiratory pressure, expired ventilation, and vital capacity between weaning success and weaning failure patients. The presence of left venticular dysfunction was a predictor of greatly prolonged mechanical ventilation, as was positive fluid balance, low serum albumin, and the number of drugs being used to treat heart failure. Prolonged bed rest and inactivity, which is a characteristic of many of these ventilator-dependent patients, is a

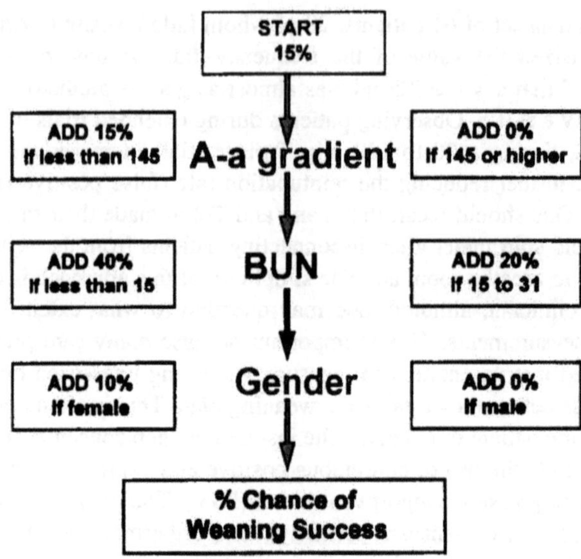

Figure 1 The A+B+G score is calculated using a patient's $P(A\text{-}a)O_2$ (mm Hg), blood urea nitrogen (BUN) (mg/dl), and gender. The sum of the percentages at each step equals the percent chance of successful weaning. For simplicity's sake, it is left unstated that nothing is added for a BUN value greater than 31. (From Ref. 20.)

key factor. Prolonged bed rest produces muscle atrophy and loss of muscle strength and endurance. In addition, prolonged bed rest leads to loss of antigravity reflexes and loss of general muscle strength, which greatly complicates rehabilitation and reconditioning and can greatly prolong ventilator dependence (23–25).

Results from weaning parameter studies on long-term mechanically ventilated patients suggest that respiratory failure is often a manifestation of general disability and multiorgan dysfunction. Viewed in that light, it is not surprising that measures of renal function and nutritional status capture dimensions that correlate with the persistence of respiratory failure. Although this may introduce uncertainty and complicate weaning assessments, it is worth remembering that the penalty for making the wrong prediction in someone with a tracheostomy is not nearly as great as it is in a patient who is prematurely extubated. Tracheostomies are usually left in place for many days after successful liberation from ventilator assistance. In contrast, orotracheal and nasotracheal tubes are often removed within 2 hr following a "successful" T-piece trial. In the latter instance, errors in clinical judgment bring about the risk associated with reintubation. In several recent series, the mortality of patients who failed extubation and needed to be reintubated approached 40% (15,16,26). To what extent reintubation is a marker of disease severity as opposed to an independent risk factor of morbidity and mortality cannot be ascertained from these studies.

Predicting ventilator dependence in a patient ventilated long-term requires a careful assessment of more than the respiratory system. The transition from mechanical ventilation to spontaneous breathing is an exercise test during which the added respiratory workload mandates an appropriate cardiovascular response. An increasing number of case series have underscored the need to consider cardiac limitation in the differential diagnosis of weaning failure (27–30). Although the responsible physiologic mechanisms can be readily appreciated in concept, cardiac weaning failure is difficult to diagnose at the bedside. Epstein (27) suggested that patients with weaning-induced heart failure (as opposed to patients with overt heart failure) have a normal rapid shallow breathing index, but that they develop rapid shallow breathing soon after cessation of machine support. Because a diagnosis of cardiac weaning limitation has important management implications, it can be helpful to formally assess a patient's hemodynamic response to weaning using a pulmonary artery catheter. Of course, in doing so one must be careful to avoid misinterpreting respiratory artifacts as evidence of pulmonary venous hypertension. Tachypneic patients invariably recruit expiratory muscles, thereby raising end-expiratory pleural, esophageal, and pulmonary artery occlusion pressure. Weaning-induced left ventricular failure should be suspected only when there is a substantial increase in pulmonary artery occlusion pressure throughout the respiratory cycle.

IV. Which of the Many Weaning Strategies Is Most Efficacious?

In principle, there are three different techniques used to wean patients from mechanical ventilation: (1) T-piece with or without the addition of CPAP, (2) synchronized intermittent mandatory ventilation (SIMV), and (3) pressure support ventilation (PSV). T-piece based weaning modalities consist of the sudden, complete withdrawal of machine support for increasing lengths of time, in contrast to techniques that involve the gradual withdrawal of machine support, such as SIMV and PSV. During T-piece weaning, the patient's cardiorespiratory response patterns can be assessed without the confounding influence of machine settings. Using the time to extubation as a primary end point, the three weaning techniques have been compared in several largle multicenter trials. On the surface, these trials have yielded conflicting results. In one such trial, intermittent T-piece breathing proved to be the most effective weaning strategy (19); in another, pressure support was superior (18); whereas the third study showed little difference between the PSV and T-piece modes (31). Synchronized intermittent mandatory ventilation performed worse than either of the other two modes. Most experts who have scrutinized the three large prospective multicenter trials agree that those studies in which one weaning mode appeared superior over another were biased in favor of that particular mode. For example, Brochard et al. (18) delayed extubation in patients assigned to the T-piece arm, while Esteban et al. (19) followed an exceedingly conservative and time-consuming pressure support withdrawal protocol.

In the late 1970s and early 1980s, there was considerable debate among intensivists whether gradual SIMV weaning was superior to intermittent T-piece trials (32). The proponents of SIMV argued that intermittent "T-piece sprints" might be fatiguing, which implied that the sudden, as opposed to gradual, withdrawal of machine support might cause maladaptive responses in breathing strategy. Not only do recent prospective clinical trials not support these predictions, but also a few caveats about SIMV are in order. First, the inexperienced physician may be tempted to seek assurances through frequent blood gas analyses during SIMV weaning, thereby prolonging and adding unnecessary cost to the weaning process. Second, SIMV with low backup machine rates may obscure the presence of impending ventilatory pump failure by blood gas criteria. This is because even an occasional large breath may augment alveolar ventilation and carbon dioxide (CO_2) elimination enough to prevent frank acidemia.

Pressure support ventilation has become a popular weaning mode for adults. In the PSV mode, a target pressure is applied to the endotracheal tube, which augments the inflation pressure exerted by the inspiratory muscles (Pmus) on the respiratory system (33). As the lungs inflate, inspiratory flow begins to decline because airway pressure and Pmus are opposed by rising elastic recoil forces. When inspiratory flow reaches a threshold value (this value differs among manufacturers), the machine switches to expiration. For a long time it was assumed that PSV was a useful means to compensate for the added resistance* of endotracheal tubes (34,35). Conceptually, this is not correct because during PSV airway pressure does not vary with flow. Furthermore, several authors have now demonstrated that pulmonary resistance (and by inference the resistance of the upper airway) remains elevated after extubation (36,37). This finding suggests that the extubated upper airway may be edematous and offers just as high a

* The term resistance describes the relationship between the pressure and flow and in the simplest case (as described by Ohm's law) is a constant. In endotracheal tubes, the pressure–flow relationship is nonlinear and is usually approximated by a quadratic equation (i.e., two constants). In other words, any increase in flow requires a disproportionate increase in driving pressure. For a mechanism or ventilator to eliminate resistive work (or to "overcome the tube resistance"), its pressure output must be repeatedly adjusted to flow. In contrast to PSV, in which the ventilator is programmed to generate a constant pressure, some newer modes (such as automatic tube compensation and proportional assist ventilation) have incorporated such pressure–flow scaling algorithms.

resistive load as a #8 endotracheal tube. This undermines the long-held notion that breathing through a T-piece is an overly burdensome challenge for a diaphragm that is prone to fatigue.

In our chronic ventilator unit we have used a variant of the T-piece trial for the past 10 yr. We use a Bivona (Bivona Medical Technologies, Gary, IN) TTS adult tracheostomy tube with a low-profile cuff that when deflated allows the patient to breathe around the tracheostomy tube (Fig. 2). This tube can be capped (see Fig. 2) and oxygen supplemented via nasal prongs. Capping of the tracheostomy reestablishes the normal physiologic glottic retard mechanism and allows the patient to speak. The ability to speak is especially helpful because patients can express their fears and concerns. In our practice, we drill a hole in the cap and place the supplemental oxygen catheter directly into the cap (38). This allows us to deliver oxygen without an appliance in the patient's face and reduce flow to approximately one-half the flow rate used transnasally. In the majority of our patients, the ability to swallow is maintained with the cuff deflated and capped. Given the high prevalence of aspiration in this group of patients, grape juice tests and formal barium swallow evaluations are almost routinely performed. Only those patients who have demonstrated that they can protect their airways receive oral food or liquids. However, we do not consider evidence of barium penetration during a swallow evaluation to be a contraindication for de-

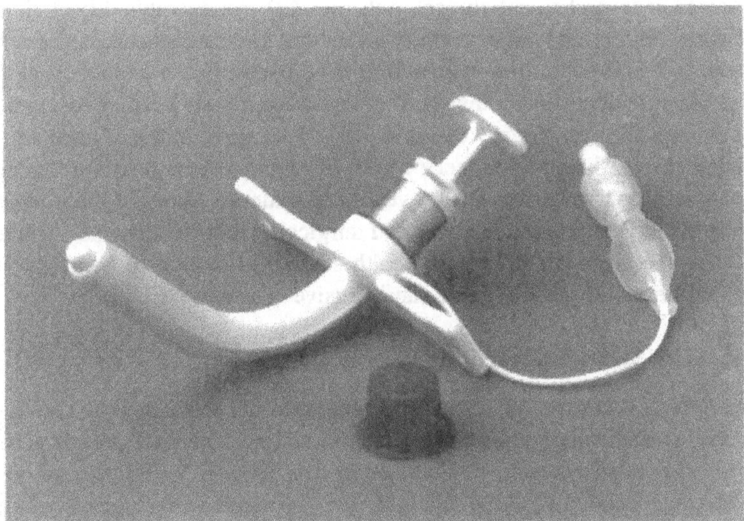

Figure 2 Bivona low-profile cuff tracheostomy tube (Bivona Medical Technologies, Gary, IN).

flating the tracheostomy tube and capping it during spontaneous breathing trials. We try to cap the tracheostomy tube for progressive periods during the day and support the patients' breathing at night with CPAP and low levels of intermittent positive inspiratory pressure. At that stage of their weaning process, patients may display episodic apnea or periodic breathing during sleep, which generally implies overassistance with pressure support as opposed to intrinsic disease. During sleep or heavy sedation, even small amounts of pressure support can raise a patient's tidal volume beyond that demanded by the ventilatory control system, producing relative hypocapnea and unstable breathing (39). Once a patient has been successfully removed from the ventilator for several days, we place a tracheostomy button. If the patient remains stable for several more days, we remove the button. We do not decannulate a patient who has persistent swallowing dysfunction, even if the patient is liberated from the ventilator. Usually, these patients ultimately recover swallow function unless they have bulbar dysfunction or upper airway damage.

V. An Organized Approach to Weaning from Long-Term Mechanical Ventilation

A. A Protocol-Driven Approach

Possibly more important than the choice of weaning mode is the benefit derived from an organized, protocol-driven team approach to weaning. This has been underscored in several recent clinical trials (40–42). For example, Ely et al. (41) reported that physicians who were made aware that their patients had successfully completed a 2-hr T-piece trial were more likely to remove the endotracheal tube and wean their patients than if they had conducted their own weaning assessment. In Ely's hands, this respiratory therapist–driven weaning protocol resulted in a shortening of ventilator dependence by 36 hr. Again, these observations need not apply to long-term mechanically ventilated patients. Many of them recover gradually from catastrophic medical and surgical insults so that the ventilator may simply be a marker of overall health status as opposed to being the one device that keeps the patient tied to an intensive care unit (ICU).

B. The Setting: Specialized Weaning Units

An ever-growing number of institutions recognize the advantage of caring for long-term mechanically ventilated patients in a setting separate from the general ICU (43). So-called chronic ventilator-dependent units (CVDU) seek to create an environment conducive to the rehabilitation of patients with respiratory failure and at the same time lower the cost of providing care for them (1,2). The weaning strategy of the long-term mechanically ventilated patient cannot be discussed without considering the overall care that is being delivered in such units. The CVDU in our institution is a self-contained area in the hospital with a dedicated medical and paramedical staff. A physician, 20.2 full-time equivalent registered nurses with expertise in and devotion to the care of patients with respiratory diseases, and a lead respiratory therapist are permanently assigned to the 9-bed CVDU. Additional personnel with shared responsibilities for other hospital services include pharmacists, respiratory therapists, physical and occupational therapists, dietitians, speech therapists, and a social worker. The unit takes a holistic approach to patient care with a strong emphasis on physical rehabilitation. Patients with respiratory failure are admitted to the CVDU only if two or more successive ventilator weaning attempts are unsuccessful and if patients are in a state of health that, in the opinion of the CVDU physician, precludes liberation from mechanical ventilation in the foreseeable future. A tracheostomy and hemodynamic stability are required because neither electrocardiographic nor hemodynamic monitoring is available in the CVDU. We do not accept patients with potentially life-threatening dysrhythmias because we believe that a patient who requires electocardiographic monitoring should not be in a CVDU. In the 9 yr of the unit's existence, we have not felt that the lack of ECG monitoring has been detrimental to patient care.

The caloric needs of patients are assessed upon admission to the CVDU and resting energy expenditure is measured in many instances. We prefer enteral over intravenous feedings and usually place a feeding tube unless the patient is able to eat. If tube feeding requirements are prolonged, a percutaneous endoscopic gastrostomy feeding tube is placed. Patients are freed from all intravenous and urinary catheters are soon as possible to reduce the risk of infection and to help with mobilization. Patients are scheduled for the various occupational and physical therapy programs and other activities during the day so that they can sleep at night.

Our experience with caring for ventilator-dependent patients in a CVDU has been very rewarding. While caution is required when basing inferences about outcomes compared with historical controls, we did report that the opening of the CVDU in our institution seemingly improved the survival of specific patient populations. In our opinion, there are several reasons for this improvement. Some can be directly attributed to the CVDU; others reflect a change in treatment philosophy that, nevertheless, was reinforced by our early CVDU experience. The staff of "regular intensive care units" are accustomed to dealing with critically ill patients who either respond to therapy and leave the ICU in a few days or who succumb to their illness. There is considerable pressure to intervene with invasive tests and procedures if day-to-day progress is slow, and inherently aggressive resident physicians and surgeons often lose hope and perspective when improvement does not occur within the usual time frame of ICU care. The physicians, nurses, and respiratory therapists are frequently too busy to spend the time required to physically or mentally rehabilitate the "chronic" ventilator-dependent patient. Furthermore, the intensive care unit environment is not conducive to rehabilitating medically stable patients whose only reason for being there is ventilator dependency. Such patients often become confused and sleep deprived from noise, frequent vital sign checks, inappropriate analgesic and sedative management, and lack of stimulation through one-on-one interactions. Patients who, other than respiratory failure, have adequate end-organ function are all too often subjected to the ICU monitoring routine that requires indwelling urinary and rectal catheters, arterial lines, central venous catheters, and nasogastric tubes. During their stay in the ICU they are exposed to a microbial environment that includes drug-resistant organisms, which places them at increased risk for nosocomial infections.

In contrast, the CVDU is staffed with professionals who bring a different perspective to the care of ventilator-dependent patients. This staff is less likely to become impatient when progress is slow and are not compelled to work up every potential problem with costly and invasive tests. Emphasis is placed on minimizing the use of sedatives, spending time with patients to meet their emotional as well as physical needs, and pursuing an intensive program targeted toward respiratory rehabilitation and improving whole-body strength. The ventilator weaning program is tailored to the individual patient's capacity and prognosis and differs from general ICU practice more in terms of day-to-day consistency than in use of specific technologies and support modes. There is no standard weaning protocol in our CVDU for the long-term ventilator-dependent patient. Each patient is individually assessed and a weaning approach specific to that patient and that patient's particular needs and potential problems is formulated. All of these activities are supported by extensive education programs for patients and their families.

C. Sedation and Weaning

A common problem encountered in patients being transferred to chronic ventilator units from intensive care units is withdrawal from sedatives and narcotics. In our experience, narcotic withdrawal is not as common a problem as is benzodiazepine withdrawal. Midazolam withdrawal in particular needs to be managed with long-acting benzodiazepines, such as chlordiazepoxide hydrochloride or lorazepam, given on a tapering schedule. In some patients, psychological assessment and treatment may be necessary. Depression is common in ventilator-dependent patients and antidepressant medications are frequently helpful. In addition, inability to sleep is a major problem and is frequently associated with depression. In these patients, trazadone given at bedtime is a very helpful sleeping medication and antidepressant.

D. Physical Therapy and Rehabilitation

Most long-term ventilator-dependent patients have been confined to bed for considerable periods of time and are profoundly deconditioned. We try to maintain a structured progressive program of weaning and physical activity. Progressive ambulation and general muscle strengthening are important for successful liberation from mechanical ventilation. We begin to walk our patients while assisting them with a portable ventilator as soon as they are medically stable and can maintain antigravity cardiovascular reflexes.

E. Swallowing Dysfunction

Swallowing dysfunction is extremely common in patients with tracheostomies. A very high percentage of patients aspirate when given liquids and solids by mouth. The association between tracheostomy and swallowing dysfunction is not well understood. Prolonged or repeated translaryngeal intubation, age, poor swallowing synchronization while on mechanical ventilation, nutritional depletion, the effects of tracheostomy on the swallow mechanism, sedation, and severe weakness have all been suggested as contributing factors (43). A recent study by Tolep et al. (44) of 35 patients receiving mechanical ventilation showed that bedside swallow evaluations were abnormal in 31% of the patients with a neuromuscular disorder and 37% of patients without a neuromuscular disorder. Appreciation of the high risk of aspiration in ventilator-dependent patients is important because aspiration of oral feedings will only further complicate the problem.

VI. Impact of Specialized Weaning Units on Outcomes

The extent to which special care units contribute to the long-term survival rate of ventilator-dependent patients is unclear. Morganroth et al. (45) reported a 70% hospital survival and a 30% 1-yr survival in 11 patients requiring 30 to 100 days of mechanical ventilation. Spicher and White (46) reported a hospital mortality of 60.8% and a 1- and 2-yr survival rate of 28.6% and 22.5%, respectively, among patients who required mechanical ventilation for at least 10 days. In contrast, in our experience only 8.7% of 206 patients (who had been mechanically ventilated on average for 44 days) died after admission to the CVDU (47). The posthospital survival was 69%, 60%, 56%, and 53% at 1, 2, 3, and 4 yr, respectively (Fig. 3). Seventy-seven percent of the 206 patients returned home, as opposed to being "kept alive" in a chronic care facility. Another institution that also participated in the HCFA demonstration project reported similar results (43). Many of our patients look to the CVDU as a source of information and support long after their discharge. Of the 186 patients discharged, 153 (82%) had been liberated from the mechanical ventilator. Twenty-four patients (13%) were discharged on

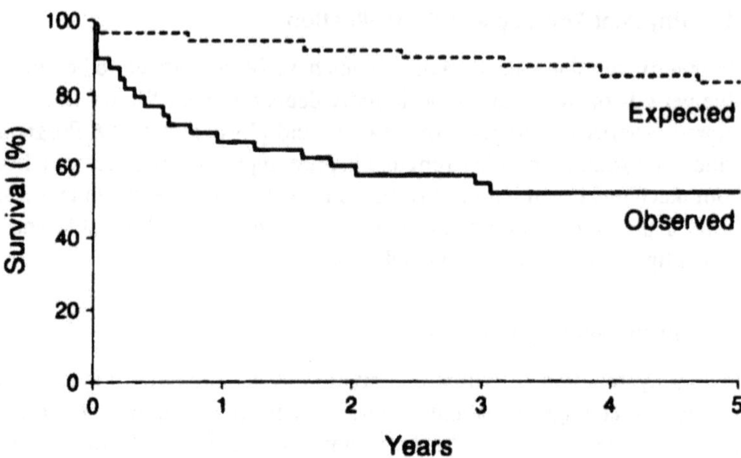

Figure 3 Comparison of 5-yr follow-up of observed and expected survival (based on Minnesota life tables) of patients in the Mayo Clinic's Ventilator-Dependent Rehabilitation Unit. (From Ref. 47.)

nocturnal mechanical ventilation and seven (4%) on continuous mechanical ventilation. Postoperative patients had a significantly greater possibility of being weaned from the ventilator ($p < 0.001$) than patients with non–surgically related ventilator dependence. Shorter stays in intensive care units before transfer to the CVDU were also related to significantly greater success in weaning from mechanical ventilation ($p < 0.002$). Ninety-six percent of postoperative patients were liberated from the ventilator, as opposed to 60% of patients with prior lung disease and 62% of patients with other medical problems (such as neurologic or cardiac disease).

Both Swinburne et al. (48) and Cohen et al. (49) suggest that the outcome of ventilator-dependent patients over age 80 is extremely poor. Swinburne et al. (48) reported a 7% hospital survival rate among ventilator-dependent octogenarians with preexisting renal disease, liver disease, cancer, systemic illness, or chronic gastrointestinal disease with malnutrition, and a 29% survival rate for patients younger than age 80 with the same premorbid conditions. Only 38% of octogenarians without premorbid conditions survived hospitalization, while 49% of those younger survived. Overall, in Swinburne's series of elderly patients who required more than 15 days of mechanical ventilation, the mortality was 91%, whereas it was 64% for younger patients. Cohen et al. (49) found a 78% mortality rate in octogenarians who were mechanically ventilated for more than 3 days in a combined medical-surgical intensive care unit at a large community teaching hospital. Our experience does not support the temptation to make management decisions or withhold therapy in ventilator-dependent patients solely on the basis of age. Of the 11 women and 6 men in the CVDU who were older than age 80, only 1 expired. More importantly, 10 of the 16 survivors went home and the rest went to nursing homes, all without mechanical ventilators.

VII. Conclusion

Management and outlook for the long-term ventilator-dependent patient have changed dramatically in the past decade. The economic pressures to limit ICU resources to patients with acute reversible catastrophic illnesses have led to the creation of intermediate care facilities in which long-term ventilator-dependent patients receive problem-focused care and rehabilitation. It is no longer justified to categorically withhold ventilatory support from a patient out of concern for creating long-term ventilator dependence. Indeed, the vast majority of patients who require ventilatory assistance for more than 3 wk either succumb to their underlying illness or can be successfully weaned and returned to family and home.

Acknowledgments

The authors would like to thank the staff of the Mayo Clinic's Chronic Ventilator Dependency Unit for making the unit so successful; we also thank L. L. Oeltjenbruns for preparing the manuscript. Supported by grants from the National Institutes of Health (HL-57364) and the Health Care Financing Administration Demonstration Project (29-P-99424/1).

References

1. Gracey DR, Gillespie DG, Nobrega F, Naessens JM, Krishan I. Financial implications of prolonged ventilator care of Medicare patients under the prospective payment system: A multicenter study. Chest 1987; 91:424–427.
2. Gracey DR, Nobrega FT, Naessens JM, Krishan I. Financial implications of prolonged ventilator care under DRGs 474 and 475. Chest 1989; 96:193–194.
3. Roussos C, Macklem PT: The respiratory muscles. N Engl J Med 1982; 307:786–797.
4. Bolton CF, Laverty DA, Brown JD, Witt NJ, Hahn AF, Sibbald WJ. Critically ill polyneuropathy: Electrophysiological studies and differentiation from Guillain-Barre syndrome. J Neurol Neurosurg Psychiatry 1986; 49:563–573.
5. Zochodne DW, Bolton CF, Wells GA, Gilbert JJ, Hahn AF, Brown JD, Sibbald WA. Critical illness polyneuropathy: A complication of sepsis and multiple organ failure. Brain 1987; 110:819–841.

6. Maher J, Rutledge F, Remtulla H, Parkes A, Bernardi L, Bolton CF. Neuromuscular disorders associated with failure to wean from the ventilator. Intens Care Med 1995; 21:737–743.
7. Anzueto A, Peters JI, Tobin MJ, de los Santos R, Seidenfeld JJ, Moore G, Cox WJ, Coalson JJ. Effects of prolonged controlled mechanical ventilation on diaphragmatic function in healthy adult baboons. Crit Care Med 1997; 25:1187–1190.
8. Wijdicks EFM, Lichty WJ, Harrison BA, Gracey DR. The clinical spectrum of critical illness polyneuropathy. Mayo Clin Proc 1994; 69:955–959.
9. Barrientos-Vega R, Mar Sanchez-Soria M, Morales-Garcia C, Robas-Gomez A, Cuena-Boy R, Ayensa-Rincon A. Prolonged sedation of critically ill patients with midazolam or propofol: Impact on weaning and cost. Crit Care Med 1997; 25:33–40.
10. Schiffman PL, Trontell MC, Mazar MF, Edelman NH. Sleep deprivation decreases ventilatory response to CO_2 but not load compensation. Chest 1983; 84:695–698.
11. Doekel RC, Zwillich CW, Scoggin CH, Kryger M, Weil JV. Clinical semistarvation: Depression of hypoxic ventilatory response. N Engl J Med 1976; 295:358–361.
12. Stroetz RW, Hubmayr RD. Tidal volume maintenance during weaning with pressure support. Am J Respir Crit Care Med 1995; 152:1034–1040.
13. Nava S, Ambrosino N, Clini E, Prato M, Orlando G, Vitacca M, Brigada P, Fracchia C, Rubini F. Noninvasive mechanical ventilation in the weaning of patients with respiratory failure due to chronic obstructive pulmonary disease: A randomized, controlled trial. Ann Intern Med 1998; 128:721–728.
14. Yang KL, Tobin MJ. A prospective study of indexes predicting the outcome of trials of weaning from mechanical ventilation. New Eng J Med 1991; 324:1445–1450.
15. Epstein SK. Etiology of extubation failure and the predictive value of the rapid shallow breathing index. Am J Respir Crit Care Med 1995; 152:545–549.
16. Epstein SK. Independent effects of etiology of failure and time to reintubation on outcome for patients failing extubation. Am J Respir Crit Care Med 1998; 158:489–493.
17. Chatila W, Jacob B, Guaglione D, Manthous CA. The unassisted respiratory rate-tidal volume ratio accurately predicts weaning outcome. Am J Med 1996; 101:61–67.
18. Brochard L, Rauss A, Benito S, Conti G, Mancebo J, Rekik N, Gasparetto A, Lemaire F. Comparison of three methods of gradual withdrawal from ventilatory support during weaning from mechanical ventilation. Am J Respir Crit Care Med 1994; 150:896–903.
19. Esteban A, Frutos F, Tobin MJ, Alía I, Solsona JF, Valverdú I, Fernández R, de la Cal MA, Benito S, Tomás R, Carriedo D, Macías S, Blanco J, for the Spanish Lung Failure Collaborative Group. A comparison of four methods of weaning patients from mechanical ventilation. N Engl J Med 1995; 332:345–350.
20. Scheinhorn DJ, Hassenpflug M, Artinian BM, LaBree L, Catlin JL. Predictors of weaning after 6 weeks of mechanical ventilation. Chest 1995; 107:500–505.
21. Leitch EA, Moran JL, Grealy B. Weaning and extubation in the intensive care unit: Clinical or index-driven approach. Intens Care Med 1996; 22:752–759.
22. Clochesy JM, Daly BJ, Montenegro HD. Weaning chronically critically ill adults

from mechanical ventilatory support: A descriptive study. Am J Crit Care 1995; 4: 93–99.
23. Hung J, Goldwater D, Convertino VA, McKillop JH, Goris ML, DeBusk RF. Mechanisms for decreased exercise capacity after bed rest in normal middle-aged men. Am J Cardiol 1983; 51:344–348.
24. Convertino V, Hung J, Goldwater D, DeBusk RF. Cardiovascular responses to exercise in middle-aged men after 10 days of bedrest. Circulation 1982; 65:134–140.
25. Greenleaf JE, Van Beaumont W, Convertino VA, Starr JC. Handgrip and general muscular strength and endurance during prolonged bedrest with isometric and isotonic leg exercise training. Aviat Space Environ Med 1983; 54:696–700.
26. Torres A, Gatell JM, Aznar E, el-Ebiari M, Puig de la Bellacasa J, Gonzales J, Ferrer M, Rodriguez-Roisin R. Reintubation increases the risk of nosocomial pneumonia in patients needing mechanical ventilation. Am J Respir Crit Care Med 1995; 152: 137–141.
27. Epstein SK. Etiology of extubation failure and the predictive value of the rapid shallow breathing index. Am J Respir Crit Care Med 1995; 152:545–549.
28. Richard C, Teboul JL, Archambaud F, Hebert JL, Michut P, Auzepy P. Left ventricular function during weaning of patients with chronic obstructive pulmonary disease. Intens Care Med 1994; 20:181–186.
29. Lemaire F, Teboul JL, Cinotti L, Giotto G, Abrouk F, Steg G, Macquin-Mavier I, Zapol WM. Acute left ventricular dysfunction during unsuccessful weaning from mechanical ventilation. Anesthesiology 1988; 69:171–179.
30. Jubran A, Mathru M, Dries D, Tobin MJ. Continuous recordings of mixed venous oxygen saturation during weaning from mechanical ventilation and the ramifications thereof. Am J Respir Crit Care Med 1998; 158:1763–1769.
31. Esteban A, Alía I, Gordo F, Fernández R, Solsona JF, Valverdú I, Macías S, Allegue JM, Blanco J, Carriedo D, León M, de la Cal MA, Taboada F, Gonzalez de Velasco J, Palazón E, Carrizosa F, Tomás R, Suarez J, Goldwasser RS, for the Spanish Lung Failure Collaborative Group. Extubation outcome after spontaneous breathing trials with T-tube or pressure support ventilation. Am J Respir Crit Care Med 1997; 156: 459–465.
32. Weisman IM, Rinaldo JE, Rogers RM, Sanders MH. Intermittent mandatory ventilation. Am Rev Respir Dis 1983; 127:641–647.
33. Hubmayr RD, Irwin RS. Mechanical ventilation: Initiation. In: Irwin RS, Cerra FB, Rippe JM, eds. Intensive Care Medicine. 4th ed. Vol I. Philadelphia, PA: Lippincott-Raven, 1999; 727–741.
34. Brochard L, Rua F, Lorino H, Lemaire F, Harf A. Inspiratory pressure support compensates for the additional work of breathing caused by the endotracheal tube. Anesthesiology 1991; 75:739–745.
35. Fiastro JF, Habib MP, Quan SF. Pressure support compensation for inspiratory work due to endotracheal tubes and demand continuous positive airway pressure. Chest 1988; 93:499–505.
36. Ishaaya AM, Nathan SD, Belman MJ. Work of breathing after extubation. Chest 1995; 107:204–209.
37. Straus C, Louis B, Isabey D, Lemaire F, Harf A, Brochard L. Contribution of the

endotracheal tube and the upper airway to breathing workload. Am J Respir Crit Care Med 1998; 157:23–30.

38. Gracey DR. Options for long-term ventilatory support. Clin Chest Med 1997; 18: 563–576.
39. Tobert DG, Simon PM, Stroetz RW, Hubmayr RD. The determinants of respiratory rate during mechanical ventilation. Am J Respir Crit Care Med 1997; 155:485–492.
40. Kollef MH, Shapiro SD, Silver P, St John RE, Prentice D, Sauer S, Aherns TS, Shannon W, Baker-Clinkscale D. A randomized, controlled trial of protocol-directed versus physican-directed weaning from mechanical ventilation. Crit Care Med 1997; 25:567–574.
41. Ely EW, Baker AM, Dunagan DP, Burke HL, Smith AC, Kelly PT, Johnson MM, Browder RW, Bowton DL, Haponik EF. Effect on the duration of mechanical ventilation of identifying patients capable of breathing spontaneously. New Engl J Med 1996; 335:1864–1869.
42. Ely WE, Bennet PA, Bowton DL, Murphy SM, Florance AM, Haponik EF. Large scale implementation of a respiratory therapist-driven protocol for ventilator weaning. Am J Respir Crit Care Med 1999; 159:439–446.
43. Make BJ, Hill NS, Goldberg AI, Bach JR, Criner GJ, Dunne PE, Gilmartin ME, Heffner JE, Kacmarek R, Keens TG, McInturff S, O'Donohue WJ Jr, Oppenheimer EA, Robert D. Mechanical ventilation beyond the intensive care unit: Report of a consensus conference of the American College of Chest Physicians. Chest 1998; 113:289S–344S.
44. Tolep K, Getch CL, Criner GJ. Swallowing dysfunction in patients receiving prolonged mechanical ventilation. Chest 1996; 109:167–172.
45. Morganroth ML, Morganroth JL, Nett LM, Petty TL. Criteria for weaning from prolonged mechanical ventilation. Arch Intern Med 1984; 144:1012–1016.
46. Spicher JE, White DP. Outcome and function following prolonged mechanical ventilation. Arch Intern Med 1987; 147:421–425.
47. Gracey DR, Hardy DC, Naessens JM, Silverstein MD, Hubmayr RD. The Mayo Ventilator-Dependent Rehabilitation Unit: A 5-year experience. Mayo Clin Proc 1997; 72:13–19.
48. Swineburne AJ, Fedullo AJ, Bixby K, Lee DK, Wahl GW. Respiratory failure in the elderly: Analysis of outcome after treatment with mechanical ventilation. Arch Intern Med 1993; 153:1657–1662.
49. Cohen IL, Lambrinos J, Fein IA. Mechanical ventilation for the elderly patient in intensive care: Incremental charges and benefits. JAMA 1993; 269:1025–1029.

17

Rehabilitation of Long-Term Mechanically Ventilated Patients

MONICA AVENDANO and ROGER S. GOLDSTEIN

West Park Hospital
University of Toronto
Toronto, Ontario, Canada

ROSA GUELL

Hospital Santa Creu I Sant Pau
Barcelona, Spain

I. Introduction

Over the last 10 years there have been marked improvements in our ability to provide mechanical support over prolonged periods for those with ventilatory failure, almost irrespective of their diagnostic classification. Over the same period, respiratory rehabilitation has been subjected to controlled clinical trials in which valid, reproducible, and interpretable outcome measures have provided the essential evidence of effectiveness. The development of outcome measures that reflect health-related quality of life contributes to our understanding of the patient's perspective on the impact of their underlying condition (1). These developments have progressed more or less in parallel. They do, however, interface in two interesting and important ways: 1) the challenge of returning to the community those individuals who become clinically stable but remain ventilator dependent and 2) the challenge of providing ventilatory support as part of a rehabilitation program for individuals with ventilatory failure. In this chapter, we comment on clinical issues associated with these two clinical interfaces. In both instances, it is important for the health care providers to have skills in respiratory rehabilitation as well as in mechanical ventilation.

II. Definition of Respiratory Rehabilitation

Respiratory rehabilitation has been defined as a multidimensional continuum of services directed to persons with pulmonary disease and their families usually by an interdisciplinary team of specialists with the goal of achieving and maintaining the individual's maximum level of independence and functioning within the community (2).

Respiratory rehabilitation consists of a comprehensive approach to the management of patients with respiratory impairments. However, attention must also be paid to the management of any other associated nonrespiratory problems, especially if respiratory failure is the consequence of a primary multisystem disease (3). The ventilator-dependant patient, as is often the case among all patients with long-standing respiratory conditions, has special needs that must be addressed. For example, once the immediate respiratory needs are met, muscle deconditioning, nutritional support, and psychosocial requirements must be addressed.

Given the variety of diagnoses and different ways in which the conditions evolve with time, respiratory rehabilitation should be individualized. In order to do so it is useful to characterize the patients in terms of their "impairment, disability, and handicap" (4). The following World Health Organization (WHO) definitions are in frequent use:

> *Impairment* is a loss or abnormality of psychological, physiologic, or anatomic structure or function. It is usually determined by a laboratory measurement. For example, in chronic respiratory conditions, the primary impairment may be reflected by a change in lung volumes, flow rates, or diffusing capacity. Secondary impairments, which often occur, may be reflected by changes in peripheral muscle strength or endurance.
>
> *Disability* (ability is also used) refers to the inability to perform an activity in the usual manner or within the normally expected range. For example, in respiratory conditions, disability is assessed using measures of functional or laboratory exercise capacity in which walking time or power output is measured together with symptoms such as dyspnea or leg effort.
>
> *Handicap* (participation is also used) represents the disadvantage resulting from an impairment or disability within the context of the individual's performance in society or in fulfilling expected roles. Individuals with similar levels of impairment and disability may have quite different levels of handicap depending on their expected roles within society. Examples of handicap include withdrawal from self-care, family and leisure activities, or employment.

An understanding of the individual patient's primary and secondary impairments, disabilities, and handicaps is useful in establishing the goals of the rehabilitation program.

III. Respiratory Rehabilitation Program

Most patients referred for respiratory rehabilitation have chronic obstructive pulmonary disease (COPD). However, patients with nonobstructive respiratory impairments are also referred and admitted. Programs generally include education, breathing strategies, energy conservation, supervised exercise training, psychosocial support, and behavioral modifications (5–9). Clearly, the components of the program will vary according to the underlying diagnostic categories of the patients. It may involve modest goals and be limited to patient and family education or it may include a fully supervised exercise program.

A. Goals

The main goals of respiratory rehabilitation are to maximize independent functioning and to improve health-related quality of life (HRQL). To achieve these goals, rehabilitative approaches frequently focus on optimizing pulmonary function and reducing symptoms such as dyspnea and fatigue. Improvements in functional exercise capacity as well as in psychosocial issues such as anxiety and depression will help the individual to participate more in physical and social activities, thereby improving their health-related quality of life (5–7). The goals should also take into consideration a realistic appraisal of the patient's potential for improvement. Some patients receiving long-term mechanical ventilation have very limited potential to improve exercise capacity, yet their ability to participate in social activities may be greatly enhanced by mounting their ventilator on an electric wheelchair.

B. The Interdisciplinary Team

As in many aspects of rehabilitation, patient care is best organized with an interdisciplinary team in which each member has a specific role (6–8). Although better-funded organizations might have separate individuals for each of the nonphysician health professional functions, another way to think of the team is in terms of skill sets, rather than individual staff, with each skill set being represented. It is essential that the team meet at regular intervals. The first meeting must be soon after admission in order for a comprehensive care plan to be established. Subsequent meetings review progress and update the team on any relevant issues. The patient and caregivers are periodically included in these meetings. Prior to discharge, members of the home care team are also included. The main responsibilities of each discipline are briefly presented below.

Physician

The physician provides medical leadership for the rest of the team, being responsible for the medical assessment and the medical management of the patient. The physician confirms the diagnosis and identifies the severity of the main symptoms. The physician enquires as to the impact of the condition on the overall lifestyle of the patient and the family. The physician is responsible for ensuring the prescription of the most appropriate treatment as well as supervising the delivery of this treatment. The prescription includes not only medical therapies and oxygen, but also selection of an appropriate ventilator system and settings.

Nurse

At the time of admission, in addition to the customary nursing assessment of the patient, the nurse explores the patient's impressions of the program and ensures that the patient has reasonable and achievable expectations. The nurse has very frequent contact with the patient and thus plays an important role in reinforcing the plan of care. At night, the nurse may be the only health professional whose constant presence reassures both those electively ventilated and those who have come from an intensive care environment. The nurse is responsible for coordinating the general education of the patient as well as developing routine care plans both in the hospital and during the transition to the home.

Physical Therapist

The physical therapist is responsible for the exercise aspects of the program. The initial assessment by the therapist includes the determination of baseline functional status, breathing pattern (accessory muscle use, pursed-lip breathing), and cough effectiveness. Functional exercise is measured using walking tests (6 min walk test or shuttle test) that include scales of dyspnea and leg effort. The exercise routine varies depending on patient mobility, ranging from simple bed exercises to a comprehensive interval training program.

Occupational Therapist

The occupational therapist is responsible for the assessment of activities of daily living and the provision of necessary assistive devices to improve functional independence at home. The occupational therapist assesses the home to ensure that it is appropriate for the installation and use of the required devices. The occupational therapist also addresses vocational and leisure activities, which for some patients will result in their return to the workforce.

Respiratory Therapist

The respiratory therapist has the knowledge and experience to assess the ventilatory needs of the patient. The respiratory therapist is responsible, in concert with physician orders, for establishing the most appropriate ventilatory support system and for ensuring that the interface is effective as well as comfortable for the patient. In addition, the respiratory therapist provides training of patients and caregivers in the management of oxygen, ventilatory equipment, and tracheostomy care.

Social Worker

The social worker assesses the family dynamics, cultural and religious influences, housing facilities, community support, financial situation, employment, and placement. The social worker participates with the patient and family in identifying ways that will enhance the social environment.

Psychologist

The psychologist is available to conduct a psychological assessment (perceptions and reactions of the patient and family) and provide psychological support if needed.

Home Care Coordinator

The home care coordinator coordinates any further support necessary for a successful transition to the community. This includes nonrespiratory equipment as well as attendant care.

C. Model Programs

Respiratory rehabilitation programs can be located in the hospital (inpatient or outpatient) or in the community (8). It should, however, be recognized that the intensive phase of rehabilitation represents only the initial part of what needs to become a lifestyle change. To be effective, rehabilitation must include issues specific to the respiratory system as well as general health care habits. Therefore, the majority of the rehabilitation (maintenance phase) should be thought of as occurring in the community setting. Accordingly, regular follow-up is an integral part of the program. More formal outcome measures may also be helpful in monitoring progress.

Most respiratory rehabilitation programs admit outpatients, whereas approximately one quarter also include an inpatient capability. In Canada, for example, most outpatient programs enroll patients for a duration of 8.3 (range 2 to 26) wk, and most inpatient programs enroll for 4.6 (range 1 to 8) wk (10). Hospital-based programs offer a more structured, intensive, and supervised program. For most of those who require ventilatory support, an inpatient program will be the modality of choice, at least in the initial stages, when the patient is being assessed and trained in the use of the ventilator. Once the patient's ventilatory support is well established, the other components of the program could be community based, or home based.

Hospital-based programs cost more than community-based programs (11). The latter also have the disadvantage of less direct supervision. This means that a higher level of patient motivation as well as more primary care physician (family doctor) involvement is necessary. For patients with COPD, inpatient, outpatient, and home-based programs have been shown to be effective (12,13). For those with neuromuscular conditions or thoracic restriction, there have been no prospective controlled randomized trials of comparable quality. However, a number of reports have detailed improvements in function that were sustained for many years (14–19).

IV. Rehabilitation in Ventilator-Assisted Individuals

There are important differences between general respiratory rehabilitation and rehabilitation for ventilator-assisted individuals (VAIs). Members of the respiratory rehabilitation team who wish to treat VAIs will require additional training to manage the combination of rehabilitation and ventilation. For example, the timing for the initiation of the various components of rehabilitation must be linked to the patient's respiratory status. Also, the educational needs of the patient and caregivers must include ventilator management and training in the use of all the necessary equipment. In addition, an individual discharged to the community with a life-support system has a particular set of psychosocial issues that must be addressed. In some cases, these issues will determine the success of the program.

A. Patient Selection

Patients are selected using both clinical and nonclinical criteria. The former includes the diagnosis, the presence of associated medical or psychosocial conditions, clinical stability, and the absence of smoking. In practice, it is often the non clinical components, such as reasonable comprehension, motivation, expectations and an appropriate home situation, including caregiver support and financial resources, that will determine the success of the rehabilitation program.

Ventilator-assisted individuals undergoing rehabilitation are not a homogeneous group. They include:

1. Patients referred for respiratory rehabilitation in whom optimization of treatment requires the elective implementation of ventilatory support as part of their rehabilitation.
2. Patients already on ventilator support who have the potential to benefit from rehabilitation. This group includes patients in whom the ventilator status might change as a result of weaning, decannulation, or changes in their ventilatory requirements (continuous vs. nocturnal ventilation).

These are discussed separately below.

Patients Referred for Rehabilitation in Whom Optimization of Treatment Includes the Elective Implementation of Ventilatory Support as Part of Their Rehabilitation

Patients with chronic hypercapnic respiratory failure are increasingly referred for respiratory rehabilitation. Most such individuals (with the exception of those with primary alveolar hypoventilation) have long-standing changes in ventilatory mechanics and coexisting alterations in central respiratory control often related to chronic hypoxia and hypercapnia. Many such individuals referred for respiratory rehabilitation have been noted during their initial assessment to exhibit signs of severe hypoventilation.

In healthy individuals, sleep is accompanied by changes in the pattern of breathing and respiratory drive. Responses to hypoxia and hypercapnia become blunted during sleep. It is therefore not surprising that, when changes in mechanics and control of breathing induced by sleep are superimposed on a ventilatory system that has underlying abnormalities of mechanics and control, such patients are especially vulnerable at night (20–24).

The presenting clinical history is frequently one of a prolonged period of stability punctuated by episodic hypercapnia in association with respiratory infections or ill-advised administration of a respiratory depressant drug. When chronic hypercapnia develops, the course is often one of cyclical emergency intubations followed by weaning and a successful return to the community. The background on which this cycle occurs is often one of deteriorating daytime arterial blood gases and increasing disability as cardiorespiratory function declines. These alterations in blood gases, pulmonary hypertension, and cor pulmonale are aggravated by exercise or by relatively minor respiratory infections (25,26).

Medical management that includes oxygen therapy will often aggravate the gas exchange abnormalities (27–29). Several reports have suggested that nightly ventilatory support, by protecting patients from the nocturnal alterations in arterial blood gases, can result in less frequent episodes of acute respiratory failure and can stabilize the disease process (14,17, 29–33). This clinical improvement is associated with an improvement in daytime arterial blood gases and a greatly enhanced level of functioning during the day. For such individuals, elective ventilatory support, initially only at night, will optimize their daytime clinical condition and allow them to participate in an exercise rehabilitation program. Rehabilitation will therefore include the initiation of elective ventilation.

Accordingly, our approach to the rehabilitation of patients in whom respiratory failure is present is to commence rehabilitation by stabilizing the disease process with elective nocturnal mechanical ventilation. The individuals can then participate in a supervised program of exercise training to further improve function.

Criteria for Elective Ventilation

It is desirable to establish clear criteria for initiation of elective ventilation as part of a respiratory rehabilitation program (14,33,34). However, there have been no prospective controlled trials that delineate the influence of elective ventilation on quality of life, morbidity, mortality, and resource requirements so firm, validated criteria have not been established. Criteria for elective ventilation might include a diagnosis of respiratory failure, a history of stability punctuated by episodic acute respiratory failure requiring emergency ventilatory support, or a history of progressive deterioration with symptoms consistent with sleep-related alterations in gas exchange. Although elective nocturnal ventilation has an important role in the management of such patients, it remains to be determined at what level of $Paco_2$ ventilation should be introduced and which measurements of pulmonary mechanics will assist the clinician in making this decision. Obviously one of the objectives of elective ventilation is to avoid emergency intubation and ventilation in the intensive care unit (ICU) (35,36). Elective ventilation in the nonacute situation has proved effective for those who have a nonobstructive ventilatory defect (14–19,30–34,37). Among such individuals, the improvement in nocturnal gas exchange, daytime function, and daytime arterial blood gases has been associated with a sustained improvement in symptoms, inspiratory muscle function, and functional exercise capacity (37). There is currently considerable interest in elective ventilation for those with COPD. However, clinical trials have so far yielded equivocal results (30–32,38,39).

Patients Already on Ventilatory Support Who Have the Potential to Benefit from Rehabilitation

Many such individuals are located in an intensive care unit, an inappropriate environment that emphasizes the intensive management of acutely ill or unstable patients and, by lacking any rehabilitative focus, actually fosters dependence (14).

A major goal for clinically stable VAIs is to achieve their maximum functional potential in preparation for the transition back to the community. Other goals include their being able to carry out or direct their daily care requirements and participate in social activities. Whereas many patients with neuromuscular conditions may not achieve self-care, they can still benefit from education and support that will increase their independence. Although rehabilitation will often include providing necessary assistive devices in the home, it is important not to create the equivalent of the intensive care unit at home.

VAIs are usually referred for rehabilitation in either of the following two circumstances.

1. Patients with chronic respiratory conditions (obstructive or nonobstructive), who require a period of protracted ventilation following an episode of acute respiratory failure. Such individuals are unable to be

weaned and usually have a tracheostomy. In many instances, following a "transitional" period of ventilation, they can be weaned totally, although medical or psychological issues often slow the process. For such individuals, rehabilitation includes a regular assessment of their ventilatory status with a view to a reduction in ventilatory support and decannulation. The ventilator may be withdrawn completely after a period of noninvasive ventilation or continued to provide ongoing support at night only. While these adjustments are being made, patients can participate fully in a comprehensive respiratory rehabilitation program.

2. Patients whose underlying diagnosis is usually a neuromuscular condition. For such individuals, rehabilitation involves an ongoing assessment of their ventilatory requirements, especially their need for a tracheostomy. As their condition progresses, their ventilatory requirements are likely to increase. Although their condition renders them almost totally dependent on caregivers, we attempt to maximize their functional independence. Whenever possible, we ventilate at night only, with periods of support during the day as required. Although we prefer noninvasive ventilation, removal of the tracheostomy tube may not always be possible. Decannulation can only be considered provided the airways can be adequately protected. It is more likely to be successful if the patient can manage to breathe without mechanical support for at least 6 hr. Standard criteria for decannulation are detailed in Table 1 (40).

B. General Approaches to Ventilation During the Rehabilitation Program

In general, the preferred mode for elective ventilation is noninvasive using a nasal mask or pillows, or an oronasal mask as an interface. Both intermittent

Table 1 Current Criteria for Removal of a Tracheostomy Tube

1. A mentally competent, cooperative patient
2. Minimal or no need for supplemental oxygen
3. Sa_{O_2} maintained >90% with aggressive airway secretion elimination
4. Adequate bulbar muscle function for swallowing
5. No history of substance abuse or uncontrollable seizures
6. Unassisted or manually assisted peak cough expiratory flows (PCEFs) that exceed at 3 l/sec
7. No conditions that interfere with the use of noninvasive ventilation interfaces (i.e., facial fractures or malformations)

Source: Ref. 40.

positive pressure volume ventilation and bilevel pressure ventilation have been reported as effective in the management of chronic respiratory failure in patients with either neuromuscular or thoracic restrictive disease (14–19,29). Good oxygen saturation can be achieved with overnight ventilation and patients will maintain better arterial blood gases during the day. For the majority of individuals positive pressure ventilation is more effective than negative pressure ventilation (plus it reduces the likelihood of upper airway obstruction), although for a few, negative pressure ventilation remains an option (41,42). For patients who have a tracheostomy, intermittent positive pressure ventilation (IPPV) with a portable ventilator might be an initial approach. Further management depends on the underlying reason for the tracheostomy. It might be related to the requirements for ventilation, to recurrent aspiration, or to the need for intensive bronchial hygiene. When a tracheostomy is unavoidable, the patients and the caregivers receive education and training in tracheostomy care to avoid the development of associated medical or psychosocial issues.

Our preference is to introduce noninvasive ventilation and then to decannulate whenever possible. For those in whom decannulation is not possible, the emphasis is on maintenance of communication and, therefore, we prefer an uncuffed tube to allow speech, accepting the leak and increasing the inspired tidal volume accordingly.

C. Patient Assessment

A comprehensive (medical and nonmedical) assessment of the patient is carried out by the rehabilitation team (8,9). As with any patient, the diagnosis is confirmed by history, physical examination, and a review of any relevant investigations. Disease severity and its impact on the patient and caregivers are further characterized by the use of general or specific health-related quality of life questionnaires. If necessary, cognitive function is also assessed. Particular attention is paid to the assessment of respiratory and peripheral muscle strength, swallowing, nutrition, and communication. Those who are ventilator dependent will only be able to undergo successful respiratory rehabilitation when their ventilatory support is effective and well established, as well as accepted by the patient, who must feel comfortable and have adequate relief of dyspnea. Daytime arterial blood gases are measured and their trends monitored noninvasively, both during unassisted ventilation and during mechanical support. Nighttime assessments vary from noninvasive screening with pulse oximetry and transcutaneous carbon dioxide monitoring to a full respiratory polysomnographic study. For ambulatory patients, an assessment of functional exercise capacity is useful.

The nonmedical assessment includes the patient's ability to carry out self-care and other activities of daily living or, if they are markedly impaired, their ability to direct their caregivers. Family dynamics, the home situation, community support, and any outstanding financial issues are also evaluated. Throughout the assessment the patient's motivation and level of knowledge are noted.

D. Program Components

The program usually includes education, breathing strategies, training in activities of daily living, exercise training, and psychosocial support. For those with severe neuromuscular conditions, the exercise training component may need to be modified or omitted entirely. The initial phase of the program is better suited to an inpatient facility, as during this phase, ventilatory support may require more frequent adjustments.

Education

A smooth transition from the hospital to the home is facilitated by the patient and the family or caregivers having a good understanding of the indications for ventilatory support. The nurse and respiratory therapist conduct group teaching sessions on a weekly basis, supplemented by individual sessions according to the special needs of the patient. Written and audiovisual materials are also used. Topics include general health, medications, nutritional habits, information related to specific conditions, and recognition of intercurrent medical conditions. All ventilator-dependent individuals and their caregivers receive training in the use of the equipment, airway hygiene, and emergency measures. Prior to their return to the community, the patients and caregivers must demonstrate competence in the use of the ventilator and its accessories. This is particularly important for those with a tracheostomy, especially if they are totally dependent on the ventilator for respiratory support. The knowledge and skills that patients and caregivers require prior to discharge are listed in Table 2.

The patients are considered to be the principal caregivers and are trained to perform or direct their own care. For patients who are totally dependent for all their needs, i.e., quadriplegics, several caregivers are trained to ensure appropriate care during the day and at night. Caregivers include family members, licensed health care professionals and non professional paid caregivers (43,44). Training proceeds at a pace comfortable enough to enable a full understanding of the information. In addition to issues of ventilation, training is broadened to include general care items, such as management of feeding tubes, safe transfers, etc.

Breathing Strategies and Chest Physiotherapy

Breathing strategies include pursed-lip and diaphragmatic breathing techniques aimed at decreasing the respiratory rate, the work of breathing, and the sensation of dyspnea (45). Such techniques may also help the patient by providing an approach to the sensation of panic (9,45).

Table 2 Knowledge and Skills That Ventilator-Dependent Patients and Caregivers Need to Know Prior to Discharge

Ventilator functioning and troubleshooting
Maintenance of ventilatory support by manual ventilation (bagging)
Maintenance and care of circuits and accessories (connections to avoid leaks and cleaning of equipment)
Airway maintenance (in tracheostomized patients), suctioning, cleaning, and changing the tracheostomy tube
Personal care (toileting, dressing, safe transfers, oral feeding or other routes)
Full range of motion to avoid contractures
Positional changes to avoid tissue trauma
Bladder and bowel routines
Management of medications
Management of the emergency situation (what to do, who to call)
Communication techniques (speech therapist may be especially helpful for speech and swallowing assessment and training among those with a tracheostomy)

Chest physical therapy is used to assist with secretion clearance (45) and has been shown to benefit those with bronchiectasis and cystic fibrosis during an exacerbation. In patients with neuromuscular conditions, expectoration is assisted with expiratory muscle aids, such as manually assisted coughing, in-exsufflation, or mechanical oscillation techniques (46).

A very useful breathing strategy, especially for those who are totally ventilator dependant, is glossopharyngeal breathing (GPB). This technique involves the use of tongue and pharyngeal muscles to aid inspiratory efforts by projecting (gulping) boluses of air past the glottis. The glottis closes with each "gulp." One breath usually consists of six to nine gulps of 60 to 100 mL each (46). This life-saving technique can provide complete ventilatory support for several hours. It also promotes self-confidence and independence. In addition, by inflating the thorax, GPB aids expectoration of secretions and reduces the need for suctioning.

Training in Activities of Daily Living

Energy conservation and work simplification assist activities of daily living (ADL) by reducing the limiting sensations of dyspnea and fatigue. In this way, activity tolerance may be increased. Advance planning, prioritization of activities, use of assistive devices, and dyspnea control are combined to maximize the available energy. In this way, activities may be increased.

The more ventilator-dependent patients are often those with the most limited mobility. Such individuals derive benefit from assistive technology that increases their independence. Those who require wheelchairs are trained in their safe operation. The chair is adapted to carry a ventilator. Devices that facilitate safe transfers are tried. Bathing, toileting, and dressing are practiced. Attention is paid to the best mattresses and the most convenient seating. For some patients, environmental and communication controls greatly increase their range of independent activities. These include keyboards as well as electro-ocular, voice-, or finger-activated controls that may be adapted for home use to activate electrical appliances. Leisure activities are included in the rehabilitation program as is computer training for personal, recreational, and educational tasks (47).

Exercise Training

Exercise training has been shown to be effective for those with COPD (12,13,48) and should be considered for all VAIs who have preserved mobility. Our approach, in agreement with others, is to alternate periods of physical activity with rest, avoiding any exhausting sets of exercise (49).

Specific ventilatory muscle training remains controversial (13,50,51) although some authors have suggested that those who are quadriplegic or have progressive neuromuscular conditions may benefit from it (51). The hope for ventilatory muscle training is that it would better equip the patient for independent breathing and improve the ability to respond to the increased ventilatory loads associated with infectious exacerbations.

Psychosocial Support

The psychosocial sequelae of chronic illness have a large impact on patients and their families (52,53) and must be addressed as part of a comprehensive rehabilitation program. A multidisciplinary approach facilitates the management of these issues. Encouraging the patient and family to participate in decision making, as well as providing relaxation exercises, panic control, and counselling as necessary, will increase the patient's sense of mastery with regard to their condition. Depression and anxiety may be helped by relaxation techniques and stress control. Group activities incorporate breathing control with good posture and positioning to minimize shortness of breath. Counseling (group or individual) and sexuality assessments are also important. Consultation with the psychologist and the occasional use of an antidepressant or anxiolytic is sometimes necessary.

The social needs and concerns regarding housing, funding, and role changes within the family are important influences on mood and emotional state, especially among individuals with neuromuscular conditions, with limited mobility, and pronounced dependence on mechanical aids. These issues should be acknowledged and addressed whenever possible in order to assist with a return to the community.

E. Program Organization

A written summary of the relevant issues should accompany the referral of subjects for rehabilitation. A customized referral form sent by the rehabilitation team to the referring physician or facility helps to ensure that key pieces of information are available. Depending on the underlying diagnosis, the complexity, and the stability of the patient, direct communication between members of the rehabilitation team and the referring facility may also be helpful. A direct assessment follows at the physician's office, the hospital ward, or the intensive care unit, including both the patient and the patient's family. The idea of rehabilitation is discussed during this initial assessment, as it is important for patients to understand the approach taken to improve their health-related quality of life. The patient also needs to acknowledge that ventilatory support might well be long term.

Those patients referred from the ICU need time to prepare themselves for a new environment. The ICU environment does not serve the medically stable individual well, especially if their only reason for remaining there is that they require ventilation. The reduction in nursing care that occurs with transfer may arouse patient feelings of insecurity. We therefore begin the rehabilitative process gradually in collaboration with the ICU team prior to transfer to a rehabilitation facility. The process includes the following:

- The ventilator system needs to be changed from a typical ICU model to one that is portable, simple to manage, and more "home user friendly."
- The tracheostomy tube should be changed to one that will allow the patient to speak.
- Routine care, such as suctioning and manual ventilation, can begin to include the patient and family. Once this has been achieved, the patient and the family should be encouraged to leave the ICU for outings around the grounds of the hospital.
- Mobilization should be encouraged as soon as rehabilitation is being considered.
- Nutritional status should be maximized. If the patient has an insufficient oral intake, a percutaneous and enteral tube should be used rather than a nasogastric tube.
- The home situation can be explored in preparation for any required modifications and renovations. These are often time consuming and should not delay the patient's eventual discharge from the rehabilitation unit.

Home ventilation training is nearly always initiated during the inpatient phase in the rehabilitation unit. In this phase, there is an ongoing assessment of the ventilatory needs (time spent on the ventilator, the ventilator settings, the potential for decannulation), as these requirements might change during the rehabilitation program. The goal is to achieve the most effective and comfortable mode of ventilation. Although the rehabilitation program is usually initiated in the hospital, in many cases, the patient can return home to complete the program on an outpatient basis. For a smooth transition between the hospital and the home, a progressive discharge schedule should be implemented early in the management of the patient with short trial periods at home prior to the final discharge (14,54,55). (For a more detailed discussion, see Chapter 14.)

After leaving the rehabilitation unit, the adequacy of ventilatory support and the overall functioning of the patient and the family require ongoing follow up. We often readmit the patient regularly, during which physiologic measures (arterial blood gases, pulmonary function tests) as well as functional exercise capacity and health-related quality of life are assessed. Nighttime ventilation is also evaluated. The first such admission is usually 2 to 3 mo after discharge, with subsequent admissions at 6- to 12-mo intervals depending on the level of stability and the degree of independence. We also follow subjects with regularly scheduled telephone calls that link the patient with the rehabilitation/home ventilation team. Such ongoing contacts, in addition to identifying problems, also enhance compliance with the principles of rehabilitation and self-care.

F. Outcome Measures and Benefits of Rehabilitation

As a discipline, respiratory rehabilitation has made considerable progress in the evaluation of outcomes both of the program as a whole and of specific components within the program. The introduction of valid, relevant, and interpretable outcomes has added scientific evidence to clinical impressions (1,56–59). Patients with COPD (nonventilated), who comprise the majority of those referred for rehabilitation, experience a decrease in dyspnea and an improvement in mastery as well as in their functional exercise capacity (12,13). Similar outcomes have been reported for those whose programs are inpatient, outpatient, or home based.

For patients who require ongoing ventilatory support (invasive or noninvasive), important improvements in daytime and nighttime arterial blood gases, respiratory muscle function, and functional exercise capacity have been demonstrated (15–19,30–32,37,60–62). Such changes have been associated with an improved sense of well-being and, in many instances, a return to meaningful activities at home or in the workforce. Many such individuals express positive life satisfaction, although dissatisfaction with their general health and sex life remain ongoing issues (63). A number of uncontrolled trials have suggested that long-term ventilatory support improves survival, especially among those with neuromuscular conditions (17,19,60–62).

To establish the user's perceptions of the impact of ventilation on their lives (64) we administered an open-ended questionnaire to 98 (48 male, 50 female) VAIs ages (mean ± SD) 47.4 ± 19.5 with chronic obstructive pulmonary disease (9%), thoracic restrictive disease (43%), and neuromuscular disease (48%) who had received home mechanical ventilation for 59.5 ± 58.3 mo. Of those surveyed, 53% were ventilated electively. Ventilator use was continuous (18%), at night only (37%), or at night with occasional daytime use (45%). Some (28%) were totally independent, and others (33%) partially dependent on caregiver assistance for daily activities. The impact of home mechanical ventilation was overwhelmingly positive (87%), although patients with a tracheostomy volunteered fewer positive statements than those ventilated noninvasively ($p < 0.05$). Just over half (53%) of the ventilator users indicated that they had experienced initial difficulties in coping with the ventilator, but only 11% identified this as an issue at the time of the survey (Table 3). Some were employed full- or part-time (19%) and some (12%) were students or homemakers (10%). Only 16% were retired due to age. Those actively looking for work constituted 22%, whereas 19% were retired due to their disability (2% unclassified). Over one-quarter of ventilator users age 19 or older believed that their health status had been a barrier to obtaining employment.

More formal assessments of participation (independence, employment, and leisure activities) together with physiologic measures of impairment and disability will help those involved in rehabilitation to set realistic achievable goals be-

Table 3 Number of Patients Volunteering Positive and Negative Statements

	Positive statements		
	Life-sustaining treatment	Mobility and freedom	Improved symptoms
COPD	1 (11%)	4 (44%)	7 (78%)
TRD[a]	10 (24%)	19 (45%)	36 (86%)
NMD[b]	15 (32%)	23 (49%)	26 (55%)
Total	26	46	69
	Negative statements		
	Limits mobility and freedom	Equipment concerns	Social implications
COPD	6 (67%)	0	0
TRD[a]	21 (50%)	11 (26%)	3 (7%)
NMD[b]	22 (47%)	10 (21%)	18 (38%)
Total	49	21	21

[a] TRD, Thoracic restrictive disease.
[b] NMD, Neuromuscular disease.
Source: Ref. 64.

yond just returning to the community. Such outcomes will also be valuable in establishing more precise evidence of the effectiveness of respiratory rehabilitation for the ventilator user.

V. Summary

The rehabilitation of VAIs has four main goals: restoring function, facilitating independence, returning people to the community, and optimizing the allocation of health care resources. Whereas some VAIs are referred for rehabilitation after initiation of ventilation, others who have ventilatory failure require initiation of elective ventilation as part of their rehabilitation program. In both cases, the attending team requires skills that include ventilator management and respiratory rehabilitation. Although respiratory rehabilitation has been shown to be effective, there have been no prospective randomized controlled trials of rehabilitation specifically for the VAI. Notwithstanding this, it is recognized that ventilation will stabilize nighttime and daytime blood gases as well as improve functional exercise. It seems likely that further benefits will accrue from adding rehabilitation. In addition, surveys that evaluate the patient's perception of ventilator assistance may be useful for establishing specific goals and directions for the rehabilitation program.

References

1. Lacasse Y, Wrong E, Guyatt GH, Goldstein RS. Health status measurement instruments in chronic obstructive pulmonary disease. Can Respir J 1997; 4(3):152–1664.
2. Pulmonary Rehabilitation Research—NIH Workshop Summary. Am J Crit Care Med 1994; 149:825–833.
3. Bach JR. Neuromuscular and skeletal disorders leading to global alveolar hypoventilation. In: Bach JR. Pulmonary rehabilitation. The Obstructive and Paralytic Conditions. Philadelphia, PA: Hanley and Belfus, 1996; 257–273.
4. World Health Organization. International Classification of Impairments, Disabilities, and Handicaps. Geneva, Switzerland: World Health Organization, 1980.
5. Ries AL. Position paper of American Association of Cardiovascular and Pulmonary Rehabilitation: Scientific basis of pulmonary rehabilitation. J Cardiopulm Rehabil 1990; 10:418–441.
6. Tiep BL. Pulmonary rehabilitation program organization. In: Casaburi R, Petty Th. Principles and Practice of Pulmonary Rehabilitation. Philadelphia, PA: Saunders, 1993; 302–316.
7. Hodgkin JE, Connors GL, Bell CW. Pulmonary Rehabilitation: Guidelines to Success. Philadelphia, PA: Lippincott, 1993.
8. Goldstein RS, Avendano MA. Model program development and outcomes in chronic obstructive pulmonary disease. In: Bach JR, Haas F. Pulmonary Rehabilitation.

Physical Medicine and Rehabilitation Clinics of North America. Philadelphia, PA: Saunders, 1996; 353–366.
9. Lareau SC, ZuWallack R, Carlin B, et al. Pulmonary rehabilitation—1999. Chest 1999; 159:1666–1682.
10. Brooks D, Lacasse Y, Goldstein RS. Pulmonary rehabilitation programs in Canada: National survey. Can Respir J 1999; 6(1):55–63.
11. Goldstein RS, Gort EH, Guyatt GH, Feeny D. Economic analysis of respiratory rehabilitation. Chest 1997; 112:370–379.
12. Lacasse Y, Wrong E, Guyatt GH, King D, Cook D, Goldstein RS. Meta-analysis of respiratory rehabilitation in chronic obstructive pulmonary disease. Lancet 1996; 348:1115–1119.
13. ACCP/AACVPR Pulmonary Rehabilitation Guidelines Panel. Pulmonary rehabilitation: Joint ACCP/AACVPR evidence-based guidelines. Chest 1997; 112:1363–1396.
14. Make BJ, et al. Report of a consensus conference of the American College of Chest Physicians: Mechanical ventilation beyond the intensive care unit. Chest 1998; 113(5):289S–344S.
15. Ellis ER, Bye PTP, Bruderer JW, Sullivan CE. Treatment of respiratory failure during sleep in patients with neuromuscular disease. Am Rev Resp Dis 1987; 135:148–152.
16. Segall D. Non-invasive nasal mask assisted ventilation in respiratory failure of Duchenne muscular dystrophy. Chest 1988; 93:1298–3000.
17. Leger P, Jennequin J, Gerard M, et al. Home positive pressure ventilation via nasal mask for patients with neuromuscular weakness or restrictive lung or chest-wall disease. Respir Care 1989; 34:73–77.
18. Bach JR, Alba AS. Management of chronic alveolar hypoventilation by nasal ventilation. Chest 1990; 97:52–57.
19. Simonds AK, Muntoni F, Heather S, Fielding S. Impact of nasal ventilation on survival in hypercapnic Duchenne muscular dystrophy. Thorax 1998; 53:949–952.
20. Phillipson EA. Control of breathing during sleep. Am Rev Resp Dis 1978; 118:909–939.
21. Ballard R, Clover CW, Suh BY. Influence of sleep on respiratory function in emphysema. Am J Respir Crit Care Med 1995; 151:945–951.
22. Hejdra YF, Dekjuijzen PNR, van Herwaarden CLA, Folgering H Th M. Nocturnal saturation and respiratory muscle function in patients with chronic obstructive pulmonary disease. Thorax 1995; 50:610–612.
23. McNicholas WT. Impact of sleep in respiratory failure. Eur Respir J 1997; 10:920–933.
24. Becker HF, Piper AJ, Flynn WE, McNamara SG, Grunstein RR, Peter JH, Sullivan CE. Breathing during sleep in patients with nocturnal desaturation. Am J Respir Crit Care Med 1999; 159:112–118.
25. Weitzemblum E, Vandevenne A, Hirth C, Parini JP, Roeslin N, Oudet P. L'hemodynamique pulmonaire au cours de l'exercice musculaire chez les bronchiteaux chroniques. Effets de l'oxygenation et de la repetition de l'exercice. Respiration 1973; 30:64–88.
26. Kessler R, Faller M, Fourgaut G, Mennecier B, Weitzemblum E. Predictive factors

of hospitalization for acute exacerbation in a series of 64 patients with chronic obstructive pulmonary disease. Am J Respir Care Med 1999; 159:158–164.
27. Sassoon C, Hassell K, Mahutte C. Hyperoxic-induced hypercapnia in stable chronic obstructive pulmonary disease. Am Rev Respir Dis 1987; 135:907–911.
28. Dunn WF, Nelson SB, Hubmayr RD. Oxygen-induced hypercapnia in COPD. Am Rev Respir Dis 1991; 144:526–530.
29. Masa JF, Celli B, Riesco JA, Sanchez de Cos J, Disdier C, Sojo A. Noninvasive positive pressure ventilation and not oxygen may prevent overt ventilatory failure in patients with chest wall diseases. Chest 1997; 112:207–213.
30. Strumpf DA, Millman RP, Carlisle CC, et al. Nocturnal positive pressure ventilation via nasal mask in patients with severe chronic obstructive pulmonary disease. Am Rev Respir Dis 1991; 144:1234–1239.
31. Elliot MW, Simonds AK, Carroll MP, Wedzicha JA, Branthwaite MA. Domiciliary nocturnal nasal intermittent positive pressure ventilation in hypercapnic respiratory failure due to chronic obstructive lung disease: Effects on sleep and quality of life. Thorax 1992; 47(5):342–348.
32. Meechan Jones JD, Paul EA, Jones PW, Wedzicha JA. Nasal pressure support ventilation plus oxygen compared with oxygen therapy alone in hypercapnic COPD. Am J Respir Crit Care Med 1995; 152:538–544.
33. Consensus Conference IV: Noninvasive positive pressure ventilation. Respir Care 1997; 42(4):364–369.
34. Robert D, Willig TN, Paulus J. Long-term nasal ventilation in neuromuscular disorders: Report of a consensus conference. Eur Respir J 1993; 6:599–606.
35. Brochard L, Mancebo J, Wysocky M, et al. Noninvasive ventilation for acute exacerbatiions of chronic obstructive pulmonary disease. N Engl J Med 1995; 333: 817–822.
36. Meduri GU, Turner E, Abou-Shala N, et al. Non-invasive positive pressure ventilation via face mask. First-line intervention in patients with acute hypercapnic and hypoxemic respiratory failure. Chest 1996; 109:179–193.
37. Goldstein RS, De Rosie JA, Avendano MA, Dolmage TE. Influence of non-invasive positive pressure ventilation on inspiratory muscles. Chest 1991; 99:408–415.
38. Restrick LJ, Fox NC, Braid G, Ward EM, Paul EA, Wedzicha JA. Comparison of nasal pressure support ventilation with nasal intermittent positive pressure ventilation in patients with nocturnal hypoventilation. Eur Respir J 1993; 6:364–370.
39. Hill NS. Non-invasive ventilation. Does it work, for whom, and how? Am Rev Respir Dis 1993; 147:1050–1055.
40. Bach JR, Saporito LR. Indications and criteria for decannulation and transition from invasive to noninvasive long-term ventilatory support. Respir Care 1994; 39(5):515–531.
41. Hill NS. Clinical applications of body ventilators. Chest 1986; 90:897–905.
42. Shneerson JM. Non-invasive and domiciliary ventilation: Negative pressure techniques. Thorax 1991; 46:131–135.
43. Goldberg AI, Alba AA, Oppenheimer EA, et al. Caring for mechanically ventilated patients at home. Chest 1990; 98:1543.
44. Bach JR, Intintola P, Alba AS, et al. The ventilator-assisted individual: Cost analysis

of institutionalization vs. rehabilitation and in-home management. Chest 1992; 101: 26–30.
45. Faling LJ. Controlled breathing techniques and chest physical therapy in chronic obstructive pulmonary disease and allied conditions. In: Casaburi R, Petty Th. Principles and Practice of Pulmonary Rehabilitation. Philadelphia, PA: Saunders, 1993; 167–182.
46. Bach JR. Prevention of morbidity and mortality with the use of physical medicine aids. In: Bach JR. Pulmonary Rehabilitation. Philadelphia, PA: Hanley and Belfus, 1996; 303–329.
47. Valenza JP, Guzzaardo SL, Bach JR. Functional interventions for persons with neuromuscular disease. In: Bach JR. Pulmonary Rehabilitation. Philadelphia, PA: Hanley and Belfus, 1996; 371–394.
48. Lacasse Y, Guyatt GH, Goldstein RS. The components of a respiratory rehabilitation program: A systematic overview. Chest 1997; 111:1077–1088.
49. Kilmer DD. The role of exercise in neuromuscular disease. In: Kraft GH. Rehabilitation of Neuromuscular Disease. Physical Medicine and Rehabilitation Clinics of North America. Philadelphia, PA: Saunders, 1998; 115–125.
50. Smith K, Cook D, Gordon H. Respiratory muscle training in chronic airflow limitation: A meta-anylisis. Am Rev Respir Dis 1992; 145:533–539.
51. Gross D. The role of ventilatory muscle training in persons with neuromuscular disease. In: Bach JR. Pulmonary Rehabilitation. Philadelphia, PA: Hanley and Belfus, 1996; 347–351.
52. McSweeny AJ, Grant I, Heaton RK, Adams KM, Timms RM. Life quality of patients with chronic obstructive pulmonary disease. Arch Intern Med 1982; 142:473–478.
53. Kaplan RM, Eakin EG, Ries A. Psychosocial issues in the rehabilitation of patients with chronic obstructive pulmonary disease. In: Casaburi R, Petty Th. Principles and Practice of Pulmonary Rehabilitation. Philadelphia, PA: Saunders, 1993; 351–365.
54. O'Donohue WJ, Giovannoni RM, Goldberg AI, Keens TG, Make BM, Plummer AL, Prentice, WS. Long-term mechanical ventilation: Guidelines for management in the home and at alternate community sites. Chest 1986; suppl 90(1):1S–37S.
55. Smith CE, Mayer LS, Parkhurst C, Perkins SB, Pingleton SK. Adaptation in families with a member requiring mechanical ventilation at home. Heart Lung 1991; 20:349–356.
56. Mahler DA, Guyatt GH, Jones PW. Clinical measurement of dyspnea. In: Mahler DA, ed. Dyspnea. New York: Marcel Dekker, 1997; 149–198.
57. Buthland RJA, Pang J, Gross ER, Woodcock AA, Geddes DM. Two-, six- and 12-minute walking tests in respiratory disease. Br Med J 1982; 284:1607–1608.
58. Singh SS, Morgan MDL, Scott S, et al. Development of a shuttle walking test of disability in patients with chronic airways obstruction. Thorax 1992; 47:1019–1024.
59. Jones NL. Clinical exercise testing. 4th ed. Philadelphia, PA: Saunders, 1997.
60. Make B, Gilmartin M, Brody JS, Snider GL. Rehabilitation of ventilator-dependent subjects with lung diseases: The concept and initial experience. Chest 1984; 86(3): 358–365.
61. Hill NS, Eveloff SE, Carlisle CC, Goff SG. Efficacy of nocturnal nasal ventilation in patients with restrictive thoracic disease. Am Rev Respir Dis 1992; 145:365–371.

62. Leger P, Bedicam JM, Cornette A, Reybet-Degat O, Langevin B, Polu JM, Jeannin L, Robert D. Nasal intermittent positive pressure ventilation: Long-term follow-up in patients with severe chronic respiratory insufficiency. Chest 1994; 105:100–105.
63. Bach JR, Campagnolo DI, Hoeman S. Life satisfaction of individuals with Duchenne muscular dystrophy with long-term mechanical ventilatory support. Am J Phys Med Rehabil 1991; 70:129–135.
64. Goldstein RS, Psek JA, Gort EH. Home mechanical ventilation. Demographics and user perspectives. Chest 1995; 108:1581–1586.

18

Outcomes of Long-Term Mechanical Ventilation

ANITA K. SIMONDS

Royal Brompton and Harefield National Health Service Trust
London, England

I. Introduction

The outcome of long-term mechanical ventilation (LTMV) can be evaluated most constructively by examining its effects on survival, the natural history of the underlying disease, respiratory and cardiac function, morbidity, and the health status and quality of life of the recipient. The socioeconomic consequences of LTMV for the family or caregivers and the community as a whole should also be considered as part of the wider impact of this technological growth area.

The results of LTMV need to be set against a background of evolving ventilatory techniques, a gradual change in patient selection and indications over the last few decades, and growing public debate on the ethics of life-saving therapies. In this chapter, the outcome of different modes of LTMV in COPD, stable neuromusculoskeletal disorders, progressive neuromuscular disease, and diffuse parenchymal lung disease in adults and children is compared. As the impact of any intervention cannot be understood without an understanding of the natural history of the underlying disease; the clinical course of obstructive and restrictive disorders in the *absence* of ventilatory assistance is considered alongside the results of LTMV using both invasive and noninvasive ventilatory modes.

II. Aims of Long-Term Mechanical Ventilation

The goals of LTMV include 1) extending life, 2) improving physical and physiologic function, 3) reducing morbidity, 4) delivering LTMV in an environment that enhances an individual's potential, and 5) providing cost-effective care (1). Any analysis of outcome should assess how effectively these objectives are met. While all goals may be straightforward to achieve in conditions such as stable chest wall disease, the emphasis shifts to extending good quality of life, rather than protracting the terminal phase of a disease, in progressive disorders such as amyotrophic lateral sclerosis (ALS).

III. Outcome Measures

A. Survival

One of the problems in assessing the survival of recipients of LTMV is that there is no consensus on the period of ventilation that constitutes long-term support. Using a definition of ventilatory assistance for more than 2 days, mortality rates of 36 to 59% are usually found. In these studies, a crucial determinant of survival is the severity of the illness—patients with an Apache II score of 21 to 25 have significantly worse mortality compared with those who scored 11 to 15 (77 vs. 10%) (2). The nature of the index disease is also important, with both COPD and malignancy acting as poor prognostic factors. Indeed, patients with malignant disease who develop respiratory failure have a 90 to 100% death rate.

However, intensive care unit (ICU) patients are clearly not in a steady-state situation for various acute medical reasons that affect the outcome to a far greater extent than the level of ventilatory support provided. For the purposes of this discussion, LTMV will be taken as ventilatory support for more than 30 days (3). In this group, a relatively good outcome can be achieved in selected patients. For example, Criner et al. (4) showed that in 77 patients of average age 61 ventilated for a mean of 68 days, 93% were discharged and 61% were alive at 1 yr. Twenty percent required continued ventilatory support.

Natural History of Untreated Disorders

Chronic Obstructive Pulmonary Disease

It is well established that life expectancy in chronic obstructive pulmonary disease (COPD) is strongly correlated with the extent of airflow obstruction. In patients who do not receive oxygen therapy there is an association between survival and the degree of polycythemia, hypercapnia, and pulmonary hypertension (5). For patients receiving long-term oxygen therapy (LTOT) in the Medical Research Council (MRC) trial (5) and Nocturnal Oxygen Therapy Trial (NOTT)

(6), the most important determinants of survival were forced expiratory volume in 1 sec (FEV_1), transfer coefficient for carbon monoxide, and the rise in Pa_{O_2} in response to oxygen therapy. Overall, 1-, 3-, and 5-yr survival rates in LTOT recipients are approximately 88, 52, and 44%, respectively. Cor pulmonale is a very poor prognostic sign, as following the development of peripheral edema two-thirds of COPD patients will be dead within 5 yr.

The situation regarding Pa_{CO_2} as a predictor of survival is complex. This is of particular relevance if the mechanism by which LTMV operates is via correction of nocturnal and diurnal hypercapnia. While the MRC trial (5) showed poorer survival in hypercapnic COPD patients, recent work has shown that a raised Pa_{CO_2} may not necessarily have an adverse effect. Aida et al. (7), in a large study of patients with COPD and pulmonary tuberculosis (TB) sequelae, found that those with a $Pa_{CO_2} > 45$ mm Hg had a better life expectancy than their normocapnic counterparts, and that in the COPD group, the presence of normocapnia did not worsen survival. A Belgian study (8) has shown that COPD survivors tend to have a bronchitic rather than emphysematous profile. These workers advocate that hypercapnic patients should be divided into two categories—those with ventilatory pump failure and those in whom hypercapnia is a terminal phase due to parenchymal lung failure. In confirmation of this notion, Aida et al. (7) showed significantly higher mortality in patients in whom Pa_{CO_2} increased by more than 5 mm Hg in the 12-month study period suggesting that they belonged to the terminal lung failure group. Cooper et al. (9) also found that P_{CO_2} rise accelerates in many cases in the 3 years before death. In addition to a chronic decline, a proportion of COPD patients will die during acute exacerbations and any intervention that alters the frequency or outcome of these events will affect overall survival.

Restrictive Chest Wall Disease

Right ventricular failure was the cause of death in over 100 patients with untreated idiopathic thoracic scoliosis followed over 50 years (10), with death occurring at a mean age of 46. Age of onset of the spinal deformity is also important. In a longitudinal study (11) of scoliotics who developed their curve before the age of 5, 10 of 15 progressed to chronic ventilatory failure in middle age. Ventilatory decompensation was much less common when the scoliosis arose in later childhood, and extremely rare in adolescent onset scoliosis (unless other cardiorespiratory conditions were also present). Nachemson (12) has shown that unfused congenital, thoracogenic and neurogenic curves have a poor prognosis.

Survival in thoracoplasty patients is likely to depend on the extent of the chest wall resection. Factors influencing mortality adversely in patients with severe thoracic deformity on the Swedish Oxygen register were age >65 and additional pulmonary pathology such as COPD (13). Although patients with uncomplicated chest wall deformity receiving LTOT survived longer than obstructive lung disease patients, an increasing number required assisted ventilation with time.

Neuromuscular Disease

For patients with neurologic or neuromuscular disorders, mortality from ventilatory decompensation will depend on the degree of respiratory and bulbar muscle involvement and the rate of progression of the condition. In some diseases, respiratory muscle involvement is inevitable (e.g., Duchenne muscular dystrophy [DMD]) and in others highly variable (e.g., limb girdle muscular dystrophy). A cardiomyopathy may complicate the picture in Duchenne muscular dystrophy, glycogen storage disorders such as Pompe's disease, or dystrophia myotonica. In patients with previous poliomyelitis, a history of requiring ventilatory support at the time of the acute illness may predict ventilatory decompensation in later life. Most DMD patients die of respiratory complications, with around 10% succumbing to a cardiomyopathy. Once daytime hypercapnia develops, average survival is around 9 to 10 months without ventilatory support (14).

Impact of Tracheostomy Intermittent Positive Pressure Ventilation on Survival

Selection criteria for long-term tracheostomy intermittent positive pressure ventilation (T-IPPV) have changed significantly over the last few decades. In the 1960s and 1970s T-IPPV was the main long term ventilatory approach, as negative pressure ventilation was rarely employed in COPD, and nasal intermittent positive pressure ventilation (NPPV) only became available in the 1980s. Consequently, T-IPPV was originally applied in a heterogeneous population of patients with COPD and neuromusculoskeletal disorders. Following the introduction of nasal intermittent positive pressure ventilation, T-IPPV is now reserved for patients with bulbar weakness, extreme ventilator dependency, or excessive secretions. Clearly, this newer clientele will have a quite different outcome compared with those with stable restrictive disorders using noninvasive ventilation, making historical comparisons of T-IPPV vs. noninvasive techniques inappropriate. Currently, T-IPPV is the most common mode of ventilation for children and adults with high spinal cord injury and progressive neurologic disease (e.g., amyotrophic lateral sclerosis/motor neuron disease [ALS/MND]) complicated by bulbar dysfunction. It is usually required in subjects undergoing diaphragm pacing. Survival in all these circumstances is largely dependent on the natural history of the underlying disease. However, complications of T-IPPV, such as accidental disconnection, hemorrhage, and acute airway obstruction, may add to mortality and morbidity in hospital, and at home.

Obstructive and Restrictive Ventilatory Disorders

Robert et al. (15) showed 3- and 5-yr survival rates of 55 and 34% in COPD patients receiving T-IPPV, which contrasts with 5-yr survival rates of 95% in postpolio patients and 70% in those with TB sequelae. Only 15% of COPD T-IPPV patients were alive at 7 years and there were no survivors after 5 years in bronchiectasis patients. Other French groups have reported similar results (16,17).

As an update to Robert et al.'s study (15), Muir (18) has retrospectively analyzed the ANTADIR French central database of T-IPPV users with COPD. Seventy percent of patients were alive at 2 years, 44% at 5 years, and 20% at 10 years. Favorable prognostic factors were age less than 65, use of an uncuffed tracheostomy tube, and a PaO_2 value of more than 55 mm Hg measured 3 mo after starting T-IPPV.

Neurologic and Neuromuscular Disease

Spinal Cord Injury. Overall survival in patients with high spinal cord injury (SCI) has improved in the last 20 years for several key reasons, most of which are unrelated to the ventilatory support provided. During the initial hospital admission, mortality is dependent on the age of the patient, the level of spinal cord lesion and extent of associated injuries. Improvements in acute care that may reduce the incidence of complete cord transection combined with comprehensive specialized rehabilitation programs provided by spinal injury units have had a major impact. A survey (19) of over 2000 SCI patients from 1955 to 1965 showed a 1-year mortality of 17 to 19% in young tetraplegics, but a 50% mortality in patients ages 35 to 44. For C1 to C4 tetraplegics, 1-year mortality was 60%, but in C5 to C7 tetraplegics, this is only 30%. An analysis of T-IPPV–dependent quadripelgic patients in 1986 (20) showed a 1-year survival of 90%, however, by 5 year, survival had fallen to 33%. More recently, Viroslav et al. (21) has found a 1-year survival of 90% in SCI T-IPPV–dependent patients compared with 100% in those who were not ventilator-dependent. Survival rates for ventilator users vs. nonusers at 3 and 5 years were 57 vs. 90% and 33 vs. 85%, respectively.

Splaingard et al. (22) have examined a 20-year experience of T-IPPV in the home from 1962 to 1983. Among over 40 adults and children in their series; the majority had spinal cord injury (SCI), DMD, spinal muscular atrophy (SMA), or central hypoventilation syndrome; none had COPD. Three-year survival was 63% for SCI patients and 74% for the other diagnoses combined. Nine patients were ultimately weaned from ventilatory support and two died following accidental disconnection from the ventilator. There was no survival difference between patients cared for by their families and those with qualified nurse attendants.

Duchenne Muscular Dystrophy. The effect of T-IPPV on survival is difficult to assess because many centers (particularly in France), use a progressive respiratory support plan starting with noninvasive techniques and then transferring to T-IPPV when vital capacity (VC) falls below 15% predicted or when bulbar problems supervene, whereas other units prefer T-IPPV from the outset. Several studies (23,24) have employed sequential noninvasive positive pressure, switching to T-IPPV in cases of NIPPV failure or if VC falls below 300 mL.

Average survival in these cases was 4 to 10 years from initiation of ventilatory support. Contrary to popular belief, bulbar involvement is usually a late feature in DMD compared with other progressive conditions such as ALS/MND.

Soudon (25) has reported results on the use of T-IPPV in a variety of congenital neuromuscular diseases, although the majority of patients had DMD (19 of 31). Mean age at introduction of T-IPPV in the DMD group was 18.5, with a VC of approximately 570 mL and $Paco_2$ > 7.3 kPa in all. Mean length of time receiving T-IPPV at the time of reporting was 3.6 years. It is notable that 10 of 19 patients remained in hospital receiving T-IPPV, and 5- were 24-hr ventilator-dependent. Volume preset ventilators were used in all patients via an uncuffed tracheostomy tube.

Amyotrophic Lateral Sclerosis/Motor Neuron Disease. Data from the Kaiser Permanente series (26) (n = 101) in California from 1985 to 1992 show a 1-year survival of 87%, 3-year survival 58%, and 5-year survival of 33% in ALS patients using T-IPPV exclusively. Most of these patients remained in hospital or subacute facilities.

Pediatric T-IPPV

The most common pediatric indications for LTMV are congenital neuromuscular disease (particularly spinal muscular atrophy, myopathies, and muscular dystrophies), central hypoventilation syndromes, spinal cord injury, and bronchopulmonary dysplasia.

Spinal Muscular Atrophy. Children with type I SMA usually present at birth or shortly after with gross muscle weakness and respiratory difficulties. Pulmonary atresia, swallowing problems, and aberrant vasomotor control can complicate the picture. If resuscitation is carried out, these individuals are likely to receive T-IPPV. Ventilatory support in severe SMA remains a controversial area, but reasonable survival results have been achieved by Barois and Estournet-Mathiaud (27) in a series of children with type I, intermediate, and type II SMA, although the majority of younger children appear to have intermediate SMA. Type III SMA patients usually present with ventilatory problems in adulthood. In the Belgian series of T-IPPV (25), six SMA II patients ages 7 to 20 and average VC 630 ml had a mean survival of 2.6 years at the time of reporting.

Others have recorded prolonged survival in six SMA patients with T-IPPV (28), although numbers are small. Three individuals had SMA I, two SMA II, and one SMA III. Survival was 4 to 8 years in SMA I patients and 4 to 27 years in types II and III. However, it should be noted that five of six of the patients remained hospitalized long term.

In a University of Michigan series (29), of 89 children treated with home ventilation, 71% received T-IPPV using synchronized intermittent positive pressure ventilation mode (SIMV) and 11% used bilevel pressure support ventilation via tracheostomy. A small number received mask ventilation. Thirty of the children had SCI, and 19 had myopathy. Overall mortality for the period 1978 to 1993 was 13%.

Congenital Central Hypoventilation Syndrome. The long-term outcome in children with congenital central hypoventilation syndrome (CCHS) has been reviewed recently (30,31). Children with CCHS have a negligible ventilatory response to hypercapnia and variable responses to hypoxia during wakefulness and sleep. As a result, they invariably require ventilatory support. In the Chicago series (30), 32 children were treated with a combination of T-IPPV and diaphragm pacing, 12 requiring 24-h ventilatory support and 10 requiring support during sleep. Twenty-two survived at the time of the report and 10 had died (five in the early years of the program). Most died of cor pulmonale, pneumonia, or aspiration, although there was one death due to technical ventilator-related problems. Median age of the surviving patients was 7 (0.5 to 14.8) after nearly 6 years of follow-up. A tracheostomy is usually required in patients receiving diaphragm pacing to obviate upper airway obstruction caused by desynchrony of upper airway and diaphragm activation. For the same reason, negative pressure ventilation should be less efficient than positive pressure methods, although there are anecdotal reports of successful use in CCHS (32,33).

Impact of Nasal Intermittent Positive Pressure Ventilation on Survival

COPD

So far there have been no long-term randomized studies of LTOT vs. nasal intermittent positive pressure ventilation (NPPV) plus LTOT in COPD patients with survival as the main end point, although several such trials are in progress. Some guidance can be gained, however, from a number of large uncontrolled series.

In a French cohort of NPPV users, Leger et al. (24) reported on 50 COPD patients treated with home LTMV. Twenty-six of these received NPPV because of chronic ventilatory failure and 24 following acute on chronic exacerbations. Mean age at initiation of ventilatory support was 63, with an FEV_1 of 39% predicted. It should be noted that 88% received LTOT in addition to NPPV. A relatively high proportion (44%) of patients discontinued NPPV, and 16% died. Overall the probability of continuing NPPV at 3 years was 53%. The authors suggest that an improvement in this result might have been achieved had NPPV been introduced earlier in the natural history of the disease.

A United Kingdom (U.K.) single center series (34) has reported closely comparable results, although management differed in that most patients received NPPV alone, without supplemental O_2. Here the 5-year probability of continuing NPPV in COPD patients was 43%. Six of 33 patients died of respiratory failure, and five (15%) withdrew from therapy because of poor tolerance. Outcome from NPPV is shown compared with survival using LTOT and T-IPPV in Figure 1.

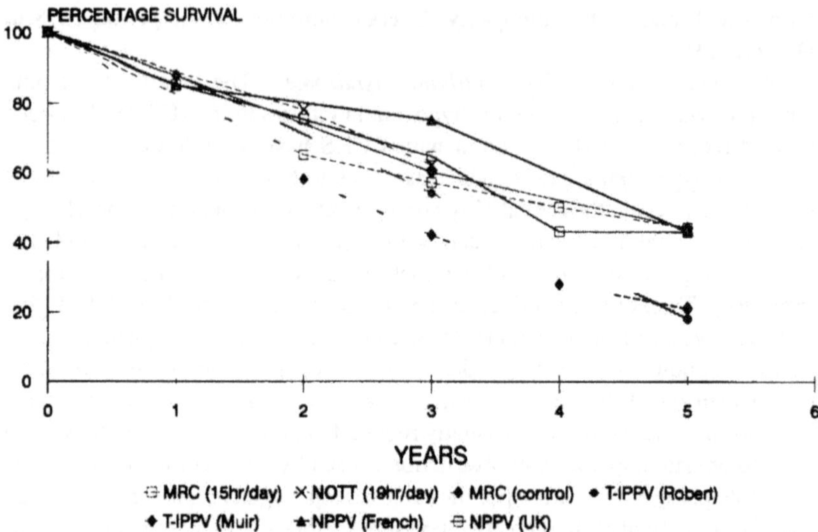

Figure 1 Five-year survival in patients receiving long-term oxygen therapy in MRC study (5) and NOTT study (6), compared with 5-year survival with tracheostomy ventilation (TIPPV) (15) and probability of continuing nasal intermittent positive pressure ventilation (NPPV) (24,34) in COPD.

In a series of 26 consecutive COPD patients who had failed LTOT due to worsening hypercapnia, 1- and 3-year survival rates using NPPV were 92 and 68%, respectively, with a mean annualized death rate of 10.8% (35). In a further group of 11 stable hypercapnic COPD patients, median survival was 2.5 yr (range 1.9 to 3.4 years) (36). Several crossover studies of LTOT vs. NPPV + LTOT have been carried out, but these are generally short term and do not have sufficient statistical power to assess mortality.

Bronchiectasis. Twenty-five patients with bronchiectasis were included in the French multicenter series (24). Three-year survival was 48%, much better than the U.K. series in which most bronchiectasis patients were dead after 2 years of NPPV (34). This can be explained by the fact that U.K. patients were sicker at the initiation of NPPV with a mean Pa_{O_2} of 42 mm Hg and Pa_{CO_2} of 68 mm Hg. Many had been referred for heart-lung transplantation, but were unsuitable for the transplant program because of nonrespiratory co-morbidity. A case control study (37) suggests that a marginal increase in survival may be seen (46 vs. 40 months in controls), but the main benefit of NPPV in bronchiectasis is probably a reduction in morbidity and downward trend in hospital admissions (see later section on health resource utilization and morbidity). Survival rates for the actively treated group were the most optimistic obtained so far at 96, 73, 63, and 31% at 1, 3, 5, and 10 years, respectively.

Cystic Fibrosis. The long-term effect of NPPV on survival in cystic fibrosis (CF) patients is not clear, as NPPV is either used as a bridge to transplantation (38), or as a palliative measure in extreme end stage disease. Piper et al. (39) treated four hypercapnic CF patients, who had failed to respond to intensive conventional therapy, with NPPV for up to 18 months. All survived, indicating that NPPV does have a role in extending life and/or bridging an individual to heart–lung transplantation. The main limitation to this approach is the scarcity of donor organs. However, it remains true that the outcome in CF patients admitted to the intensive care unit for conventional intubation and ventilation is very poor (40), even if weaning is attempted using NPPV (41).

Restrictive Chest Wall Disorders/Stable Neuromuscular Disease. Both the French (24) and U.K. series (34) provide data on survival in restrictive groups treated with NPPV (Fig. 2). In this area too, no randomized controlled studies exist, but as there is no other effective therapy for decompensated hypercapnic failure in restrictive patients, and the prognosis is dismal once cor pulmonale has developed, such trials are almost certainly unethical and unlikely to be carried out. Encouragingly, the studies available show concordant results. The French series comprised 105 patients with kyphoscoliosis and 80 with post-TB lung dis-

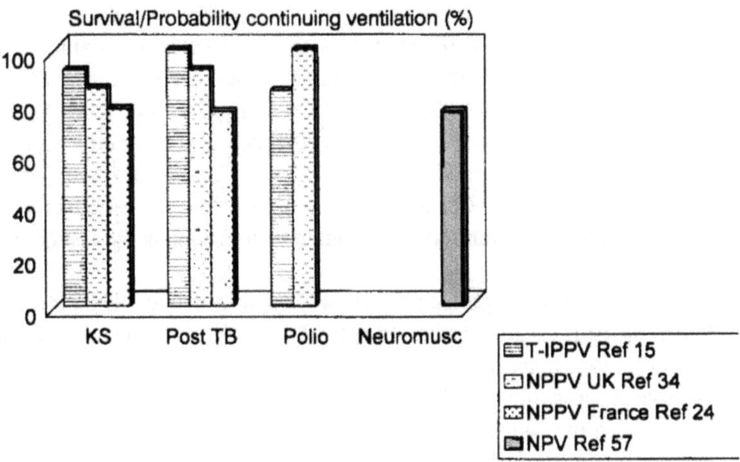

Figure 2 Five-year survival with tracheostomy ventilation (T-IPPV) (15), and probability of continuing nasal intermittent positive pressure ventilation (NPPV) in kyphoscoliosis (KS), posttuberculous (Post TB) lung disease, and postpolio (Polio) patients (24,34). Neuromusc = 5-year survival in mixed group of neuromuscular patients receiving negative presssure ventilation (NPV) (57).

ease. The U.K. Royal Brompton series contains 47 patients with idiopathic scoliosis, 30 with previous poliomyelitis, 20 with post-TB lung disease, and 29 with neuromuscular disease. The probability of continuing NIPPV in the French series was 76% at 3 years for scoliosis and post-TB disease. In the U.K. group, the probability of continuing NPPV at 5 years was 79% (CI 66 to 92%) for scoliosis, 100% for postpolio patients, and 94% (CI 83 to 100%) for those with TB lung disease (Fig. 2). In these series, continuation on NPPV represents survival, as only one patient with scoliosis withdrew from therapy. Five scoliosis patients died of respiratory failure and all these were referred late for NPPV and had developed severe pulmonary hypertension. The remaining deaths were due to unrelated malignant disease.

It should be noted that there are some differences between the series, as patients in the French series tended to be older, have a higher $Pa{O_2}$ and a lower $Pa{CO_2}$ on initiation of NPPV, and were more likely to receive supplemental O_2 than patients in the U.K. series.

Progressive Neuromuscular Disease

Duchenne Muscular Dystrophy. Rideau and Delaubier (42) pioneered NPPV to treat DMD patients. As indicated previously, assessment of the outcome of NPPV alone is difficult, as many DMD patients receive NPPV initially and then transfer to T-IPPV. In the 16 patients with DMD in the French cohort (24), five transferred to T-IPPV and the probability of continuing NPPV at 3 years was 36%.

More recently, NPPV has been used as the sole mode of ventilatory support in a consecutive series of 23 DMD patients with hypercapnic ventilatory failure (mean $Pa{CO_2}$ 10.3 kPa) (43). One-, three- and five-year survival rates were 85% (CI 69 to 100%), 73% (53 to 94%), and 73% (53 to 94%), respectively. Although a control group was not included, as this was considered to be unethical, it does seem that NPPV can extend survival in DMD by at least 5 to 7 years, and in some cases for longer periods. For the majority of this time the patients required only nocturnal support, with ventilator dependency increasing in the last 6 months of life.

The use of assisted cough techniques (44) combined with NPPV or mouth intermittent positive pressure ventilation (MPPV) is probably crucial to the success of noninvasive modes in DMD patients, particularly in those with peak cough flow rates of less than 160 L/min. By facilitating sputum clearance, insufflation–exsufflation machines may reduce the complications of a chest infection before the development of ventilatory failure. Bach et al. (45) have shown that the use of noninvasive ventilation together with cough insufflation–exsufflation devices produces similar survival to conventional T-IPPV, with reduced morbidity.

Contrary to the above results in hypercapnic patients, the use of NPPV to *prevent* the development of ventilatory failure and extend survival is not effective. In a French prospective multicenter study (46), normocapnic DMD patients with a vital capacity 20 to 50% predicted were randomized to NIPPV or a control group without ventilatory support. During a follow-up of over 4 years, no difference was seen in the onset of hypercapnic failure or decrease in VC to below 20%. Furthermore, more patients died in the NPPV group (8 vs. 2 in control group). It has been suggested that these results may be attributable to the possibility that provision of NPPV may cause families to delay seeking medical help at the time of acute exacerbations. In addition, NPPV was poorly tolerated and therefore treatment *efficacy* was not assessed. This speculation notwithstanding, there is no evidence to recommend the early introduction of NPPV before the development of ventilatory failure.

Amyotrophic Lateral Sclerosis/Motor Neuron Disease. In addition to a few anecdotal reports, there has been only one small randomized study of NPPV in ALS/MND patients (47). Bilevel pressure support was provided to a group with a mean VC 70% predicted and P_{CO_2} 5.3 kPa. A significant survival advantage was seen in the group using pressure support ($p < 0.004$). Importantly, older patients seemed to derive at least as much benefit as younger patients. Aboussouan et al. (48) have examined the characteristics that determine the ability of ALS patients to tolerate NPPV. In their series of 39 ALS patients with orthopnea and/or hypercapnia, 46% were able to tolerate NPPV (defined as ability to use NPPV during sleep for at least 4 consecutive hours). Bulbar symptoms partly contributed to intolerance, but did not preclude successful NPPV use. Overall, ALS patients who tolerated NPPV survived longer than individuals intolerant of ventilatory support.

In a comparison of T-IPPV provided mainly in the hospital and noninvasive ventilation provided mainly at home for patients with ALS/MND, no difference in survival was found (49). However, patients were not stratified for bulbar or nonbulbar disease.

Pediatric Nasal Intermittent Positive Pressure Ventilation

It is ironic that despite early reports suggesting that young children would be unable to tolerate masks (50), pediatric NPPV is now one on the fastest growth areas of LTMV. In fact, NPPV has largely replaced T-IPPV in congenital myopathies, muscular dystrophies, types II and III SMA, spina bifida, craniofacial disorders, obesity hypoventilation syndromes, and in some cases of CCHS. In most studies, bilevel positive pressure devices have been used (51,52). Significant improvement in diurnal and nocturnal blood gas tensions with long-term survival are reported (51,52).

Impact of Negative Pressure Ventilation on Survival

Chronic Obstructive Pulmonary Disease

Although anecdotal work (53) has indicated physiologic improvement, the consensus of opinion is that negative pressure ventilation (NPV) is less effective in

COPD than in neuromusculoskeletal disease. Controlled trials of NPV in COPD (54–56) have been short term and focused on physiologic end points, such as respiratory muscle strength, arterial blood gas tensions, and exercise tolerance, rather than mortality. As there is little demonstrative effect on these measures and NPV is poorly tolerated by COPD patients, it seems unlikely that NPV has a favorable impact on survival. However, Corrado et al. (57) have reported favorable mortality rates among COPD patients treated with a combination of short-course NPV for acute exacerbations followed by LTOT.

Restrictive Chest Wall Disorders

In contrast to the work in COPD, there is a long track record of NPV in restrictive disorders. In a report of 20 years' experience with tank ventilation in neuromuscular disease (58), survival varied from 6 months to 19 years, with 5- and 10-year survival rates of 76 and 61%, respectively. The few patients who failed NPV tended to be younger (less than age 3) and suffered from recurrent pneumonia or atelectasis. In the older age group, NPV failed in individuals with severe thoracocervical scoliosis that impeded the neck seal of the tank ventilator. One patient died of electrical power failure. Excellent results (58–60) have also been obtained by other groups skilled in negative pressure techniques, although this expertise remains limited to relatively few centers wordwide. This lack of technical skills, combined with the fact that negative pressure devices are bulky and inconvenient, means that NPPV has largely superseded NPV.

Pediatric NPV

Long-term NPV (either tank ventilation or cuirass) has been widely used in children, particularly those with neuromuscular disease (33). Extended survival is possible, although most studies are descriptive and contain small numbers of patients. In a recent U.K. survey (61) of children receiving home ventilation, only 10% were using NPV.

Mouth Ventilation

Mouth ventilation (MPPV) used alone or combined with other modes of noninvasive ventilation has been employed in over 250 patients with neuromuscular disease (62). Commercial or customized mouthpieces were used. Significant numbers of patients in this series had negligible vital capacity, yet it was possible to fully support ventilation long term without the need for tracheostomy. Sixty-one patients successfully used MPPV for more than 10 years. There has been no direct comparison of MPPV with NPPV or NPV. Mouth ventilation probably should be seen as suitable for the sole support of some patients, and as a complementary technique for others. However, its role outside of neuromuscular disease is limited.

B. Physiologic Outcome

Diurnal Arterial Blood Gas Tensions

COPD

Results from crossover studies of the effect of NPPV on arterial blood gas tensions (ABGs) in COPD are mixed, and likely to be closely related to patient selection. Lin (63) showed no improvement in arterial Po_2, Pco_2, bicarbonate (HCO_3) or pH in COPD patients after 2 weeks of O_2 therapy, NPPV, or the combination of NPPV+LTOT. Not surprisingly, baseline and mean SaO_2 did improve on O_2 and NPPV+O_2 compared with NPPV alone. As this study was short in duration, it is possible that full acclimatization to NPPV was not achieved. Furthermore, the level of pressure support employed (mean 12 cm H_2O) may have been insufficient.

A 3-month controlled trial of NPPV vs. sham ventilatory support has been carried out by Gay et al. (64). Compliance was poor in that only four of seven patients tolerated bilevel support and just one demonstrated a significant fall in $Paco_2$. An earlier crossover study of NPPV also demonstrated poor tolerance and no change in arterial blood gas tensions (65). By contrast, two groups have shown significant improvements in Pao_2 and $Paco_2$. In a crossover trial of LTOT vs. LTOT+NPPV (66), Pao_2 and $Paco_2$ improved significantly compared with values on LTOT alone. On average there was a rise in Pao_2 of 5.9 mm Hg and a fall in $Paco_2$ of 4.5 mm Hg in NPPV. These results are in line with an observational study that showed an increase in Pao_2 of 5 mm Hg and a decrease in $Paco_2$ of 7 mm Hg (67). Interestingly, these arterial blood gas levels continued to improve over 12 to 18 months, indicating that long-term assessment may be more reliable than short-term studies.

Additional support for these findings comes from an observational study of 11 COPD patients (36), which shows a mean improvement in Pao_2 from 45 (7) to 56 (9) mm Hg and a fall in $Paco_2$ from 60 (10) to 48 (9) mm Hg after 12 mo of domiciliary NPPV.

In the French multicenter series (24), Pao_2 rose from 49 to 52 mm Hg (p = NS) and $Paco_2$ fell from 54 to 46 mm Hg ($p < 0.02$) at 12 mo and these values were sustained at 2 years. Approximately 88% of patients received supplemental O_2. The U.K. Royal Brompton Hospital series (34) showed that from a baseline Pao_2 of 46 (6) mm Hg and $Paco_2$ of 62 (13) mm Hg in COPD, a mean increase in Pao_2 of 6 mm Hg and decrease in $Paco_2$ of 7 mm Hg was obtained after 1 year of NPPV (Fig. 3).

In bronchiectasis patients, NPPV may improve arterial blood gas tensions marginally (68) or slow their deterioration (37).

Restrictive Disorders

Improvements in ABGs during spontaneous breathing after initiation of NPPV in those with restrictive disorders are almost always more impressive than in those

Physiological effects of long term NPPV in restrictive and obstructive disorders

	Scoliosis	Post TB	Polio	DMD	COPD	Bronchiec
Baseline PaO2 mmHg [24,34]	50 54	45 52	53	75	46 54	42 56
Change in PaO2 on NPPV mmHg [24,34]	+8	+8	+13	+10	+6	-7
Baseline PaCO2 mmHg [24,34]	61 53	63 54	59	52	62 54	68 56
Change in PaCO2 on NPPV mmHg [24,34]	-10	-7	-10	-12	-7	-8
SaO2 on NPPV[24,66,73]	⇑	⇑	⇑	⇑	⇑	⇑
PaCO2 on NPPV [24,66,73]	⇓	⇓	⇓	⇓	⇓	⇓
Sleep quality[34,64-66]	⇑	⇑	⇑	⇑	+/-	+/-
Lung function [24,34,73]	No change	No change	No change	No change	No change	No change
Resp muscle function [73,77]	+/?	+/?	+/?	NK	No change	NK
Exercise[66]	⇑	NK	NK	NK	NK	NK
Baseline pulmonary artery pressure[63]	⇑	⇑	NK	NK	⇑	NK
Change with NPPV[63]	⇓	⇓	NK	NK	No change	NK
Quality of life[34,43,66]	⇑	⇑	⇑	⇑	+/-	+/-
Annual hospital days Pre NPPV[24]	34	31	NK	18	49	41
Post NPPV 1 year[24]	6	10	NK	7	17	No change

Figure 3 Physiological effects of long-term nasal intermittent positive pressure ventilation (NPPV) in restrictive and obstructive disorders. Exercise = exercise endurance, Resp muscle function = respiratory muscle function, NK = not known or preliminary results only, +/? = studies suggest benefit but not confirmed.

with obstructive lung disease. The main problem of alveolar hypoventilation in restrictive disorders is more easily corrected by LTMV, because the additional problems of ventilation-perfusion ratio (V/Q) mismatch and diffusion disturbance seen in obstructive lung disease are usually absent.

Equivalent improvements in ABGs can be obtained in those with progressive disorders such as DMD (43). Similar data are not available for ALS/MND, but anecdotal evidence suggests that ABGs can be well maintained here too, at the cost of increased ventilator dependency over time.

Negative Pressure Ventilation

While NPV may correct severe acidosis and hypercapnia in acute exacerbations of COPD (69), the large Montreal sham controlled study (56) of domiciliary NPV together with two other short-term trials (54,55) showed no significant change in ABGs in chronic COPD patients. This is in conflict with data obtained using intermittent weekly NPV in an uncontrolled study (70). These intermittent NPV results have not been duplicated in a controlled trial. The difference in outcome may also be explained by different patient selection.

Conversely, NPV in restrictive disorders may produce comparable improvements in ABGs to NPPV and TIPPV (71). However, in one group of restrictive patients transferred from NPV to NPPV, arterial blood gas tensions improved further, suggesting NPPV may be the more mechanically efficient technique (34).

Nocturnal Arterial Blood Gas Tensions/Sleep Architecture/Sleep Quality

Tracheostomy Intermittent Positive Pressure Ventilation

There are few data on the effect of T-IPPV on nocturnal and diurnal blood gas tensions or sleep quality in obstructive and restrictive disorders. Among patients swapped from T-IPPV to noninvasive ventilation, the vast majority preferred noninvasive techniques for sleep quality (72).

Nasal Intermittent Positive Pressure Ventilation

Meecham-Jones et al. (66) showed a significant improvement in mean overnight transcutaneous carbon dioxide ($Tcco_2$) with LTOT+ NPPV compared with LTOT alone in patients with COPD. The mean increment in Pco_2 on NPPV+LTOT was 2.6 (1.8) mm Hg, compared with an increase of 8.2 (4.5) mm Hg on O_2 alone. Nocturnal Sao_2 increased and the frequency of hypopneas decreased in both treatment arms. The improvement in daytime $Paco_2$ was correlated with the decrease in nocturnal Pco_2 ($r = 0.69$, $p = 0.01$). Sleep efficiency was 81% on NPPV+O_2, compared with 69% on O_2 alone and 51% during the baseline study, when the patients breathed air spontaneously. The distribution of rapid eye movement/non–rapid eye movement (REM/NREM) sleep did not change on treatment.

However, other workers have shown no change in sleep efficiency during NPPV (65) or even a decrease (64). These differences may be attributable to the fact that the Meecham Jones et al. study was 6 months in duration whereas the Lin study (63) was short term. Thus, acclimatization to NPPV may be an important factor. In addition, patient selection and the ventilator settings employed are likely to be crucial. The Strumpf et al. study (65) enrolled patients with an average $Paco_2$ of 46 mm Hg, whereas in the similarly designed Meecham Jones et al. study average $Paco_2$ was 56 mm Hg. This indicates that patients with marked hypercapnia fare better, especially if NPPV is targeted at minimizing nocturnal hypoventilation, and overnight Pco_2 control is confirmed. This will often require an inspiratory positive airway pressure (IPAP) setting in excess of 14 cm H_2O.

There are few polysomnographic studies of the effects on NPPV of sleep architecture. In a study looking at breathing during sleep after at least 6 months of domiciliary nocturnal NPPV, Piper et al. (73) showed that the fall in Sao_2 from baseline value during REM and NREM sleep was considerably reduced with the patients breathing spontaneously off NPPV, and CO_2 retention was also reduced. This carryover effect after discontinuing ventilatory support suggests that mechanisms such as improvement in hypercapnic drive and arousal reflex may be important. It also demonstrates that restrictive patients can cope with a night off NPPV should equipment problems occur or use of the device proves inconvenient. Interestingly, 4 of the 14 patients were unable to maintain REM sleep while breathing spontaneously. All aroused from sleep on desaturation, indicating a heightened arousal reflex. Improvements in nocturnal hypoventilation were similar in chest wall disease and stable neuromuscular patients.

Using a similar approach, NPPV was withdrawn for 1 week in restrictive patients who had previously used nocturnal respiratory support for at least 6 months (74). Daytime symptoms of somnolence, headache, and dyspnea returned rapidly, and nocturnal monitoring during spontaneous ventilation showed a greater degree of desaturation than during respiratory support. This nocturnal deterioration occurred in the face of unchanged daytime arterial blood gas tensions, pulmonary function, and respiratory muscle strength, confirming the impression that the main mechanism of action of NPPV is via correction of nocturnal hypoventilation.

In general, NPV may be less efficient at correcting nocturnal blood gas tensions than NPPV, as it can cause upper airway collapse leasing to obstructive apneas and desynchronization may be promoted by fixed-rate negative pressure pumps.

Self-reported sleep quality tends to be improved with noninvasive ventilation where the aim has been to control nocturnal hypoventilation rather than rest the respiratory muscles. In patients with restrictive and obstructive disorders who had used domiciliary nocturnal NPPV for 6 months to 7 years, 67% reported average sleep quality, 21% very good sleep quality, and only 5% described poor sleep quality (34).

Pulmonary Function

There is little evidence that LTMV using any mode influences FEV_1 in COPD. Likewise no change in FVC was seen in several long-term studies of NPPV (24,34,73) in chest wall and neuromuscular disease.

Respiratory Muscle Strength

The short-term effects of ventilatory support on respiratory muscle strength are better documented than the long-term impact. Interpretation of data is limited by the fact that simple mouth pressures are usually used, and these are dependent on patient cooperation and motivation. Almost all studies have focused on the impact of noninvasive modes rather than T-IPPV.

One of the main hypotheses underpinning the use of ventilatory support in hypercapnic respiratory failure is that the respiratory muscles become fatigued and require "rest." The presence of fatigue has not, however, been convincingly documented (75). Nonetheless, respiratory muscle weakness is clearly present in those with neuromuscular disease, and the mechanical efficiency of these muscles is impaired by chest wall distortion, and as a result of hyperinflation in COPD (76).

Examining the mechanisms by which diurnal blood gas tensions improve in COPD patients receiving NPPV, Elliott et al. (77) demonstrated that this was unlikely to be attributable to improved respiratory muscle function as there was no increase in inspiratory or expiratory muscle strength over 6 to 12 months. This is in contrast to results from short-term studies. However, a reduction in P_{CO_2} was correlated with a decrease in gas trapping and residual volume, suggesting that a diminution in respiratory load may be important.

More positive effects on respiratory muscle strength have been obtained following NPPV in restrictive disorders, although some caveats remain regarding the reliability of mouth pressures. An overall increase in $P_{I}max$ from 41 to 65% predicted and $P_{E}max$ from 58 to 83% predicted ($p < 0.01$) was seen after at least 6 months NPPV in chest wall disease and neuromuscular patients (73). There was no correlation between change in respiratory muscle strength or vital capacity and awake Pa_{CO_2}. However, there was an negative correlation between minimum REM arterial oxygen saturation and change in $P_{I}max$ % predicted ($r = 0.63, p < 0.05$).

Negative pressure ventilation may also have favorable effects on respiratory muscle function—indeed early studies of the effect of tank ventilators on diaphragm activity provided the rationale for NPV in chronic lung disease (78,79). Short-term trials suggest that NPPV may be more effective than NPV in offloading the respiratory muscles (80), although it is not clear whether this is of clinical relevance.

Ventilatory Drive

Hypercapnic drive is depressed in patients with chronic hypercapnia and may be further decreased by sleep deprivation and fragmentation. Primary drive disorders are a feature of some central neurologic conditions, and also occur in conjunction with respiratory muscle weakness in patients with myotonic dystrophy and bulbar polio. Use of NPPV can correct secondary depression of hypercapnic drive, as it has been shown that the fall in $Paco_2$ following NPPV in COPD correlates with increased minute ventilation at an end-tidal CO_2 of 60 mm Hg—suggesting enhanced chemosensitivity (77).

Renal Hemodynamics

It is a common finding that diuretic therapy can be reduced following the initiation of ventilatory support in hypercapnic respiratory failure, and that progression of ventilatory failure to cor pulmonale can be prevented. The mechanism by which this occurs is unclear. Recent work suggests that edema is precipitated in hypercapnic patients as a result of a reduction in renal reserve (81), as cardiac function seems well preserved. By correcting hypercapnia, NPPV may have a favorable effect on renal hemodynamics (82).

Pulmonary Hypertension

There have been few studies on the impact of LTMV on pulmonary artery pressure subsequent to the early observation that NPV can improve pulmonary hemodynamics significantly in restrictive chest wall disease (83). However, Schonhofer et al. (84) have recently measured pulmonary artery pressure (PAP) before and after 1 year of domiciliary NPPV in patients with restrictive and obstructive lung disease. Restrictive patients tended to have a higher baseline PAP at rest and during exercise than those with COPD, and PAP fell significantly after a year of NPPV. By contrast, initial PAP was lower in the COPD patients, but was not altered by NPPV therapy. Intriguingly, there was no relationship between improvement in Pao_2 and $Paco_2$, and fall in PAP in the restrictive group.

Left Ventricular Function

Sleep-disordered breathing is a prominent feature of cardiac failure and, notably, patients with Cheyne-Stokes respiration (CSR) have a higher mortality than those without sleep-disordered breathing. There are conflicting reports on the efficacy of nasal continuous airway pressure (CPAP) in congestive cardiac failure (85,86), and preliminary work suggests that NPPV may be more effective (87). This hypothesis requires careful confirmation, not least because recent use of bilevel positive pressure therapy in acute pulmonary edema produced an excess of myocardial infarctions, despite the fact that $Paco_2$ fell more rapidly than in CPAP users (88).

Exercise Tolerance and Endurance

A controlled study (89) has shown that exercise tolerance in scoliosis patients using domiciliary NPPV increased considerably. It is not established whether this is due to an improvement in arterial blood gas tensions, respiratory muscle strength, or a reconditioning effect on peripheral muscles, but several mechanisms probably play a part.

Use of inspiratory pressure support during exercise improves walking distance and reduces breathlessness (90). It is therefore plausible that the application of NPPV during pulmonary rehabilitation exercise regimens may augment benefit, although this remains to be proven.

C. Health Resource Utilization and Morbidity

The MRC LTOT trial (5) produced no change in overall hospital admissions in oxygen users compared with the control group. In LTMV patients, morbidity data are usually based on hospital admissions, as there is little information on outpatient consultations and home visits.

Tracheostomy Intermittent Positive Pressure Ventilation

Muir et al. (18) have shown that in COPD patients receiving T-IPPV, days in hospital fell from 72 in the 12 months preceding tracheostomy to 41 for the first year of T-IPPV, 30/year for the second year, and 23/year for the third year of T-IPPV.

Nasal Intermittent Positive Pressure Ventilation

Hospital admissions before and after 1 year of NPPV were reduced from 49 to 17 days in COPD patients, from 34 to 6 days in scoliosis patients, and from 31 to 10 days in those with post-TB lung disease (24). Indeed, even patients treated with a short course of NPPV for an acute exacerbation may also derive long-term benefit in terms of reduced intensive care unit utilization in the subsequent year compared with a group managed without NPPV (91).

Bronchiectasis patients often place major demands on hospital beds. In the French multicenter study (24) hospital days for bronchiectasis patients before LTMV were on average 48 (55) and this fell to 10 days in the year after NPPV was initiated. This reduction in morbidity has been confimed by Garcia Tejero et al. (68) who showed a reduction in annual episodes of respiratory failure from 3.5 (3) pre-NIPPV to 2 (2) while receiving NPPV.

For U.K. DMD patients receiving NPPV, average admission rate was

0.64/year, with each stay lasting an average of 4 days (43). Values were not available for the year preceding ventilatory decompensation. Leger et al. (24) found hospital days reduced from 18 in the year preceding NPPV to 7 in the first year of ventilatory support. In a comparison of pulmonary morbidity in DMD patients receiving T-IPPV, part-time noninvasive ventilation, or 24-hour noninvasive ventilation, Bach et al. (45) have shown that hospitalization was significantly reduced using noninvasive methods, as were days in hospital per year, excluding admissions for initiation of ventilatory support.

It is clear that the tracheostomy in itself is a cause of morbidity, with some hospital admissions required to deal with hemorrhage, granulomata, inspissated secretions, stricture formation, or to perform surgical revision.

NPPV is not free of side effects, but these are generally not life-threatening in nature. One of the most important is nasal bridge pressure sores, which usually necessitate an adjustment in mask size or interface. Another common problem is gastric distension, which may respond to a swap from volume preset to pressure preset ventilator, adjustment of the level of pressure support, or simply a change in sleeping position. Rhinitis may occur in up to 50% of patients (24).

Negative Pressure Ventilation

Patients using negative pressure equipment complain of back pain, discomfort, and often feel cold using the pneumojacket, tank ventilator, or cuirass in the winter.

Mouth Ventilation

The mouthpieces employed to deliver mouth ventilation have been observed to cause quite marked dental deformity, and should not be used full-time in children with growing dentition.

D. Health Status and Quality of Life

Physiologic outcome measures do not tell us the whole story of the impact of a disease and its treatment on an individual's life. Thus, patients with the same FEV_1 or PO_2 may experience quite a different level of health impairment and disability. Tools to assess health status and quality of life have been refined in the last decade and therefore there are few comparative data on, for example, T-IPPV vs. NPPV in COPD. It is also obvious using current protocols that patients requiring T-IPPV are likely to have more disability than those receiving NPPV. Most studies of quality of life employ generic measures, such as the Short Form 36 (SF-36), Nottingham health profile, or Sickness Impact Profile, which allow comparisons across disease groups. The disease-specific St. George's Hospital Questionnaire is commonly used in COPD patients.

In a crossover study of NPPV+O_2 vs. O_2 alone in COPD, total symptom score and disease impact using the St. George's Respiratory Questionnaire were improved compared with results on O_2 alone, where a small deterioration was seen (66). This is in keeping with the lack of improvement in quality of life shown in most other studies of LTOT. A trend to improvement was also seen in the 6- to 12-month study of NPPV in COPD by Elliott et al. (77).

Health status measured by the SF-36 in NPPV users with restrictive and obstructive lung disease has been shown to be equivalent to other groups with chronic disease such as U.S. ambulatory patients with heart failure or diabetes mellitus (34) (Fig. 4). This contradicts the popular view that the health status of ventilator users is likely to be significantly worse than nonventilator groups with chronic health problems.

Perhaps the greatest area of concern is the quality of life in patients with progressive neurologic disease who are provided with ventilatory support. Here the aim is to palliate symptoms and extend life which is worthwhile to the individual, and emphatically not to protract the process of death. No controlled trials exist of T-IPPV in ALS/MND or DMD. A comparison of ALS/MND patients

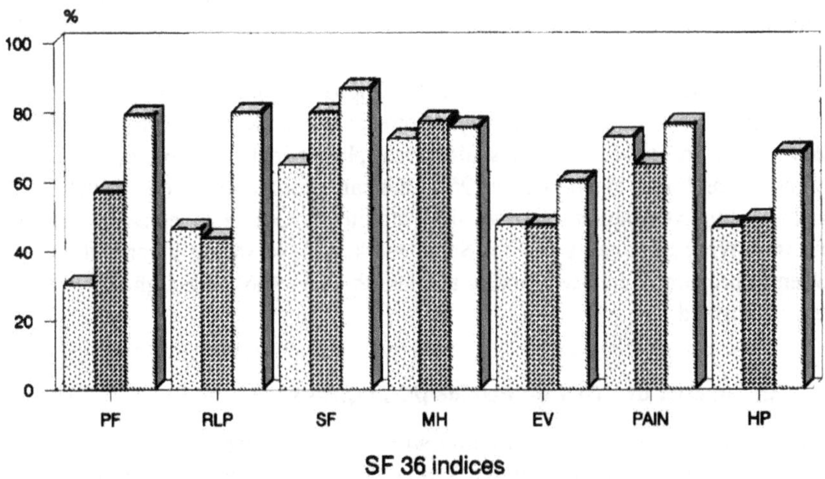

Figure 4 Health status measured by the Short Form 36 (SF-36) generic questionnaire in patients receiving domiciliary nasal intermittent positive pressure ventilation (NPPV), in a U.S. group with chronic diseases and in U.K. age-matched normal subjects (Healthy Life Survey, [HLS UK]). PF = physical function, RLP = role limitation related to physical factors, SF = social function, MH = mental health, EV = energy and vitality, Pain = total pain, HP = health perception. 0 = minimum score, 100 = maximum score. (Redrawn from Ref 34.)

using T-IPPV and NPPV (92) showed that far more patients with NPPV could be managed at home, and 100% of NPPV users were satisfied with their mode of ventilation compared to only 72% of T-IPPV users. However, these groups were not equivalent in that NPPV was started electively, whereas in most cases, T-IPPV was instituted as an emergency without the opportunity for advance decision making. Preparation for ventilatory support and advance directives are clearly helpful for patients and their families. In ALS/MND patients randomized to bilevel pressure support, an early trend to improvement in quality of life occurred, but this did not reach significance (47).

In an overview of NPPV users, DMD patients scored SF-36 values that were comparable to those with nonprogressive disorders in terms of health perception and social aspects, despite a lower level of physical function (43). In Sweden neuromuscular patients have been shown to have lower quality of life scores than scoliosis and post-TB lung disease patients (93), but this cohort was heterogeneous.

It has been pointed out that health professionals may consistently underestimate the quality of life of patients with progressive disorders (94). Only 12.5% DMD patients receiving LTMV reported dissatisfaction with their lives in general. Decisions concerning ventilatory support should therefore be based on the individual's own perception of the quality of their life, not on assumptions made by the health care team.

The mechanism(s) by which LTMV improves quality of life is not clear. NIV patients report a reduction in symptoms of nocturnal hypoventilation. Sickness Impact Profile scores in muscular dystrophy patients are adversely affected by fatigue and poor sleep quality (95). One can hypothesize that a reduction in nocturnal hypoventilation improves sleep architecture, thereby decreasing fatigue and improving the quality of life. Some workers have shown a correlation between improvement in sleep quality and health status (66), although this has not been confirmed.

E. Impact of LTMV on Families/Caregivers

Twenty-four hour invasive ventilation will obviously have a greater impact on family life than nocturnal nasal ventilation (55,96). It is also evident that carers prefer noninvasive ventilation to T-IPPV if this is a realistic proposition (72).

Many families form part of the care rota for their ventilator-dependent relative. Aday et al. (97) have examined the concerns of families with 24-hour T-IPPV–dependent children. These were found to be focused on the child's continued health and long-term development, financial worries, and being restricted to the house. Privacy is a problem, and issues arising out of parental authority vs. professional nursing advice can cause conflict. Families who had less than 36 hour/week nursing help often felt unprepared for the relentless nature of the caring role, and experienced a sensation of isolation and abandonment following their child's discharge from hospital. Many families reported a significant decrease in peer relationships and recreational activities (96).

Siblings of the ventilated child and other family members inevitably receive less attention, but tend to be protective of the ventilator-assisted individual and find it hard to express negative feelings. Most families have to get used to living with a degree of uncertainly since the long-term outcome of mechanical ventilation is not always clear in individual cases (98). Despite these very real difficulties, life satisfaction scores for both patients and families are surprisingly high (96) and the vast majority do not regret the decision to carry out LTMV at home.

F. Community Impact and Economics

Society demands that health care resources are used appropriately. At the same time, health workers have a responsibility to provide the best quality of life possible for the mechanically ventilated patient. Most LTMV patients would prefer to be at home if this is feasible. The cost of nocturnal home NIPPV is around $3000 to $3500/year compared with an annual cost of approximately $200,000 for an individual requiring domiciliary 24-hour T-IPPV. Most of this sum is needed to cover personnel costs rather than equipment costs, and is reduced if nonlicensed caregivers are employed. These expenses compete with other community health needs in an economic climate in which fixed or decreasing health budgets are the norm. While the marked growth in NPPV is likely to reduce average cost of LTMV per patient, an analysis of trends (99) shows that total patient numbers will inevitably rise.

One positive outcome of the increase in LTMV is that reports (100,101) suggest that community attitudes to disability are influenced favorably by the placement of ventilator-dependent children in mainstream schools and adults in routine occupational environments.

Site of Care

It is clear that it is neither cost effective nor appropriate for a LTMV user to remain in an intensive care unit or acute facility once stability has been achieved and long-term needs established. In recent years, there has been a growth in regional intermediate care or weaning centers. Encouraging results in discontinuing ventilation and optimizing long-term ventilatory care have been reported by some of these centers (102–104), although appropriate patient selection is crucial and comparative trials of outcome have not yet been carried out. It is important to realize that not all patients will be suitable for long-term home care, and not all families are able to take on this responsibility. Regional intermediate centers have a useful role in this respect, as they are almost certainly less costly than acute care alternatives.

The Future

One of the most pressing needs is for more efficient worldwide data collection on the provision and outcome of LTMV in adults and children. Comprehensive central agencies that are responsible for data collection exist in some countries (105,106), but these few and far between. Over the next few years, it is likely that appropriate guidelines for using domiciliary NPPV in COPD will be established. Studies in progress are also likely to clarify the indications for LTMV in progressive neuromuscular disease and establish more clearly the impact of respiratory support on health-related quality of life in patients and their families. Work on the role of NPPV in chronic cardiac failure may lead to exciting opportunities to change the natural history of ventricular failure. The value of LTMV during pulmonary rehabilitation needs to be determined.

A recent survey in Minnesota (99) shows that the most rapid expansion in LTMV is in the provision of noninvasive ventilation, which accounts for 47% of the increase in ventilator-dependent patients from 1992 to 1998. This is likely to reflect developments elsewhere in the United States and Europe, and is a trend that is likely to continue. It is hoped that NPPV, in particular, will become available more equitably throughout the world. This spread should be facilitated by the publication of outcome analyses and increasing familiarity with noninvasive techniques by anesthestists and acute medical teams.

Technically, modification of ventilatory modes will continue to be explored and smaller, more portable ventilators will become available. The interface remains the Achilles' heel of NPPV, and simpler-to-construct customized masks made of newer synthetic materials and other innovative interfaces are on the horizon.

References

1. Report on a Consensus Conference of the American College of Chest Physicians. Mechanical ventilation beyond the intensive care unit. Chest 1998; 113(5):292S.
2. Knaus WA. Prognosis with mechanical ventilation: The influence of disease, age, and chronic health status on survival from an acute illness. Am Rev Respir Dis 1989; 140(suppl):S8–S13.
3. Make BJ. Indications for home ventilation in critical care unit patients. In: Robert D, Make BJ, Leger P, et al., eds. Home Mechanical Ventilation. Paris: Arnette Blackwell, 1995; 229–240.
4. Criner GJ, Kreimer DT, Pidlaoan L. Patient outcome following prolonged mechanical ventilation via tracheostomy (Abstr). Am Rev Respir Dis 1993; 147:A874.
5. Medical Research Council Working Party Report. Long term domiciliary oxygen therapy in chronic hypoxic cor pulmonale complicating chronic bronchitis and emphysema. Lancet 1981; 1:681–685.
6. Nocturnal Oxygen Therapy Trial Group. Continuous or nocturnal oxygen therapy

in hypoxaemic chronic obstructive lung disease. Ann Intern Med 1980; 93:391–398.

7. Aida A, Miyamoto K, Nishimura M, Aiba M, Kira S, Kawakami Y. Prognostic value of hypercapnia in patients with chronic respiratory failure during long-term oxygen therapy. Am J Resp Crit Care Med 1998; 158:188–193.
8. Dubois P, Jamart J, Machiels J, Smeets F, Lulling J. Prognosis of severely hypoxaemic patients receiving long-term oxygen therapy. Chest 1994; 105:469–474.
9. Cooper CB, Waterhouse J, Howard P. Twelve year clinical study of patients with hypoxic cor pulmonale given long term domiciliary oxygen therapy. Thorax 1987; 42:105–110.
10. Freyschuss V, Nilsonne U, Lundgren KD. Idiopathic scoliosis in old age. 1. Respiratory function. Arch Med Scand 1968; 184:365.
11. Branthwaite MA. Cardiorespiratory consequences of unfused idiopathic scoliosis. Br J Dis Chest 1986; 80:360–369.
12. Nachemson A. A long term follow up study of non-treated kyphoscoliosis. Acta Orthop Scand 1968; 39:466–476.
13. Strom K, Pehrsson K, Boe J, Nachemson A. Survival of patients with severe thoracic spine deformities receiving domiciliary oxygen therapy. Chest 1992; 102: 164–168.
14. Vianello A, Bevilacqua M, Salvador V, Cardaioli C, Vincenti E. Long-term nasal intermittent positive pressure ventilation in advanced Duchenne's Muscular Dystrophy. Chest 1994; 105:445–448.
15. Robert D, Gerard M, Leger P, Buffat J, Jennequin J, Holzapfel L, Mercatello A, Salamand J, Bertoye A. Domiciliary ventilation by tracheostomy for chronic respiratory failure. Rev Fr Mal Resp 1983; 11:923–936.
16. Bertrand A, Milane J, Dufranc P. Traitement au long cours de insuffisance respiratoire chronique par ventilation endotracheale a domicile chez 118 patients tracheotomises. Rev Fr Mal Resp 1985; 2:91–95.
17. Dudeffant P, Manier G, Gbikpi-Benissan G, Cardinaud P. Devenir des insuffisants respiratoire chroniques traites a domicile par tracheostomie et ventilation assistee. Rev Fr Mal Resp 1985; 2:145–150.
18. Muir J-F, Girault C, Cardinaud P, Polu JM, and the French Cooperative Group. Survival and long-term follow-up of tracheostomized patients with COPD treated by home mechanical ventilation. Chest 1994; 106:201–209.
19. Messord MPH, et al. Survival after spinal cord trauma. Arch Neurology 1978; 35: 78–83.
20. Wicks AB, Menter RR. Long term outlook in quadriplegic patients with initial ventilator dependency. Chest 1986; 90:406–410.
21. Viroslav J, Rosenblatt R, Tomazevic SM, et al. Care, life expectancy and quality of life in respiratory tetraplegics. In: Robert D, Make BJ, Leger P, et al., eds. Home Mechanical Ventilation. Paris: Arnette Blackwell, 1995; 241–247.
22. Splaingard ML, Frates FC, Harrison GM, et al. Home positive pressure ventilation. Twenty years experience. Chest 1983; 84:376–382.
23. Rideau Y, Delaubier A, Guillou C, Renardel-Irani A. Treatment of respiratory insufficiency in Duchenne's muscular dystrophy: Nasal ventilation in the initial stages. Monaldi Arch Chest Dis 1995; 50:235–238.

24. Leger P, Bedicam JM, Cornette A, Rybet-Degat O, Langevin B, Polu JM, Jeannin L, Robert D. Nasal intermittent positive pressure ventilation. Long term follow-up in patients with severe chronic respiratory insufficiency. Chest 1994; 105:100–105.
25. Soudon P. Mechanical ventilation by tracheostomy in neuromuscular diseases: Experience and evaluation. Eur Respir Rev 1993; 3:300–304.
26. Oppenheimer EA. Amyotrophic lateral sclerosis: Care, survival and quality of life on home mechanical ventilation. In: Robert D, Make BJ, Leger P, et al., eds. Home Mechanical Ventilation. Paris: Arnette Blackwell, 1995; 249–260.
27. Barois A, Estournet-Mathiaud B. Spinal muscular atrophy: Respiratory management as a function of clinical aspects. In: Robert D, Make BJ, Leger P, et al., eds. Home Mechanical Ventilation. Paris: Arnette Blackwell, 1995; 261–275.
28. Wang T-Y, Bach JR, Avilla C, Alba AS, Yang G-FW. Survival of individuals with spinal muscular atrophy on ventilatory support. Am J Phys Med Rehabil 1994; 71: 207–211.
29. Nelson VS, Carroll JC, Hurvitz EA, Dean JM. Home mechanical ventilation of children. Dev Med Child Neurol 1996; 38:704–715.
30. Weese-Mayer DE, Silvestri JM, Menzies LJ, Morrow-Kenny AS, Hunt CE, Hauptman SA. Congenital central hypoventilation syndrome: Diagnosis, management and long term outcome in thirty two children. J Pediatr 1992; 120:381–387.
31. Gaultier C, Trang H. Congenital central alveolar hypoventilation. Long term ventilatory support. In: Robert D, Make B, Leger P., et al., eds. Home Mechanical Ventilation. Paris: Arnette Blackwell; 1995; 277–284.
32. Hartmann H, Jawad MH, Noyes JP, Samuels MP, Southall DP. Negative extrathoracic pressure ventilation for infants with central hypoventilation syndrome. Pediatr Pulmonol 1992; 14:255.
33. Samuels MP, Southall DP. Negative extrathoracic pressure in the treatment of respiratory failure in infants and young children. Br Med J 1989; 299:1253–1257.
34. Simonds AK, Elliott MW. Outcome of domiciliary nasal intermittent positive pressure ventilation in restrictive and obstructive disorders. Thorax 1995; 50:604–609.
35. Sivasothy P, Smith IE, Shneerson JM. Mask intermittent positive pressure ventilation in chronic hypercapnic respiratory failure due to chronic obstructive pulmonary disease. Eur Respir J 1998; 11:34–40.
36. Jones SE, Packham S, Hebden M, Smith AP. Domiciliary nocturnal intermittent positive pressure ventilation in patients with respiratory failure due to severe COPD: Long term follow-up and effect on survival. Thorax 1998; 53:495–498.
37. Benhamou D, Girault C, Faure C, Portier F, Muir JF. Nasal mask ventilation in acute respiratory failure: Experience in elderly patients. Chest 1992; 102:912–917.
38. Hodson ME, Madden BP, Steven MH, Tsang VT, Yacoub MH. Non-invasive mechanical ventilation for cystic fibrosis patients—a potential bridge to transplantation. Eur Respir J 1991; 4:524–527.
39. Piper AJ, Parker S, Torzillo PJ, Sullivan CE, Bye PT. Nocturnal nasal IPPV stabilizes patients with cystic fibrosis and hypercapnic respiratory failure. Chest 1992; 102:846–850.
40. Swami A, Evans TW, Morgan CJ, et al. Conventional ventilation as a bridge to heart-lung transplantation in cystic fibrosis (abstr). Eur Respir J 1991; 4:188s.

41. Cadiergue V, Philit F, Langevin B, Sab JM, Thouret JM, Heyer L, Guerin C, Robert D. Outcome of cystic fibrosis patients admitted in intensive care unit for respiratory failure: Role of noninvasive ventilation. Eur Respir J 1998; 12(suppl 28):129s.
42. Rideau Y, Delaubier A. Management of respiratory neuromuscular weakness. Muscle Nerve 1988; 11:407–408.
43. Simonds AK, Muntoni F, Heather S, Fielding S. Impact of nasal ventilation on survival in hypercapnic Duchenne muscular dystrophy. Thorax 1998; 53:949–952.
44. Bach JR. Mechanical insufflation-exsufflation. Comparison of peak expiratory flows with manually assisted and unassisted coughing techniques. Chest 1993; 104: 1553–1562.
45. Bach JR, Ishikawa Y, Kim H. Prevention of pulmonary morbidity for patients with Duchenne muscular dystrophy. Chest 1998; 112:1024–1028.
46. Raphael J-C, Chevret S, Chastang C, Bouvet F. Randomised trial of preventive nasal ventilation in Duchenne muscular dystrophy. Lancet 1994; 343:1600–1604.
47. Pinto AC, Evangelista T, Carvalho M, Alves MA, Sales Luis ML. Respiratory assistance with a non-invasive ventilator (BiPAP) in MND/ALS patients: Survival rates in a controlled trial. J Neurol Sci 1995; 129(suppl):19–26.
48. Aboussouan LS, Khan SU, Meeker DP, Stelmach K, Mitsumoto H. Effect of noninvasive positive-pressure ventilation on survival in amyotrophic lateral sclerosis. Ann Intern Med 1997; 127:450–453.
49. Moss AH, Oppenheimer EA, Casey P, Cazzoli PA, Roos RP, Stocking CB, Siegler M. Patients with amyotrophic lateral sclerosis receiving long-term mechanical ventilation. Advance care planning and outcomes. Chest 1996; 110:249–255.
50. Heckmatt JZ, Loh L, Dubowitz V. Night-time nasal ventilation in neuromuscular disease. Lancet 1990; 335:579–582.
51. Teague WG. Pediatric application of noninvasive ventilation. Respir Care 1997; 42:414–423.
52. Simonds AK, Ward S, Heather S, Bush A, Rosenthal M, Muntoni F. Outcome of domiciliary nocturnal non-invasive mask ventilation in paediatric neuromusculoskeletal disease. Thorax 1998; 53(suppl 4):A10.
53. McClement J, Christianson LC, Hubaytor RT. The body type respirator in the treatment of chronic obstructive pulmonary disease. Ann NY Acad Sci 1965; 121: 748.
54. Zibrak JD, Hill NS, Federman EC, Kwa SL, O'Donnell C. Evaluation of intermittent long term negative-pressure ventilation in patients with severe COPD. Am Rev Respir Dis 1988; 138:1515–1518.
55. Celli B, Lee H, Criner G, Bermudez M, Rassulo J, Gilmartin M, Miller G, Make B. Controlled trial of external negative pressure ventilation in patients with severe chronic airflow limitation. Am Rev Respir Dis 1989; 140:1251–1256.
56. Shapiro SH, Ernst P, Gray-Donald K, Martin JG, Wood-Dauphinee S, Beaupre A, Spitzer WO, Macklem PT. Effect of negative pressure ventilation in severe chronic obstructive pulmonary disease. Lancet 1992; 340:1425–1429.
57. Corrado A, De Paola E, Messori A, Bruscoli G, Nutini S. The effect of intermittent negative pressure ventilation and long-term oxygen therapy for patients with COPD. Chest 1994; 105:95–99.
58. Splaingard ML, Frates RC, Jefferson LS, Rosen CL, Harrison GM. Home negative

pressure ventilation: Report of 20 years experience in patients with neuromuscular disease. Arch Phys Med Rehab 1985; 66:239–242.
59. Kinnear WJM, Shneerson JM. Assisted ventilation at home: Is it worth considering? Br J Dis Chest 1985; 79:313–351.
60. Sawicka EH, Loh L, Branthwaite MA. Domicilary ventilatory support: An analysis of outcome. Thorax 1988; 43:31–35.
61. Jardine EJ, Wallis C. A survey of UK children receiving long-term ventilatory support at home. Thorax 1997; 52(suppl 6):A23.
62. Bach JR, Alba AS, Bohatiuk G, Saporito L, Lee M. Mouth intermittent positive pressure ventilation in the management of postpolio respiratory insufficiency. Chest 1987; 91:859–864.
63. Lin C-C. Comparison between nocturnal nasal positive pressure ventilation combined with oxygen therapy and oxygen monotherapy in patients with severe COPD. Am J Respir Crit Care Med 1996; 154:353–358.
64. Gay PC, Hubmayr RD, Stroetz RW. Efficacy of nocturnal nasal ventilation in stable severe chronic obstructive pulmonary disease during a 3 month controlled trial. Mayo Clin Proc 1996; 71:533–542.
65. Strumpf DA, Millman RP, Carlisle CC, Grattan LM, Ryan SM, Erickson AD, Hill NS. Nocturnal positive-pressure ventilation via nasal mask in patients with severe chronic obstructive pulmonary disease. Am Rev Respir Dis 1991; 144:1234–1239.
66. Meecham Jones DJ, Paul EA, Jones PW, Wedzicha JA. Nasal pressure support ventilation plus oxygen compared to oxygen therapy alone in hypercapnic COPD. Am J Respir Crit Care Med 1995; 152:538–544.
67. Elliott MW, Simonds AK, Carroll MP, Wedzicha JA, Branthwaite MA. Domiciliary nocturnal nasal intermittent positive pressure ventilation in hypercapnic respiratory failure due to chronic obstructive lung disease: Effects on sleep and quality of life. Thorax 1992; 47:342–348.
68. Garcia-Tejero MT, Petitjean T, Langevin B, Philit F, Gerard M, Zaoui M, Robert D. Long term noninvasive ventilation in adult patients with diffuse bronchiectasis. Eur Respir J 1998; 12(suppl 28):309s.
69. Corrado A, De Paola E, Gorini M, Bruscoli G, Nutini S, Tozzi D, Ginanni R. Intermittent negative pressure ventilation in the treatment of hypoxic hypercapnic coma in chronic respiratory insufficiency. Thorax 1996; 51:1077–1082.
70. Gutierrez M, Beroiza T, Contreras G, Diaz O, Cruz E, Moreno R, Lisboa C. Weekly cuirass ventilation improves blood gases and inspiratory muscle strength in patients with chronic airflow limitation and hypercarbia. Am Rev Respir Dis 1988; 138: 617–623.
71. Jackson M, Hockley S, King MA, et al. A comparison of the physiological results of treatment with NIPPV or cuirass ventilation (abstr). Am Rev Respir Dis 1991; 143:A585.
72. Bach J. A comparison of long-term ventilatory support alternatives from the perspective of the patient and care-giver. Chest 1993; 104:1702–1706.
73. Piper AJ, Sullivan CE. Effects of long term nocturnal nasal ventilation on spontaneous breathing during sleep in neuromuscular and chest wall disorders. Thorax 1996; 9:1515–1522.
74. Hill NS, Eveloff SE, Carlisle CC, Goff SG. Efficacy of nocturnal nasal ventilation

in patients with restrictive thoracic disease. Am Rev Respir Dis 1992; 145:365–371.

75. Similowski TS, Yan A, Gauthier AP, Macklem PT, Bellemare F. Contractile properties of the human diaphragm during chronic hyperinflation. N Engl J Med 1991; 325:917–923.
76. Polkey MI, Kyroussis D, Hamnegard C-H, Mills G, Green M, Moxham J. Diaphragm strength in chronic obstructive pulmonary disease. Am J Respir Crit Care Med 1996; 154:1310–1317.
77. Elliott MW, Mulvey DA, Moxham J, Green M, Branthwaite MA. Domiciliary nocturnal nasal intermittent positive pressure ventilation in COPD: Mechanisms underlying changes in arterial blood gas tensions. Eur Respir J 1991; 4:1044–1052.
78. Rochester DF, Braun NM, Laine S. Diaphragmatic energy expenditure in chronic respiratory failure. Am J Med 1977; 63:223–231.
79. Braun NM, Marino WD. Effect of daily intermittent rest of respiratory muscles in patients with severe chronic airflow limitation (CAL) (abstr). Chest 1984; 85:59s–60s.
80. Belman MJ, Soo Hoo GW, Kuei JH, Shadmehr R. Efficacy of positive vs negative pressure ventilation in unloading the respiratory muscles. Chest 1990; 98:850–856.
81. Sharkey RA, Mulloy EMT, Kilgallen IA, O'Neill SJ. Renal functional reserve in patients with severe chronic obstructive pulmonary disease. Thorax 1997; 52:411–415.
82. Baudouin SV. Oedema and cor pulmonale revisited. Thorax 1997; 52:401–402.
83. Garay SM, Turino GM, Goldring RM. Sustained reversal of chronic hypercapnia in patients with alveolar hypoventilation syndromes. Am J Med 1981; 70:269–274.
84. Schonhofer B, Wenzel M, Barchfeld T, Kohler D. Long-term effects of non-invasive mechanical ventilation on pulmonary hemodynamics in patients with chronic respiratory insufficiency. Eur Respir J 1999 (in press).
85. Bradley TD, Holloway RM, McLaughlin PR, et al. Cardiac output response to continuous positive airway pressure in congestive heart failure. Am Rev Respir Dis 1992; 145:377–382.
86. Davies RJO, Harrington KJ, Ormerod OJM, et al. Nasal continuous positive airway pressure in chronic heart failure with sleep disordered breathing. Am Rev Respir Dis 1993; 147:630–634.
87. Naughton MT. Heart failure and central apnoea. Sleep Med Rev 1998; 2:105–116.
88. Mehta S, Jay GD, Woolard RH, et al. Randomized prospective trial of bilevel versus continuous positive airway pressure in acute pulmonary edema. Crit Care Med 1997; 25:620–628.
89. Schonhofer B, Wallstein S, Kohler D, et al. Effect of noninvasive mechanical ventilation on endurance performance in patients with chronic ventilatory insufficiency (abstr). Eur Respir J 1998; 12(suppl 28):310s.
90. Keilty SEJ, Ponte J, Fleming TA, Moxham J. Effect of inspiratory pressure support on exercise tolerance and breathlessness in patients with severe stable chronic obstructive pulmonary disease. Thorax 1994; 49:990–994.
91. Confalonieri M, Parigi P, Scartabellati A, Aiolfi S, Scorsetti S, Nava S, Gandola L. Noninvasive mechanical ventilation improves the immediate and long-term out-

come of COPD patients with acute respiratory failure. Eur Respir J 1996; 9:422–430.
92. Cazzolli PA, Oppenheimer EA. Home mechanical ventilation for amyotrophic lateral sclerosis: Nasal compared to tracheostomy intermittent positive pressure ventilation. J Neurol Sci 1996; 139:123–128.
93. Pehrsson K, Olofson J, Larsson S, Sullivan M. Quality of life in patients treated by home mechanical ventilation due to restrictive ventilatory disorders. Respir Med 1994; 88:21–26.
94. Bach JR, Campagnolo DI, Hoeman S. Life satisfaction of individuals with Duchenne muscular dystrophy using long-term mechanical ventilatory support. Am J Phys Med Rehabil 1991; 70:129–135.
95. Ahlstrom G, Gunnarsson L-G, Kihlgren A, Arvill A, Sjoden P-O. Respiratory function, electrocardiography and quality of life in individuals with muscular dystrophy. Chest 1994; 106:173–179.
96. Robins Miller J, Colbert AP, Osberg JS. Ventilator dependency: Decision-making, daily functioning and quality of life for patients with Duchenne muscular dystrophy. Dev Med Child Neurol 1990; 32:1078–1086.
97. Aday LH, Wegener DH, Anderson RM, Aitken MJ. Home care for ventilator-assisted children. Health Aff 1989; Summer:137–147.
98. Robins Miller J, Colbert AP, Schock NC. Ventilator use in progressive neuromuscular disease: Impact on patients and their families. Dev Med Child Neurol 1988; 20:200–207.
99. Adams AB, Shapiro R, Marinii JJ. Changing prevalence of chronically ventilator-assisted individuals in Minnesota: Increases, characteristics, and the use of non-invasive ventilation. Respir Care 1998; 43:635–636.
100. Russ D. A Family's Perspective. In: Driver LE, Nelson VN, Warschausky SA, eds. The Ventilator-Assisted Child. A Resource Guide. Texas: Communication Skill Builders, 1997; 181–192.
101. Juntunen D. Transitions: A Personal Perspective. In: Driver LE, Nelson VS, Warschausky SA, eds. The Ventilator-Assisted Child. A Practical Resource Guide. Texas: Communication Skill Builders, 1999; 171–179.
102. Scheinhorn SJ, Artinian BM, Catlin JL. Weaning from prolonged mechanical ventilation. The experience at Regional Weaning Center. Chest 1994; 105:534–539.
103. Gracey DR, Naessens JM, Viggioano RW, Koenig GE, Silverstein MD, Hubmayr RD. Outcome of patients cared for in a ventilator dependent unit in a general hospital. Chest 1995; 107:494–499.
104. Smith IE, Shneerson JM. A progressive care programme for prolonged ventilatory failure: Analysis and outcome. Br J Anaesth 1995; 75:399–404.
105. Chailleux E. ANTADIR [Association Nationale pour le Traitement A Domicile de l'Insuffisance Respiratoire Chronique] Observatory. Data of January 1 1996 Trends. Paris: ANTADIR, 1997.
106. ANTADIR [Association Nationale pour le Traitement A Domicile de l'Insuffisance Respiratoire Chronique]. Activity of the Association System. Abstracts. Paris: ANTADIR, 1994.

19

Measurement of Health Status in Patients on Long-Term Mechanical Ventilation

PAUL W. JONES

St. George's Hospital Medical School
London, England

MAURO CARONE and GIORGIO BERTOLOTTI

IRCCS Istituto di Riabilitazione
Veruno, Italy

I. Introduction

With chronic ventilatory failure the underlying disease process is rarely reversible and usually progresses despite treatment. Whilst increasing life expectancy is an important objective in managing chronic disease, optimization of the quality of a patient's life is also an important objective of care. This becomes especially important when it is considered that treatments are often symptomatic and their most important impact may be on quality of life.

Chronic ventilatory failure has both direct and indirect effects upon the health of the patient. Some of the direct effects may be related to the underlying disease process in the lungs, chest wall, or diaphragm, manifested largely by breathlessness. Other effects may be associated with disturbances of lung gas exchange, causing hypoxia and hypercapnia. Indirect effects may be due to secondary consequences on other organ systems. These would include cardiovascular deconditioning, and muscle wasting, resulting in weakness and fatigue. These may be as important as the direct effects, as evidenced by the observation that patients with chronic obstructive pulmonary disease (COPD) judged questionnaire items related to fatigue to be more important than those related to breathlessness (1). Furthermore, leg fatigue is as important a determinant of exercise limitation as breathlessness (2). Indirect psychosocial effects, such as depression due to restriction of activities and anxiety or panic due to high levels of breathlessness, can have a major impact on the patients' sense of well-being.

Health and well-being are measured using questionnaires. Such instruments are often called "quality of life" questionnaires, but this is a misnomer. Quality of life is unique to the individual. Even the restricted term "health-related quality of life" is inappropriate since ill health can affect the quality of an individual's life in many different ways. Human existence is extremely varied and rich in variety. It is not possible to capture in a single questionnaire the many ways in which disability and handicap may affect a patient's life. Furthermore, this would not be desirable. The principal reason for measuring health is the need to make comparisons among groups of patients and types of treatment. This requires that each patient is assessed in the same way. For this reason, health status questionnaires usually have individuality removed. To ensure that a questionnaire is not biased more toward some individuals than others, the questionnaire writers go to some lengths to ensure that the questions are relevant to all patients with the targeted condition. Thus, a health status questionnaire measures disease effects that form a common denominator among patients. It treats each patient as a "typical" patient, thereby denying individuality to each. For this reason, the term "health status measurement" will be applied throughout this chapter when discussing any formal standardized method of quantifying the impact of disease on a patient's life and well-being. The concept of "quality of life" is extremely important in medicine, but at the level of individual patient care. Techniques for measuring individual "quality of life" are developing, but are not yet suitable for routine use in clinical research.

II. Utility Scales

This type of scale is potentially the most useful way in which health status is measured since it attempts to quantify the utility, preference or value placed upon a health state. Using such instruments, different health states can be compared on an absolute scale that runs from perfect health to death. Furthermore, death can be incorporated as a health state. This has particular advantages in diseases such as chronic ventilatory failure in which death may occur during a study period. Even if deaths do occur, the health status of the entire intention-to-treat population can still be measured at the end of the study using a utility scale. This would not be possible with other scales that do not include death, since the measurements would be confined to the survivors—overestimating the apparent health gain due to the treatment.

Two utility instruments have found quite wide application, one of which is the Quality of Well-Being Scale (QWB). This is a generic health status instrument with utility weights. It has been validated in patients with airways disease (3) and has been used in pulmonary rehabilitation (4), but it does not have sufficient sensitivity to detect changes in health status despite clear improvements in exercise performance and breathlessness during daily life. A second instrument that is being increasingly used because it is easy to use is the EuroQol EQ-5D (5,6). This has not yet been validated in patients with severe chronic lung disease.

There are two main problems associated with the use of this type of questionnaire to measure the health of patients requiring long-term mechanical ventilation. To convert responses to the questionnaire items into a utility scale that ranges from perfect health to death, weights are attached to each item. These are derived empirically and there is always debate about which weights should be used, those derived from patients or those from the normal population. Health economists argue that it should be the latter. Such arguments become particularly pertinent in patients requiring chronic ventilation. They are often in a condition that is almost inconceivable to most healthy people who would, in all probability, find such conditions to be equivalent to or worse than death. Against this is the experience of such patients and their carers who consider their lives worthwhile and fulfilling despite major restrictions. Interestingly, however, even physicians and other healthcare workers (i.e., healthy people knowledgeable about the disease) tend to overestimate the loss of quality of life of patients with neuromuscular disorders (7,8). Clearly, physically disabled persons adapt their lifestyles to their physical limitations. It is probable that under such conditions, a phenomenon known as response-shift occurs in which patients reset their internal norms of what is tolerable or acceptable to them. There is evidence that this shift may occur even in mild to moderate asthma (9).

A further problem with utility scales is that, like most general health status instruments, they may lack sufficient sensitivity to detect effects of specific treatments for specific conditions. Nonetheless, the utility scale approach has much to offer, particularly in the setting of chronic illness, although much more evaluation will be necessary before this type of instrument can be applied with confidence in patients requiring long-term mechanical ventilation.

III. Generic Questionnaires

These instruments were designed to address the impact of a wide range of diseases on health status. Three different generic instruments have been used in severe respiratory diseases, the Sickness Impact Profile (SIP) (10), the short form of the Medical Outcome Study Questionnaire (SF-36) (11) and the Nottingham Health Profile (NHP) (Table 1).

Table 1 Summary of Health Status Questionnaires

Instrument	Type	Validated in COPD	Comments
Sickness Impact Profile (SIP)	Generic	yes	Does not correlate with Po_2
Short Form-36 (SF-36)	Generic	yes	Limited discriminative ability for COPD vs. respiratory failure
Nottingham Health Profile (NHP)	Generic	yes	
Chronic Respiratory Questionnaire (CRQ)	Specific for COPD	yes	
St. George's Respiratory Questionnaire (SGRQ)	Specific for COPD	yes	Correlates with level of hypoxia, but not hyper-capnia
MRF-28	Specific for respiratory failure	yes	Correlates with SGRQ, but gives wider range of scores and should dis-criminate better between levels of function

A. Sickness Impact Profile

The SIP is a valid measure of impaired general health in chronic airflow limitation, particularly in patients with a $FEV_1 < 50\%$ predicted (12–14), although SIP scores have not been shown to correlate with hypoxemia (15–17). Until recently it was not known whether this lack of correlation was due to insensitivity of the questionnaire, or the absence of an effect of hypoxia on health status, but a correlation between arterial Po_2 and health status has been reported when health status was measured using a disease-specific instrument (17). It is noteworthy that in the same study, no correlation was found between level of hypoxia and SIP score. For this reason, there is some concern about the SIP as being a suitable measure for patients with respiratory failure.

B. Short Form 36

The SF-36 (18) has been applied in severe respiratory patients in two different studies. Simonds and Elliott (19) studied patients with hypercapnic chronic respiratory failure caused by obstructive or restrictive diseases. Smith and Shneerson (20) administered the SF-36 to a group of severe patients with acute or acute on chronic respiratory failure 1 year after successful discharge from an intensive

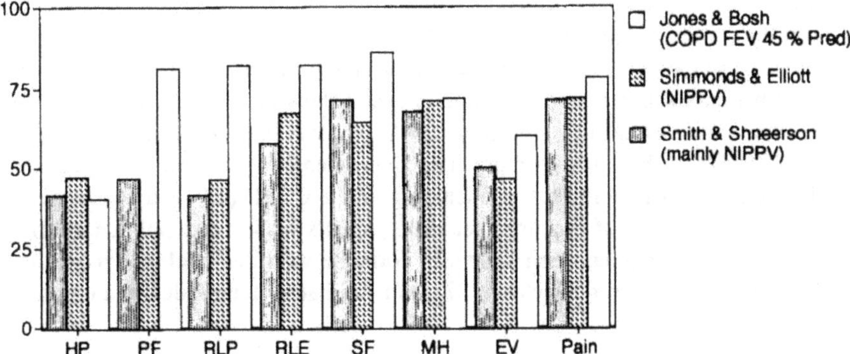

Figure 1 SF-36 scores from three studies, one performed in patient with moderate-severe COPD, but not receiving ventilation (21), one in patients on NIPPV (19), and one in patients mainly on NIPPV (20). HP, general health perception; PF, physical function; RLP, role physical limitation; RLE, role emotional limitation; SF, social function; MH, mental health; EV, energy and vitality.

care unit. The scores differed from those of healthy subjects, but formal tests of the discriminative properties of the SF-36 have not been performed in patients with respiratory failure. Combining the results from different studies suggests an overall pattern to the impact of respiratory failure. Compared with patients with moderate to severe COPD (21), patients receiving ventilatory support register more severe impairment of their physical capabilities, but their general and mental health ratings are similar (Fig. 1). Of course, this does not tell us whether decreased physical function is due to greater impairment of lung function or a consequence of respiratory failure.

C. Nottingham Health Profile

In a large cross-sectional study on COPD patients (22), the NHP distinguished between different degrees of severity assessed in terms of FEV_1, although not quite as well as the St. George's Respiratory Questionnaire (SGRQ)—a disease-specific questionnaire for COPD (23). In an uncontrolled study of domiciliary ventilation in COPD, the NHP showed significant improvement in total score, physical mobility, emotional reactions, and energy compared with the run-in period (24).

IV. Disease-Specific Measures Developed for COPD

Two disease-specific questionnaires developed for use in COPD have been used in patients with chronic respiratory failure (see Table 1). The Chronic Respiratory

Questionnaire (CRQ) has been applied to patients with severe airway obstruction (mean FEV_1 39% predicted), but blood gases were not reported so it is not clear whether these patients had chronic respiratory failure (25). The SGRQ has been used in patients with respiratory failure (17) and shown to be responsive to nocturnal ventilation using bilevel positive airway pressure in patients with hypercapnic COPD (26). This questionnaire has been extensively validated in patients with diseases of airflow limitation, including severe COPD (23), and does appear to be a valid measure of impaired health in patients with severe pulmonary impairment. The SGRQ has been shown to correlate with the level of hypoxia in COPD (Fig. 2) (17), bronchiectasis (27), and ventilatory failure due to a number

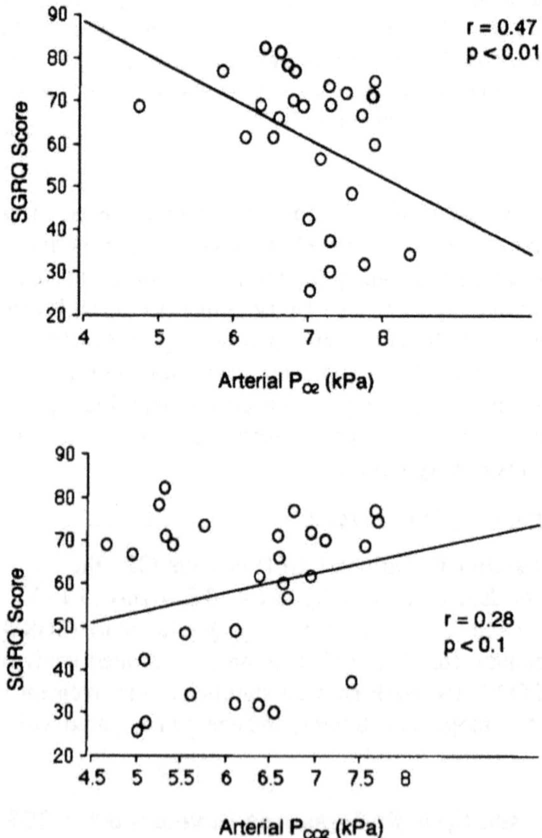

Figure 2 Correlation between health status measured using the St. George's Respiratory Questionnaire (SGRQ) and arterial Po_2 and Pco_2 in patients with COPD. (From Ref. 31.)

of causes (28). In contrast, no correlation was seen between hypercapnia and SGRQ score in any of these three studies (Fig. 2). The mechanism of the link between hypoxia and health status is not clear, but a multivariate analysis of data from patients with bronchiectasis (27) showed that arterial Po_2 and exercise performance were both independent correlates of the SGRQ score. This suggests that the link between hypoxemia and health status is not mediated through exercise limitation. A direct effect of cerebral hypoxia on the perception of well-being remains a possibility, although there is no evidence for or against such a mechanism.

V. MRF-28: A Specific Questionnaire for Respiratory Failure

While there is evidence that health status questionnaires developed for COPD may have some validity for use in patients with respiratory failure, there are concerns about their application in this setting. Neither the CRQ nor the SGRQ was developed in severe chronic respiratory failure (CRF) patients. Such patients lie at the very end of the usable scoring range of these questionnaires. This may be important, especially in long-term follow-up studies, since they may not be able to detect deterioration over time. Both questionnaires were developed in patients with COPD, but many patients with lung disease severe enough to require long-term ventilatory support have other diseases, such as kyphoscoliosis. Furthermore, the metabolic consequences of chronic respiratory failure may have additional effects, such as disturbance of cognitive function, that may not be detected by existing questionnaires. For this reason, a recent study set out to identify a core set of questionnaire items common to CRF patients irrespective of age, gender, and underlying disease (29).

Initially, 152 items were identified from a wide range of sources, including semi-structured interviews with patients. These were reduced to 28 items using a structured hierarchical approach described by O'Leary and Jones (30). Principal components analysis identified three main factors: one that could be titled "Daily Activity," a second called "Cognitive Function" that addressed issues around memory and concentration, and a third factor that could be labeled "Invalidity." The remaining eight items did not form any recognizable single factor. This questionnaire, named the MRF-28 (29), correlated with SGRQ (Fig. 3) and SIP scores, but showed a wider scoring range than either of these two instruments (Fig. 4). This suggests that it will provide better discrimination among different levels of impaired health compared with the existing questionnaires.

One of the most important aspects of this new questionnaire is the cognitive function component, which concerns memory function and concentration. Unlike laboratory tests of cognitive function, these questionnaire items address the im-

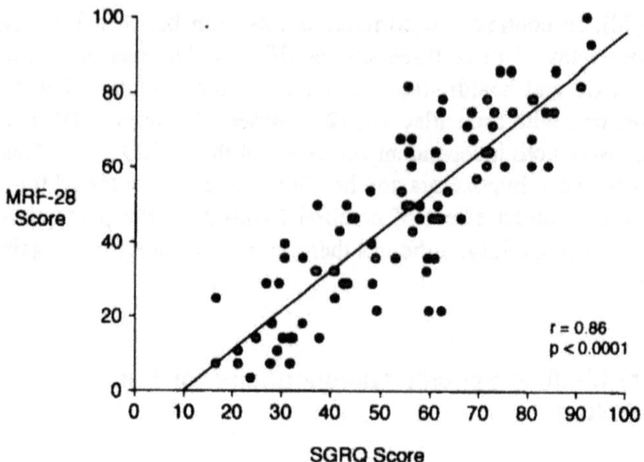

Figure 3 Correlation between the SGRQ (a COPD disease-specific questionnaire) and the MRF-28 (a questionnaire developed specifically for patients with respiratory failure). Data obtained from patients on long-term ventilatory support and/or long-term oxygen therapy. (From Ref. 29.)

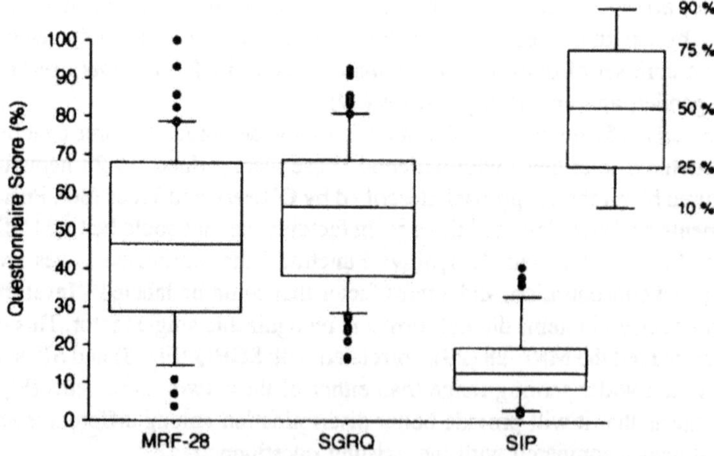

Figure 4 Box plots of scores for a generic questionnaire (SIP), a COPD-specific questionnaire (SGRQ), and a respiratory failure questionnaire (MRF-28), obtained in patients on long-term ventilation and/or long-term oxygen therapy. (From Ref. 29.)

pact of impaired cognitive function on daily life, not just the existence of impairment. Another new feature of the MRF-28 is the grouping of items that have been termed invalidity. This term was selected because the dominant item in this factor identified by principal components analysis during the questionnaire's development was: "Because of my lung disease I have become an invalid." Other items in this component are related to an inability of patients to exert themselves, the experience of social isolation, and dependency on others. While isolated examples of similar items may be found in other questionnaires, this study has shown that a sense of general invalidity is a fairly specific component of poor health due to severe respiratory failure.

Longitudinal validation of this new questionnaire is still in progress, but there is evidence that it does have good discriminative ability, i.e., the ability to distinguish among different levels of disease. The total score correlated with physiologic variables such as exercise tolerance and arterial Po_2, clinical factors such as oxygen flow requirements at rest and with exercise, breathlessness in daily life, and mood disturbance (29). In contrast, the cognitive component correlated only with anxiety, and depression, whereas the invalidity component correlated largely with disability due to breathlessness, anxiety and depression. The study has shown that the health of patients with respiratory failure is different from that of patients with less severe lung disease in terms of both quantity and quality. This justifies the development of a health status questionnaire designed specifically for use in patients with respiratory failure.

VI. Effect of Long-Term Ventilation on Health Status

There have been relatively few studies of long-term ventilation that have used health status questionnaires developed specifically for use in patients with chronic lung disease. One of the most comprehensive is that carried out by Meecham-Jones et al. (26) in which hypercapnic, hypoxemic patients with COPD were recruited to a randomized crossover study of nasal pressure support ventilation (NPSV) through a bilevel positive airway pressure device. After a 1-mo run-in period, these patients either remained on long-term oxygen (LTOT) or continued to receive their LTOT and also used nocturnal NPSV. During the period on NPSV, daytime arterial Po_2 on room air was 5.9 mm Hg higher and Pco_2 was 4.5 mm Hg lower than when patients were treated with LTOT alone. This physiologic improvement was highly statistically significant ($p < 0.0001$), but it is not clear what benefits an increase in Po_2 from 44 mm Hg to 50 mm Hg offered the patients other than the numerical improvement. Data obtained with the SGRQ show that this improvement was associated with a clinically significant improvement in health status that exceeded the threshold for a minimum clinically significant difference with this questionnaire (Fig. 5). Similar results were obtained in an

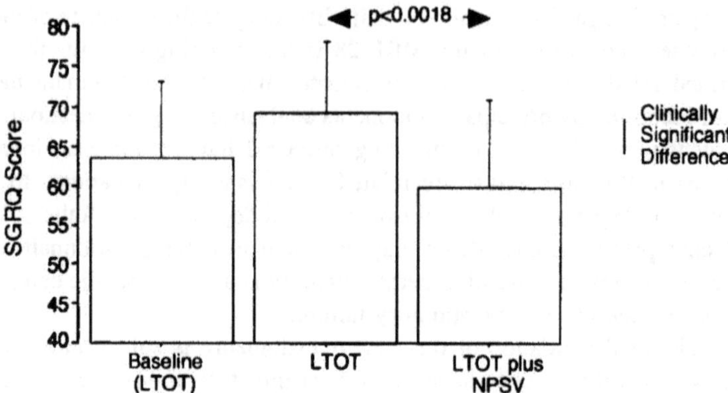

Figure 5 Effect of long-term oxygen therapy (LTOT) and long-term oxygen plus nasal pressure support (NPSV) in patients with hypoxic hypercapnic COPD. (From Ref. 26.)

uncontrolled 6-month study in which the SGRQ score improved by a clinically significant amount compared with baseline (24).

The mechanism for the improvement in health status in the Meecham-Jones study is not entirely clear, but improved oxygenation is a possibility. The within-patient improvements in Po_2 and SGRQ associated with use of NPSV paralleled the between-patient relationship between Po_2 and SGRQ (see Fig. 2). However, the correlation between improvements in Po_2 and SGRQ was not statistically significant ($p > 0.1$). This may have been due to a "type 2" error, because only 14 patients completed the study. Another possible mechanism may have been improved sleep; a 30% increase in total sleep time was observed after NPSV compared with LTOT alone in the 10 patients who underwent polysomnography after each phase of the study. Unfortunately, there were again too few patients to provide a reliable test of any correlation between sleep and health status. Although it is not possible to identify the specific mechanism for the improvement in the patients' health status with NPSV treatment, it is worth noting that this discussion is only possible because health status measurements detected differences.

In the two studies that have used the SGRQ, the psychosocial impacts component showed the largest and most consistent change. Changes in the symptoms and activity components of the SGRQ were not so large or consistent between studies (24,26). Interestingly, the NHP showed a similar pattern following domiciliary nasal ventilation; the biggest improvements were in the emotional reactions and energy components (24)—precisely the areas covered by the impacts component of the SGRQ.

VII. Summary and Conclusions

Health status measurements have been applied to patients with ventilatory failure in only a few studies so far. Useful but limited information has been derived from generic questionnaires or those developed for patients with less severe chronic lung disease. However, some features of the health impairment of patients needing long-term ventilation may be unique, necessitating use of a condition-specific instrument if these features are to be assessed. Studies using existing questionnaires show that long-term ventilation may produce worthwhile benefits to patients. They are also beginning to point to mechanisms that need to be explored further, such as the link between hypoxia and health.

Mortality is arguably the most important outcome of studies of long-term ventilatory support, but it is reasonable to suggest that health status constitutes another key clinical outcome of studies that set out to demonstrate benefit from this treatment. Hence, studies on long-term ventilation should use health status outcome measures specifically tailored for patients with chronic respiratory failure.

References

1. Guyatt GH, Berman LB, Townsend M, Pugsley SO, Chambers LW. A measure of quality of life for clinical trials in chronic lung disease. Thorax 1987; 42:773–778.
2. Killian KJ, Leblanc P, Martin DH, Summers E, Jones NL, Campbell EJM. Exercise capacity and ventilatory, circulatory and symptom limitation in patients with chronic airflow limitation. Am Rev Respir Dis 1992; 146:935–940.
3. Kaplan RM, Atkins CJ, Timms R. Validity of a quality of well-being scale as an outcome measure in chronic obstructive pulmonary disease. J Chron Dis 1984; 37: 85–95.
4. Ries AL, Kaplan RM, Limberg TM, Prewitt LM. Effects of pulmonary rehabilitation on physiologic and psychosocial outcomes in patients with chronic obstructive pulmonary disease. Ann Int Med 1995; 122:823–32.
5. EuroQol Group. EuroQol—a new facility for the measurement of health-related quality of life. Health Policy 1990; 20:329–332.
6. Brooks R, EuroQol Group. EuroQol: The current state of play. Health Policy 1996; 37:53–72.
7. Bach JR, Campagnolo DI, Hoeman S. Life satisfaction of individuals with Duchenne's muscular dystrophy using long-term mecahnical ventilatory support. Am J Phys Med Rehabil 1991; 70:129–135.
8. Bach JR, Campagnolo DI. Psychosocial adjustment of postpoliomyelitis ventilator-assisted individuals. Arch J Phys Med Rehabil 1992; 73:934–939.
9. Barley EA, Quirk FH, Jones PW. A comparison of diary cards vs. health status questionnaires as measures of the severity and impact of asthma. Eur Respir J 1999.

10. Bergner M, Bobbitt RA, Carter WB, Gilson BS. The Sickness Impact Profile: Development and final revision of a health status measure. Med Care 1981; 19:787–805.
11. Stewart AL, Hays R, Ware JE. The MOS short-form general health survey. Reliability and validity in a patient population. Med Care 1988; 26:724–732.
12. Williams SJ, Bury MR. Impairment, disability and handicap in chronic respiratory illness. Soc Sci Med 1989; 29:609–616.
13. Jones PW, Baveystock CM, Littlejohns P. Relationships between general health measured with the Sickness Impact Profile and respiratory symptoms, physiological measures and mood in patients with chronic airflow limitation. Am Rev Respir Dis 1989; 140:1538–1543.
14. Jones PW. Quality of life measurement for patients with diseases of the airways. Thorax 1991; 46:676–682.
15. Prigatano GP, Wright EC, Heaton RK, Adams KM, Timms RM. Quality of life and its predictors in patients with mild hypoxemia and chronic obstructive pulmonary disease. Arch Intern Med 1982; 144:1613–1619.
16. McSweeny J, Grant I, Heaton RK, Adams KM, Timms RM. Life quality of patients with chronic obstructive pulmonary disease. Arch Intern Med 1982; 142:473–478.
17. Okubadeyo AA, Jones PW, Paul EA, Wedzicha JA. Does long-term oxygen therapy affect quality of life in patients with chronic obstructive pulmonary disease and severe hypoxaemia? Eur Respir J 1996; 9:2335–2339.
18. Ware JE, Sherbourne CA, Davies AR. The MOS short-form general health survey. Publication P-7444. Santa Monica, CA: Rand Corporation, 1988.
19. Simmonds AK, Elliott MW. Outcome of domiciliary nasal intermittent positive pressure ventilation in restrictive and obstructive disorders. Thorax 1995; 50:604–609.
20. Smith IE, Shneerson JM. A progressive care programme for prolonged ventilatory failure: Analysis of outcome. Br J Anaesth 1995; 75:399–404.
21. Jones PW, Bosh TK. Changes in quality of life in COPD patients treated with salmeterol. Am J Resp Crit Care Med 1997; 155:1283–1289.
22. Ferrer M, Alonso J, Morera J, et al. Chronic obstructive pulmonary disease stage and health-related quality of life. Ann Intern Med 1997; 127:1072–1079.
23. Jones PW, Quirk FH, Baveystock CM, Littlejohns P. A self-complete measure for chronic airflow limitation—the St George's Respiratory Questionnaire. Am Rev Respir Dis 1992; 145:1321–1327.
24. Perrin C, El Far Y, Vandenbos F, et al. Domiciliary nasal intermittent positive pressure ventilation in severe COPD: Effects on lung function and quality of life. Eur Respir J 1997; 10:2835–2839.
25. Wegner RE, Jörres RA, Kirsten DK, Magnussen H. Factor analysis of exercise capacity, dyspnoea ratings and lung function in patients with severe COPD. Eur Respir J 1994; 7:725–729.
26. Meecham-Jones DJ, Paul EA, Jones PW, Wedzicha JA. Nasal pressure support ventilation plus oxygen compared with oxygen therapy alone in hypercapnic COPD. Am J Respir Crit Care Med 1995; 152:538–544.
27. Wilson CB, Jones PW, O'Leary CJ, Cole PJ, Wilson R. Validation of the St George's Respiratory Questionnaire in bronchiectasis. Am J Respir Crit Care Med 1997; 156: 536–541.
28. Schönhofer B, Ardes P, Geibel M, Köhler D, Jones PW. Evaluation of a movement

detector to measure daily activity in patients with chronic lung disease. Eur Respir J 1997; 10:2814–2819.

29. Carone M, Bertolotti G, Anchisi F, Zotti AM, Donner CF, Jones PW. Analysis of factors that chraracterize health impairment in patients with chronic respiratory failure. Eur Respir J 1999; 13:1293–1300.
30. O'Leary CJ, Jones PW. The influence of decisions made by developers on health status questionnaire content. Qual Life Res 1998; 7:545–550.
31. Okubadejo A, Jones PW, Wedzicha J. Quality of life in patients with chronic obstructive pulmonary disease and severe hypoxaemia. Thorax 1996; 51:44–47.

AUTHOR INDEX

Italic numbers give the page on which the complete reference is cited.

A

B

C

D

E

F

G

H

I

J

K

L

M

N

O

P

S

T

U

Y

Z

SUBJECT INDEX

A

B

F

G

H

N

O

P

Q

R

S

T

U

V

W

Milton Keynes UK
Ingram Content Group UK Ltd.
UKHW021929071024
449327UK00022B/1746

9 780367 398163